Physiology *of* Exercise

For Physical Education, Athletics and Exercise Science

Physiology *of* Exercise

For Physical Education, Athletics and Exercise Science

Fifth Edition

Herbert A. deVries

University of Southern California

Terry J. Housh

University of Nebraska-Lincoln

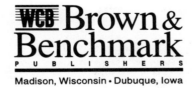

WCB Brown & Benchmark

PUBLISHERS

Madison, Wisconsin • Dubuque, Iowa

Book Team

Executive Editor *Ed Bartell*
Editor *Scott Spoolman*
Production Editor *Michelle M. Campbell*
Designer *Kristyn A. Kalnes*
Art Editor/Processor *Carla Goldhammer*
Photo Editor *Shirley Lanners*
Permissions Coordinator *Vicki Krug*
Visuals/Design Developmental Consultant *Marilyn A. Phelps*
Visuals/Design Freelance Specialist *Mary L. Christianson*
Publishing Services Specialist *Sherry Padden*
Marketing Manager *Steven Yetter*
Advertising Manager *Brett Apold*

Brown & Benchmark

A Division of Wm. C. Brown Communications, Inc.

Executive Vice President/General Manager *Thomas E. Doran*
Vice President/Editor in Chief *Edgar J. Laube*
Vice President/Sales and Marketing *Eric Ziegler*
Director of Production *Vickie Putman Caughron*
Director of Custom and Electronic Publishing *Chris Rogers*

Wm. C. Brown Communications, Inc.

President and Chief Executive Officer *G. Franklin Lewis*
Corporate Senior Vice President and Chief Financial Officer *Robert Chesterman*
Corporate Senior Vice President and President of Manufacturing *Roger Meyer*

Cover photo © Eugen Gebhardt/FPG International

Line art created by Precision Graphics, Champaign, IL.

Copyedited by Bonnie Guen

Freelance permissions editor Karen Dorman

Consulting Editor A. Lockhart

A Times Mirror Company

Library of Congress Catalog Card Number: 92–76074

ISBN 0–697–10097–9

Printed in the United States of America by Wm. C. Brown Communications, Inc.,
2460 Kerper Boulevard, Dubuque, IA 52001

10 9 8 7 6 5 4 3 2 1

Contents

Preface   xv

part 1
Basic Physiology Underlying the Study of Physiology of Exercise   1

1   The Why of Physiology of Exercise   3

Why Physical Fitness? 4
Improving Human Athletic Performance 4
Professionalism in Physical Education and Athletics 5
"Get Some Exercise" 6
Gender and Age Differences in Response to Training 6
Scientific Method 7
Overview of Text 8

2   Structure of Muscle Tissue   10

Gross Structure of Skeletal Muscle 11
Microscopic Structure of Skeletal Muscle 11
Structure of the Muscle Cell or Fiber 12
Muscle Fiber Types 15
Structure of the Myofibril and the Contractile Mechanism 17
Blood Supply and Lymphatics 23
Nerve Supply 23

3   Energetics of Muscular Contraction and Adaptations to Training at the Cellular Level   28

Energetics of Muscular Contraction 29
Adaptations to Training and Conditioning at the Cellular Level 34
Energy Substrate and Training 39

4   The Physiology of Muscle Contraction   46

Physiology of Gross Muscle Contraction 47
Electromyography in Analysis of Muscle Function 56

5 The Nervous System and Coordination of Muscular Activity 68

The Neuron and the Motor Unit 69
The Reflex Arc and Involuntary Movement 70
Intersegmental and Suprasegmental Reflexes 71
Proprioception and Kinesthesis 72
The Alpha and Gamma Systems for Muscular Control 78
Higher Nerve Centers and Muscular Control 82
Posture, Balance, and Voluntary Movement 84
Perception of Effort 85
Use-Disuse Phenomena in the Nervous System 85
Does Viscerosomatic Motor Inhibition Limit Exercise? 86
Practical Considerations 86

6 The Heart and Exercise 93

Review of the Cardiac Cycle 94
The Cardiac Output 95
Coronary Circulation and Efficiency of the Heart 103
Factors Affecting the Heart Rate 105
The Heart Rate during and after Exercise 106
Effects of Athletic Training on the Heart 109
Training Effects at the Cellular Level 109
The Cardiac Reserve Capacity 110
Heart Murmurs 110

7 The Circulatory System and Exercise 115

Hemodynamics: Principles Governing Blood Flow 116
The Microcirculation: Blood Flow through the Capillary Bed 118
Control of Blood Distribution 120
Blood Distribution in Rest and Exercise 121
Blood Pressure 122
Arterial Blood Pressure during Exercise 125
Blood Flow in Exercising Muscles 126
Blood and Fluid Changes during Exercise 129
Blood and Fluid Changes from Training 129

8 The Lungs and External Respiration 136

Anatomy of External Respiration 137
Mechanics of Lung Ventilation 137
Nomenclature for the Lung Volumes and Capacities 139
Respiratory Control 139

Importance of Breathing Pattern 142
Efficiency of Breathing 145
Improving Performance by Better Breathing 146
Training Effects on Pulmonary Function 146
Respiratory Phenomena 147
Unusual Respiratory Maneuvers 148
Effects of Air Pollution on Respiration 150
Smoking—Self-Induced Air Pollution 151

9   Gas Transport and Internal Respiration 156

Properties of Gasses and Liquids 157
Gas Transport by the Blood 159
Internal Respiration 160
Regulation of Acid-Base Balance 162
Acid-Base Balance as a Factor Limiting Performance 165
Changes in Lung Diffusion in Exercise 165
Use of Oxygen to Improve Performance 166
What Sets the Limits of Aerobic Power? 167

10   The Endocrine System and Exercise 172

Nature of Hormones 173
Importance of Hormones in Exercise and Sports 175
Endocrine Effects on Performance-Related Parameters 176
Pituitary-Adrenocortical Axis and Stress Theory 177
Effect of Exercise on Endocrine Function 180

11   The Immune System and Exercise 192

The Immune System 193
Nonspecific Immune Mechanisms 193
Specific Immune Mechanisms 196
The Effects of Exercise and Immune Function 199
Clinical Implications of Exercise and Immune Function 202

12   Exercise Metabolism 207

Definition of Terms 208
Methods for Standardizing and Measuring Exercise Loads 210
Methods for Measuring Energy Consumption 214
Oxygen Deficit and Recovery Oxygen 216
New Concepts Concerning Recovery Oxygen 218

Training Effect on Anaerobic Metabolism and Recovery
      Oxygen 221
Intermittent Work (Interval Training) 221
Maximal O_2 Consumption as a Measure of Physical Fitness 222
Respiratory Quotient 223
The Anaerobic Threshold Controversy 224
Theoretical Problems with the Anaerobic Threshold Concept 225
Negative Work 226

part 2
Physiology Applied to Health and Fitness 233

13 Health Benefits: Prophylactic and Therapeutic Effects of Exercise 235

Physical Activity, Physical Fitness, and All-Cause Mortality 236
The Cardiovascular System and Exercise 237
Lipid Metabolism and Exercise 241
Pulmonary Function Effects 242
Oxygen Transport Effects 242
Effects on Bones, Joints, and Connective Tissue 242
Effects of Exercise on Cancer 243
The "Tranquilizer Effect" 244
Effect of Exercise on Psychiatric State 245

14 Physical Fitness Testing 252

Measurement of Physical Working Capacity (PWC) by Maximum
      O_2 Consumption 254
Estimation of PWC from Heart Rate at Submaximal Loads 260
Measurement of Anaerobic Capabilities 273
New Concepts in Measuring Physical Fitness 275
Motor Fitness Tests 280
The New AAHPERD Health Related Physical Fitness Test 282
Physical Fitness Evaluation as a Function of Age Groups 282

15 Physical Conditioning for Health and Fitness (Prescription of Exercise) 287

Principles Involved in Scientific Prescription of Exercise 289
Need for Medical Evaluation and Exercise Testing Prior to
      Participation in Endurance Exercise 289
Training Curves 292

Interval Training versus Continuous Exercise 292
Recommendations of the American College of Sports Medicine
(ACSM) for Developing Cardiorespiratory Fitness in Healthy
Adults 293
Mode of Exercise (ACSM Recommendation: Aerobic in
Nature) 293
Intensity of Exercise 295
Duration of Exercise (ACSM Recommendation: Twenty to Sixty
Minutes of Continuous Aerobic Exercise) 297
Frequency of Exercise (ACSM Recommendation: Three to Five
Days per Week) 300
Exercise Prescription 301
Effects of Gender and Age on Training Adaptations 305
Specificity of Training 305
Potential Physiological Changes Resulting from Training 305
Training as a Stressor 306

16 Exercise Physiology in the Prevention and Rehabilitation of Cardiovascular Disease 311

Anatomy and Physiology of the Coronary Arteries 313
Nature of Coronary Heart Disease (CHD) 314
Theories Regarding Causation of CHD 315
The Risk Factor Concept in CHD 317
Physiological Bases for Use of Exercise in CHD Prevention 317
Exercise Physiology in Cardiac Rehabilitation 319
Principles of Exercise Testing in Cardiac Rehabilitation 320
Exercise Prescription for Cardiac Rehabilitation 324
Weight Training for Cardiac Rehabilitation 325
Program Development 326

17 Metabolism and Weight Control 334

Body Weight and Health 335
Physiology of Weight Gain and Weight Loss 335
What Is Normal Weight? 337
Methods for Estimating Body Composition 338
Gaining Weight 346
Reducing Weight 346
Water Retention in Weight Reduction Programs 353
Spot Reducing 354
The Long-Haul Concept of Weight Control 354

18 Growth, Development, and Exercise in Children and Adolescents 360

Growth, Development, and Maturation 361
Normal Growth Patterns 362
"Making Weight" in Athletics 364
Exercise and Aerobic Fitness 365
Exercise and Anaerobic Fitness 368
Strength 371
Weight Training versus Weight Lifting versus Body Building 371
Weight Training during Prepubescence and Postpubescence 372
Potential Hazards of Weight Training 374
Characteristics of a Weight Training Program 375

19 Age and Exercise 380

Age Changes in Muscle Function 383
Age and the Cardiovascular System 387
Changes in Pulmonary Function 388
Age and Physical Working Capacity (PWC) 389
Age and the Nervous System 391
Age and Body Composition 392
Effects of Physical Conditioning on Losses in Functional Capacities Caused by Aging 392
Principles for Conduct of Conditioning Programs for Older Men and Women (over Sixty) 396
Implications for Physical Education and Athletics 399

20 Neuromuscular Fatigue 409

Historical Perspective 410
Importance of Neuromuscular Fatigue 411
Physiology of Fatigue 413
Electromyographic Observations of Fatigue 417
Psychological Effect of Fatigue (Staleness) 418

part 3
Physiology of Training and Conditioning Athletes 423

21 Physiology of Muscle Strength 425

Physiology of Strength 426
Methods for Measurement and Training of Strength 432
Effect of Various Factors on Strength 439

22 Development of Muscular and Circulorespiratory Endurance 447

Endurance as a Factor in Human Performance 448
Local or Muscular Endurance 449
General or Circulorespiratory Endurance 455

23 Efficiency of Muscular Activity 467

Aerobic versus Anaerobic Efficiency 470
Running Economy 470
Effect of Speed on Efficiency 472
Effect of Work Rate on Efficiency 474
Effect of Fatigue on Efficiency 475
Diet and Efficiency 475
Effects of Environmental Temperature 475
Effect of Wind on Running Efficiency 475
Effect of Obesity on Efficiency 476
The Looseness Factor 476
Acceleration–Deceleration versus Smooth Movement 476
Pace and Efficiency 477
Efficiency of Positive and Negative Work 478

24 Speed 484

Intrinsic Speed of Muscle Contraction 485
Force–Velocity Relationship 486
Specificity of Speed 487
Strength and Speed 488
Flexibility and Speed 489
Body Mechanics and Speed in Running 489
Body Mechanics and Speed in Swimming 490
Physiological Considerations in the Design of Running Tracks 490

Gender Differences in Speed of Movement 490
Variation of Speed with Distance in Running and Swimming 492
Limiting Factors in Speed 492
Methods for Improving Sprint Speed 494

25 Flexibility 498

Physiology of Flexibility 499
Measuring Flexibility 501
Methods for Improving Range of Motion 503
Weight Training and Flexibility 507
Factors Affecting Flexibility 507

26 Physiology of Muscle Soreness—Cause and Relief 511

Immediate versus Delayed Muscle Pain 512
Theoretical Basis for Delayed Onset Muscle Soreness (DOMS) 512
Attempt at Unification and Simplification: Practical Aspects for
    Coach and Athlete 518
Physiology Underlying Static Stretching 519
Prevention of Muscular Soreness 520
Relief of Muscular Soreness 521
Severe Muscle Problems 522

27 Warming Up 527

Practice Effect versus Physiological Warm-Up 528
Physiology of Warming Up 528
Types of Warm-Up 531
Effect of Warm-Up on Various Athletic Activities 532
Duration of the Warm-Up Effect 534
Recovery between Events 534
Warm-Up and Prevention of Muscle Injury 535
Warm-Up and Heart Function 535

28   Environment and Exercise   540

Physiology of Adaptation to Heat and Cold   541
Exercise in the Cold   542
Exercise in the Heat   544
Human Limitations in the Heat   546
Acclimatization to Hot Environments   551
Fluid and Electrolyte Replacement   554
Exercise at High Altitudes   555

29   Nutrition for Athletes   562

Long-Term Dietary Considerations and Requirements   563
Suggested Training Rules for Good Nutrition   574
Effect of Exercise on the Function of the Stomach   575
Pre-Event Objectives   577
Pregame Procedure   577
Glycogen Supercompensation (Carbohydrate Loading) for
    Endurance Events   578

30   Special Aids to Performance   583

Alkalinizers   584
Phosphate Loading   586
Amphetamines (Benzedrine)   586
Anabolic Steroids   587
Aspartates   587
Blood Doping (Erythrocythemia)   588
Blood Doping with Erythropoietin   589
Caffeine   590
Carbohydrate Feeding (Glucose, Fructose, and Glucose
    Polymer)   591
Improving Lactate Tolerance by Lactate Ingestion   592
Oxygen and Vitamins   592
Wheat-Germ Oil   592

31 The Female in Athletics 599

Structural Gender Differences 600
Physiological Gender Differences 601
Female Limitations in Athletics 602
Physiological Adaptations to Training in Females 604
Adaptations to Strength Training in Females 606
The Menstrual Cycle and Athletics 610
Pregnancy, Childbirth, and Athletics 612
Athletic Injuries 615
Emotional Factors 615

Index 621

Preface

Over the years of working with undergraduate and graduate students in the physiology of exercise laboratory, I've noticed that theory and practice are not always related in the student's mind. Too often, the scientific method remains an ivory tower concept, never applied. Unfortunately, some coaches base their practices on the methods of a highly successful athlete, whose success may be totally unrelated to the fads used in his or her training. Because of such practices and conditions, I have made an effort to bring theory and practice closer together—adding the *how to* approach while at the same time respecting scientific investigations that provide the *why* for the *how to*.

Physiology of Exercise for Physical Education and Athletics is concerned with human responses and adaptations to muscular activity. The text provides a basis for the study of physical fitness and athletic training. It is written primarily for the upper-division undergraduate student who has a background in basic anatomy and general physiology. A knowledge of physics, chemistry, or mathematics beyond the high school level is not necessary. In addition, those who aspire to be athletic coaches will find within these pages the scientific basis for their profession. Since emphasis is placed upon the holes in our patchwork quilt of knowledge and since a substantially updated and expanded bibliography is provided at the end of each chapter, the text can also assist the graduate student who wishes to chip away at the frontiers of knowledge in this discipline. Those who use exercise as a therapeutic modality will also find guiding principles in this text.

Ever since the first edition this textbook has been divided into three parts, because I realize that students enter this field with greatly diverse backgrounds in the basic sciences. Thus, Part 1 selectively reviews the most pertinent areas of basic physiology. In classes where the students' background in general physiology is strong, the instructor can emphasize applications that are presented in Parts 2 and 3. We have maintained this organization because of its basic pedagogic soundness and its obvious advantages where homogeneity of lower-division preparation is not common.

In the third edition a clearer division and better definition of the second and third parts was possible. In the years since the second edition, it had become clear that physical fitness can contribute substantially to lifelong good health. The body of evidence that was previously only suggestive had rapidly become compelling. Therefore, the text was reorganized to recognize that the study of exercise physiology has two major interests for the physical educator. The first is the enhancement of health and physical fitness for the general population, and the second is optimization of performance in the various types and levels of competitive athletics. Thus, the third and fourth editions were organized quite naturally into three parts. The first deals with the basic physiology that provides the groundwork for application to our field. Although this is organized on a systemic basis, the potential applications are pointed out and emphasized. Recognizing the basic differences in interest between those who are primarily teachers of health and physical education and those whose future lies largely in the coaching of athletics, the second section deals with the physiology of exercise directed toward health and fitness, while the third section is devoted to the scientific improvement of athletic performance.

The foregoing is how I introduced the fourth edition of this text. I now have a much more important introduction to make. I have prevailed upon Dr. Terry J. Housh to join me in writing this fifth edition. It is with great pleasure and satisfaction that I welcome Dr. Housh to the rewarding task of communicating the body of knowledge in exercise physiology to the new generations of physical education teachers and coaches. He is, at a young age, already Director of the Human Performance Laboratory at the University of Nebraska-Lincoln. He has achieved eminence in our field and has had wide experience with both undergraduate and graduate students who are impressed with his enthusiasm as well as his erudition. Those who are familiar with the earlier editions will readily recognize the improvement that our collaboration has brought about in this fifth edition.

Herbert A. deVries
Laguna Beach, California

In the fifth edition we have added three new chapters. In the first section we have included a chapter (chap. 11) titled "The Immune System and Exercise." Anecdotal evidence suggests that exercise enhances an individual's resistance to infection, but coaches are often concerned about an increased number of infectious episodes particularly near the end of the competitive season. These conflicting testimonials indicate a need to discuss such important questions as: 1) the effect of acute and chronic exercise upon immune function; 2) the relationship of intensity, duration, and frequency of exercise and immune function; and 3) what clinical implications result from the foregoing relationships?

In the second section we have added a chapter (chap. 18) titled "Growth, Development, and Exercise in Children and Adolescents." The interest and participation of children and adolescents in recreational and competitive sports has increased dramatically in recent years. Therefore, professionals in our field must be knowledgeable in the areas of normal growth and development as well as the effects of exercise on young competitors. Chapter 18 attempts to satisfy this need.

In the world of physical education and most especially in the realm of athletic performance, we are constantly involved directly or indirectly with the concept of fatigue. In all events in which time or distance are criteria of success, we are of necessity concerned with an endpoint largely determined by this entity we call "fatigue." Since neuromuscular fatigue is so basic to performance we have added a new chapter (chap. 20) on this subject to the second section of the text.

The fifth edition contains many new and updated figures. In some instances, however, we chose to retain classic figures from older references. When communication could be improved, existing figures from the fourth edition were modified or new figures were added. However, when updating figures from more recent citations did not add to the clarity of presentation, we chose to retain the well established figures from the past. We believe that the primary responsibility of this text is to communicate, in the best possible way, with students who are studying to become physical educators, coaches, and exercise scientists. Part of our commitment to those students is to maintain a link with the rich heritage of exercise physiology, while also providing the most up-to-date information available. One way to provide an understanding of the chronology of developments in exercise physiology is to include the classic works in the area along with the most modern citations and utilize some of the excellent diagrams and figures from the pioneer scientists in our discipline.

We are grateful to the hundreds of scientists around the world who have made this text possible. While it is not possible to acknowledge every contributor to this work we would like to recognize the following scientists who have been influential in the course of our professional lives: Martha Coryell, Stroudsburg State University; Roger J. Williams, University of Texas; J. Pat Meehan and Aileene Lockhart at University of Southern California; Glen O. Johnson, University of Nebraska-Lincoln; and William G. Thorland, Washington State University.

We also wish to thank our editors, Chris Rogers and Scott Spoolman of Brown & Benchmark Publishers, for their generous support.

Herbert A. deVries,
Laguna Beach, California

Terry J. Housh,
Lincoln, Nebraska

PART **1**

Basic Physiology Underlying the Study of Physiology of Exercise

The Why of Physiology of Exercise

Why Physical Fitness?
Improving Human Athletic Performance
Professionalism in Physical Education
    and Athletics
"Get Some Exercise"
Gender and Age Differences in Response
    to Training

Scientific Method
Overview of Text
    Basic Physiology of Exercise
    *Physiology Applied to Health
        and Fitness*
    *Physiology of Training and
        Conditioning Athletes*

The undergraduate student in physical education often regards physiology of exercise as one of the more difficult and rigorous courses in the curriculum. He or she may well ask, "Is all this scientific preparation really necessary so that I can teach physical education and coach track, swimming, football, and so on?" This is a fair question. In this chapter we answer that question as well as give an overview of intensely interesting, provocative, and highly practical material on the physiological basis of all human movement, whether performed for work, for play, for physical conditioning, or for training for athletic competition.

Physiology of exercise is a subdivision of general physiology and is concerned largely with the improvement of human functional capacities. This can involve the enhancement of health and physical fitness for the general population or the optimization of performance in the various types and levels of competitive athletics.

Why Physical Fitness?

As little as twenty to thirty years ago, discussions about physical fitness frequently evolved into arguments about definition. The discussion often ended with this question: Physical fitness for what? The implication of that question, which not all of us accepted even then, was that we need only be fit enough to meet the necessary physical challenges of our workaday world, with maybe a little bit left over for good measure! Since most of us in this overly mechanized and industrialized civilization meet very few physical challenges, low levels of functional capacity (fitness) were acceptable. Applying the concept of "pursuit of excellence" to optimizing physical fitness awaited the knowledge boom of the past three decades. We now have enough scientific evidence to answer the question, Physical fitness for what?, with this simple statement: Optimal levels of physical fitness are conducive to lifelong good health. The second section of the text presents much of the important scientific evidence that supports this statement.

Improving Human Athletic Performance

With respect to the development of the best possible performance in our athletes, we must recognize that coaching is both art and science. The art lies in the application of sound psychological and sociological principles in the development of motivation and in the ingenuity displayed in designing workouts to gain desired ends without inducing boredom or unhappiness in athletes. But no matter how good an artist the coach may be, all is for naught if he or she does not have a sound grounding in exercise physiology, which teaches the nature of the body's responses to training stimuli, both immediate (acute response) and long-term (chronic adaptation).

If a coach has overworked (commonly called overtrained) the athletes for a period of time, no amount of art will prevent staleness from setting in. Conversely, ignorance of the physiological bases of good training practice, such as progressive resistance training for power or interval training for endurance, will prevent the athletes from realizing their full potential and will probably result in a poor win-loss record!

Even more important than the win-loss record, however, is the maintenance of good health in athletes. Well-trained professional coaches must know the physiological effects of environmental factors such as heat and cold on their charges. Every year several athletes die on the football field from heatstroke. Most of these deaths could be prevented if all coaches were thoroughly trained in the basics of environmental physiology. Also important for the health of the athlete is good nutritional practice. Too many coaches, even today, rely on conventional wisdom instead of scientific evidence about the diet of their athletes.

The use of drugs to improve performance is a hazardous practice at best, and it is doubly deplorable because the hazard is rarely accompanied by any significant improvement in performance. Athletes have died in ignorance because they used amphetamines while bicycle racing on a hot day. With the seeming ease of access for the athlete to a variety of drugs, the coach must not only be aware of the manifestations of these drugs in their athletes but must also be aware of their health hazards. As the list of banned substances increases and as drug testing is becoming increasingly available and mandated by school athletic organizations, the coach or physical education instructor will have to become the knowledge base from which the athlete is guided.

Professionalism in Physical Education and Athletics

During World War II we trained lay members of the army (enlisted men who had been well-known players in baseball, football, or other sports) to be noncommissioned physical training leaders in six to eight weeks. These soldiers functioned quite well in leading calisthenics programs and athletic competitions. Were they equivalent to physical education professionals? Most definitely not! While they knew the what of the program, they did not in most cases understand the why. They had not had professional training in the basic exercise sciences, such as exercise physiology, kinesiology, and motor learning. Thus they depended on commissioned officers who were professionally trained physical educators to develop the overall training program and to guide its implementation. This practice of utilizing nonprofessional exercise leaders is still common today in the current exercise revolution. Due to the public's demand for access to exercise, health clubs, industrial fitness programs, and even clinically supervised conditioning and rehabilitation programs have turned to the well-motivated and reasonably skilled, yet academically unprepared exercise leader, a trend that is gradually changing as professional organizations are beginning to require certification and/or licensure for their individual disciplines or professions.

The difference between a professional and a lay person is that the member of a profession has "professed" a commitment to a learned discipline with a well-defined body of knowledge. This profession implies, in turn, the application of the scientific method to the professional body of knowledge, usually within a well-structured college or university curriculum. Thus the professional physical educator learns basic principles that are grounded in the scientific method. All practice then (to the extent that scientific data are available) is based on scientifically derived principles. Untrained lay persons can only practice what has been handed down to them, since they do not understand the underlying principles that should govern their practice. For example, lay coaches can only do what they have seen their coaches (or other athletes) do, whether right or wrong.

While the lay person can only function at the cookbook level, that is, follow the instructions of a professionally trained individual, the person trained in the basic sciences, such as exercise physiology, proceeds from first principles. We, as members of a learned profession, must always seek out the mechanisms underlying our practice. In doing so, we derive at least four practical advantages: 1) we can better predict results; 2) we can better control the conditioning and training process, thus protecting the health of our charges; 3) we grow more efficient in terms of results gained per unit of time spent; and 4) we may even satisfy our intellectual curiosity with respect to cause-and-effect relationships in our field (this, of course, is research).

"Get Some Exercise"

Most of us have heard a physician or a well-meaning friend advise: "Jack, what you need is some exercise." Implicit in such a prescription is that it makes no difference whether one lifts weights for an hour, swims a mile, or jogs three miles. It is long past time for our profession to grab the reins of leadership in this domain. Let's educate the public and the health-related professions, too, to understand that the admonition "get some exercise" is analogous to a physician's writing a prescription that simply says, "Administer some drugs." Just as there are many drugs to choose from when prescribing aspirin for a headache, so are there many exercise training and conditioning modalities, each of which can be modified or administered in terms of intensity, frequency, and duration. Many of us at work in our exercise physiology research laboratories are developing dose-response relationships for the various types of exercise. Physical education students must learn what is presently available in our pharmacopoeia of exercise. We must learn the scientific answers to how much is enough, how much is too much, and how much is best for any given individual. What is presently known in this area is presented in chapter 15.

The future holds great promise for expanding the physical education profession from one that at present limits its audience largely to schoolchildren to one that will cater to the needs of people of all ages and both genders. Who in a sales position would voluntarily limit his or her clientele to a small percentage of the total population (persons six to eighteen instead of birth to seventy)? Interestingly, the public's acceptance of the need for adult fitness seems to have advanced far more rapidly than our profession's leadership in training the personnel for such programs. Obviously, such personnel must be well grounded in exercise physiology to prevent hazardous situations from arising among middle-aged and older people who may have unrecognized disease problems as well as flabby muscles and poor cardiovascular function as a result of sedentary living.

Gender and Age Differences in Response to Training

Only in recent years have females begun to participate to any great extent in physical conditioning programs or competitive athletics. Women's athletics worthy of the name did not exist prior to World War I, and women did not begin Olympic competition until 1928. Because of women's very recent entry into the sports world, professionals are only now beginning to accumulate data in their laboratories about the similarities and differences in response between males and females to the stimuli of exercise and heavy training regimens. It has been a long, slow process, but we now know that females respond similarly to men to a conditioning program and derive the same health benefits. With respect to high-level competition, women come much closer to the men's records than men would have supposed only a few years ago. Yet, there are some dramatic differences in female responses. For example, women had long avoided weight training for fear of developing bulging and unsightly muscles. However, the truth of the matter is that the female's response to weight training is very different from the male's, probably because of endocrine differences. Intense weight training at a level that brings about large and well-defined muscles in the male only serves to enhance the strength and power of the female, with only slight increases in muscle bulk. The conventional wisdom that prohibited heavy weight training for women because it would lead to masculineness was probably the result of someone observing that some highly successful female athletes were unusually muscular. What probably happened was that women who were extremely muscular by genetic endowment (mesomorphs) were more likely to pursue and succeed in athletic careers.

The issue of pregnancy further complicates the problem of physical conditioning and/or sports training in women. The ramifications of exercise to the mother and fetus are only now being addressed in research and will ultimately become a very serious concern for the physical education instructor and coach at both the secondary and collegiate levels. Today we are able to conclude from the research literature that 1) mild to moderate exercise is probably not harmful to the normally active pregnant woman, and 2) independent of pregnancy, there are probably no gender differences in the ability to benefit from strenuous physical activity.

With respect to age, as recently as two decades ago it was assumed on insufficient scientific evidence that an older person was virtually untrainable! How old was "older"? Would you believe forty? Evidence from our own laboratory dispels this myth. We have shown that seventy- and eighty-year-olds, if healthy, have the same relative capacity for training as the young. That is to say, the percentage improvement in performance with training is every bit as good in the elderly as in the young. Our findings have now been corroborated by several other investigators and will be discussed in detail in chapter 19.

Scientific Method

Physical educators or coaches who claim membership in the profession are morally bound to base their practice on the best (most reliable and authoritative) information available. Obviously, hearsay evidence is not in the same class with evidence derived from application of the scientific method in controlled experiments. The credibility of various sources of evidence can be ordered from poorest to best as follows:

1. Hunch or guess.
2. Hypothesis—a tentative supposition (based on hunches or guesses) provisionally adopted to explain certain facts and to guide the investigation of others. A hypothesis is set up to be tested and accepted or rejected on the basis of further observation or experiment.
3. Theory—based on some scientific evidence but insufficiently verified to be accepted as fact. Theories provide the basis for developing principles.
4. Principle—a settled rule of action based on theories that are well supported by research findings. Principles are the guidelines for making decisions in our professional activities.

True professionals are set apart from lay practitioners in their ability and inclination to challenge the source of information. For example, the lay coach hears that a certain athlete, who has broken the world record for the 1,500-meter run, is a confirmed vegetarian. Not having been trained in the application of the scientific method and also unable or unwilling to read the available research literature, the coach assumes a cause-and-effect relationship between the outstanding performance and the athlete's vegetarian habits. The coach then attempts to make vegetarians out of all athletes. The professionally trained coach sees this explanation of superior performance for what it is—no better than a hunch or guess, at best. This coach goes to the professional literature, consulting reliable sources in physiology, biochemistry, and nutrition. Finding no support for a cause-and-effect relationship between superior running ability and a vegetable diet, the coach rejects the hunch that the record performance was causally related to the athlete's vegetarianism.

In the long run, coaching practice that is based on scientifically derived principles rather than on unproven hunches or personal opinions will be considerably more successful. For this reason, this text will present the pertinent sources of research information in the hope that students will learn to be discerning consumers of information about physical education and coaching practices.

Overview of Text

This text is organized into three parts. The first part deals with the basic physiology that provides the groundwork for application in our field. Although the information is organized by systems of the body, the potential applications are pointed out and emphasized.

Recognizing the basic differences in interest between those who are primarily teachers of health and physical education and those who will be involved largely in the coaching of athletics, the second part of the book deals with the physiology of exercise in relation to health and fitness. The third part is devoted to the scientific improvement of athletic performance.

Basic Physiology of Exercise

Of all the tissue composing the human body, by far the greatest proportion is muscle, which makes up about 40% of body weight. Furthermore, all movement must be implemented through the skeletal muscles. Therefore we begin with a study of muscles. Since a knowledge of structure (anatomy) is necessary for understanding function (physiology), the second chapter deals with gross, microscopic, and submicroscopic structure. Recent evidence obtained through the electron microscope even allows us to explore the fascinating relationship between structure and function.

The third chapter tells the story of how energy from the food we eat is made available to individual muscle cells. Recent research has made it abundantly clear how important this information is to the best possible preparation of athletes for competition.

Chapter 4 covers the physiology of gross muscle contraction, dealing with such practical problems as muscle fatigue, muscle length and tension, and speed and force of contraction in relation to power output, a concern in all physical activity. Even the design of derailleur bicycles is based on the principles presented here.

Nervous control of the muscles, which is responsible for the beautifully coordinated movements possible in champion athletes, is discussed in chapter 5. The groundwork is laid here for understanding such practical problems as how strength is limited, how muscle sense is developed, and why some forms of stretching are superior to others.

The next two chapters (6 and 7) describe how the heart and circulation act as the transport system for bringing in necessary oxygen and nutrients and removing the products of metabolism. Here the groundwork is laid for understanding how training affects the heart and blood vessels and how different types of exercise affect the work of the heart.

Chapters 8 and 9 deal with breathing function and the transport of gases by the blood, including such practical matters as the best breathing patterns, second wind, the use of hyperventilation in athletics, the effects of smoking on wind, and aerobic capacity.

Chapter 10 deals with the effects of the

endocrine system during exercise and competition and the effects of physical conditioning on the endocrines.

Chapter 11 is a new chapter that presents information about the effect of exercise on immune function. Activity has always been considered a prudent modality in improving one's health. The actual impact of exercise on health may be related, in large part, to the ability of the immune system to respond favorably to training.

Chapter 12 pulls together all the foregoing chapters to provide the terminology and information necessary to utilize scientific principles in applying physiology to health and fitness and to the training of athletes.

Physiology Applied to Health and Fitness

In chapter 13, in the second section of the book, we discuss the large, new body of knowledge that spells out the potential health benefits of physical fitness.

Chapter 14 describes in some detail the methods used in exercise physiology laboratories around the world in the measurement of aerobic power, aerobic capacity, and in stress testing.

Chapter 15 applies this basic knowledge to the prescription of exercise.

While the incidence of cardiovascular disease is seemingly on the decline, it still constitutes the major cause of premature mortality in this country. Chapter 16 is devoted exclusively to the potential ways in which physical conditioning may prevent cardiovascular disease and rehabilitate its victims.

Chapter 17, on metabolism and weight control, provides the scientific bases for successful weight maintenance and reduction and discusses the conventional wisdom and misinformation that have made obesity such a problem in the United States. Nutrition is discussed, and simple means for evaluating one's diet are provided.

Chapter 18 is a new chapter that introduces the topic of growth and development. Exercise has always been considered important for the development of bones and muscle in children. This chapter provides the background material related to the role of exercise in growth and its importance in physiological development.

Chapter 19 on age and exercise presents available evidence on the physiological effects of aging, together with evidence that suggests that much of what has been accepted as the effect of aging is really the result of our sedentary lifestyle, which leads to atrophy of muscles and other tissues and dysfunction in general.

Chapter 20 is a new chapter on neuromuscular fatigue. Fatigue affects our ability to perform all types of physical activity. This chapter discusses the physiological mechanisms underlying muscle fatigue and the implications for athletes and industrial workers.

Physiology of Training and Conditioning Athletes

In this section, all available scientific evidence that can be applied to the problems of coaching is culled selectively and presented in the form of a structured approach to systematic improvement of athletic performance. To do this sport by sport would be to revert to a cookbook philosophy; moreover, generalization would be difficult. Therefore we adopt a more scientific approach in which we discuss the individual elements of human performance. Thus the section is organized into chapters dealing with strength, endurance, muscular efficiency, speed, flexibility, muscle soreness, warming up, environmental factors, nutrition, special aids, and female athletes.

So, now that you have briefly glimpsed what lies ahead and you understand the need for exposure to the physiology of exercise, you are ready to press on to the study of one of the most fascinating and intriguing subdivisions of physiology: human physiological responses, both immediate and long-term, to the demands of exercise.

2

Structure of Muscle Tissue

Gross Structure of Skeletal Muscle

Microscopic Structure of Skeletal Muscle

Structure of the Muscle Cell or Fiber

Muscle Fiber Types

Structure of the Myofibril and the Contractile Mechanism

Blood Supply and Lymphatics

Nerve Supply

All human activity, whether in work or sport, depends ultimately on the contraction of muscle tissue for its driving forces. There are three types of muscle tissue in the human body:

1. Smooth, nonstriated muscle, which is found in the walls of the hollow viscera and blood vessels.
2. Striated, skeletal muscle, which provides the force for movement of the bony leverage system.
3. Cardiac muscle, which is found only in the heart.

Smooth muscle receives its innervation from the autonomic nervous system and ordinarily contracts independently of voluntary control. The fibers of smooth muscle are usually long, spindle-shaped bodies, but their external shape may change somewhat to conform to the surrounding elements. Each fiber usually has only one nucleus.

Skeletal muscle, which is innervated by the voluntary or somatic nervous system, consists of long, cylindrical muscle fibers. Each fiber is a large cell with as many as several hundred nuclei and is structurally independent of its neighboring fiber or cell. Skeletal, or striated muscle, as the name implies, is most easily distinguished by its cross-striations of alternating light and dark bands (fig. 2.1).

Cardiac muscle in all vertebrates is a network of striated muscle fibers. It differs structurally from the other two types of muscle tissue mainly in the interweaving of its fibers to form a network, called a syncytium, that differentiates it from skeletal muscle, which is also striated. It further differs from smooth muscle in that it has cross-striations, which smooth muscle does not have. Cardiac muscle contracts rhythmically and automatically, without outside stimulation. Whereas skeletal muscle is made up of discrete fibers that can contract individually (but with other members of its motor unit), cardiac muscle is composed of a network of fibers that responds to innervation with a wavelike contraction that passes through the entire muscle.

Gross Structure of Skeletal Muscle

If we dissected a limb such as the upper arm and removed the skin, subcutaneous adipose tissue, and the superficial fascia, we would lay bare the biceps brachii muscle and note that it is covered in its entirety by a deep layer of fascia that binds the muscle into one functional unit. This outermost sheath of connective tissue is called the epimysium, and it merges at the ends of the muscle with the connective tissue material of the tendon. Thus the force of muscular contraction is transmitted through the connective tissues, binding the muscle to the tendon, then through the tendon to the bony structures, to bring about movement. The importance of the fascial tissues has been shown by a recent experiment in which a small slit in the epimysium resulted in a 15% loss in muscle strength (9).

In cross section, one can see that the interior of the muscle is subdivided by septa into bundles of muscle fibers (fig. 2.2). Each bundle contains upwards of a dozen, possibly as many as several hundred, fibers. Each bundle is called a fasciculus and has a more or less complete connective tissue sheath called the perimysium. The structures discussed so far are visible to the naked eye.

Microscopic Structure of Skeletal Muscle

A microscope is needed for more detailed study—in order to see the structure of an individual fiber and how the fibers form fasciculi

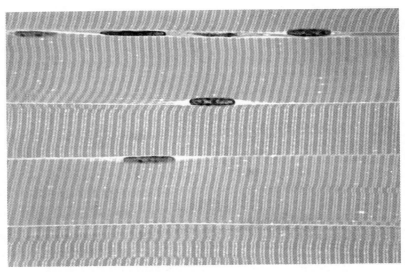

Three skeletal muscle fibers showing the characteristic cross-striations. © Edwin Reschke.

(fig. 2.2). Each fiber is surrounded by a flimsy sheath called the endomysium. The need for these connective tissue sheaths—endomysium around the single fiber, perimysium around the fasciculus, and epimysium about the whole muscle—is explained by the fact that one fiber may not run through the whole length of a muscle, or even through a fasciculus (fig. 2.3). Therefore it becomes necessary to transmit the force of contraction from fiber to fiber to fasciculus, and from fasciculus to fasciculus (since these sometimes do not run through the length of a large muscle either) to the tendons, which act upon the bones. This is a function of the connective tissues described above.

The dimensions of individual fibers vary, according to most investigators, from 10 to 100 microns (1,000 microns = 1 mm) in diameter and from 1 mm to the length of the whole muscle. Thus the thickness of a large fiber is roughly comparable to that of a fine human hair, while the smaller fibers cannot be seen by the unaided eye. Each fiber constitutes one muscle cell. Each muscle has fibers of characteristic size, and the thickness of each fiber is related to the forces involved in the function of the muscle. Thus the fibers of the extrinsic ocular muscles are small in diameter, whereas those of the quadriceps femoris are large.

Structure of the Muscle Cell or Fiber

The cell membrane of the muscle cell is called the sarcolemma. This membrane is extremely thin and seems almost structureless, even under the electron microscope (fig. 2.4). Inside the sarcolemma are the many nuclei, mainly situated peripherally, close to the sarcolemma. Corresponding to the cytoplasm of other cells is the sarcoplasm, which is the more fluid part of the cell. Running longitudinally within the sarcoplasm are slender columnlike structures called myofibrils, which have alternating segments of light and dark color. The presence of the myofibrils imparts to the fiber as a whole

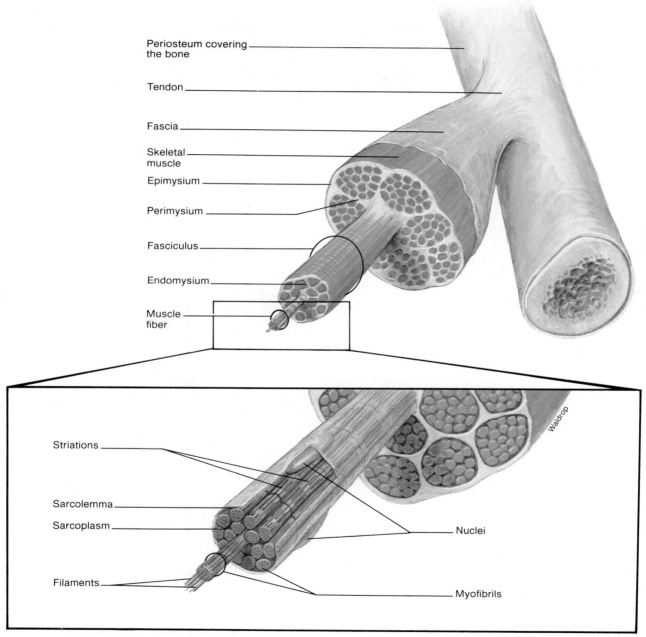

Periosteum covering the bone

Tendon

Fascia

Skeletal muscle

Epimysium

Perimysium

Fasciculus

Endomysium

Muscle fiber

Striations

Sarcolemma

Sarcoplasm

Filaments

Nuclei

Myofibrils

Waldrop

Figure 2.2   The relationship between muscle fibers and the connective tissues of the tendon, epimysium, perimysium, and endomysium. Close-up shows an expanded view of a single muscle fiber. (From J. W. Hole, Jr., *Human Anatomy and Physiology,* 5th edition. Copyright © 1990 Wm. C. Brown Communications, Inc., Dubuque, Iowa. All rights reserved. Reprinted by permission.)

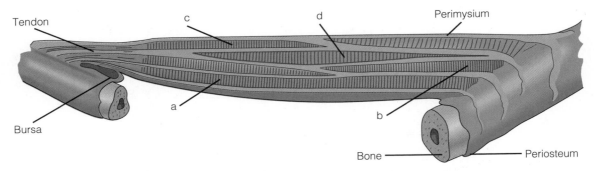

Figure 2.3   Diagram of attachment of muscle to skeleton and relation of fibers to each other within a fasciculus: (a) fiber extends the length of fasciculus; (b) fiber begins at periosteum but ends in muscle; (c) fiber begins at tendon but ends in muscle; (d) both ends of fiber within the muscle (redrawn from Braus). (From Copenhaver, W. M.; Bunge, R. P.; and Bunge, M. B. *Bailey's Textbook of Histology*, 1971. Courtesy of Williams & Wilkins Company, Baltimore.)

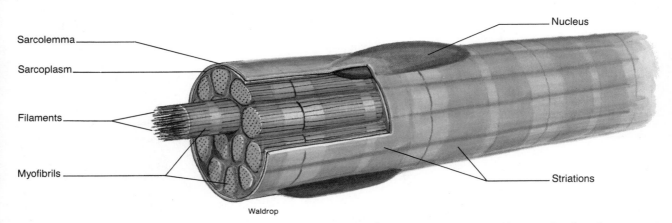

Figure 2.4   A skeletal muscle fiber is composed of numerous myofibrils that contain the filaments of actin and myosin. Skeletal muscle fiber is striated and multinucleated. (From Stuart Ira Fox, *Human Physiology*, 4th edition. Copyright © 1993 Wm. C. Brown Communications, Inc., Dubuque, Iowa. All rights reserved. Reprinted by permission.)

the appearance of lengthwise striations. The cross-striations, however, are far more obvious because the dark segments of the many myofibrils are arranged in lateral alignment. All light segments are likewise aligned with one another.

Muscle Fiber Types

For many years, anatomists and histologists have classified muscles as red or white according to whether red or white fibers predominated in the makeup of the gross muscle structure. In this classification, the red fibers were considered better suited to long-term, slow contractions, as required of postural, antigravity muscles, while the white fibers were considered differentiated for speed of contraction and thus were to be found predominantly in the flexor muscles.

In recent years, with the advent of modern histochemical techniques, examination of chemical constituents at the cellular level became possible and provided the means to correlate the functional activity of individual fibers with their morphology. Thus identifying skeletal muscle fiber types has become more sophisticated and at the same time has provided laboratory-derived information that helps us understand why one person may be better suited to endurance-type athletics while another excels in sprint-type athletics.

Various workers have named from two to as many as eight different fiber types, based on the new laboratory techniques. The disparity in the number of types named has in part been caused by the fact that some investigators have used human muscle while others have used animal muscle. We now know that there are interesting differences between human and animal muscles with respect to fiber types. In addition, nomenclature was based on at least four different approaches: 1) the anatomical appearance; red versus white, and so on, 2) muscle function; fast-slow or fatigable versus fatigue-resistant, 3) biochemical properties, such as high or low aerobic capacity, and 4) histochemical properties, such as the enzyme profile of the fiber.

There seems to be agreement on a classification system based on three fiber types (table 2.1) that can best serve our purposes with respect to human muscle (7, 18). The older, fast twitch (white) versus slow twitch (red) system has become inadequate because there are two subtypes of fast twitch fibers, with both physiological and histochemical differences. Most important from the standpoint of exercise physiology, they respond differently to training. For these reasons we shall use the nomenclature of Peter (18) and coworkers as shown in table 2.1.

First, we must take up some basic considerations with respect to muscle makeup. It has been shown (2) that surgical crossing of the motor nerve supplying a fast muscle such as flexor hallucis longus with that of a slow muscle such as soleus resulted in a reversal of the muscles' contractile properties. Therefore we suspected that all muscle fibers within one motor unit were of the same fiber type. That has been verified (3). While the percentages of the three fiber types present in the various muscles of one person may be quite different, the fiber type (with respect to fast or slow twitch, at least) for any one muscle is established early in life and probably does not change thereafter (5, 6). Some recent investigators have suggested the possibility of converting fast twitch fibers to slow twitch and vice versa (12, 17, 20). In any event, training can bring about considerable improvement in both aerobic capacity and glycogen content of the muscle, as will be discussed in the next chapter. Also there appears to be no difference between genders with respect to fiber-type percentages (5).

Table 2.1	Classifications and Characteristics of Human Skeletal Muscle Fibers		
A. Nomenclature			
1. Dubowitz and Brooke (7)	Type I	Type IIa	Type IIb
2. Peter et al. (18)	Slow, oxidative (SO)	Fast, oxidative, glycolytic (FOG)	Fast, glycolytic (FG)
3. Older systems	Red slow twitch (ST)	White Fast Twitch (FT)	
B. Characteristics			
1. Speed of contraction	Slow	Fast	Fast
2. Strength of contraction	Low	High	High
3. Fatigability	Fatigue-resistant	Fatigable	Most fatigable
4. Aerobic capacity	High	Medium	Low
5. Anaerobic capacity	Low	Medium	High
6. Size	Small	Largest	Large
7. Capillary density	High	High	Low

The significance of the fiber-type composition for athletics becomes readily apparent from a consideration of table 2.1. The individual endowed with a high percentage of slow twitch (ST) fibers, which are slow but highly fatigue-resistant, would be a good candidate for distance running or other endurance events. On the other hand, a person whose genetic makeup produced high percentages of fast twitch (FT) fibers would be predisposed toward success in power and sprint events. These expectations have been supported by recent laboratory work in which samples of muscle tissue in different persons under varying conditions were taken with biopsy needles. Early work in this area by Gollnick and associates (10) showed interesting relationships between successful performance in endurance athletic events and the percentage of slow, oxidative (SO) fibers. More recent work by Costill and colleagues (6) supported

these findings. They found that the gastrocnemius muscles of fourteen championship-caliber distance runners were characterized by high percentages of (SO) fibers (79%), while the same muscles in trained middle distance runners had only 62%, only slightly more than untrained men at 58%. Interestingly, they also found that the SO fibers of the elite runners were 22% larger than their FT fibers, the opposite of what is usually found (table 2.1). This is probably a selective training effect resulting from the heavy use of the type SO fibers.

In the studies of human muscle using only two categories of fibers, slow twitch (ST) and fast twitch (FT), there is agreement that these two categories do not change their relative proportions as the result of training; only their size and oxidative capacities improve. However, work (19) using the newer classification of three muscle types (table 2.1) suggests that changes within the FT fibers are the important responses to training. Thus research suggests that humans can adapt to different muscular activities by way of a shift from fast twitch, glycolytic (FG) fibers to fast twitch, oxidative, glycolytic (FOG) fibers in response to distance running, and from FOG muscles to FG muscles in response to weight training. This is an attractive hypothesis in that it would bring human adaptive responses in line with those observed in lower mammals by several different groups of investigators.

Only recently have we found evidence that intact human skeletal muscle behaves in a fashion related to the behavior of animal skeletal muscle with respect to fiber types. Thorstensson and coworkers (21, 23) in Sweden have shown significant correlations of .48 and .50 between the percentage of FT fibers an athlete has in the knee extensor muscles and the maximal torque produced (a measure of strength). Similar correlations were observed between percentage of FT fibers and the speed of muscle contraction. Furthermore, the Thorstensson studies (22) showed an even stronger correlation (.86) between the percentage of FT fibers and the rate at which fatigue sets in.

With respect to fiber type, our genetic endowment determines to a large extent whether we should pursue endurance-type sports or sports that demand sprint or power in their performance. In either case, ultimate success depends on many other factors such as training, conditioning, and dedication.

Structure of the Myofibril and the Contractile Mechanism

The advent of the electron microscope and its wide use in recent years has provided greater insight into both the structure and function of the myofibril. Though the story is not complete in all details, the sliding filament model of muscle contraction is now widely accepted as the best explanation of all the experimental data (16).

The sarcomere is the functional unit of the myofibril, and it extends from Z line to Z line, as shown in figures 2.5 and 2.6. Each sarcomere is composed of two types of interdigitating parallel filaments that run the length of the myofibril. One type (myosin) is about twice as thick as the other, and its length is equal to the length of the A band (the dark band seen as part of the striation effect). The second (actin) and thinner type of filament is longer and extends inward from both Z membranes, almost to the center of the sarcomere. The amount by which the two ends of the thin filament fail to meet constitutes a lighter band within the dark A band that is called the H zone. The area between the ends of the thick filaments is less dense and therefore gives the light band appearance of the striation effect, which is known as the I band. Thus the light and dark striped effect of striated muscle rests on a rational basis of bands of greater and lesser optical density, as can be seen in figure 2.5. The cross-sectional views show the relationship of each thick filament to a hexagon of six thin filaments, each hexagon, however, being shared by three thick filaments (fig. 2.5).

Chemical extraction of the muscle protein myosin results in the disappearance of the dark A band (fig. 2.6), while extraction of the muscle protein actin similarly affects the I band. These facts are very strong evidence that the thick filaments consist of myosin and the thin filaments of actin and also tropomyosin.

A sliding movement of the actin and myosin filaments during contraction of the myofibril has been well demonstrated. It seems that the A bands remain the same length, while the I bands change only in shortening below 90% of the myofibrils' resting length (fig. 2.7). The exact nature of the changes in the H zone are not as yet clearly understood, although the

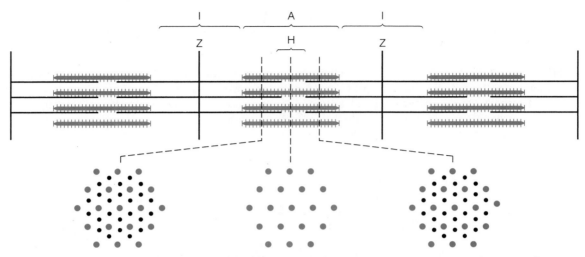

Figure 2.5   Diagrammatic representation of the structure of striated muscle, showing overlapping arrays of actin- and myosin-containing filaments, the latter with projecting cross-bridges on them. For convenience of representation, the structure is drawn with considerable longitudinal foreshortening. With filament diameters and side spacings as shown, the filament lengths should be about five times the lengths depicted. (From Huxley, H. E. "The Structural Basis of Muscular Contraction," in *Proceedings of the Royal Society of London* 178:131, 1971. Courtesy of the Royal Society of London.)

disappearance of the H zone during contraction is well established. The contractile process depends on the presence of adenosine triphosphate (ATP) and its splitting by dephosphorylation into adenosine diphosphate (ADP) and phosphate. This splitting of an ATP bond furnishes large amounts of energy.

Now we must account for the mechanics involved in bringing about the sliding of the filaments and the biochemical events that initiate and provide the energy for this interdigitation of the actin and myosin filaments. The most acceptable explanation for the process of contraction at the cellular level is as follows:

1. An electrical impulse conducted by the motor nerve activates the motor end plate of the muscle fiber, which in turn brings about the release of a substance that depolarizes the resting muscle membrane. This depolarization is what is recorded and measured by electromyographic methods as muscle action potentials.

2. The action potential in turn sets off two independent electrical currents, one of which is a weak longitudinal current, the other a transverse current that moves inward into the fiber along a system of tubules (fig. 2.8).

3. The inwardly invading current releases internal, tightly bound calcium (13).

4. In the fiber's resting state, inactivity is maintained because a complex of two other proteins, troponin and tropomyosin, when in combination with actin, prevents the normal course of interaction between actin and myosin filaments. When the calcium ions are released because of the electrical excitation, they bind strongly to the

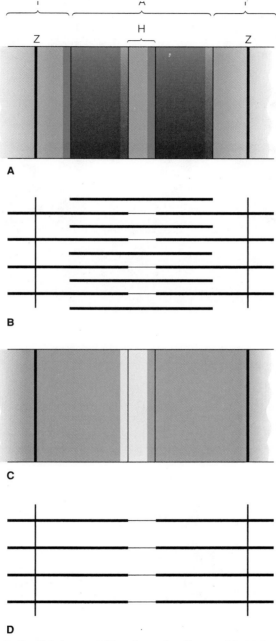

Figure 2.6   Diagram illustrating the changes taking place when the muscle protein myosin is extracted chemically. Differences in optical density before and after extraction are shown in **a** and **c,** with a logical schematic explanation in **b** and **d.** (From Huxley, H. E., and Hanson, J., in *The Structure and Function of Muscle,* G. H. Bourne, ed., 1960. Courtesy of the Academic Press, Orlando.)

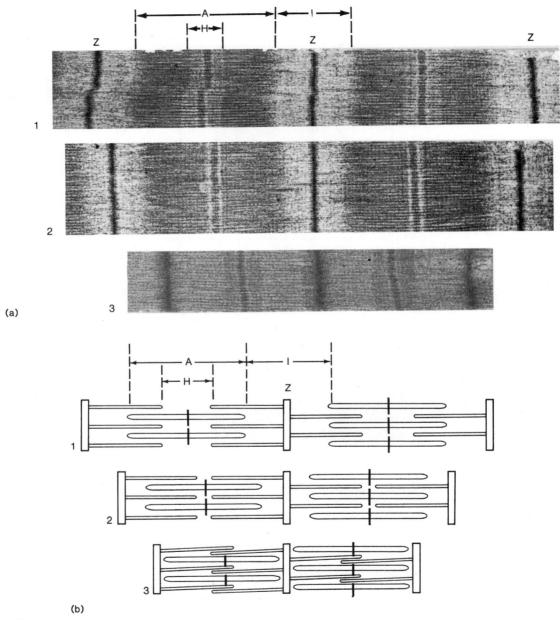

Figure 2.7   The sliding filament model of contraction. As the filaments slide, the Z lines are brought closer together. The A bands remain the same length during contraction, but the I and H bands get progressively shorter and may eventually become obliterated. (a) and (b) © H. E. Huxley.

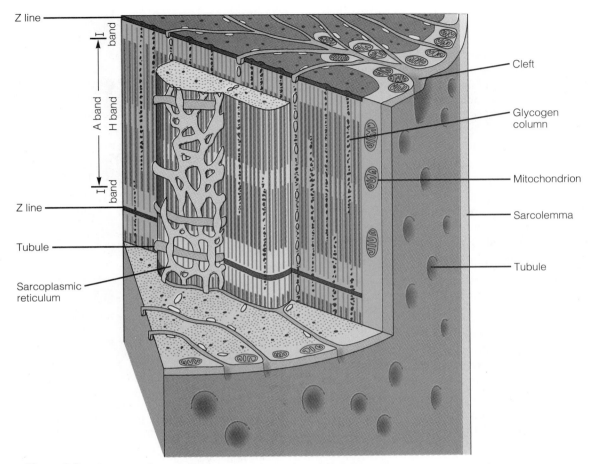

Z line

I band

A band

H band

I band

Z line

Tubule

Sarcoplasmic reticulum

Cleft

Glycogen column

Mitochondrion

Sarcolemma

Tubule

Figure 2.8   Structure of muscle fiber consists of a number of fibrils, which in turn are made up of orderly arrays of thick and thin filaments of protein. A system of transverse tubules opens to the exterior of the fiber. The sarcoplasmic reticulum is a system of tubules that does not open to the exterior. The two systems, which are evidently involved in the flow of calcium ions, meet at a number of junctions called dyads or triads. Mitochondria convert food to energy. The sarcolemma is a membrane surrounding the fiber. (From Hoyle, G. *How Is Muscle Turned On and Off?* Copyright © 1970 by Scientific American, Inc. All rights reserved.)

troponin-tropomyosin complex and thus suppress the inhibitory action upon the interaction of the actin and myosin, which are then free to combine.

5. The combination of actin-myosin acts as an enzyme (catalyst), which is called actomyosin adenosine-triphosphatase, or actomyosin ATPase. Actomyosin

ATPase catalyzes the breakdown of ATP to ADP + P, which in turn furnishes the energy for contraction (8).

6. Having defined the contractile structure and its source of energy, we now need to explain the mode of action of the cross-bridges in making the filaments slide to shorten the sarcomere and thus the

myofibril—the fiber and the whole muscle. The most plausible explanation is offered by H. E. Huxley (16), who was involved in the original formulation of the sliding filament theory (11), along with the independent work of A. F. Huxley (14). Figure 2.9 illustrates the process referred to as the swinging cross-bridge model.

7. When the nerve impulse ceases, relaxation occurs because the calcium no longer binds to the troponin-tropomyosin complex and the inhibitory function on the actin-myosin interaction is restored, thus ending the contraction process.

Earlier in vitro experiments had shown that three necessary elements of muscle function—relaxation, contraction, and rigor mortis—could be explained as follows:

1. In the presence of ATP (unsplit), actomyosin breaks down into a noncontractile state of dissociated actin and myosin, thus causing relaxation.

2. When ATP splits to form ADP + P, actomyosin threads reform, and the reformed threads contract in the presence of more ATP.

3. If the reformed actomyosin thread is removed from the presence of ATP, it resists extension.

These in vitro observations seem to explain the facts observed in vivo:

1. Relaxation, in the presence of unsplit ATP.

2. Contraction, in the presence of unsplit ATP, when some ATP is undergoing dephosphorylation.

3. Rigor mortis, caused by total dissipation of ATP after its splitting has already caused the precipitation of inextensible actomyosin threads.

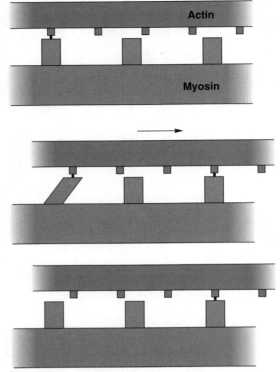

Figure 2.9   Diagram showing, very schematically, possible mode of action of cross-bridges. A cross-bridge attaches to a specific site on the actin filament, then undergoes some configurational change, which causes the point of attachment to move closer to the centre of the A band, pulling the actin filament along in the required manner. At the end of its working stroke, the bridge detaches and returns to its starting configuration, in preparation for another cycle. During each cycle, probably one molecule of ATP is dephosphorylated. Asynchronous attachment of other bridges maintains steady force. (From Huxley, H. E. "The Structural Basis of Muscular Contraction," in *Proceedings of the Royal Society of London* 178:131, 1971. Courtesy of the Royal Society of London.)

Blood Supply and Lymphatics

In keeping with the high level of metabolic activity of muscle tissue, muscle is extremely well supplied with capillaries. Each muscle fiber is supplied with several capillaries. To furnish this rich vascularization, larger branches of arteries penetrate the muscle by following the paths of the septa between fasciculi (in the perimysium). The arteries furnish arterioles to the fasciculi, and the arterioles give off capillaries at sharp angles to individual fibers. The veins typically follow the arteries, and even the smallest veins have valves. Lymphatic capillaries are found only at the fascicular level of organization.

Nerve Supply

Because each muscle fiber represents a single cell and is a discrete functioning unit, it must be innervated individually. This is not to say, however, that one nerve cell (motor neuron) may not innervate more than one muscle cell by sending branches from the same nerve fiber to several or many muscle fibers (fig. 2.10). The cell bodies of the neurons (nerve cells) lie in the ventral horns of the spinal cord. The axons of these cells form the nerve fibers of the efferent fibers of the peripheral nerves, which innervate the muscles. Each nerve, as seen grossly in dissection, represents the association of many axons or nerve fibers, just as a gross muscle represents many muscle fibers. The nerve fibers, like the arterioles, travel in the perimysium and branch several times, thus permitting one neuron to innervate more than one muscle fiber.

The ratio of nerve fibers to muscle fibers varies with the degree of precision required of the muscle. In one of the muscles that moves the eye, a ratio of one nerve fiber to one muscle

fiber has been found. However, one nerve cell may innervate as many as several hundred muscle fibers.

The neuron and its axon (or nerve fiber) with its branches, plus the muscle fibers supplied by all the branches, form the basic neuromuscular unit: the motor unit. The intersection of the branches of the nerve fiber and the muscle fiber is called the neuromuscular junction or myoneural junction. The branches of the nerve fiber and a specialized portion of the sarcolemma of the muscle fiber called the motor end plate are separated by a small space known as the neuromuscular cleft or synaptic cleft. Within the nerve fibers at the neuromuscular junction are vesicles (called synaptic vesicles), which contain the neurotransmitter acetylcholine.

The muscle fibers making up one motor unit do not lie contiguously; they are usually scattered throughout a considerable volume of the gross muscle structure (fig. 2.11). Thus muscle fibers innervated by twigs of the same motor neuron may be positioned in several different fasciculi. This fact has important implications for our discussion of electromyography in a later chapter.

Summary

1. Three types of muscle tissue are present in the human body.

   a. Smooth, nonstriated: usually found in viscera and blood vessels

   b. Skeletal, striated: found in the somatic muscles

   c. Cardiac, striated syncytium: found only in the heart

2. Gross structure of skeletal muscle is at three levels.

   a. Whole muscle, surrounded by epimysium

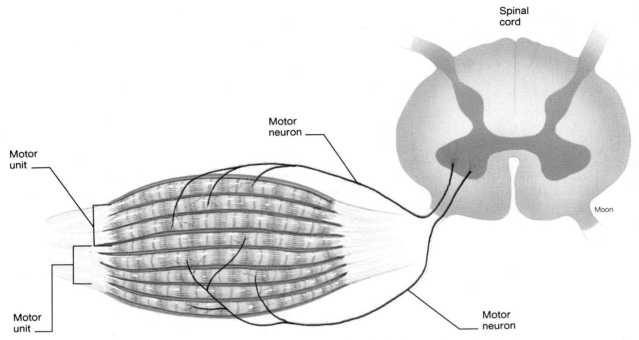

Figure 2.10   A diagram illustrating the innervation of muscle fibers by different motor units. (Actually, many more muscle fibers would be included in a single motor unit than is shown in this drawing.) (From Stuart Ira Fox, *Human Physiology*, 4th edition. Copyright © 1993 Wm. C. Brown Communications, Inc., Dubuque, Iowa. All rights reserved. Reprinted by permission.)

b. Muscle bundle or fasciculus, surrounded by perimysium, which constitutes the septum seen grossly in cross section

c. Muscle fiber, surrounded by endomysium

3. In the microscopic structure of skeletal muscle, fiber diameter is roughly related to the load of work the muscle ordinarily performs.

4. Each skeletal muscle fiber represents one multinucleated cell in which the sarcolemma is the cell membrane and the sarcoplasm roughly corresponds to the cytoplasm of other cells.

5. Newer systems of classification for human muscle fiber types include three basically different skeletal muscle fibers: a) slow twitch, oxidative (SO), b) fast twitch, oxidative, glycolytic (FOG), and c) fast twitch, glycolytic (FG). Genetic endowment determines the proportion of slow twitch to fast twitch fibers (SO to FOG + FG). But available evidence suggests that endurance training may cause a shift from FG to FOG, and power training may cause a shift from FOG to FG.

6. There is an abundant supply of capillaries to muscle tissue to support the large metabolic demands of exercise.

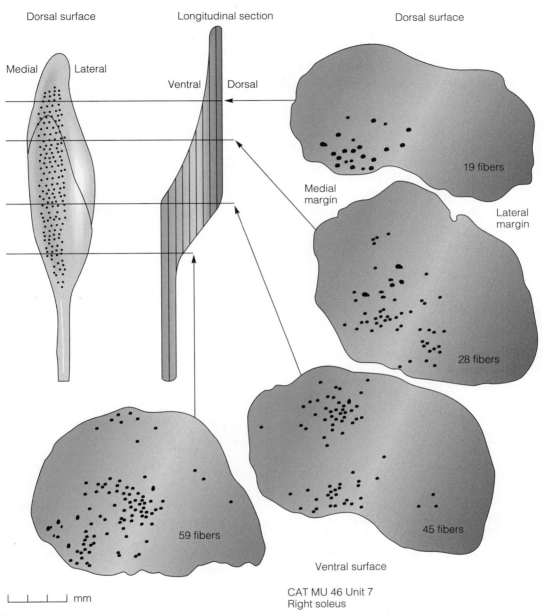

Dorsal surface

Medial   Lateral

Longitudinal section

Ventral   Dorsal

Dorsal surface

Medial margin

Lateral margin

19 fibers

28 fibers

59 fibers

45 fibers

Ventral surface

mm

CAT MU 46 Unit 7
Right soleus

Figure 2.11   Distribution of muscle fibers in a motor unit. The diagrams on the upper left represent the whole soleus muscle as seen from the dorsal surface and in longitudinal section. The extent of the ventral aponeurosis of origin and of the dorsal aponeurosis of insertion are indicated by heavier lines on the longitudinal section, and the arrangement of primary fiber fasciculi is denoted by the parallel lines. Crosshatched area represents the approximate territory of the muscle unit projected onto the muscle outline. Cross sections taken through various levels along the longitudinal axis of the muscle are shown in outline tracings. Muscle fibers belonging to the studied unit have been plotted as dots. The approximate levels of sectioning are indicated on the whole muscle diagrams. Fiber counts are given on each section. (From Burke, R. E., et al., in *Journal of Physiology* 238:503–14. © Cambridge University Press, London. Reprinted by permission.)

7. When a neuron in the ventral horn of the spinal cord is stimulated, its axon, all of the axon's branches, and all of the muscle fibers supplied by the branches function together simultaneously as a motor unit.

8. A motor unit may consist of one neuron with its axon (nerve fiber) innervating one muscle fiber, or it may consist of one neuron with its axon branching and innervating as many as several hundred muscle fibers.

9. Although the muscle fibers of one motor unit function together, they do not constitute a unified structure. In fact, in many cases they are distributed throughout a considerable volume of muscle tissue.

References

1. Bailey, Kenneth. Muscle protein. *Br. Med. Bull.* 12:183–87, 1956.

2. Buller, A. J., Eccles, J., and Eccles, R. Interactions between motor neurons and muscles in respect of the characteristic speeds of their responses. *J. Physiol.* 150:417–39, 1960.

3. Burke, R. E., Levine, D. N., Tsairis, P., and Zajac, F. E. Physiological types and histochemical profiles in motor units of the cat gastrocnemius. *J. Physiol.* 234:723–48, 1973.

4. Burke, R. E., Levine, D. N., Saloman, M., et al. Motor units in cat soleus muscle: physiological, histochemical and morphological characteristics. *J. Physiol.* 238:503–14, 1974.

5. Costill, D. L., Daniels, J., Evans, W., Fink, W., Krahenbuhl, G., and Saltin, B. Skeletal muscle enzymes and fiber composition in male and female track athletes. *J. Appl. Physiol.* 40:149–54, 1976.

6. Costill, D. L., Fink, W. J., and Pollock, M. L. Muscle fiber composition and enzyme activities of elite distance runners. *Med. Sci. Sports* 8:96–100, 1976.

7. Dubowitz, V., and Brooke, M. H. *Muscle Biopsy: A Modern Approach.* Philadelphia: W. B. Saunders Company, 1973.

8. Ebashi, S., and Endo, M. Calcium ion and muscular contraction. *Prog. Biophys. Mol. Biol.* 18:125–83, 1968.

9. Garfin, S. R., Tipton, C. M., Mubarak, S. J., Woo, S. L., Hargens, A. R., and Akeson, W. H. Role of fascia in maintenance of muscle tension and pressure. *J. Appl. Physiol.* 51:317–20, 1981.

10. Gollnick, P. D., Armstrong, R. B., Saubert, C. W., Piehl, K., and Saltin, B. Enzyme activity and fiber composition in skeletal muscle of untrained and trained men. *J. Appl. Physiol.* 33:312–19, 1972.

11. Hanson, J., and Huxley, H. E. The structural basis of contraction in striated muscle. *Symp. Soc. Exp. Biol. Med.* 9:228–64, 1955.

12. Howald, H., Billeter, R., and Jenny, E. Transitional fibers in middle distance runners. *Experientia* 36:747, 1980.

13. Hoyle, G. How is muscle turned on and off? *Sci. Am.* 222:84–93, 1970.

14. Huxley, A. F. Muscle structure and theories of contraction. *Prog. Biophys. Chem.* 7:257–318, 1957.

15. Huxley, H. E. The ultrastructure of striated muscle. *Br. Med. Bull.* 12:171–73, 1956.

16. Huxley, H. E. The structural basis of muscular contraction. *Pro. R. Soc. Med.* 178:131–49, 1971.

17. Jansson, E., Sjodin, B., and Tesch, P. Changes in muscle fiber type distribution in man after physical training. *Acta Physiol. Scand.* 104:235–37, 1978.

18. Peter, J., Barnard, R., Edgerton, V., Gillespie, C., and Stempel, K. Metabolic profiles of three fiber types of skeletal muscle in guinea pigs and rabbits. *Biochemistry* 11:2627–33, 1972.

19. Prince, F. P., Hikida, R. S., and Hagerman, F. C. Human muscle fiber types in power lifters, distance runners and untrained subjects. *Pfluegers Arch.* 363:19–26, 1976.

20. Schmidtbleicher, D., and Haralambie, G. Changes in contractile properties of muscle after strength training in man. *Eur. J. Appl. Physiol.* 46:221–28, 1981.

21. Thorstensson, A., Grimby, G., and Karlsson, J. Force-velocity relations and fiber composition in human knee extensor muscles. *J. Appl. Physiol.* 40:12–16, 1976.

22. Thorstensson, A., and Karlsson, J. Fatigability and fibre composition of human skeletal muscle. *Acta Physiol. Scand.* 98:318–22, 1976.

23. Thorstensson, A., Larsson, L., Tesch, P., and Karlsson, J. Muscle strength and fiber composition in athletes and sedentary men. *Med. Sci. Sports* 9:26–30, 1977.

3

Energetics of Muscular Contraction and Adaptations to Training at the Cellular Level

Energetics of Muscular Contraction
    Regeneration of ATP Energy from
    Carbohydrate Food
    Regeneration of ATP Energy from
    Fat and Protein
Adaptations to Training and Conditioning
    at the Cellular Level

Endurance Training (Aerobic
    Metabolism)
Sprint Training (Anaerobic
    Metabolism)
Strength and Power Training
Energy Substrate and Training
    Training Effects on Cellular Energy
    Substrate Level

Energetics of Muscular Contraction

As described in the chapter 2, the breakdown of adenosine triphosphate (ATP) to adenosine diphosphate (ADP), $ATP \rightarrow ADP + P +$ approximately 8,000 calories of energy (or 8 kcal), furnishes the immediate source of energy for the contractile mechanism. This chapter discusses the processes by which ingested food energy is converted and utilized to regenerate the energy of the high energy bonds of the ATP, which ultimately make the muscle cell (fiber) contract.

In the past, considering the biochemistry of muscular contraction in depth did not seem justified because these theoretical concepts could not be applied as down-to-earth physical education and athletic training principles. However, there are now several compelling reasons for the physical educator and coach to become familiar with at least the rudiments of muscle contraction at the cellular level.

1. There is evidence that some very important effects of athletic training occur at the cellular level of organization in terms of modification of intracellular structure and the enzyme systems that are so important to energy supply.
2. There is now excellent laboratory data bearing on the need for diet modification to maximize the athlete's cellular energy supply.
3. Researchers in physical education have become sophisticated in the use of the electron microscope and biochemical procedures, and understanding their research reports will require our professional readership to have more background in this area.

In short, the material in this chapter is now essential to a scientifically based program of physical education and athletic training.

The metabolic processes that supply the energy needs of muscle contraction ordinarily take place in the presence of adequate O_2 to oxidize the carbohydrate sources of energy completely to CO_2 and H_2O. This constitutes *aerobic* muscle activity, which in general is exercise that is low enough in intensity to be carried on for at least five minutes or longer. Energy for exercise that is so intense that exhaustion ensues within one to two minutes or less must be supplied largely by *anaerobic* processes (without O_2), because O_2 cannot be transported via the lungs and cardiovascular system rapidly enough to supply such a demand.

In general, four processes occurring within the muscle cell have to do with the chemistry of muscle contraction, and three of them are common to aerobic and anaerobic contraction. The first three reactions are reversible. That is to say, the reactions are such that as some molecules of ATP are being broken down to provide energy for muscle fiber contraction, other molecules of ADP and P are being regenerated (at a cost of energy provided by the next reaction down, $CP \rightarrow C + P$). A balance obviously must be struck between the rate of breakdown and the rate of regeneration or the muscle effort would run out of gas. Thus each reaction in the chain depends on energy supplied from reactions below to remain in balance while supplying energy to the reaction above. Or we may say that each succeeding reaction supplies energy for the reversal of the preceding reaction, as follows:

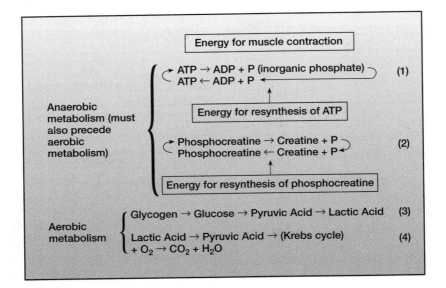

This diagram is a great oversimplification in that it does not show the intermediate reactions and enzyme systems that are necessary. Figure 3.1 provides more detail for the reader interested in biochemistry.

Aerobic and anaerobic metabolism share the common paths of *glycogenolysis* and *glycolysis.* Glycogenolysis is defined as the breakdown of the large glycogen molecule into many glucose molecules, while glycolysis is defined as the splitting of the glucose molecule into two pyruvic acid molecules. In the absence (or relative shortage) of O_2, the reactions can proceed only through equation 3 in the diagram with the production of lactic acid as the end product, plus the freeing of small amounts of energy. The fourth reaction, with its oxidative (therefore aerobic) pathway, provides greater amounts of energy.

Regeneration of ATP Energy from Carbohydrate Food

We may think of the overall conversion of carbohydrate in our food to energy in terms of the following simple equation, which summarizes the diagram found in figure 3.1.

$$C_6H_{12}O_6 + 6O_2 \rightarrow 6CO_2 + 6H_2O + Energy$$
Glucose   Oxygen   Carbon   Water
                     dioxide

While this is indeed straightforward, it could only happen in such direct fashion by raising the temperature very high and actually *burning* the carbohydrate in a very hot flame, a process that is not consistent with living tissue. To bring about the conversion of food energy to ATP energy for muscle contraction at body temperature, many intermediate steps catalyzed by enzyme systems are necessary. The above equation is quite correct in that it summarizes the whole process, but it tells us nothing about how this process is actually accomplished. It is the enzyme systems that promote the stepwise chemical breakdown of the foodstuffs at body temperature to provide the energy for muscle contraction. Enzymes are proteins that have the ability to promote specific chemical reactions without themselves being degraded or changed in the process. Thus

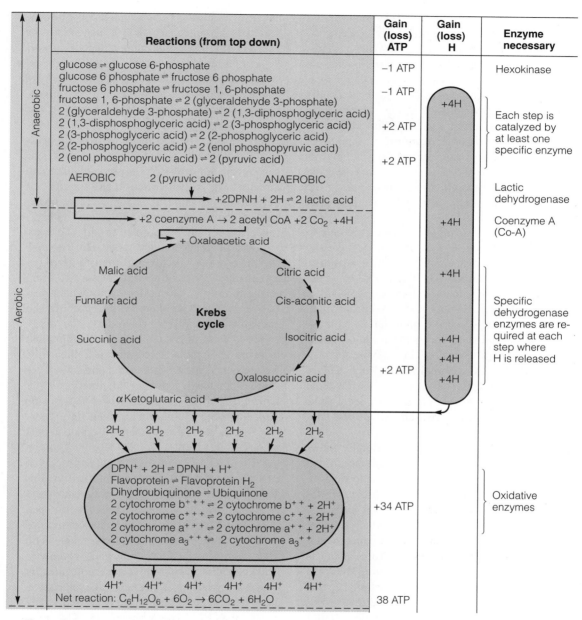

Figure 3.1   The breakdown of glucose (basic building block of all carbohydrates) to furnish the energy for regeneration of ATP.

the same enzyme protein can function over and over again in the same metabolic process.

The final products of carbohydrate digestion in the alimentary tract are the *monosaccharides* (6-carbon-atom sugars) *glucose, fructose,* and *galactose.* These are the results of the breakdown of such larger carbohydrate molecules as starch and the usual sugars included in the diet (*disaccharides*). The three monosaccharides are interconvertible, and as they pass through the liver they are converted almost entirely to glucose for transport in the blood to the muscle cells and other tissues of the body.

As the glucose molecule enters the muscle cell through the sarcolemma, a process greatly aided by the presence of insulin, it is immediately phosphorylated. That is to say, the 6-carbon-atom monosaccharide picks up a phosphate radical on its number 6 carbon atom and becomes glucose-6-phosphate. Note in figure 3.1 that this process of phosphorylation requires the presence of the enzyme *hexokinase,* as well as the breakdown of one ATP to form ADP + P. Since our discussion has to do with formation of ATP, this would seem to be a step in the wrong direction, but we will wait for the whole story.

Once phosphorylated, the glucose molecule is trapped in the muscle cell because it requires the enzyme *phosphatase* to dephosphorylate the glucose and the muscle cell has no phosphatase, although the liver cells and some other tissues do. This is immediately important from the practical standpoint in that we now know that the energy stored away in one muscle is not available to another that may be in the process of exhausting its energy due to locally heavy work. We will return to this concept later in the consideration of muscular endurance.

The glucose-6-phosphate, once in the cell, can be either utilized directly for energy, as shown in figure 3.1, or stored, depending on

cell activity levels. To be stored it must be converted to glycogen, which is a large chain or network of glucose molecules called a *polymer.* The polymerization process involves several steps and requires several enzymes. The glycogen is deposited as granules in glycogen columns as shown in figure 2.8. Storage in the form of large, polymerized molecules is necessary so that the intracellular osmotic pressure is not unduly raised, which it would be if carbohydrate were stored as glucose units. The amount of glycogen stored in the muscle cell determines its endurance for exercise under certain conditions, as we will discuss later in this chapter. The breakdown products of protein and fat digestion and lactic acid can also be converted to glucose and then to glycogen for storage. We shall now direct our attention to the more detailed pathways by which carbohydrate can be broken down to produce the energy necessary for rebuilding the ATP, which is what is needed by the myofilaments to bring about muscle contraction. Basically, we are concerned with aerobic and anaerobic sources of energy. However, we must resist the temptation to think of muscular activity as *either* aerobic or anaerobic. Even light exercise brings both mechanisms into play, as will be described later.

Figure 3.1 illustrates the whole process of carbohydrate metabolism schematically. Glucose becomes available as an energy substrate either by the glycogenolysis of glycogen stored in the muscle fiber or by the transportation of blood glucose into the muscle fiber. The glucose molecule first undergoes glycolytic breakdown into two pyruvic acid molecules, as shown in figure 3.1. The enzyme hexokinase is necessary to add a phosphate (PO_4 or P) radical to make glucose-6-phosphate. This process costs the breakdown of one ATP to ADP + P. Each of the further steps of glycolysis is also catalyzed by at least one enzyme specific to that step, and one more ATP is broken down to add the second P to form fructose-1, 6-phosphate (the 1, 6 means that there are two phosphates in the molecule, one at the number 1 carbon atom and one at the number 6 carbon atom). Note, however, that the cost of breaking down two ATPs is recouped with a net total gain of two ATP molecules during the process of glycolysis, which results in formation of two molecules of pyruvic acid. In the absence of O_2 (or insufficient O_2), the end products of glycolysis—pyruvic acid and H atoms—combine to form lactic acid. This last step is important because, if the end products of a reaction accumulate, the reaction is ended before all of the energy substrate can be used.

In the presence of sufficient O_2, the system does not back up at the pyruvic acid step, because pyruvic acid can now continue on its aerobic course by entering the mitochondria and proceeding through a metabolic system called the *Krebs cycle* (also called *citric acid cycle* or *tricarboxylic acid cycle*). The course of aerobic metabolism is much more advantageous, because up to this point the anaerobic route has netted us only two ATP molecules generated from one molecule of glucose. As will be seen, complete aerobic breakdown will provide at least thirty-eight molecules of ATP per molecule of glucose.

The next stage in glucose breakdown requires the conversion of the two pyruvic acid molecules into two molecules of acetyl coenzyme A (acetyl CoA). Acetyl CoA combines with the oxaloacetic acid to become citric acid, and the Krebs cycle is underway. The net result of the Krebs cycle is to degrade the acetyl portion of the acetyl CoA to CO_2 and H atoms. The steps of the Krebs cycle depend upon specific enzymes called *dehydrogenases* to break off the H atoms, which are subsequently oxidized, liberating large amounts of energy for formation of ATP molecules. Note that although only two ATP molecules are regenerated from one molecule of glucose in the Krebs cycle itself, twenty H atoms are released.

The H atoms that are released must be converted to H ions (written $H+$) before they can react with O_2 to form water and large amounts of energy. This is accomplished by the oxidative enzymes of the respiratory chain (also called the electron transport system). (These enzymes and those of the Krebs cycle reside in the mitochondria of the cell.) This is schematized at the bottom of figure 3.1, which shows the final breakdown of the glucose molecule. The net chemical reaction for the whole aerobic process depicted in figure 3.1 is as follows:

$$C_6H_{12}O_6 + 6O_2 + 38ADP + 38P \rightarrow$$
$$6CO_2 + 6 H_2O + 38ATP$$

Since each high-energy phosphate bond represents about 8 kcal and each gram molecular weight of glucose (180 gm) has an ultimate energy value of about 4 kcal/per gram, the efficiency of this process of storing energy as ATP is about

$$\frac{38 \times 8}{180 \times 4} = \frac{304}{720} = 42\%.$$

Regeneration of ATP Energy from Fat and Protein

As will be seen in later discussion, exercise of intensities up to about 70% of maximum proceeds largely by way of energy gained from fat metabolism. Thus the regeneration of ATP energy from fat is quite important in exercise physiology. Energy can also be provided for work by protein metabolism, but this becomes important in exercise physiology only in a state of negative energy balance (starvation or the semistarvation of rigorous weight reduction). Recent findings, however, suggest that prolonged exercise is analogous to short-term starvation in that as much as 10% of total calorie cost may be the result of protein breakdown (27). Figure 3.2 shows the derivation of energy from the metabolism of fat, carbohydrate, and protein.

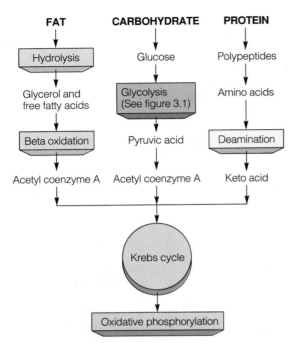

Figure 3.2   Derivation of energy from the metabolism of the three basic foodstuffs by way of the final common path: the Krebs cycle and oxidative phosphorylation.

Use of Protein for Energy

Proteins are very large complex molecules and consist of from 20 to 100,000 amino acids, which are the basic building blocks of all proteins. The digestive enzymes of the stomach start the breakdown of protein. It is carried further in the small intestine to the polypeptide level (combination of several amino acids) and completed to the amino acid level in passing through the wall of the small intestine into the blood. The amino acids are then deaminated in the liver (removal of the ammonia radical), becoming keto acids. These resulting keto acids are then converted into substances that can enter the Krebs cycle and then proceed to complete degradation and energy formation as has been described for carbohydrate.

It is important to recognize that just as all three foodstuffs can be utilized for energy, they are also convertible into fat for storage when the food ingested exceeds the need. In the case of protein, some amino acids must first go through gluconeogenesis to become carbohydrate before being deposited as fat pads.

Adaptations to Training and Conditioning at the Cellular Level

Only in recent years have we begun to realize how very specific are the cellular adaptations to training or conditioning. During the course of evolution, different muscles have developed different abilities. For example, muscle composed largely of fast twitch (FT) fibers can work hard and quickly but cannot maintain forces efficiently, whereas muscles with a large complement of slow twitch (ST) fibers work somewhat slower but have great ability to maintain a force for a long period.

Furthermore, we have learned that even the nature of the required energy substrate

Use of Fat for Energy

Fat is basically a combination of three fatty acids, each of which is attached to one of the three carbon atoms of a glycerol molecule. Chemically this combination (fat) is called a *triglyceride*.

The first step in the utilization of fat for energy is the hydrolysis into the original components, glycerol plus three fatty acids. The glycerol is easily changed by enzymic action into glyceraldehyde, which can be used for energy via the phosphogluconate pathway that occurs in the liver or in the fat cells, but not in muscle. The fatty acids undergo a process called *beta oxidation,* which involves a stepwise breakdown of the long-chain fatty acid molecule into acetyl CoA molecules, which then enter the Krebs cycle and proceed just as the acetyl CoA from carbohydrate.

varies with the intensity-duration characteristics of the exercise. Thus, when exercise is continued for many hours, the limits are set by the supply of adequate food in the form of fat and carbohydrate. For somewhat more intense work that is to be maintained for one to three hours, the limit is set by the level of glycogen stored within the muscle at the start of exercise. The glycogen may be used either relatively slowly via complete oxidation (aerobic metabolism) to form CO_2, water, and many molecules of ATP, or it may be used very quickly and anaerobically to make much less ATP per molecule of glucose. In the latter case, lactic acid accumulates, which can so increase the acidity of the tissues that intermediate metabolic processes are severely limited by the increased hydrogen ion concentration. For shorter periods—a few minutes up to thirty minutes—availability of O_2 may be the limiting factor. For very heavy workouts that can be maintained only a matter of seconds, the rate of creatine phosphate breakdown is probably limiting. But the ultimate maximum speed of a muscle is set by the rate at which actomyosin ATPase can break down ATP.

For these reasons, we shall discuss cellular adaptations to conditioning in three different areas: 1) endurance exercise, 2) sprint or speed-type exercise (involving anaerobic metabolism), and 3) strength and power training.

Endurance Training (Aerobic Metabolism)

Cardiovascular-respiratory system adaptations to training have occupied the interest of exercise physiologists for many years, but we now recognize that endurance exercise also induces major adaptations in the skeletal muscle, which helps explain the improvement shown with training in capacity for prolonged work.

Myoglobin

Animal studies have shown that endurance exercise increases the concentration of myoglobin in the skeletal muscle. In rats, this increase amounts to 80% (27). Myoglobin probably facilitates O_2 utilization in muscle by enhancing O_2 transport through the cytoplasm (sarcoplasm) to the mitochondria in this species (16). However, this factor may not be important in humans since heavy endurance training for eight weeks was reported to cause no significant increase in myoglobin (37).

Mitochondrial Enzymes

A number of investigators working with both rodents and humans have found that the enzymes of the respiratory chain (fig. 3.1) increase some twofold in skeletal muscle in response to endurance exercise (16). The enzymes of the Krebs cycle also increase significantly but by differing amounts ranging from 35% to 100%. Thus the protein composition of the mitochondria changes with training, since the enzymes (protein) do not all increase proportionately. These changes are related to the daily work load and the total training time (3).

There are also major increases in the levels of enzymes involved in the activation, transport, and beta oxidation of long-chain fatty acids, which thus improve the organism's ability to utilize fat as an energy source. As might be expected, these enzymic changes approximately double the capacity of trained muscles to oxidize a variety of energy substrates (16).

Mitochondrial Size and Number

Probably the most important training effect of endurance exercise is the increase in mitochondrial protein, which has been reported by several different groups of investigators (2, 5, 9, 25). Both the size and the number of mitochondria in the muscle cell are increased as the result of training if the intensity of the training stimulus is sufficiently severe. It will be recalled from the preceding discussion of muscle metabolism that the very important enzymes of both the Krebs cycle and the respiratory chain reside in the mitochondria of the muscle cell. Holloszy (15) has shown that training rats on a treadmill produces a twofold increase in their capacity to oxidize pyruvate. Oxidation of pyruvate represents the entire aerobic portion of the muscle cell's metabolic process; this tells us that the cell is now able to work at double the load, since the glycolytic pathway is probably not a limiting factor.

Differences in Response by Fiber Type

In animals, endurance exercise has been shown to result in increases in mitochondrial enzyme levels in all three fiber types. The capacity of FT muscle (white) for oxidative metabolism increases, and recent animal experiments have suggested the possibility of converting FT fibers to ST fibers. As for human muscles, recent evidence suggests that endurance training brings about a shift from FG (fast twitch, glycolytic) to FOG (fast twitch, oxidative, glycolytic) fiber types (32). This increase in oxidative capacity would, of course, serve to improve aerobic performance (endurance).

Glucose-Alanine-Glucose Cycle

In figure 3.1 only two routes are shown for the removal of the pyruvate with its consequent energy production and formation of ATP. However, recent evidence (7) has shown the importance of a third route. Pyruvate can be converted in muscle tissue to the amino acid alanine in the presence of the enzyme alanine transaminase. The alanine is transported by the blood to the liver where its carbon skeleton is reconverted to glucose, which becomes available as energy at a later time in the form of blood sugar (glucose). Since endurance exercise increases alanine transaminase in trained muscles 50% to 80% (30), it is possible that this adaptation could result in conversion

of a greater proportion of pyruvate to alanine and less to lactate, thus creating a more favorable environment for muscle contraction.

Glycolytic Enzymes

Endurance exercise results in only small and probably physiologically insignificant changes in the glycolytic enzymes, with the exception of hexokinase, which tends to vary directly with respiratory capacity. It is thought that the glycolytic process (labeled anaerobic in fig. 3.1) is not limiting in endurance exercise, although the supply of glycogen for energy substrate may be. The limits appear to be set at the level of the Krebs cycle, and the respiratory chain and the training adaptations with respect to enzyme response are consistent with this concept.

Energy Substrate Availability

The supply of muscle glycogen available in the muscle fiber for endurance exercise can be greatly enhanced by a combination of appropriate exercise and diet. This will be discussed in greater detail later in this chapter.

Preferential Use of FFA as Energy Substrate

It has been suggested that, at the same relative work load, trained men "preferentially" use FFA as an energy source (6). This would, of course, provide a carbohydrate sparing effect and increase muscular endurance. This hypothesis is supported by other investigators who have found lower respiratory exchange ratios in trained subjects (35), which also reflects a greater utilization of fat for energy.

Physiological Implications of Cellular Adaptations

As Holloszy (16) has pointed out: "It now seems clear, as skeletal muscle adapts to endurance exercise it becomes more like heart muscle in its mitochondrial and cytoplasmic enzyme patterns." Thus, in addition to greater glycogen stores there is a slower depletion of glycogen, lower lactate levels, and a greater oxidation of free fatty acids during exercise.

The significance of increased oxidative capacity at the cellular level has been defined by the work of Davies, Packer, and Brooks (5) who found that a 403% increase in endurance capacity (time to exhaustion) correlated highly ($r=0.92$) with cellular oxidative capacity but poorly with VO_2 max. On the other hand, VO_2 max for the whole body correlated strongly ($r=0.82$) with the maximum intensity of work load achieved. Thus we may conclude that mitochondrial factors determine the duration of an endurance activity, while aerobic capacity (VO_2 max) determines the intensity or maximum rate at which the activity can be performed.

Sprint Training (Anaerobic Metabolism)

The effects of sprint training on anaerobic metabolism are less well defined than the well-documented effects of endurance training on aerobic metabolism. In short-term, heavy exercise, the only significant energy pools available are 1) the breakdown of the phosphagens, ATP and CP, and 2) glycolysis, the breakdown of glucose to pyruvate and lactic acid as described in figure 3.1.

Limiting Factors

The energy available from the breakdown of all possible ATP and CP has been shown to be approximately equivalent to 1.2 liters of O_2 utilization (23). Thus, in an event such as the 100-meter dash, which requires supramaximal O_2 consumption rates on the order of 20 or more liters per minute, the phosphagen breakdown can support maximal effort at that speed for only about four seconds. The energy available from anaerobic breakdown of glycogen must furnish the balance.

Two separate groups of investigators (19, 23) have shown that in exercise heavy enough

to be maintained for only one to two minutes (anaerobic), the rate of phosphagen regeneration is likely to be the limiting factor. Under these conditions the CP level is completely depleted, and after that time the work can no longer be continued at the same high rate. However, under such conditions the blood lactate also builds up to very high levels, and it remains an open question whether the limits for sprint performance are set by lack of energy substrate (phosphagen depletion) or by accumulation of metabolic end products such as lactate.

Effects of Training

In a study on rats, Hickson, Heusner, and Van Huss (14) compared the effects of sprint and endurance training. Interestingly, they found that similar enzyme adaptations occurred over time with the two very different training regimens. They found no increase in the glycolytic enzymes in the rat after sprint training, and their work suggests that the preexisting levels of glycolytic capacity in the rat muscles studied were adequate to supply the energy needs even during the stress of very heavy exercise. Unexpectedly, they found an increase in mitochondrial enzymes (those involved in aerobic metabolism) in response to sprinting as well as to endurance training.

On the other hand, Gollnick and associates (10) trained six young men for five months, four days a week, one hour a day, at 75% to 95% of maximal work load. Any training that can be sustained for one hour would be expected to challenge largely the aerobic pathways, but they found a doubling in PFK activity as well as in succinic dehydrogenase. Since PFK is an enzyme that is thought to reflect glycolytic capacity best, this data suggests a considerable increase in anaerobic capacity in humans even though the exercise challenge was largely aerobic. Interestingly they also found that oxidative (aerobic) capacity was increased in both FT and

ST muscle fibers, but glycolytic capacity (anaerobic) was improved only in the FT fibers.

Russian investigators (39) have found increases in creatine phosphate, and this may be the most important training adaptation.

Strength and Power Training

It is in strength and power training that the gross effects of cellular changes are best exhibited. The hypertrophic (increase in size of the muscle) changes in response to very heavy work have been observed since time immemorial and scientifically elucidated over a period of at least a hundred years.

Hypertrophy

Most of our information with respect to cellular changes in hypertrophy has come from animal studies, largely those done on rats. The most common animal model for the study of hypertrophy has been the surgical severing of the rat gastrocnemius, which produces an overload on the remaining ankle extensors, the soleus and the plantaris, where the processes of hypertrophy can be clearly observed (8). In this type of experiment very rapid responses are common. The rat soleus typically increases in weight by 40% within six days. This rapid growth is due mostly to an enlargement of muscle fibers (hypertrophy), although occasionally muscle fiber splitting (hyperplasia) is also seen. In the rat as well as in humans, the hypertrophy is accompanied by increased muscle strength.

Muscle hypertrophy has been demonstrated in rats under these conditions even when the pituitary gland has been removed and in diabetic animals, implying that growth hormone, insulin, and even testosterone are not essential to muscle hypertrophy. This finding may not carry over to human muscle hypertrophy, however, as will be discussed in later chapters.

Another interesting finding in the rat model is that hypertrophy is still induced in the overworked muscle when the animal is fasted and other relatively unused muscles are in a process of wasting (atrophy) (8).

The increase of muscle weight reflects an increase in protein, which is largely sarcoplasmic protein in contradistinction to the enzyme and mitochondrial protein that is seen to increase in endurance conditioning. By eight hours after surgery protein synthesis in rats is enhanced, and indeed within one hour of surgery the active transport of certain amino acids is increased. The magnitude of this latter effect is related to the amount of contractile activity in the muscle.

Most interesting from a therapeutic viewpoint is the fact that simple, passive stretching of rat muscle was found to retard protein degradation and to stimulate amino acid transport. This knowledge could lead to less atrophy and better physical therapy in persons who are immobilized in a cast or by occupation (astronauts). This finding suggests that increased tension, whether active or passive, is the necessary stimulus affecting muscle protein balance. Such a hypothesis appears to be consistent with all observed facts.

Hyperplasia (Increased Number of Muscle Fibers)

Recent work (12) has shown an increase in fiber number by 20.5% in cats in response to high resistance exercise. It was suggested that for those exercises where not only increased muscle tension but rapid movement is necessary to produce maximum force, fiber splitting may be an important mechanism for improving the rate of tension development.

Biochemical Adaptations

Very interesting experiments are underway at McMaster University in Canada where the effects of weight training are being elucidated. In one experiment (29), nine college-age men were studied by needle biopsy under control conditions and before and after five months of weight training and five weeks of immobilization. Training resulted in an 11% increase in arm circumference and a 28% increase in elbow extension strength. These changes were accompanied by significant increases in the phosphagens ATP and CP by 18% and 22% respectively. Immobilization significantly reduced CP concentration by 25%. These findings bring theory and practice closer together.

Mitochondrial Density
MacDougall and coworkers (28) at Mc-Master University reported on six weight lifters before and after six months of weight training. Training resulted in a significant 26% reduction in mitochondrial volume density of the trained elbow extensors, a 25% reduction in the ratio of mitochondrial volume to myofibrillar volume (the contractile elements), and a 12% increase in volume density of the sarcoplasm. Fiber area was increased by 39% for FT and 31% for ST fibers. Thus heavy resistance training leads to dilution of the mitochondrial volume density by virtue of an increase in myofibrillar size and cytoplasmic volume.

Fiber Type and Power
Komi and colleagues (26) studied anaerobic performance capacity in eighty-nine athletes. They found that the main determinants of successful performance in explosive events like jumping were related to muscle fiber composition. The correlation between vertical velocity (measured by timing a short run up stairs) and the percentage of FT fibers was .37. However, more recent work by Schantz and colleagues (36) failed to corroborate this finding in that no significant relationship was found between maximal tension developed per unit of muscle cross-sectional area and percentage of type I fiber area. The determinant of force produced was largely the cross-sectional area of the muscle involved ($r=0.94$).

In agreement with earlier work they found no difference in tension produced per unit cross-sectional area among men, women, and body builders.

Summary of Cellular Training Adaptation
While all the answers are not yet in, the present available evidence suggests that there are three basic modes of adaptation to training at the cellular level: 1) improvement of aerobic capacity, 2) enhancement of anaerobic capacity, and 3) hypertrophy.

Endurance training at prolonged exercise of moderate intensity improves aerobic capacity mainly through increased levels of mitochondrial enzymes, increased mitochondrial size and number, larger glycogen stores, and generally greater oxidative capacity in both FT and ST fibers.

Sprint training at high speeds in intensive workouts for short periods, as commonly used in interval training, increases the enzyme PFK, which is reflective of glycolytic capacity, and most important, creatine phosphate, which is likely to limit anaerobic work.

Strength and power training involving near maximal voluntary contraction (MVC) strength increases the cross-sectional area of muscle fibers, a result also observed grossly as hypertrophy.

Energy Substrate and Training

Until quite recently our only evidence regarding the energy substrate utilized by working muscles was indirect—obtained by calculating respiratory quotients (RQ) as described in chapter 12 on exercise metabolism. In 1962 Bergstrom introduced a biopsy needle that he and Hultman and their coworkers subsequently used to good advantage in making direct observations of the level of various energy substrates remaining in an active muscle after various types, intensities, and durations of muscle work. From such studies, rates of utilization have become available that have various practical implications for athletes and coaches.

Figure 3.3 shows the rate of glycogen depletion in working muscle cells when they are fatigued by bicycle exercise at various work loads (35). When the individual is working at 70% to 80% of maximal aerobic power ($\dot{V}O_2$ max), exhaustion occurs when the muscle fiber's glycogen supply is depleted. This suggests that at such work loads the muscle can utilize only glycogen stored in the muscle cells for its energy substrate, although at lighter loads glucose and free fatty acids transported by the blood form the source of energy. At maximal work loads, the load cannot be sustained long enough to bring about glycogen depletion. At lighter loads of 60% or less of aerobic power, the limiting factor is probably the availability of blood-borne glucose and free fatty acids (FFA). Under the conditions of lighter loading, the liver store of carbohydrate may become an important factor (34). It must be understood that only the duration of the effort is set by the energy stores available; the rate of work that can be maintained depends upon O_2 transport and possibly on rate-limiting enzymic processes.

Although glycogen depletion and muscular exhaustion are closely related in bicycle work, this is not the case in distance running. Costill and coworkers (4) have shown that complete glycogen depletion is not seen after intense distance running even though the maximal O_2 requirement may be 80% to 90%. The most likely explanation for this interesting difference between running and cycling is probably a difference in muscle fiber recruitment, since the Costill group also found marked depletion of ST fibers with very little depletion of FT fibers. Thus, although total muscle glycogen during running was depleted by only 56%, there was a 93% decline in periodic acid-Schiff (PAS) dark-stained ST fibers

(measure of glycogen storage). Apparently the FT fibers cannot be fully recruited in running as they are in cycling with respect to the vastus lateralis muscle, which the researchers sampled.

The situation is quite different with respect to isometric exercise. It has been calculated that the actual utilization of glycogen under maximum isometric contraction is only about one-tenth that available to the muscle, and consequently glycogen stores cannot be a limiting factor in isometric contraction (19). Indeed, fatigue occurring isometrically at any load above 20% of maximum cannot be explained on the basis of glycogen depletion, and loads below that are unimportant in human athletic performance (1). A more definitive answer regarding the question of isometric muscle fatigue must await further research.

Training Effects on Cellular Energy Substrate Level

Using the muscle biopsy technique, Karlsson and associates (24) have shown increased levels of ATP concentration in muscle as a result of seven months of military training, which included distance running two to three times per week. ATP concentration in muscle, of course, would be very important during periods of anaerobic work when work-load intensity is too heavy to permit O_2 transport to keep up with tissue demand.

With respect to carbohydrate energy sources, the percentage of energy that is supplied by glycogen is apparently affected to some extent by its relative availability to the muscle cell as a result of diet. Pruett (33) has shown that the percentage contribution of carbohydrate varies with diet and work load as follows:

Work load	Standard diet	High fat	High carbohydrate
50% $\dot{V}O_2$ max	40%	35%	50%
70% $\dot{V}O_2$ max	53%	50%	60%

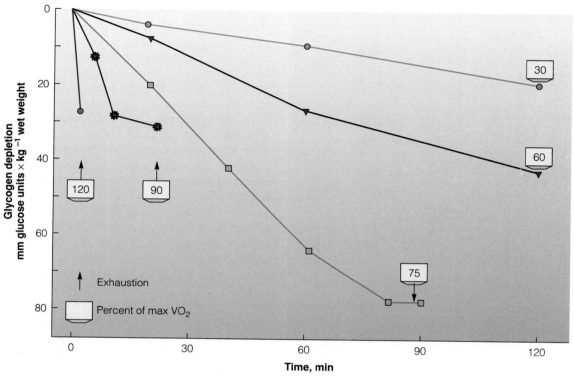

Figure 3.3   Glycogen depletion in the quadriceps muscle during bicycle exercise of different intensities. (From Saltin, B., and Karlsson, J., in *Muscle Metabolism during Exercise,* B. Pernow, and B. Saltin, eds., 1971. Courtesy of Plenum Press, New York.)

Hultman, working with Bergstrom and others, has reported some findings that are of importance to anybody concerned with endurance-type athletics (17, 18, 20, 21). Most important, he has shown that endurance under heavy aerobic work loads is determined largely by the level of glycogen storage in the muscle cells. Thus, for such work, the rate or intensity is set by O_2 transport capacity (to be discussed in following chapters), but the duration or total work that can be accomplished is set by the level of glycogen stored within the cell.

Of even greater practical interest are the data found in figure 3.4. Here one can see the very important *overshoot phenomenon.* That is, when a muscle is worked hard enough to bring about glycogen depletion, it develops the ability to store greater than normal amounts of glycogen. Second, it can be seen that recharging the stored glycogen depends greatly on the type of diet. On a carbohydrate-rich diet, glycogen resynthesis was complete in twenty-four hours, whereas on a carbohydrate-free diet of the same caloric content, resynthesis was complete only after eight to ten days. It was also shown that the glycogen content of the liver was dependent upon diet. If carbohydrate is not supplied in the diet, liver glycogen can decrease rapidly to values that will not sustain work for more than about one hour (by glycogenolysis after muscle glycogen has been depleted).

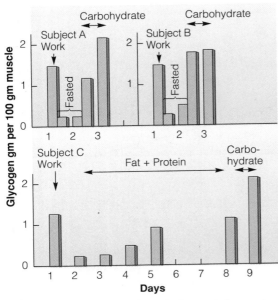

Figure 3.4   Muscle glycogen before and after work. Two subjects (upper graph) fasted for one day and got carbohydrate diet on day 2; the third subject (lower graph) got fat and protein diet during eight days, and thereafter one day of carbohydrate. (From Hultman, E. *American Heart Association Monograph Series*, no. 15, 1967, p. 106. Courtesy of the American Heart Association, Dallas.)

Unfortunately, the overshoot phenomenon works only for the muscle that has been worked, and the glycogen storage level varies considerably from muscle to muscle.

It has also been shown (38) that in rats FOG fibers have a glycogen repletion rate three times that of FG fibers and twice that of SO fibers. If this is true for human muscle also, then recovery for endurance exercise should be considerably more rapid than that for high intensity exercise such as sprints. This seems consistent with coaching experience.

A short fast of up to six hours was found to have no effect on glycogen level, so that a long wait for an athletic competition after a meal will have no adverse effects, unless stomach growls annoy teammates.

The exact mechanism of the overshoot phenomenon is not yet fully understood. Jeffress, Peter, and Lamb (22) have reported that an increase in glycogen synthetase, an enzyme necessary to the storage of glycogen, results from training, but this alone cannot fully explain the overshoot.

Training also has a *glycogen-sparing* effect in that the better trained athlete can supply more blood-borne energy substrate, primarily free fatty acids that supply the bulk of the energy for resting and low level, long duration exercise (13).

For the reader who would like more details on the subject of cellular adaptations to exercise, excellent reviews are available (9, 16, 39).

Summary

1. ATP energy, which is the immediate source of energy at the acto-myosin filament level, is replenished by the breakdown of phosphocreatine (also called creatine phosphate). The energy for regeneration of phosphocreatine is in turn supplied by *glycolysis*, the breakdown of glucose to pyruvic acid. Under *anaerobic* conditions the pyruvic acid is converted to lactic acid, whose accumulation eventually brings about cessation of exercise. Under *aerobic* conditions the first three reactions are in turn refueled by energy gained from the complete oxidation of the pyruvic acid to carbon dioxide and water.

2. Both fat and protein can also be used for energy, but only fat is important in exercise metabolism unless exercise is of very long duration.

3. The chemical breakdown of foodstuffs to supply energy for the regeneration of ATP from ADP and P is accomplished by a complex process in which many

protein enzymes are necessary as catalysts. The overall reaction describing the entire chain of events can be written as follows:

$$C_6H_{12}O_6 + 6O_2 + 38ADP + 38P \rightarrow 6CO_2 + 6H_2O + 38ATP$$

The synthesis of 38 ATP molecules represents the accumulation of about 304 kcal of energy from the oxidation of some 720 kcal of glucose (1 gm molecular weight).

4. Endurance-type training using prolonged exercise at moderate intensities improves aerobic capacity at the cell level mainly through increased levels of mitochondrial enzymes, increased mitochondrial size and number, larger glycogen stores, and in general greater oxidative capacity for both FT and ST fibers.

5. Sprint-type training, accomplished through high speed, intensive workouts for short periods such as commonly used in interval training, results in increases in the enzyme PFK, which reflects glycolytic capacity and, most important, creatine phosphate (CP), which is likely to be the limiting factor for anaerobic work.

6. Strength and power training involving near maximal voluntary contraction (MVC) strength results in increases in the cross-sectional area of muscle fibers, which are also observed grossly as hypertrophy. Recent evidence suggests that hyperplasia may also be important.

7. At heavy work loads of 70% to 80% of capacity, glycogen stored in the muscle cell provides the energy for contraction, and endurance time depends on the level of glycogen storage in the muscle at the beginning of exercise. This is not true, however, for isometric exercise.

8. At maximal work loads the work cannot be sustained long enough to deplete the stored glycogen, and the end point is probably determined by the level of lactic acid accumulation, or CP depletion.

9. When muscular work is such that glycogen is depleted, the muscle responds by large increases of glycogen storage. This response is complete within twenty-four hours on a carbohydrate-rich diet but may take eight to ten days on a carbohydrate-free diet of equal caloric content.

10. Training also has a *glycogen-sparing* effect in that better trained athletes are able to utilize more free fatty acid as energy substrate.

References

1. Ahlborg, B., Bergstrom, J., and Hultman, E. Muscle metabolism during isometric exercise performed at constant force. *J. Appl. Physiol.* 33:224–28, 1972.

2. Barnard, R. J., Edgerton, V. R., and Peter, J. B. Effect of exercise on skeletal muscle: 1. Biochemical and histological properties. *J. Appl. Physiol.* 28:762–66, 1970.

3. Benzi, G. et al. Mitochondrial enzymatic adaptation of skeletal muscle to endurance training. *J. Appl. Physiol.* 38:565–69, 1975.

4. Costill, D. L., Gollnick, P. D., Jansson, E. D., Saltin, B., and Stein, E. M. Glycogen depletion pattern in human muscle fibers during distance running. *Acta Physiol. Scand.* 89:374–83, 1973.

5. Davies, K. J. A., Packer, L., and Brooks, G. A. Biochemical adaptations of mitochondria, muscle, and whole animal

respiration to endurance training. *Arch. Biochem. and Biophy.* 209:539–54, 1981.

6. Evans, W. J., Bennett, A. S., Costill, D. L., and Fink, W. J. Leg muscle metabolism in trained and untrained men. *Res. Q.* 50:350–59, 1979.

7. Felig, P., and Wahren, J. Amino acid metabolism in exercising man. *J. Clin. Invest.* 50:2703–14, 1971.

8. Goldberg, A. L., Etlinger, J. D., Goldspink, D. F., and Jablecki, C. Mechanism of work-induced hypertrophy of skeletal muscle. *Med. Sci. Sports* 7:185–98, 1975.

9. Gollnick, P. D. Biochemical adaptations to exercise: anaerobic metabolism. In *Exercise and Sport Sciences Reviews,* ed. J. H. Wilmore. New York: Academic Press, 1973.

10. Gollnick, P. D., Armstrong, R. B., Saltin, B., Saubert, C. W., Sembrowich, W. L., and Shepherd, R. E. Effect of training on enzyme activity and fiber composition of human skeletal muscle. *J. Appl. Physiol.* 34:107–11, 1973.

11. Gollnick, P. D., Ianuzzo, C. D., and King, D. W. Ultrastructural and enzyme changes in muscles with exercise. In *Muscle Metabolism during Exercise,* eds. B. Pernow and B. Saltin, pp. 69–71. New York: Plenum Press, 1971.

12. Gonyea, W. J. Role of exercise in inducing increases in skeletal muscle fiber number. *J. Appl. Physiol.* 48:421–26, 1980.

13. Havel, R. J. Influence of intensity and duration of exercise on supply and use of fuels. In *Muscle Metabolism during Exercise,* eds. B. Pernow and B. Saltin, pp. 315–25. New York: Plenum Press, 1971.

14. Hickson, R. C., Heusner, W. W., and Van Huss, W. D. Skeletal muscle enzyme alterations after sprint and endurance training. *J. Appl. Physiol.* 40:868–72, 1976.

15. Holloszy, J. O. Effects of exercise on mitochondrial oxygen uptake and respiratory enzyme activity in skeletal muscle. *J. Biol. Chem.* 242:2278–82, 1967.

16. ———. Adaptation of skeletal muscle to endurance exercise. *Med. Sci. Sports* 7:155–64, 1975.

17. Hultman, E. Physiological role of muscle glycogen in man with special reference to exercise. In *Am. Heart Assoc. Monograph,* no. 15, pp. 99–112, 1967.

18. ———. Muscle glycogen stores and prolonged exercise. In *Frontiers of Fitness,* ed. R. J. Shephard, pp. 37–60. Springfield: Charles C. Thomas, 1971.

19. Hultman, E., Bergstrom, J., and McLennan-Anderson, N. Breakdown and resynthesis of phosphorylcreatine and adenosine triphosphate in connection with muscular work in man. *Scand. J. Clin. Lab. Invest.* 19:56–66, 1967.

20. Hultman, E., Bergstrom, J., and Roch-Norlund, A. E. Glycogen storage in human skeletal muscle. In *Muscle Metabolism during Exercise,* eds. B. Pernow and B. Saltin, pp. 273–88. New York: Plenum Press, 1971.

21. Hultman, E., and Nilsson, L. H. Liver glycogen in man; Effect of different diets and muscular exercise. In *Muscle Metabolism during Exercise,* eds. B. Pernow and B. Saltin, pp. 143–51. New York: Plenum Press, 1971.

22. Jeffress, R. N., Peter, J. B., and Lamb, D. R. Effects of exercise on glycogen synthetase in red and white skeletal muscle. *Life Sci.* 7:957–60, 1968.

23. Karlsson, J., Diamant, B., and Saltin, B. Muscle metabolites during submaximal and maximal exercise in man. *Scand. J. Clin. Lab. Invest.* 26:385–94, 1971.

24. Karlsson, J., Nordesjo, L. O., Jorfeldt, L., and Saltin, B. Muscle lactate, ATP, and CP levels during exercise after physical training in man. *J. Appl. Physiol.* 33:199–203, 1972.

25. Kiessling, K. H., Piehl, K., and Lundquist, C. G. Effect of physical training on ultrastructural features in human skeletal muscle. In *Muscle Metabolism during Exercise,* eds. B. Pernow and B. Saltin, pp. 97–101. New York: Plenum Press, 1971.

26. Komi, P. V., Rusko, H., Vos, J., and Vihko, V. Anaerobic performance capacity in athletes. *Acta Physiol. Scand.* 100:107–14, 1977.

27. Lemon, P. W. R., and Mullin, J. P. Effect of initial muscle glycogen levels on protein catabolism during exercise. *J. Appl. Physiol.* 48:624–29, 1980.

28. MacDougall, J. D., Sale, D. G., Moroz, J. R., and Howald, H. Mitochondrial volume density in human skeletal muscle following heavy resistance training. *Med. Sci. Sports* 11:164–66, 1979.

29. MacDougall, J. D., Ward, G. R., Sale, D. G., and Sutton, J. R. Biochemical adaptation of human skeletal muscle to heavy resistance training and immobilization. *J. Appl. Physiol.* 43:700–703, 1977.

30. Mole, P. A., Baldwin, K. M., Terjung, R. L., and Holloszy, J. O. Enzymatic pathways of pyruvate metabolism in skeletal muscle: adaptations to exercise. *Am. J. Physiol.* 224:50–54, 1973.

31. Pattengale, P. K., and Holloszy, J. O. Augmentation of skeletal muscle myoglobin by a program of treadmill running. *Am. J. Physiol.* 213:783–85, 1967.

32. Prince, F. P., Hikida, R. S., and Hagerman, F. C. Human muscle fibre types in power lifters, distance runners, and untrained subjects. *Pfluegers Arch.* 363:19–26, 1976.

33. Pruett, E. D. R. Glucose and insulin during prolonged work stress in men living on different diets. *J. Appl. Physiol.* 28:199–208, 1970.

34. Rowell, L. B. The liver as an energy source in man during exercise. In *Muscle Metabolism during Exercise,* eds. B. Pernow and B. Saltin, pp. 127–41. New York: Plenum Press, 1971.

35. Saltin, B., and Karlsson, J. Muscle glycogen utilization during work of different intensities. In *Muscle Metabolism during Exercise,* eds. B. Pernow and B. Saltin, pp. 289–99. New York: Plenum Press, 1971.

36. Schantz, P., Randall-Fox, E., Hutchison, W., Tyden, A., and Astrand, P.O. Muscle fiber type distribution, muscle cross-sectional area, and maximal voluntary strength in humans. *Acta Physiol. Scand.* 117:219–26, 1983.

37. Svedenhag, J., Henriksson, J., and Sylven, C. Dissociation of training effects on skeletal muscle mitochondrial enzymes and myoglobin in man. *Acta Physiol. Scand.* 117:213–18, 1983.

38. Terjung, R. L., Baldwin, K. M., Winder, W. W., and Holloszy, J. O. Glycogen repletion in different types of muscle and in liver after exhausting exercise. *Am. J. Physiol.* 226:1387–91, 1974.

39. Yakovlev, N. N. Biochemistry of sport in the Soviet Union: beginning, development and present status. *Med. Sci. Sports* 7:237–47, 1975.

4

The Physiology of Muscle Contraction

Physiology of Gross Muscle Contraction
*The Muscle Twitch and Its
Myogram*
*Summation of Contractions and
Tetanus*
*Temperature Effects on Muscle
Contraction*
The All-or-None Law
Gradation of Response
Muscle Fatigue
Types of Contraction
*Mechanical Factors in Muscular
Activity*

Electromyography in Analysis of Muscle
Function
*Basic Concepts of Electrical
Phenomena and
Electromyography*
*Applications of EMG to
Physiological Problems*
Estimation of Strength
Muscle Tonus
Resting Muscle Tonus

Physiology of Gross Muscle Contraction

Muscle tissue is specifically differentiated for the purpose of contraction; thus its most important physiological property is *contractility*. However, it possesses other properties common to protoplasm in general: *irritability* and *conductivity*. Irritability indicates that muscle tissue responds to adequate stimuli with its typical response, contraction. Conductivity means that an adequate stimulus will be propagated throughout any one muscle fiber in skeletal muscle, and from fiber to fiber in smooth and cardiac muscles for reasons described in chapter 2.

Excised muscle may be stimulated electrically, chemically, and mechanically. The intact muscle is normally stimulated by its motor nerve only, but it can also be stimulated electrically through the skin, as is frequently done by physicians and physical therapists, and mechanically, as when a bruise elicits a contracture (charley horse).

The Muscle Twitch and Its Myogram

It has been customary in elementary physiology textbooks to describe the simple muscle twitch as the basis for understanding the process of muscle contraction. This concept is likely to be helpful only if the student realizes from the outset that this is not typical of muscle contraction either in the intact body or even in an excised muscle that is normally innervated.

In the typical laboratory experiment, the gastrocnemius muscle of a frog is excised and hung from a ring stand so that its contraction, that is, the movement of its free end, is recorded on the rotating drum of a kymograph. The muscle is then stimulated electrically by a single shock to the entire sciatic nerve trunk,

or to the muscle itself, to which it responds under these conditions by a single twitch. The record of the events occurring during this contraction is called a *myogram* (fig. 4.1).

At this point the student must understand the two basic differences between the laboratory preparation and normal stimulation and contraction processes as they occur in the intact animal; otherwise conceptualizing other aspects of neuromuscular function will be difficult.

1. In the laboratory preparation, nearly all of the nerve fibers for the whole muscle are innervated simultaneously because all the fibers of the sciatic nerve are shocked at the same time, but the innervation of normal human muscle is asynchronous, motor unit by motor unit; or we might say each nerve fiber is stimulated individually at varying points in time.

2. In the laboratory preparation, the twitch is the response to a single stimulation (shock). This probably never occurs in the intact organism, for we know that innervation of human muscle is accomplished by volleys of nerve impulses, ranging from five or six per second to as many as eighty or ninety.

Having recognized the foregoing artifacts, there is still much we can learn from the myogram of the muscle twitch. After the stimulus is applied, approximately 0.01 second elapses before contraction of the frog muscle begins. This interval is called the *latent period,* and it has been found to be much shorter— 0.001 second—if the muscle is completely unloaded (recording by optics). The shortening of the muscle is called the *contraction phase,* which typically takes approximately 0.04 second in the frog gastrocnemius. The lengthening of the muscle back to its resting length

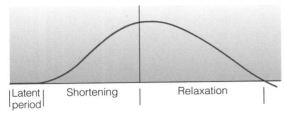

| Latent period | Shortening | Relaxation |

Figure 4.1   The muscle twitch and its myogram.

occupies about 0.05 second, and this is called the *relaxation phase.* These values, of course, vary from species to species and from muscle to muscle within the same species, as was discussed in chapter 2 in regard to fast and slow twitch muscle fibers.

Summation of Contractions and Tetanus

With the same muscle preparation discussed on the previous page, and by application of a second stimulus to the nerve trunk within the period of the single twitch, tension can be increased considerably (fig. 4.2). The best results are usually gained when the stimulus for the second contraction occurs at the high point of the first. The second contraction is very similar to the first, but it starts with the elevated level of tension (or shortening) supplied by the first contraction. The explanation for this phenomenon, *summation of contractions,* seems to be that the short duration of the single twitch does not allow sufficient time for the structural rearrangements within fibers (discussed in chapter 2) to go to completion (34).

If the same preparation is stimulated repeatedly with a series of shocks too closely spaced to allow a complete relaxation phase, a prolongation of the contraction occurs, called *tetanus* (fig. 4.3). If a relaxation phase persists, as is shown in the curves A, B, C, and D of the illustration, it is termed a *partial* or *incomplete tetanus.* If the relaxation phases are completely eliminated, as in the E curve, it is called a *complete tetanus.* In a complete tetanus the developed tension may be three to four times that of the single twitch.

Temperature Effects on Muscle Contraction

The effects of temperature on intact human muscle have been known for a long time (32, 33). The contraction time for the human gastrocnemius muscle increases with cooling by as much as 21% to 82%, depending on the temperature drop and the length of time the muscle is cooled. The relaxation time under comparable conditions of cooling increases from 51% to 150%. Heating the muscle, on the other hand, causes small but significant improvements in the speed of contraction (12%) and in the speed of relaxation (22%). It should be pointed out that the important factor here is the deep-muscle temperature.

More recent work has corroborated the early work in this area and has provided further elucidation of practical significance. Petajan and Eagan (26) have shown that exercise-induced heating is more effective than is the same amount of passive heating in improving the rate of muscular relaxation after stimulation. Furthermore, they also provided evidence that training induces an increased rate of muscle relaxation after exercise.

Also worth noting is that if the gastrocnemius muscle is cooled, the relaxation phase is slowed down two to three times as much as the contraction phase. It has been postulated that this difference may explain poor performance or muscle injury after improper or insufficient warm-up. The rationale for this hypothesis is that a slowly relaxing antagonist may be driven into its relaxation phase by a relatively faster contracting agonist. Thus there would be an opposition of forces of the paired muscles around any given joint, which might result in sore muscles or impaired performance—certainly a reasonable hypothesis.

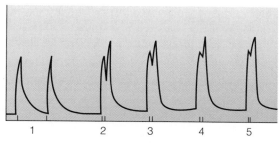

Figure 4.2   Summation of twitches. (From Zoethout. *Introduction to Human Physiology*, 1948. Courtesy of The C. V. Mosby Company, St. Louis.)

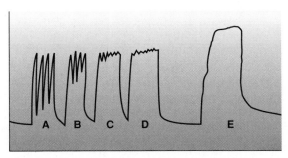

Figure 4.3   Muscle curves showing the genesis of tetanus; *A, B, C, D,* incomplete tetani; *E,* complete tetanus. Faradic shocks of the same intensity were used throughout. (From Zoethout. *Introduction to Human Physiology*, 1948. Courtesy of The C. V. Mosby Company, St. Louis.)

deVries would like to present another equally reasonable hypothesis in this vein. A representative time for one stride in sprinting is approximately 0.4 second. Tuttle's work (32) indicated a slowing of the total twitch (gastrocnemius) in cooling down to 0.54 second after 5 minutes and to 0.88 second after 20 minutes of cooling. This suggests that contraction of the agonist, or prime mover, may occur while the muscle is still in a somewhat contracted condition from the previous stimulation; this results in a summation of contractions without a relaxation phase for the muscle concerned. That this condition may

very likely result in contracture or sore muscles will be discussed in detail in chapter 26.

The words of A.V. Hill summarize the effects of temperature. "The speed of everything that can be measured in muscle is diminished two or three times by a fall in temperature of 10°C" (19). Hill also points out that mammalian muscle can be quickened approximately 20% by elevating body temperature 2°C, and he suggests that a good runner might do 100 yards in 8 seconds under these conditions.

The All-or-None Law

If a muscle fiber (or motor unit) is stimulated by a single impulse at or above threshold value, it responds by a contraction, or twitch, that is maximal for any given set of conditions of nutrition, temperature, and so on. In other words, stimulation by impulses much larger than threshold value will result in no increase in either the shortening or the force of contraction. This is referred to as the *all-or-none law* of muscle contraction. Obviously this law applies to the motor unit, since all its component fibers are innervated by the same nerve fiber and impulse. (It does not, of course, apply to whole muscles.)

The all-or-none law, however, has been widely misinterpreted to mean that a muscle fiber or motor unit is capable of producing no more force than that exhibited following stimulation by a single impulse at or above the threshold for contraction. This interpretation is clearly in error given that successive stimuli can result in increased force production by a muscle fiber or motor unit due to summation of contractions.

Gradation of Response

Because of the all-or-none law for the contraction of motor units and muscle fibers, other explanations must be sought for the fact that whole muscles are capable of exquisitely fine gradations in speed and in force of contraction. There are two methods by which the nervous system brings this about: 1) *recruitment,* which means varying the number of motor units innervated, and 2) *rate coding,* which means increasing or decreasing the rate of firing for the motor units involved.

To begin with, we have known for some time that smaller motor units and those composed of slow twitch, oxidative fibers in particular have the lowest thresholds for voluntary activation and are therefore selectively involved in low intensity contractions. When recruitment is involved, increasingly forceful contractions are achieved by the recruitment of progressively larger motor units, including those with fast twitch glycolytic fibers. This is called the *size principle* (8, 18).

On the other hand, motor units already active can discharge at higher frequencies (rate coding) and thereby generate greater tensions, as discussed earlier in this chapter. Work in this area suggests that the method for generating increasing forces in humans varies from muscle to muscle (3). For example, recruitment was found to be the major mechanism in the deltoid for increasing force of contraction from 40% to 80% of maximal voluntary contraction (MVC), while in a small muscle of the finger, rate coding played the major role (7).

Of interest to physical educators and physiologists are the incredible feats performed by humans under great stress and during hypnotic states. Some investigators have found that electrical stimulation under conditions of maximal voluntary contraction brings about further increase of force, while other investigators have not. Findings of unfused motor units at 80% MVC in the deltoid muscle, which primarily uses recruitment for increasing force, suggests that rate coding has a tremendous potential for increasing force up to (and even beyond) MVC. If the central nervous system were to increase firing rates in the large, fast twitch motor units of the deltoid such as it does in the finger muscle, extraordinary force levels could be achieved for short periods of time (7).

Muscle Fatigue

It has long been known that when a muscle is caused to contract repeatedly and with very short rest intervals (one to two seconds), a decrement in response can be seen both in the intact muscle and in the excised muscle. Figure 4.4 illustrates this fatigue phenomenon in the excised muscle. The first few contractions demonstrate the treppe effect (in a rested muscle); then, after a period of normal contractions, the response of the muscle grows less—both in the contraction and the relaxation phase—until finally no visible reaction to further stimulation is obtained.

This points to several factors of practical importance to the physical educator and the coach. First, the effect on the relaxation phase is larger in magnitude than the effect on the contraction phase. This lack of relaxation is referred to as *contracture* and plays an important role in the discussion of muscle cramping. Second, it has been reported (23) that at the point of complete fatigue, where there is no further visible response from the stimulation, the muscle action potentials may be undiminished. This indicates that the nervous transmission of the impulse through the myoneural junction can be absolved of blame for fatigue in this experiment. Furthermore, nerve fibers have been found to be practically indefatigable, and thus the site of fatigue seems to be either in the muscle contractile mechanism or in the coupling of the action potential to the contraction process. Although older work seemed to indict the myoneural junction as the site of fatigue, at least in excised muscle, the finding of undiminished action potentials by Merton (23) (when the muscle is no longer capable of response) is strong evidence to the contrary.

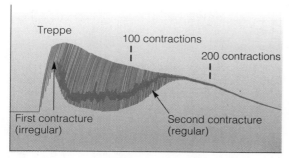

Figure 4.4 Effect of repeated stimulation. The muscle was stimulated electrically at intervals of one second. Note the effect of fatigue on the ability of the muscle to "relax." (From Howell. *A Textbook of Physiology*, 11th ed., 1930. Courtesy of W. B. Saunders Company, Philadelphia.)

Our discussion refers only to *local muscular fatigue* in one muscle or in one functional muscle group. General fatigue of the entire organism must be considered from a different vantage point, much greater in scope. This will be discussed at greater length in chapter 20.

Types of Contraction

Muscular contraction is an unfortunate term in that it implies shortening. In actuality, innervation of a muscle often results in an expenditure of energy to produce force that is used either in maintaining a held position or in opposing lengthening as a muscle resists a superior force or slows down the effect of gravity. The nomenclature for these various types of muscular contraction is not standard, and therefore at least five terms are necessary for the study of exercise physiology.

Isometric Contraction

Isometric contraction (also called static contraction) involves producing tension without movement at the joint or shortening of the muscle fibers. Examples of isometric contractions are squeezing a hand grip dynamometer or pushing against an immovable object.

Isotonic Contraction

Isotonic contraction involves moving a constant resistance through a range of motion. Unlike an isometric contraction, it includes movement at a joint. Technically, the term isotonic is incorrect because the amount of tension produced within the muscle changes as the joint angle changes. Therefore, to more precisely describe the fact that the external resistance is constant throughout the range of motion, the phrase *dynamic constant external resistance* (DCER) exercise is gaining popularity, although the term isotonic is still widely used. Examples of activities that utilize isotonic contractions are training with free weights and the sports of power and olympic lifting.

Isokinetic Contraction

Isokinetic contraction involves the contraction of a muscle at a constant velocity. This is normally accomplished by instrumentation that allows for the selection of a predetermined contraction velocity. Isokinetic contractions are commonly used in rehabilitative settings.

Concentric versus Eccentric Contraction

Concentric and eccentric differentiate between shortening and lengthening types of contraction. *Concentric contraction* is the production of force while the muscle is shortening. In *eccentric contraction,* a muscle produces force that is less than the opposing external force; although the muscle tries to shorten, it is actually lengthened during its contraction phase. Examples of this are use of the biceps brachii in letting the body down slowly from a chin-up and use of the inward rotators of the humerus in arm wrestling. The loser's inward rotators, although attempting to shorten, have been forced to lengthen by the superior force of the opponent.

It is customary to measure the mechanical work output of muscular contraction by the method of the physicist: $W = F \times D$; W is the work done, and F is the force acting through a distance, D. Thus the computation of the work load for a concentric contraction in lifting a 100-pound weight 2 feet is $W = 100 \times 2$, or $W = 200$ foot-pounds of work done. In isometric or static contraction, however, since no movement is involved and $D = 0$, no mechanical work is done, although "physiological" work is performed because tension is produced and ATP is utilized. In eccentric contraction, where the 100-pound weight is slowly lowered 2 feet—through the forced stretching of muscles resisting the force of gravity—it is suggested that the same formula be used and that this work load of 200 foot-pounds be termed negative work.

Mechanical Factors in Muscular Activity

For any given strength and nutritive condition of a muscle, there are at least three very practical considerations for physical educators and coaches regarding the external force that can be produced from that muscle:

1. The angle of pull of the muscle.
2. The length of the muscle at any given time.
3. The velocity of muscle shortening.

Angle of Pull

The angle between the lengthwise axis of the muscle and the lengthwise axis of the bone it is causing to move is referred to as angle *a*. In the diagram (fig. 4.5), force triangles are drawn to show the relationship of the internal muscular force exerted (side *B*), which is held the same throughout figure 4.5, to the net force available to do the work (side *A*) and to the wasted force (side *C*). The optimal value of the angle of pull is closely approximated by the condition in figure 4.5, part 2. When the muscle pulls at right angles to the bone that it is moving, sides *A* and *B* will coincide, and all

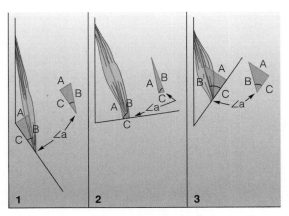

Figure 4.5   Effect of the angle of pull of a muscle upon the external force *A* provided for equal amounts of internal muscular force *B*. Side *C* in each case represents wasted internal force.

of the muscle's internal force becomes available to do useful external work. At angles of pull greater or less than the optimal value, the wasted force, side *C*, becomes larger, and the externally available force, side *A*, becomes smaller for any given value of muscular effort (side *B*).

For example, the most difficult points in a chin-up seem to be at the very bottom and top of the exercise, which are represented by parts 1 and 3 of figure 4.5, respectively. Subjects who are able to start chinning themselves can probably get past the midpoint where the angle of pull is favorable, but will have difficulty stretching their necks over the bar at the top. In addition, figure 4.6 provides a simplified example of the relationship between strength and joint angle for the forearm flexion movement. Note that the ability to produce tension to overcome external resistance is dependent upon the joint angle and, as demonstrated in figure 4.5, is a function of the angle of pull of the muscles involved.

Length of Muscle

At any given time during contraction, the length of the muscle determines how much internal force or tension it can generate. It has

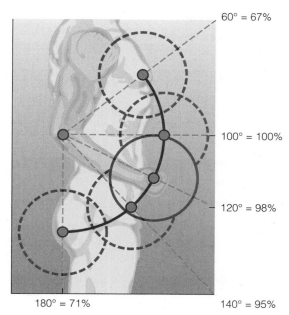

60° = 67%

100° = 100%

120° = 98%

180° = 71%   140° = 95%

Figure 4.6   Variation in strength relative to the angle of contraction, with 100 percent representing the angle at which strength is optimal. (From Jack H. Wilmore and David L. Costill, *Training for Sport and Activity*, 3d edition. Copyright © 1988 Wm. C. Brown Communications, Inc., Dubuque, Iowa. All rights reserved. Reprinted by permission.)

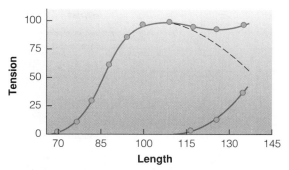

Figure 4.7   Relation between length and tension. One hundred is rest length and maximum tension. Monotonic increasing curve at lower right represents effect of passive stretch on tension. Upper solid curve is obtained from system as a whole. Broken line represents behavior of contractile elements when passive stretch curve is subtracted from upper curve. (From Zierler, Kenneth L., Mechanism of muscle contraction and its energetics. In Montcastle, Vernon B., editor: *Medical Physiology*, ed. 13, St. Louis, The C. V. Mosby Co., 1974).

been demonstrated that, in an isolated muscle fiber, the tension developed in a tetanus is maximum at the maximum resting length and decreases with greater and with lesser lengths (29). The same general conditions have been observed in intact skeletal muscle (1).

The relationship between muscle length and tension is one of the few in physiology in which cellular structure and cellular function can be shown to be related. Figure 4.8 shows the results of ingenious experiments by Gordon, Huxley, and Julian (17) to define the length-tension relationship within a single sarcomere. We can see clearly that the electron micrographs of sarcomere length nicely support the sliding filament theory discussed in chapter 2. Thus at position 1, where few cross-bridges can interact, the developed tension is near zero. As the cross-bridges attain

more binding sites, tension rises to near maximum at point 2. At points 3 and 4 the situation is still near optimal, and tension declines only slowly. Points 5 and 6, showing rapid decline in tension, are thought to result from two factors: 1) the extensive overlap of the actin and myosin filaments interferes with the formation of cross-bridges, and 2) the rigidity of the thick myosin filaments probably absorbs some of the force that is generated. Note the close agreement between the length-tension relationship in gross muscle (fig. 4.7) with the length-tension relationship in the single sarcomere as developed in figure 4.8. The small differences can probably be accounted for by the connective tissue present in the gross muscle.

Thus the principle for physical education is, "Put the muscle on stretch to obtain the greatest force of which the muscle is capable." However, the stretch factor that provides the greatest internal forces may be working at odds with the aforementioned angle of pull, which determines how much of the internal muscle force will be externally available for useful

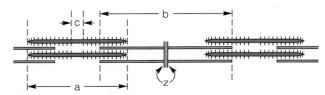

A Schematic diagram of filaments, indicating nomenclature for the relevant dimensions.

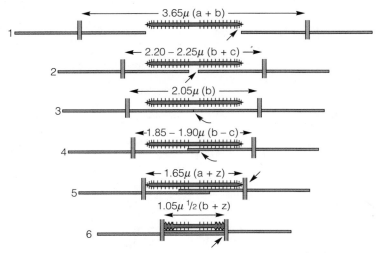

B Critical stages in the increase of overlap between thick and thin filaments as a sarcomere shortens.

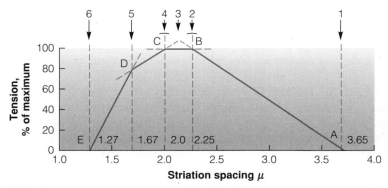

C Tension levels in sarcomere as striation spacing narrows.

Figure 4.8   Relationship of tension developed to the position of actin and myosin filaments within a sarcomere. (From Gordon, A. M.; Huxley, A. F; and Julian, F. J., in *Journal of Physiology* 184:170–92, 1966. Reprinted by permission.)

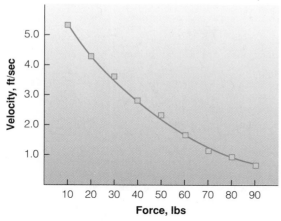

Figure 4.9   Force-velocity relationship in healthy young men. (From Damon, E. L., in *An Experimental Investigation of the Relationship of Age to Various Parameters of Muscle Strength*. Ph.D. diss., Physical Education, University of Southern California, 1971. Reprinted by permission.)

work. Thus the intelligent analyst of athletic activity must consider the interaction of both factors to achieve the best results.

Velocity of Muscle Shortening (The Force-Velocity Curve)

The velocity with which a muscle shortens affects the external force available (fig. 4.9). It has been found that as the velocity of shortening increases, the force decreases in exponential fashion (14). This indicates that force falls off disproportionately as the speed of contraction increases, and this in turn dictates an optimum speed for a needed amount of force.

Recently, the exponential shape of the force-velocity curve has been challenged (25), but the discrepant findings were the result of isokinetic testing in which fatigue may have been the cause of the deviations from the smooth exponential curve found by all previous investigators.

A.V. Hill (19) suggested the optimum speeds for muscular efficiency and power are approximately the same: 20% to 30% of the maximum speed at which the muscle can shorten under zero load. Further research is needed to determine how these figures could be applied to power events, such as the shot put.

Improvement of Force and Work Delivery by Dynamic Stretching of Muscle

Cavagna, Dusman, and Margaria (5) have provided us with some concepts in muscle physiology that have direct application to athletic performance in certain events. Having found that the efficiency of running was considerably better (40%) than that usually calculated for simple cycle ergometer work (25%), they looked for the source of this increased efficiency in the possible storage of energy in elastic tissues during negative work. This energy could be released to aid the subsequent positive contraction. Thus in running, as the extended leg strikes the ground, the quadriceps is forced into lengthening to accept the weight of the body and in so doing accumulates elastic energy, which is immediately used to augment the following positive work of striding. They found that the maximal positive work (*W'*) done by a muscle shortening immediately after being stretched is greater than the work (*W*) done when shortening from a state of isometric contraction. They further found that the improvement represented by the ratio *W'/W* increases with the speed of stretching and shortening and also with the length of the muscle. This principle holds true not only for the work produced but for the force production.

Thus for such events as the discus or the shot put the ultimate results will be better the longer and more rapid the preparatory windup. Such a windup also requires optimal development of flexibility, of course.

Electromyography in Analysis of Muscle Function

Basic Concepts of Electrical Phenomena and Electromyography

It has been known, at least since the middle of the nineteenth century, that the contraction of muscle tissue is accompanied by an electrical change that can be recorded and measured. The electrical change is called a *muscle action potential* (MAP), and the recording of muscle action potentials (or their currents) is called *electromyography* (EMG). The MAP arises at the muscle cell membrane (or sarcolemma) and passes lengthwise through the fiber in wavelike form as the fiber is stimulated to contract. The science of recording and analyzing MAPs probably received its greatest impetus in the related science of *electrocardiography*, in which the events of the cardiac cycle are recorded on electrocardiograms (ECGs) and examined for abnormality. Physicians also use electromyography clinically in the diagnosis of various types of muscular diseases such as spasticity and paralysis.

Most EMG instrumentation and procedures have been developed for the use of physicians in diagnosing abnormal neuromuscular function and may be thought of as *qualitative* rather than *quantitative* in nature since the greatest concern is with the recording and analysis of the *wave form* of the MAP from single discrete motor units.

Quantitative electromyography is the study of the amount of electrical activity that is present in a given muscle under varying conditions. Obviously it is not electrical activity per se that is of interest here; rather it is the fact that EMG recordings accurately reflect muscle activation at a level of sensitivity at which palpation and other methods fail to produce evidence.

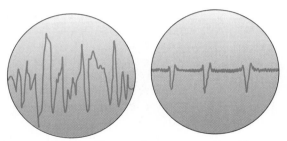

Figure 4.10   Differences between recordings of single motor-unit potentials with needle electrodes (right) and summated potentials from many motor units with surface electrodes (left).

Investigators in exercise physiology and kinesiology (sometimes physical therapy and physical medicine) are mainly concerned with occurrences in the whole muscle rather than in isolated motor units. For this reason, surface electrodes on the skin over the belly or the motor point of the muscle are used. Thus the firing of many motor units is observed simultaneously and a better statistical sampling is obtained than by the use of needle electrodes. This results, however, in a wave form that is a summation of the randomly organized activity of the many motor units observed, and it tells us nothing about any one motor unit. Also, the MAPs—in passing through the muscle tissue, fascia, subcutaneous fat, and skin—are severely attenuated (decreased in magnitude). Therefore, if we wish to know what is going on in a resting or relatively inactive muscle, we need recordings of extremely high sensitivity. (deVries has recorded meaningful differences in activity of resting muscles in which the difference between two conditions is less than 1 μv.) The difference between recordings of individual motor units with needle electrodes and recordings of summated potentials from many motor units with surface electrodes is shown in figure 4.10.

It is important to realize that when many motor units fire randomly, some will, by chance, fire simultaneously, and the size of the wave form recorded at that point will be larger.

Furthermore, as a muscle is required to produce more tension, ever greater numbers of motor units are recruited; by the laws of chance, more will fire simultaneously, and the wave form will grow larger in amplitude as more tension is produced.

The information to be gained from the pattern of motor unit spikes shown in the right-hand side of figure 4.10 is immediately obvious. We can count the spikes and measure the amplitude, but we have absolutely no quantitative knowledge of what the whole muscle is doing. We know only what is going on in one motor unit. As it turns out, the physiological significance of the electrical activity in the total gross muscle rests on the mean amplitude of the summated MAPs. The problem here can be immediately recognized by posing the question: What is the mean amplitude of the summated MAPs shown in the left side of figure 4.10? What do we measure to get a true mean value for a function that varies constantly and randomly over time as does the *interference pattern* (so-called from electronics parlance) of figure 4.10? To do this requires integration (a procedure of calculus). This concept of integration is simply depicted in figure 4.11. First, the integration process can be applied only to the electrically positive or negative halves of the spikes. Otherwise the end result would be zero, with the positive being balanced out by the negative aspects of the wave form. Thus, as the first step shown in figure 4.11B, we have eliminated the negative swinging part of the spikes. Next, we must think of the spikes as having area, as in figure 4.11C. The dimensions of this area are, vertically, microvolts of electrical activity (μv) and, horizontally, time in fractions of a second. The next step is to convert the area under the random spikes into a neat geometric figure such as a rectangle whose area equals height times length (or in this case μv times seconds). This conversion to the rectangle is accomplished by *planimetry* (tracing the curve with an engineering instrument that provides the area

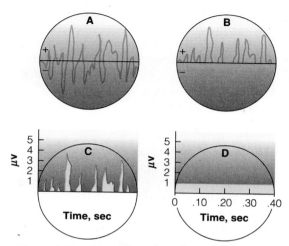

Figure 4.11   Integration of muscle action potentials to get true mean value of their amplitude.

under any curve). Now we have the area of figure 4.11D in an approximate rectangle whose dimensions are a height of 1.0 μv and a time of 0.40 seconds, yielding an area of 1.0 × 0.40, or 0.40 μv second. This is the reading we would obtain from the planimeter. To get the mean μv level, then, we need only divide as follows:

$$\frac{\mu v \times sec}{sec} \text{ or } \frac{1.0 \ \mu v \times 0.40 \ sec}{0.40 \ sec} = 1.0 \ \mu v$$

Now we can say that over the 0.40-second observation period the mean amplitude of the MAPs was 1.0 μv. Fortunately, electronic integrators are available that accomplish the whole procedure without resorting to planimetry.

Only through integration can accurate data regarding the physiological importance of the electrical activity in the muscle be evaluated. Even such a tedious process as measuring spike amplitudes is of little value for precise data because the amplitude constantly and randomly varies. To get a true mean one must know over what period of time the spike has acted. A fat spike is more important than a thin spike of equal amplitude in determining the true mean value.

Equipment was developed for deVries's laboratory that simplifies the integration procedure. This equipment will record integrated EMG potentials with a sensitivity of 0.3 μv. Using this equipment, deVries and his colleagues accumulated evidence that the electrical activity from muscle tissue—even at the lowest levels—is indeed entirely similar to that at the higher levels. Figure 4.12 shows the high relationship between muscle tension in the elbow flexors and electrical output at the very lowest tension levels when all possible care has been taken to reduce electrode resistance to an essential minimum. We have also shown a highly significant correlation of 0.58 between resting oxygen consumption and the level of EMG in one representative muscle group (the elbow flexors). These two lines of evidence confirm that even at the very lowest levels of electrical activity, it is motor unit activity that is measured (13).

Applications of EMG to Physiological Problems

Estimation of Tension Developed within a Muscle

Often in the physiology of exercise laboratory one desires to know the tension developed within a given muscle. It has been shown by Lippold (22) and coworkers that the EMG voltage is proportional to the force of contraction in isometric contraction and that in movements of constant velocity the electrical activity is proportional to the tension developed. In movements of constant tension the electrical activity is proportional to the velocity (constant velocity) (4). This work has been extended in deVries's laboratory to include accelerated movements (6), and it was found that even here the electrical activity is proportional to the *effort impulse value,* a measurement of effort suggested by Starr (31).

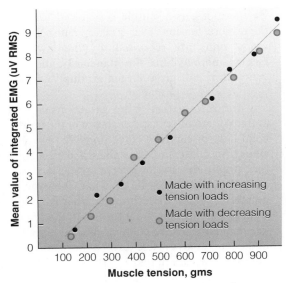

Figure 4.12   Integrated EMG output from elbow flexors as a function of muscle tension.

Thus we may conclude that in any kind of physical activity, a reasonably good estimate of the tension or effort developed within the muscle can be obtained through appropriate EMG instrumentation and techniques (integration is necessary, of course). This would be difficult if not impossible to attain by any other means.

Estimation of Strength

Where the musculature is relatively normal, measurement of maximal strength by cable tension, strain gauge, or dynamometer provides one dimension that is unquestionably related to the functional state of the tissue. As a *physiological measurement,* however, maximal strength is notoriously contaminated by psychological factors such as motivation. Muscle tonus is another dimension for evaluating muscle function. Although this term is widely used by members of all professions dealing with muscle tissue, a definition that satisfactorily encompasses all experimental evidence available does not as yet exist.

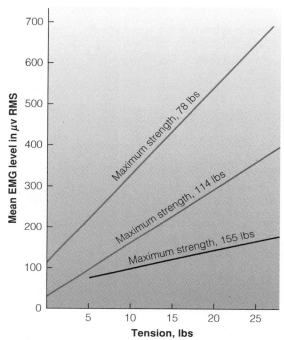

Figure 4.13 Electrical activity in a muscle as a function of the force of contraction. Note the differences of the rate of increase in activity between subjects of varying levels of strength.

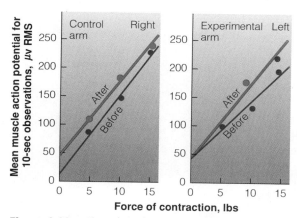

Figure 4.14 Changes in the experimental and control elbow flexors as the result of placing the left elbow flexors in a cast for four weeks. *Left:* right biceps (control arm). *Right:* left biceps (experimental arm). (From deVries, Herbert A., in *American Journal of Physical Medicine* 47:10, 1968. Courtesy of Williams & Wilkins Company, Baltimore.)

It has been proposed (11, 15) that the functional state of muscle be evaluated in terms of the *efficiency of electrical activity* (EEA). This interesting concept is illustrated in figure 4.13. It is obvious that the stronger person (flatter slope) needs less activation (electrical activity) for any given muscle loading. deVries has shown that this EMG slope, or EEA, as plotted in figure 4.13 is well related (in young subjects) to measured strength ($r = -.75$ to $-.90$). The EEA is also sensitive to hypertrophy and atrophy of muscle through use and disuse, as shown in figures 4.13 and 4.14.

EMG Evaluation of Hypertrophy versus Neural Factors in the Time Course of Strength Gain

Moritani and deVries (24) developed a method for separating the effects of 1) strength "learning" through improvement of neural factors and 2) true muscular hypertrophy. In figure 4.15 hypertrophy is reflected in a flatter slope of the EMG voltage-force relationship because fewer available motor units need be recruited at any given load. On the other hand, learning is reflected not in change of slope but in the innervation of more motor units, with an accompanying increase in the maximum EMG voltage.

Using this method, the researchers showed that young men training with weights achieve the largest part of the strength gain through learning to better innervate the muscle for the first three weeks, after which time the gains are largely attributable to hypertrophy (fig. 4.16).

EMG Estimation of Endurance— Fatigue Parameters

When a muscle contracts isometrically against constant force, the electrical activity in that muscle increases with time as shown in figure 4.17. This phenomenon is thought to be the result of the fatigue process impairment of muscle fiber function, so that additional motor

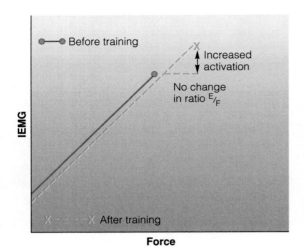

A Strength gain due to neural factors

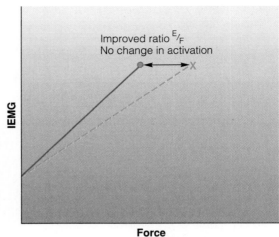

B Strength gain due to hypertrophy

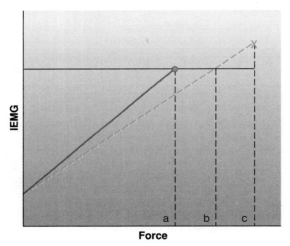

C Evaluation of percentage contributions of neural factors (NF) versus hypertrophy (MH)

$$\%MH = \frac{b - a}{c - a} \times 100$$

$$NF = \frac{c - b}{c - a} \times 100$$

Figure 4.15   Schema for evaluation of percentage contributions of neural factors (NF) and muscular hypertrophy (MH) to the gain of strength through progressive resistance exercise. *E/F* ratio is EMG voltage (IEMG) to force relationship. (From Moritani, T., and deVries, Herbert A., in *American Journal of Physical Medicine* 58: 115–30, 1979. Courtesy of Williams & Wilkins Company, Baltimore.)

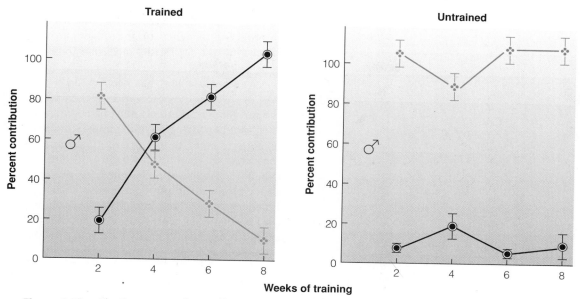

Figure 4.16   The time course of strength gain showing the percentage contributions of neural factors (❖———❖) and hypertrophy (◉———◉) in the trained and untrained arms of two male subjects. (From Moritani, T., and deVries, Herbert A., in *American Journal of Physical Medicine* 58:115–30, 1979. Courtesy of Williams & Wilkins Company, Baltimore.)

unit recruitment must take place to compensate for the constantly decreasing force available per fiber. If the fatigue process is brought about quickly with loads of 30% to 50% maximal voluntary contraction (MVC), the plot of EMG voltage as a function of time usually approximates linearity (later data in the laboratory show the curve to be an exponential with a considerable period of approximate linearity). The slope of this curve can be used under appropriate conditions for estimating the rate at which muscle fatigues (12). Test-retest reliability of such curves was found to be $r = .93$. The validity of this approach was evaluated by correlating the slope coefficient of the fatigue curve against measured maximal endurance time. The correlations were found to be $r = .79$ and $.82$ using isometric tensions of 40% and 50% of MVC, respectively. The important point to remember here is that in plotting either the EEA curve or the fatigue curve only a few data points are required, which can be obtained without the subject going beyond 25% to 50% of maximum capacity in either case. Obviously, this eliminates making the usually invalid assumption that the investigator has obtained a true maximum effort from a subject under testing conditions since motivation and other psychological factors are no longer pertinent.

Note in figure 4.17 the dramatic difference in the rate at which flexor muscles and the extensor muscles involved in posture show fatigue. This undoubtedly reflects the fiber type makeup of these muscles. The flexors generally are composed of more FG fibers, which are easily fatigued (see chaps. 2 and 3).

Observation of Other Physiological Phenomena by EMG

Many interesting physiological phenomena are mirrored in the electrical activity of the skeletal muscles. One of the more easily observed

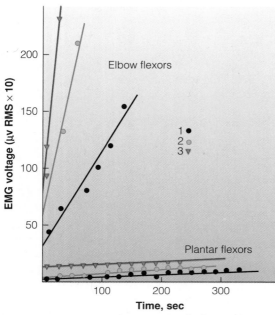

Figure 4.17   EMG fatigue curves in three test runs on the same subject with increasing fatigue of elbow flexors and plantar flexors. (From deVries, Herbert A., in *American Journal of Physical Medicine* 47:175, 1968. Courtesy of Williams & Wilkins Company, Baltimore.)

is the increase in electrical activity in irrelevant muscles when any one skeletal muscle is strained. Thus, if we load the right elbow flexor group to 50% to 75% or more of MVC, we can detect measurable activity of at least five μv in the previously inactive left elbow flexors. deVries has shown that even straining the eyes to read fine print raises the electrical activity in the elbow flexors by about 100% (9).

Another interesting phenomenon that deVries routinely demonstrates for his students is the effect of hyperventilation upon the activity of irrelevant forearm muscles. The *blowing off* of CO_2, as discussed in later chapters, raises pH and increases irritability of muscle tissue, which is displayed by twofold to fivefold increases of electrical activity (best shown in the most peripheral flexor muscles).

This, of course, is the reason for the commonly observed tendency of the fingers to curl (flex) toward a fist during moderate to severe hyperventilation.

Another use that has been made of this type of EMG is the observation of the onset of the *shivering response*. It must be noted, however, that perceiving all of the interesting phenomena referred to in this section requires a sensitivity beyond that which is ordinarily available in apparatus designed for the physician because the physician doesn't need it. Furthermore, without integration procedures, even a change in wave form that doubles the energy is not always easily discernible on the oscilloscope.

Muscle Tonus

The classic experiments of Sherrington (30) on stretch reflexes resulted in the theory that muscle tonus is the result of a partial tetanus of muscle tissue in which there is a *constant* state of activity by a small portion of the muscle fibers. This constant state of activity was thought to be the result of *myotatic* (stretch) reflexes that originate in the muscle spindles and reflexly innervate the alpha motor neurons (chap. 5). Forbes (16) speculated that this muscle tonus was brought about not by constant contraction of the same fibers, but by a *rotation of duty* among many different motor units. Thus skeletal muscles were thought never to be in a state of complete rest.

By these concepts, postural tonus results from constant feedback from a postural muscle that is stretched by slight swaying, which deforms the muscle spindles and brings about afferent impulses to the spinal cord that reflexly innervate the motor units of the stretched muscle to contract. The resulting contraction checks the sway, and balance is restored.

However, with the advent of electromyographic equipment of ultrahigh sensitivity pioneered by Jacobson (20) with the help of

Bell Telephone Laboratories, it was found that skeletal muscles in relaxed subjects (supine or sitting) could be electrically silent for minutes at a time. Since it was well known that any muscular contraction, no matter how small, is accompanied by MAPs, this required modification of the traditional concept of muscle tonus. The findings of electrical silence in relaxed, resting muscles in humans have been corroborated by many other laboratories (although not always with the same rigorous level of sensitivity). Thus Jacobson (20, p. 229), as early as 1938, suggested redefining muscle tonus in skeletal muscles as ". . . a state of slight contraction, more or less constant, or irregular, often present, but *sometimes absent in health.*"

In the light of recent research, the most acceptable definition of general muscle tonus is that of Basmajian (2, p. 41):

> . . . *the general tone of a muscle is determined both by the passive elasticity or turgor of muscular (and fibrous) tissues and by the active (though not continuous) contraction of muscle in response to the reaction of the nervous system to stimuli. Thus, at complete rest, a muscle has not lost its tone even though there is no neuromuscular activity in it.*

Resting Muscle Tonus

Over a period of many years, since electromyographic recording of MAPs has become a common laboratory procedure, many investigators have reported electrical silence in relaxed, resting muscles. However, it is an obvious truism that to demonstrate the absence of a physiological phenomenon, it is necessary to use equipment that has the capacity to render observable any and all phenomena under consideration. Obviously, the use of a magnifying glass to observe bacteria might result in the false conclusion that no such organisms exist. It is always more difficult to show the absence of an event than its presence.

Seen in this light, most evidence has not been conclusive because of deficiencies in equipment. Investigators have at times been satisfied that electrical silence existed when their sensitivity did not allow detection of anything under fifty microvolts. Furthermore, the use of needle electrodes to find electrical silence is akin to sampling the opinion of only a few persons to predict the outcome of a national election. Obviously, the smaller the sampling, the greater the potential error in the conclusion.

Nevertheless, electrical silence has been demonstrated by a few investigators such as Jacobson whose work is unimpeachable. The conclusion that muscles can indeed be entirely inactive rests upon their work. deVries has found that, without special training, ten of twenty-nine physical education students could achieve complete relaxation (electrical silence) in the right quadriceps femoris muscle for a period of two minutes. Under similar conditions, only four of the twenty-nine could achieve electrical silence in the right elbow flexors. Jacobson has demonstrated that the ability to relax voluntarily can be improved by training.

Nothing that has been said should be construed as denying the activity of the neuromuscular system as a participant in general muscle tonus. Electrical silence is achieved only by relaxed subjects under the best laboratory conditions. How often, for how long, or in how many muscles this may occur in everyday activity is quite another question. The best we can say at present is that it is possible for some persons to relax selected muscles completely on some occasions and under certain conditions. It is felt that the definition for general muscle tonus stated by Basmajian and referred to earlier is the best summation of the present state of our knowledge.

Postural Muscle Tonus

There is little agreement upon the mechanisms of postural tonus and, more specifically, upon the presence or absence of neuromuscular activity in the extensor muscles involved in maintaining the erect posture in humans.

In comprehensive reviews of the work done in this area, Ralston (27) and Ralston and Libet (28) concluded that during easy standing there is no electrical activity, even in such postural muscles as the erector spinae and lower leg muscles unless the subject sways sufficiently.

It seems rather difficult to accept the hypothesis of "hanging on the ligaments" as it were, in anything that approaches normal erect posture. Therefore, deVries reinvestigated this question with highly sensitive equipment (10). Highly significant differences were found in muscular activity in the lower leg between resting and easy standing (standing in a very relaxed fashion). All subjects showed a marked increase in activity in two lower leg muscles when they changed from the resting (seated position) to the standing position. Furthermore, no convincing evidence of electrical silence was found, even for brief periods, in either muscle in any subject. This agrees completely with the work of Jacobson (21), the only other investigator whose equipment achieved the same sensitivity. It would seem that those who found electrical silence in these muscles did so because of deficiencies in equipment.

As a consequence of these experiments (10), it would seem that the traditional concepts of postural tonus are still tenable and that the more recent research that purports to find electrical silence in postural muscles rests on insufficient evidence from equipment of insufficient sensitivity.

Effects of Exercise upon Resting Muscle Tonus

It has long been thought that one of the benefits of exercise is the improvement of muscle tonus. It has also been observed that the lack of exercise from having a cast on a fractured leg or from forced bed rest results in a degree of flaccidity. Although these statements are probably true, they seem to be unsupported by experimental evidence at this time.

Physiology of Muscle Tonus

The most logical explanation of muscle tonus, based on the research cited above, seems to rest on the existence of a *passive component* and an *active component*.

Passive Component

The passive component is composed of the elasticity of muscle and connective tissues, plus the tissue turgor, which may be defined as the pressure with which body fluids tend to distend their surrounding tissues. This factor is present regardless of the state of innervation.

Active Component

The active component rests on the gamma loop, to be discussed in chapter 5, and is in large part hypothetical. The most logical explanation that encompasses all experimental results is as follows.

1. Muscle tonus rests on a reflex basis.

2. The afferent limb of the reflex arises in the receptor of the muscle spindle and enters the spinal cord where it synapses directly with the alpha ventral horn cells.

3. A constant facilitation effect is brought about by impulses from subcortical nuclei, reticular substance, and vestibular and cerebellar pathways.

4. Firing of the alpha ventral horn cells innervates a small proportion of the motor units in all muscles concerned with posture, probably (although not demonstrably) in rotating fashion, as postulated by Forbes (16).

5. In muscles other than the postural muscles, provided the subject is

sufficiently relaxed, complete inactivity may exist at least for short periods of time.

Summary

1. The *myogram* illustrates the contraction of a whole muscle (muscle twitch) when it is artificially innervated by a single stimulus. Its response consists of a *latent period* of 0.001–0.01 second, a *contraction phase* of approximately 0.04 second, and a *relaxation phase* of approximately 0.05 second.

2. If, during one muscle twitch, a second stimulus occurs, a *summation of contractions* will occur that results in greater tension than either twitch separately.

3. A *tetanus* or *tetanic contraction* results from repeated stimulation of muscle when the intervals between stimuli are too short to allow complete relaxation. If *no* relaxation occurs between stimuli, it is a complete tetanus, and the tension developed may be three to four times that of a single twitch.

4. Low muscle temperatures result in slow contraction and relaxation phases. This effect is relatively much greater in the relaxation phase. High temperatures have a converse effect. These two facts have important implications for warm-up and the prevention of muscular distress.

5. The *all-or-none law* states that a muscle fiber (or motor unit) contracts either maximally or not at all in response to a single stimulus.

6. *Gradation of response* in muscle tissue is brought about by two methods: (a) *recruitment*, which involves varying the number of motor units innervated, and (b) *rate coding*, which means increasing or decreasing the rate of firing for the motor units involved. The mechanism used varies from muscle to muscle.

7. The *site of local muscular fatigue* seems to be peripheral and probably involves either the contractile mechanism itself or the coupling of the muscle action potential (MAP) to the contractile mechanism—or both. This conclusion remains somewhat controversial, however.

8. The *external muscular force* available for useful work is the result of three component factors: (a) the angle of pull of the muscle, (b) the length of the muscle, and (c) the velocity of shortening.

9. Whenever a muscle is innervated, one or more MAPs are produced that can be recorded and measured by *electromyography* (EMG).

10. By recording MAPs, muscle activation can be measured quantitatively. deVries refers to this use of EMG as *quantitative EMG*, in contradistinction to the methods and instrumentation commonly applied by the physician who is usually more concerned with the observation of the *wave form* of MAPs from single motor units.

11. When surface electrodes are used in EMG, the *interference pattern* observed on the oscilloscope is the result of the summation of several or many different motor units firing randomly in time.

12. To make meaningful use of EMG data from the interference pattern requires integration procedures to calculate true mean amplitudes. Integration may be accomplished by *planimetry* or by electronic integrators.

13. That the integrals so achieved (or the true mean amplitudes calculated from

them) have physiological significance has been well verified in various laboratories.

14. The methods of quantitative EMG have been applied to many aspects of exercise physiology:

    a. It has been shown that the tension developed within a muscle can be estimated (i) under isometric tension, (ii) under constant velocity movement, and (iii) under accelerated movements.

    b. Strength and functional quality of muscle tissue can be evaluated in young subjects by the slope of the EMG voltage regression on force of contraction.

    c. The endurance (or fatigue rates) of muscles can be objectively evaluated by the slope of the EMG voltage regression upon time when the subject holds an isometric contraction of 40% to 50% maximal voluntary contraction.

    d. Highly sensitive EMG instrumentation also renders visible the reactions of muscle tissue to such homeostatic displacements as occur during hyperventilation.

15. Resting muscle tonus is the result of *active* and *passive components*. The active component is due to neuromuscular activity and is not always present. The passive component is due to tissue pressure and the elastic quality of muscle and connective tissue and is continuous during the life of the organism.

16. Postural muscle tonus has been shown to have both components in all muscles that are involved in maintaining the erect posture. Investigations that have failed to show the active component probably suffered from deficient equipment.

References

1. Banus, M. G., and Zetlin, A. M. The relation of isometric tension to length in skeletal muscle. *J. Cell. Comp. Physiol.* 12:403–20, 1938.

2. Basmajian, J. V. *Muscles Alive.* Baltimore: Williams & Wilkins Co., 1962.

3. Belanger, A. Y., and McComas, A. J. Extent of motor unit activation during effort. *J. Appl. Physiol.* 51:1131–35, 1981.

4. Bigland, B., and Lippold, O. C. J. The relation between force, velocity, and integrated electrical activity in human muscles. *J. Physiol.* 123:214–24, 1954.

5. Cavagna, G. A., Dusman, B., and Margaria, R. Positive work done by a previously stretched muscle. *J. Appl. Physiol.* 24:21–32, 1968.

6. Damon, E. L. An experimental investigation on the equating of isometric, concentric, and eccentric muscular efforts. Not published.

7. DeLuca, C. J., Le Fever, R. S., McCue, M. P., and Xenakis, A. P. Behaviour of human motor units in different muscles during linearly varying contractions. *J. Physiol.* 329:113–28, 1982.

8. ———. Control scheme governing concurrently active human motor units during voluntary contractions. *J. Physiol.* 329:129–42, 1982.

9. deVries, H. A. Neuromuscular tension and its relief. *J. Assoc. Phys. Ment. Rehabil.* 16:86–88, 1962.

10. ———. Muscle tonus in postural muscles. *Am. J. Phys. Med.* 44:275–91, 1965.

11. ———. Efficiency of electrical activity as a physiological measure of the

functional state of muscle tissue. *Am. J. Phys. Med.* 47:10–22, 1968a.

12. ———. Method for evaluation of muscle fatigue and endurance from electromyographic fatigue curves. *Am. J. Phys. Med.* 47:125–35, 1968b.

13. deVries, H. A., Burke, R. K., Hopper, R. T., and Sloan, J. H. Relationship of resting EMG level to total body metabolism with reference to the origin of tissue noise. *Am. J. Phys. Med.* 55:139–47, 1976.

14. Fenn, W. O., and Marsh, B. S. Muscular force at different speeds of shortening. *J. Physiol.* 85:277–97, 1935.

15. Fischer, A., and Merhautova, J. Electromyographic manifestations of individual stages of adapted sports technique. *Health and Fitness in the Modern World,* chap. 13. Chicago: The Athletic Institute, 1961.

16. Forbes, A. Spinal reflexes. *Physiol. Rev.* 2:401, 1922.

17. Gordon, A. M., Huxley, A. F., and Julian, F. J. The variation in isometric tension with sarcomere length in vertebrate muscle fibres. *J. Physiol.* 184:170–92, 1966.

18. Henneman, E., Somjen, G., and Carpenter, D. O. Functional significance of cell size in spinal motor-neurons. *J. Neurophysiol.* 28:560–80, 1965.

19. Hill, A. V. The design of muscles. *Br. Med. Bull.* 12:165–66, 1956.

20. Jacobson, E. *Progressive Relaxation.* Chicago: University of Chicago Press, 1938.

21. ———. Innervation and tonus of striated muscle in man. *J. Nerv. Ment. Dis.* 97:197–203, 1943.

22. Lippold, O. C. J. The relation between integrated action potentials in a human muscle and its isometric tension. *J. Physiol.* 117:492–99, 1952.

23. Merton, P. A. Problems of muscular fatigue. *Br. Med. Bull.* 12:219–21, 1956.

24. Moritani, T., and deVries, H. A. Neural factors vs. hypertrophy in the time course of muscle strength gain. *Am. J. Phys. Med.* 58:115–30, 1979.

25. Perrine, J. J., and Edgerton, V. R. Muscle force-velocity and power-velocity relationships under isokinetic loading. *Med. Sci. Sports* 10:159–66, 1978.

26. Petajan, J. H., and Eagan, C. J. Effect of temperature and physical fitness on the triceps surae reflex. *J. Appl. Physiol.* 25:16–20, 1968.

27. Ralston, H. J. Recent advances in neuromuscular physiology. *Am. J. Phys. Med.* 36:94–120, 1957.

28. Ralston, H. J., and Libet, B. The question of tonus in skeletal muscle. *Am. J. Phys. Med.* 32:85–92, 1953.

29. Ramsey, R. W., and Street, S. The isometric length-tension diagram of isolated skeletal muscle fibers of the frog. *J. Cell. Comp. Physiol.* 15:11–33, 1940.

30. Sherrington, C. S. *Integrative Action of the Nervous System.* New Haven: Yale University Press, 1923.

31. Starr, I. Units for the expression of both static and dynamic work in similar terms and their application to weight lifting experiments. *J. Appl. Physiol.* 4:21–29, 1951.

32. Tuttle, W. W. The effects of decreased temperature on activity of intact muscles. *J. Lab. Clin. Med.* 26:1913–15, 1941.

33. ———. The physiologic effects of heat and cold on muscle. *Athletic J.* 24:45, 1943.

34. Wilkie, D. R. The mechanical properties of muscle. *Br. Med. Bull.* 12:177–82, 1956.

5

The Nervous System and Coordination of Muscular Activity

The Neuron and the Motor Unit

The Reflex Arc and Involuntary
    Movement

Intersegmental and Suprasegmental
    Reflexes

Proprioception and Kinesthesis

The Alpha and Gamma Systems for
    Muscular Control

Higher Nerve Centers and Muscular
    Control
    The Pyramidal System
    The Extrapyramidal System
    The Proprioceptive-Cerebellar
        System

Posture, Balance, and Voluntary
    Movement
    Posture
    Balance
    Voluntary Movement

Perception of Effort

Use-Disuse Phenomena in the Nervous
    System

Does Viscerosomatic Motor Inhibition
    Limit Exercise?

Practical Considerations
    Effects of Hypnosis and Emotional
        Excitement on Performance
    Proprioceptive Neuromuscular
        Facilitation (PNF)
    The Dynamogenic Effect of
        Concontractions
    Reaction Time and Movement Time
    Effect of Fatigue
    Motor Set versus Sensory Set

The nervous system can be divided in two principal ways. First, we can think of it as divided structurally into *central* and *peripheral* components. The central component consists of the brain and spinal cord, and the peripheral component consists of all the ganglia (groups of nerve cells not in the spinal cord) and nerve fibers (axons). Second, it is divided functionally into the *somatic* and *autonomic* systems, both of which have central as well as peripheral components. The autonomic system controls the internal environment and innervates the smooth muscles of the gastrointestinal tract, the blood vessels, and so on, as well as the endocrine glands.

The autonomic system has two divisions: 1) the *sympathetic division,* whose central outflow is from the thoracic and lumbar regions of the spinal cord, and 2) the *parasympathetic division,* which originates in the cranial nerves and in the sacral region of the spinal cord. In a very general way, these two divisions of the autonomic system are antagonistic and balance each other. The sympathetic has to do with "fight or flight" adjustments of the organism in a dangerous situation, to the stress of sport, and in other tension-producing activities. The parasympathetic, on the other hand, is related in a general way to functions that we usually do not consciously control, such as digestion.

The *somatic system* consists of the central and the peripheral components of the nervous system that have to do with peripheral reception of nervous impulses, conduction to the spinal cord or brain, organization of motor patterns, and conduction back to the skeletal muscles to bring about the desired movements.

The Neuron and the Motor Unit

The *neuron,* a single nerve cell, is the basic structural unit of the nervous system. It is specialized for its function by having a high degree of irritability and conductivity. There are billions of neurons in the nervous system, and usually several neurons are interconnected by *synapses* to form pathways for conduction of nervous impulses. The neurons that conduct sensory impulses from the periphery to the central nervous system are called *sensory* or *afferent* neurons; the neurons that conduct impulses from the central nervous system to the muscles and other effectors are called *motor* or *efferent* neurons. Although neurons are microscopic in width, one cell may extend in length from the cerebral cortex almost to the caudal end of the spinal column, or an equal distance from the spinal cord to a muscle in the foot, a distance of approximately three feet.

The typical motor neuron (fig. 5.1) has two types of processes from its cell body: 1) *dendrites,* which receive impulses and conduct them to the cell body, and 2) an *axon,* which conducts the impulses away from the cell and accounts for the great length of some neurons. The cell body of the motor neuron, which innervates skeletal muscle, lies in the gray matter in the ventral horn of the spinal cord, and its axon joins many axons from other motor neurons (and many sensory axons) to form a spinal nerve. This spinal nerve is thick enough to be seen and handled grossly in dissection.

The motor nerve, after entering the muscle through the epimysium, branches and rebranches until one axon enters a fasciculus. The axon then branches into many twigs, each of which innervates one muscle fiber. Thus the

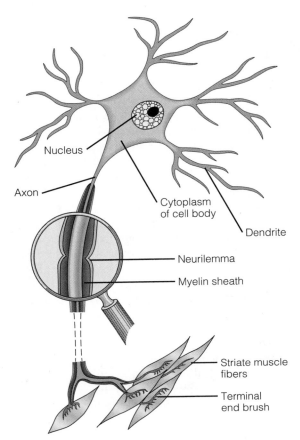

Nucleus

Axon

Cytoplasm
of cell body

Dendrite

Neurilemma

Myelin sheath

Striate muscle
fibers

Terminal
end brush

Figure 5.1   A diagrammatic drawing of a neuron. At the top is the cell body and its numerous branchings, the dendrites. They make up the soma of the neuron. The axon, of which there is only one, extends downward. The point at which the axon leaves the soma is the axon hillock. Axons, and sometimes dendrites, may be covered with a myelin sheath and, outside the nervous system, with a neurilemma. (From *Physiological Psychology* by C. T. Morgan and E. Stellar. Copyright © 1950 McGraw-Hill, Inc. Used by permission of McGraw-Hill Book Company.)

cell body in the ventral horn, plus the axon and all its twigs, together with the many muscle fibers innervated by the twigs form one *motor unit*.

The Reflex Arc and Involuntary Movement

A great deal of muscular activity is accomplished by reflex control. A *reflex* is most simply defined as an involuntary motor response to a given stimulus. An illustration is the automatic, unthinking response to touching a hot surface. In its simplest form, a reflex consists of a discharge from a sensory nerve ending, called a *receptor* or *sensory end organ,* whose impulses are propagated over the sensory nerve fiber to a *synapse,* or junction, in the spinal cord with a motor neuron. When the motor neuron is stimulated to discharge, impulses are propagated over its axon to the *effector* (muscle or gland), bringing about the reflex response. The sensory pathway is *afferent,* and the motor pathway is *efferent.*

This simple reflex arc (fig. 5.2) occurs in the *myotatic* or stretch reflex, and because there is only one synapse in the cord, it is called a *monosynaptic reflex.* Other reflexes, such as the *flexion reflex* (used in removing the hand from a hot surface), involve at least three neurons and two synapses. These are called *disynaptic reflexes* for three or more neuron arcs, or *multisynaptic* for four or more neuron arcs (fig. 5.3). The short neuron that serves to connect the sensory and motor neurons in this case is called an *internuncial* or *association* neuron.

The preceding discussion is an oversimplification of what actually occurs. For example, for the flexion reflex to proceed with dispatch, the antagonistic extensor muscle group must be prevented from acting. This inhibition of the antagonists is accomplished by kinesthetic impulses from the muscle spindles of the flexor muscle. These synapse not only with the flexor motor neurons directly but also indirectly with the motor neurons of extensor muscles of the same joint. This process is called *reciprocal inhibition.*

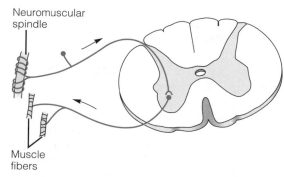

Figure 5.2   Diagram of a two-neuron reflex—from a spindle in a muscle back to other fibers of the same muscle. Arrows indicate direction of conduction. (From Gardner, E. *Fundamentals of Neurology,* 2d ed. © 1958. Reprinted by permission of the author.)

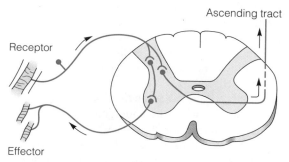

Figure 5.3   Diagram illustrating how impulses from a cutaneous receptor reach an effector (skeletal muscle) by a three-neuron arc at the level of entrance. (From Gardner, E. *Fundamentals of Neurology,* 2d ed. © 1958. Reprinted by permission of the author.)

Applying this same flexion reflex to the foot (in stepping on a sharp object), we find that not only does the reflex result in withdrawal of the foot with its concomitant reciprocal inhibition of the extensor muscle of the same leg, but it may also result in the extension of the contralateral (opposite) leg to support the body during the flexion reflex. This action of the contralateral limb is called the *crossed extensor reflex*. It is the result of *facilitation* that is also brought about by action

of the afferent neuron from the muscle spindles but upon the motor neuron of the extensor muscles of the opposite limb.

This is still not a complete account of even these simple reflexes, and the reader interested in reflexes should see a text in neurology for further discussion. Even the simplest reflex involves the organizing and integration of responses into meaningful movement patterns.

Knowing the reflex mechanism of the stretch reflex will greatly facilitate understanding the scientific principles involved in recent research in flexibility and in the muscle soreness phenomenon, which are discussed in part 3 of this text.

Intersegmental and Suprasegmental Reflexes

Reflexes are not necessarily limited to causing action at the same spinal cord level as the incoming afferent stimulus. For example, in the scratch reflex of the dog, the stimulus (a flea-bite, for example) may occur at a level where the afferent part of the reflex arc enters the cord in the upper thoracic area, and the response is brought about by the hind leg muscles, whose efferents leave the cord at the sacral level. The association neuron travels down the dog's spinal cord a considerable distance before synapsing with the motor neuron, which forms the efferent pathway to bring about the scratching response. This is illustrated in figure 5.4, which also shows the possibilities for contralateral responses as well as upward or downward conduction pathways in the spinal cord. Reflexes that involve more than one spinal segment (or level) are called *intersegmental reflexes.*

So far we have considered only spinal reflexes. Turning our attention to postural mechanisms, we see that, although these do not require conscious volitional control, they are

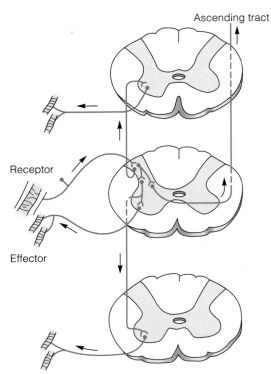

Figure 5.4 Diagram of the connections by which impulses from a receptor reach motor neurons at different cord levels. (From Gardner, E. *Fundamentals of Neurology,* 2d ed. © 1958. Reprinted by permission of the author.)

abolished in the absence of the centers and pathways of the brain. For example, in a faint or in anesthesia, postural reflexes fail. The spinal or segmental portion of the reflexes involved in posture can still be elicited with the proper stimulus.

Thus it is apparent that higher brain centers are necessary for postural reflexes, and for this reason we refer to this group of reflexes as *suprasegmental reflexes.* The stretch or myotatic reflex forms the basic component of the postural reflexes, but it depends on facilitation from higher centers for incoming sensory impulses to achieve threshold value and thus bring about total postural responses. Furthermore, higher brain centers seem to

be necessary to coordinate and control these mechanisms.

Proprioception and Kinesthesis

For the optimal coordination of motor patterns to take place in the brain and spinal cord, a constant supply of sensory information must be available to feed back the results of movement as it progresses (36). This feedback of sensory information about movement and body position is termed *proprioception.* The receptors for proprioception are of two types: vestibular and kinesthetic.

The *vestibular receptors* are found in the nonauditory labyrinths of the inner ear. Each of these two labyrinths, one on each side in the temporal bone of the skull, consists of a small chamber, the *vestibule,* which communicates with three small canals known as *semicircular canals* (fig. 5.5). Within the semicircular canals is a fluid called *endolymph.*

The inertia of the endolymph, which results in its remaining stationary at the first part of a movement of the body and also its continued movement when the body has returned to a resting position, disturbs a sensory receptor organ, the *crista.* This disturbance is transmitted to the brain by way of the vestibular branch of the eighth cranial nerve. Thus the sensory information from the cristae of the semicircular canals provides the data regarding movement—more specifically, rotational acceleration or deceleration of movement as in twisting or tumbling. Movement in itself is not recognized. For example, moving at almost the speed of sound in an airliner produces no sensation, unless a change of direction or velocity occurs.

Along with the semicircular canals, the *utricle* and *saccule* of the vestibule complete the vestibular system. Apparently, the saccule has little if any function in equilibrium or position sense; it seems to be involved in sensory

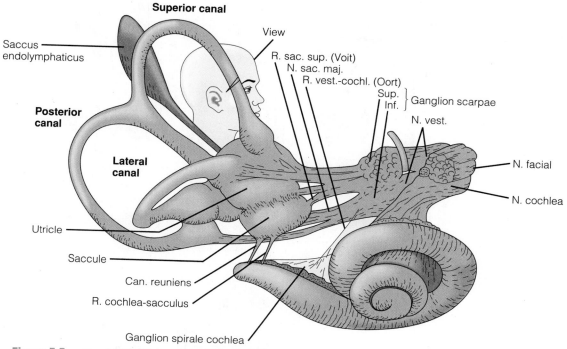

Superior canal

Saccus endolymphaticus

Posterior canal

Lateral canal

Utricle

Saccule

Can. reuniens

R. cochlea-sacculus

Ganglion spirale cochlea

View

R. sac. sup. (Voit)
N. sac. maj.
R. vest.-cochl. (Oort)
Sup. } Ganglion scarpae
Inf.
N. vest.

N. facial

N. cochlea

Figure 5.5   Drawing showing structural relations of innervation of the human labyrinth (by Max Brodel). (From *The Anatomical Record* 59:403–18, 1934 by Max Brodel.)

perception of vibration only. The utricle, however, is the sense organ that provides the data necessary for positional sense. The *otolith organ* in the utricle responds to linear acceleration and to tilting and thus seems to be the source of data that informs us of our posture in space.

Although no sensation of movement is produced in the body of a passenger in an airliner (in smooth air), the *orientation* of the body in space, as in standing upright or lying down, is clearly recognized, even with the eyes closed. This recognition of spatial orientation is the result of interpretation of sensory information received from the otolith organ in the utricle.

The kinesthetic sense and its receptors are of even greater interest (fig. 5.6). At least five types of receptors serve the muscle sense,

or *kinesthesis:* 1) the muscle spindle,* 2) the Golgi tendon organ, 3) the pacinian corpuscle, 4) Ruffini receptors, and 5) free nerve endings. It has long been known that these receptors provide the individual with muscle sense. One can tell what one's limbs or body segments are doing at any given time without having to look. For instance, the normal individual has no difficulty making accurately controlled movements, such as bringing one's finger from arm's length to touch the end of one's nose, even when blindfolded. Furthermore, one can usually make reasonably accurate guesses about the weight of an object by lifting it.

Spindle afferents, although extremely important in their sensory input to reflex behavior, do not contribute to subjective sensations.

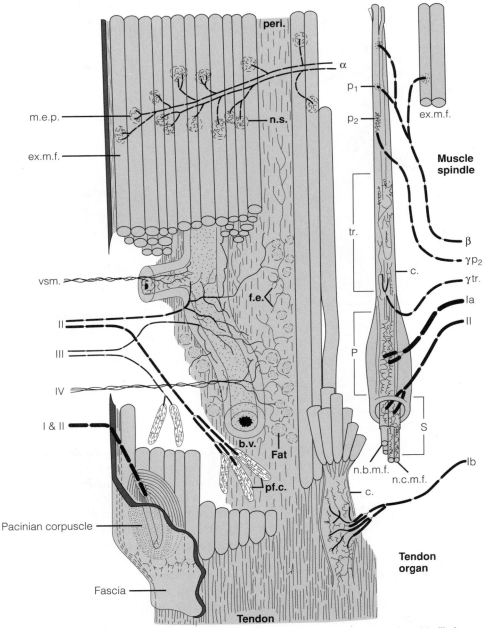

Figure 5.6   Schema of the innervation of mammalian skeletal muscle based on a study of cat hindlimb muscles. Those nerve fibers shown on the right of the diagram are exclusively concerned with muscle innervation; those on the left also take part in the innervation of other tissues. Roman numerals refer to the groups of myelinated (I, II, III) and unmyelinated (IV) sensory fibers. Greek letters refer to motor fibers. The spindle pole is cut short to about half its length, the extracapsular portion being omitted. Blood vessel (b.v.); capsule (c.); epimysium (epi.); extrafusal muscle fibers (ex.m.f.); nuclear-bag muscle fiber (n.b.m.f.); nuclear-chain muscle fiber (n.c.m.f.); nodal sprout (n.s.); motor end plate; primary ending; p_1, p_2, two types of intrafusal end plates: perimysium; paciniform corpuscle; secondary ending; trail ending; vasomotor fibers. (From Barker, D. In *Handbook of Sensory Physiology*, 1973, vol. III, pt. 2. Courtesy of Springer-Verlag, Berlin, Heidelberg, New York.)

This muscle sense, or kinesthesis as it is properly called, is important in providing sensory information for skilled movement. However, recent research indicates that this system, particularly the muscle spindle and its attendant nerve supply, may be even more important in functioning as *autogenetic governors* of motor-nerve activity (13). The muscle spindles have their own motor-nerve system, which is important enough to constitute about one-third of the total efferent fibers that enter skeletal muscle (22).

Therefore let us consider the muscle spindle first and in some detail (fig. 5.7). The spindle is large enough to be visible to the naked eye and is fusiform, as the name implies. That muscle spindles are widely distributed throughout muscle tissue is clearly illustrated by the large number of efferent fibers that serve them. However, the distribution varies from muscle to muscle. In general, the muscles used for complex movements (such as finger muscles) are abundantly supplied with up to thirty spindles per gram of muscle, while muscles involved in only very gross movements such as latissimus dorsi may have only one to two per gram. In some of the cranial muscles no spindles were found (4, 38).

Each spindle consists of a connective tissue sheath 4 to 10 mm long that contains from five to nine *intrafusal muscle fibers* (IF) in mammalian tissue. These IF fibers are quite different from the typical fibers (extrafusal or EF) of muscle described in chapter 2, which are involved in bringing about gross muscle contraction. Spindle structure is shown in figures 5.6 and 5.7. It is important to note that the spindles are always oriented parallel to the EF fibers. There are two types of IF fibers:

1. Usually there are two *nuclear bag fibers,* which are thicker and longer and in which as many as a dozen nuclei are crowded into the middle section.

2. There are three to seven *nuclear chain fibers,* which are so named because their nuclei, although also located in the midsection, are fewer in number and are arranged in single file, forming a thinner, shorter fiber.

At each end of the IF fiber are the motor poles, which are the contractile elements composed of striated myofibrils.

The sensory end organs within the spindles are of two types, the *annulo spiral ending* (also called primary ending) and the *flower spray ending* (also called secondary ending). The large annulospiral type Ia afferent nerve axon (only one per spindle) sends individual twigs to wrap around the middle of each nuclear bag fiber and other less well-developed spiral terminals to most of the nuclear chain fibers. The flower spray endings are so named because they arborize in spraylike formation from a smaller afferent nerve fiber (type II) and wrap themselves around nuclear chain fibers almost exclusively. There may be one or two flower spray endings per spindle. They attach not at the nuclear area but at one or both sides of it in the transition zone between the motor pole and the nuclear area.

Both of these endings are deformed by the stretching of the intrafusal fibers. Because these intrafusal fibers lie lengthwise, parallel with the skeletal (extrafusal) fibers, an externally applied stretch results in stretching the intrafusal as well as the extrafusal fibers. The consequent deformation of the annulospiral ending evokes an afferent discharge in its large, type Ia sensory nerve (fast-conducting). Simultaneously, the flower spray ending discharges into its type II sensory nerve (slow-conducting). This afferent discharge from the spindle results in a motor response: contraction of the muscle that was stretched. This response, called a *stretch* or *myotatic reflex,* is typified by the tendon jerk elicited when a physician strikes the patellar tendon.

The annulospiral ending responds to both phasic and static stretching, whereas the flower spray ending responds to static stretch but is relatively insensitive to phasic stretch (9).

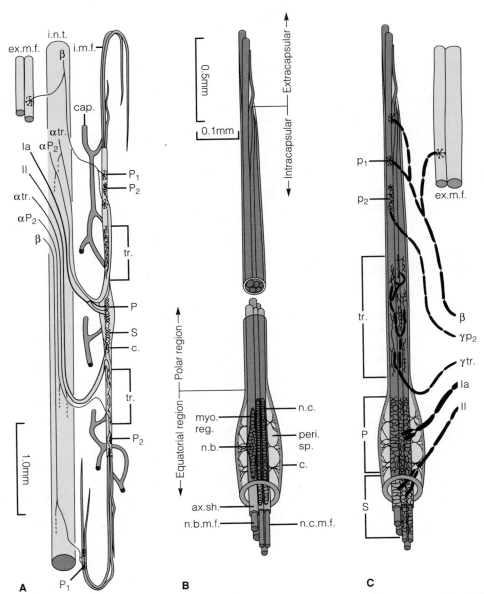

Figure 5.7   Schematic diagrams illustrating the structure and innervation of the mammalian muscle spindle as found in cat hindlimb muscles. **A** shows the general proportions of the receptor; the ends of the poles are curled round so as to fit into the figure. **B** shows the morphology of the equatorial region and about half of one pole. The same figure is used in **C** with the addition of the sensory and motor innervation. ax.sh., axial sheath; c., capsule; cap., capillary; ex.m.f., extrafusal muscle fibers; i.m.f., intrafusal muscle fibers; i.m.t., intramuscular nerve trunk; myo.reg., myotube region; n.b., nuclear bag; n.c., nuclear chain; n.b.m.f., nuclear-bag muscle fiber; n.c.m.f., nuclear-chain muscle fiber; P, primary ending; p₁, p₂, two types of intrafusal motor end plates; peri.sp., periaxial space; S, secondary ending; tr., trail ending. Sensory nerve fibers indicated by Roman numerals, motor fibers by Greek letters. (From Barker, D. In *Handbook of Sensory Physiology*, 1973, vol. III, pt. 2. Courtesy of Springer-Verlag, Berlin, Heidelberg, New York.)

The Golgi tendon organ (fig. 5.6), a somewhat simpler end organ, is found in the musculotendinous junction and throughout the perimysial connective tissues. It should be noted that this ending is in series with the skeletal muscle fibers and therefore is deformed by tension in the tendon whether by passive stretching or by active shortening of the muscle. It therefore discharges under both conditions, whereas the spindle discharges only when the muscle is stretched. The spindle ceases to fire when contraction begins because it is in parallel with the extrafusal muscle fibers and is thus unloaded as soon as the extrafusal fibers shorten in contraction (fig. 5.8).

A further difference in function between the spindle and the tendon organ is that the spindle facilitates—indeed, may cause—contraction, whereas the tendon organ seems to be a protective device, inhibitory not only to its muscle of origin but to the entire functional muscle group as well (30). The stretch reflex that originates in the muscle spindles is the basis for unconscious muscular adjustments of posture where a slight stretching of the extensor muscles at the knee, for instance, is immediately corrected by reflex shortening to prevent collapse. The tendon reflex that prevents overstressing the tissues is called the *inverse myotatic reflex*. Granit (13) points out that "the muscle machine is working under self-regulation from autogenetic governors, first aiding it to contract, then damping the discharge from its motoneurons."

The pacinian corpuscle is a large encapsulated end organ, made up of several layers of fibrous tissue in which nerve endings ramify. These receptors, although widely distributed throughout the body, do not lie within the muscle tissue proper. They are found concentrated in the region of the joints and in the sheaths of tendons and muscles and consequently are pressed upon when muscles contract. They are excited by the deformation of deep pressure and may be more important than

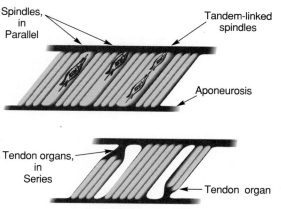

Figure 5.8   The principle of "in series" and "in parallel" arrangement of muscle receptors with reference to extrafusal (nonspindle) muscle fibers. Spindles lie between muscle fibers, either with both poles ending in interfascicular connective tissue, with one pole attached to a tendon, or in some short muscles with both poles inserting into muscle tendons or aponeuroses. In muscles with long extrafusal fasciculi, several spindles may be linked in tandem by one or more long intrafusal fibers that pass from one capsule to another. This histological distinction of series and parallel arrangements has a physiological counterpart in response characteristics of the afferent during contractions. (From "Peripheral Receptors: Their Excitation and Relation to Reflex Patterns," by Earl Eldred, M.D., *American Journal of Physical Medicine* 46:69, 1967. Courtesy of Williams & Wilkins Company, Baltimore.)

the spindles and tendon organs in detecting passive movement or position of a body segment in space.

Ruffini receptors are scattered throughout the collagenous fibers of joint capsules and are differentially activated by joint movement. Consequently, they are probably most important in sensing joint position and motion. As can be seen in figure 5.9, each individual receptor ending monitors a well-defined and restricted range of the total movement. The sensing of the complete movement is thus the result of integration by the nervous system of the bits and pieces of information provided by the many Ruffini receptors.

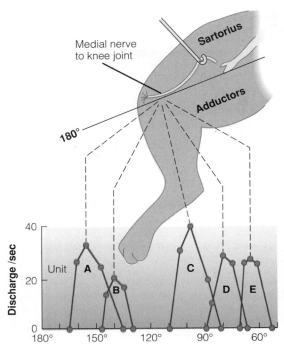

Figure 5.9   Range fractionation in signaling of joint position. Five joint receptor units were isolated from the medial nerve to the knee joint of the cat. Each unit discharged only over a restricted range of knee positions and had a maximum at one fairly sharply defined point. The discharge was constant at a stable position of the joint but became elevated during movements within the response range for that unit. (From "Peripheral Receptors: Their Excitation and Relation to Reflex Patterns," by Earl Eldred, M.D., and adapted from S. Skoglund, in *American Journal of Physical Medicine* 46:69, 1967. Courtesy of Williams & Wilkins Company, Baltimore.)

Unmyelinated, free nerve endings are thought to be widely distributed through muscles, tendons, joints, fascia, and ligaments, but the only definite histological information seems to indicate their distribution to these tissues is not direct but indirect—by serving the blood vessels that supply these tissues. Their function as kinesthetic receptors is also largely unknown.

In summary, proprioception involves sensing five aspects of muscle status:

1. *Active contraction,* by the tendon organ discharge
2. *Passive stretch,* by spindle discharge only, since tendon organ threshold is high
3. *Tension,* by tendon organ discharge
4. *Position,* by discharge of Ruffini receptors
5. *Pressure sensation* from pacinian corpuscles

The sense of limb position rests largely on the last two elements of proprioception.

The Alpha and Gamma Systems for Muscular Control

It has been shown that approximately one-third of all the efferent nerve fibers that enter a muscle have no connection with skeletal, extrafusal muscle fibers (22); rather, these nerve fibers have been demonstrated to innervate the intrafusal fibers of the muscle spindles. This is important and is of practical significance in understanding muscular control. The smaller motor-nerve fibers that make up this one-third of the total efferent nerve fibers are called *gamma efferent fibers,* in contrast to *alpha efferent fibers,* which are larger and are the motor-nerve fibers for the extrafusal or skeletal muscle fibers.

In figure 5.10 the monosynaptic response to stretch can be traced as follows:

1. Stretching the main muscle fibers of the quadriceps results in stretching the muscle spindle and its intrafusal fibers.
2. The annulospiral nerve ending in the intrafusal fibers is distorted and causes propagation of nervous impulses to the cord via the large Ia spindle afferent.

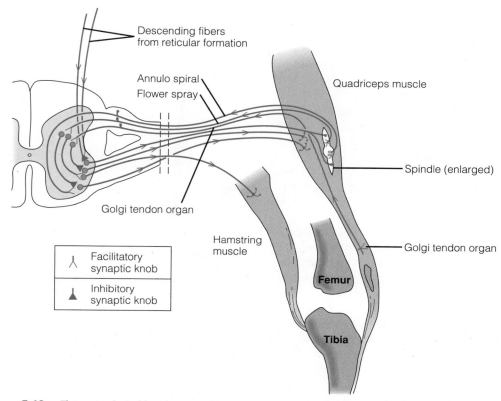

Descending fibers from reticular formation

Annulo spiral

Flower spray

Quadriceps muscle

Spindle (enlarged)

Golgi tendon organ

⅄	Facilitatory synaptic knob
▲	Inhibitory synaptic knob

Hamstring muscle

Golgi tendon organ

Femur

Tibia

Figure 5.10   The myotatic and inverse myotatic reflexes as autogenetic governors of movement at the knee joint. Note that supraspinal influence, both facilitatory and inhibitory, is brought to bear on the gamma efferent neuron, thus setting the bias of the spindle.

3. The large spindle afferent synapses directly with the large alpha efferent, which brings about muscular contraction (stretch reflex) of the quadriceps.

It will also be noted in figure 5.10 that the flower spray receptor activates its smaller, slower conducting type II afferent, which goes through an internuncial neuron to end in an inhibitory synapse with the alpha motor neuron pool. Activation of the flower spray ending also facilitates the alpha motor neuron going to the antagonistic flexor muscle, shown as the hamstring group in the diagram. Typically, the flower spray ending, if it is in an extensor muscle, facilitates contraction of the antagonistic flexors and inhibits its own extensor muscle. When this ending lies in a flexor, it helps to bring about the stretch reflex or shortening of the flexor. The threshold for stimulating the flower spray ending is much higher, so the action is usually controlled by the annulospiral ending until the stretching is considerable.

As the extrafusal fibers contract, the intrafusal fibers in the spindle go slack (figs. 5.6 and 5.8). Thus the deformation of the annulospiral ending is relieved, and consequently the innervation of the large spindle afferent ceases and the stretch reflex is over. In voluntary movement, however, the situation is somewhat more complex. As the extrafusal fibers contract, the intrafusal fibers are innervated by their motor nerves, the gamma efferents, which causes a shortening of the intrafusal fibers and a consequent resetting of the spindle length, as it were, so that they are again (and constantly) sensitive to any stretching of spindles. Thus a system is set up in which the innervation of the intrafusal fibers sensitizes the spindle, and the spindle firing causes more contraction of the extrafusal fibers. This is an alternative method for initiating movement and provides feedback information about the *length* of the muscle.

One other system (fig. 5.11) should also be noted. When the alpha efferent neuron fires, a recurrent axon collateral is also innervated, which synapses with an internuncial neuron in the cord called a *Renshaw cell*. This cell has the property of synapsing with and inhibiting other motoneurons. Its system constitutes what is termed a *feedback loop*. In other words, the fact that the alpha neuron is initiating contraction in the main muscle is *fed back* and is used to inhibit other muscle fibers from making the contraction too strong. This is negative feedback, in that action tends to limit itself from getting out of control. The process by which a physiological (or mechanical) mechanism controls itself by feeding back information that reflexly governs the action is called a *servomechanism*.

Another factor enters into the reflex control of muscular movement. You will recall from our discussion of kinesthetic receptors that the Golgi tendon endings are also sensitive to stretch. The response, however, is inhibitory in nature, and there is evidence that these endings inhibit not only the muscle from which the afferent impulse arises but the entire functional muscle group (30). The tendon endings have a higher threshold to stretch than the spindles and consequently do not fire until considerably more force is expended. However, they are very sensitive to tension brought

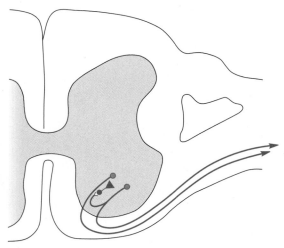

Figure 5.11   The Renshaw internuncial neuron or Renshaw cell is the short interneuron with the inhibitory synaptic knob, which is activated by a recurrent collateral from an alpha motor nerve.

about by active contraction of the muscle fibers with which they are in series. Even 0.1 gm of force results in impulse propagation from the Golgi tendon organ (GTO) (21). Consequently, the GTO is thought to be important in providing feedback information about the tension produced by the muscle. It must also be considered important as a peripheral source of inhibition to protect the muscle against too great an overload.

As has been pointed out by investigators in this area such as Granit (13), Holmgren and Merton (20), and Mountcastle (32), muscles seem to be controlled by a system of autogenetic governors. Muscular activity seemingly can be initiated by either the alpha or gamma efferents. Indeed, it is now thought that coactivation is the rule (35). A constant feedback of information by the muscle spindles and tendon organs provides the central nervous system with the data needed to control the movement as it progresses. The spindles are, in the words of Granit, "the private measuring instruments of the muscle's servomechanisms.

They do not record length so much as differences in length between the extrafusal muscle fibers and intrafusal fibers of the spindles. The tendon organs apply the brakes to muscular contraction to prevent the development of too great a tensile force, which could result in injury to muscle and/or tendon."

The work of Granit and Kaada (14) indicates that the gamma efferent system is tonically activated from central regions, such as the diencephalic reticular system, the motocortex, and the anterior lobe of the cerebellum. This tonic activity of the gamma efferents results in a degree of tonus in the muscle spindles, which in turn tonically innervates the large spindle afferents for postural reflexes and results in postural tonus of the extensor muscle groups throughout the body.

Furthermore, the stretch reflex has some interesting qualities for muscle stretching in developing flexibility or in warming up athletes. There is evidence that the stretch reflex has two components, one of which is the result of phasic (jerky) stretching and the other the result of static (maintained) stretching (22, 27, 32). The phasic response seems to be faster and stronger and is typified by synchronous discharges of the spindles, whereas the static response is slower and weaker and is typified by asynchronous discharge of the spindles.

From the practical standpoint, then, we may say that the *amount* and *rate* of response of a stretch reflex are proportional to the *amount* and *rate* of stretching. In other words, the use of bouncing or jerking movements in stretching will cause the muscle to contract with a vigor proportional to that of the bouncing and jerking. It is rather obvious that this is not desirable, either in warming up cold muscles for athletic participation or in work that is designed to improve flexibility.

There is also a difference between the stretch reflexes of the flexor and extensor muscles. The phasic component of the reflex is well developed in both, but the static stretch component is well defined only in the extensors, where it is needed for the sustained muscular activity of maintaining posture.

It would seem intelligent for the physical educator and coach to apply known principles. If muscle tissues are to be loosened up, lengthened, or relaxed, the use of a sustained pull on the muscle would tend to eliminate the phasic component of the stretch reflex. The pull should be of sufficient force to reach the threshold of the tendon organs or flower spray endings. This will then initiate the inverse myotatic reflex, which will inhibit the muscle under stretch and thus further aid in stretching the muscle.

These reflex patterns can be applied in other areas. It seems reasonable to believe, for example, that the upper limits of muscle strength and power must be set by the level of inhibition brought about centrally by the Renshaw cell and peripherally by the GTO and the flower spray endings. Learning to disinhibit may be an important part of strength training, in bringing about an increased firing rate of FT motor units as discussed in chapter 4.

In the light of the preceding discussion it is easy to see how muscle cramp can be brought about by making a maximally vigorous contraction of a muscle in a shortened position. This can be demonstrated by maximal contraction of a fully flexed biceps. What happens is that in the shortened position no tension can be placed on the tendon organ (see the length-tension diagram in chap. 4). So we have maximum innervation with minimal inhibition, and the result in a large percentage of trials is cramping. Fortunately, this newfound knowledge can be applied to relieve the cramp. One simply forces the muscle into its longest position, thereby creating tension in the tendon and the GTO, with resulting inhibition that relieves the cramp.

Higher Nerve Centers and Muscular Control

So far the discussion of muscular control has centered around the involuntary reflex systems. Now we will consider the voluntary control of muscular activity by the brain. It will be convenient to consider this in three parts: 1) the *pyramidal system,* 2) the *extrapyramidal system,* and 3) the *proprioceptivecerebellar system.* Although much is known about the function of the brain in controlling muscular activity, a much greater portion awaits further research. Furthermore, a complete discussion of what is known of the motor functions of the brain is beyond the scope of this text and unnecessary for its purposes. Therefore the discussion is somewhat brief and is confined to those aspects that are of interest to the physical educator.

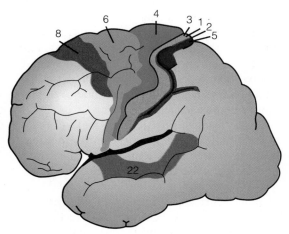

Figure 5.12   Diagram of the areas of the human cerebral cortex involved in the extrapyramidal system. In the frontal lobe are areas 4, 6, and 8. In the postcentral region are areas 1, 2, 3, and 5. Down in the temporal lobe, area 22 is concerned in the extrapyramidal pathways. (From *Physiological Psychology* by C. T. Morgan and E. Stellar. Copyright © 1950. Used by permission of McGraw-Hill Book Company.)

The Pyramidal System

The cerebral cortex has been mapped out in fair detail, over a period of time, by two methods: 1) by relating clinically observed motor defects with the lesions seen in surgery and autopsies, and 2) by electrically stimulating the cortex of experimental animals and observing the resulting motor effects. This research has resulted in cytoarchitectural maps of the human cortex. The most commonly used map is that of Brodmann. Our areas of interest are shown in figure 5.12.

The pyramidal system originates in large nerve cells, shaped like pyramids, that lie mainly in area 4 of the cortex. It was once thought that the giant Betz cells were the entire source of the pyramidal tracts, but research has indicated they are only about 2% of the total motoneurons of the pyramidal system. The axons from the motoneuron cell bodies in area 4 form large descending motor pathways, called *pyramidal tracts,* that go directly (in

most cases) to synapses with the motor neurons in the ventral horn of the spinal cord, with which we have already dealt. The neurons whose cell bodies are in the brain are commonly called *upper motor neurons,* and those in the spinal cord are called *lower motor neurons.* Seventy to 85% of the nerve fibers of the pyramidal tract cross from one side to the other, some at the level of the medulla, others at the level of the lower motoneuron.

Area 4 of the cortex is also referred to as the *motor cortex* or, because of its location, as the *precentral gyrus.* The mapping of the motor cortex clearly demonstrates a neat, orderly arrangement of stimulable areas. The area of cortex devoted to a given body part is *not* proportional to the amount of tissue served but rather to the complexity of the movement potential of the body part. It has been shown that the hands and the muscles of vocalization involve a disproportionate share of motoneurons.

It should be pointed out that the motor cortex is oriented by *movement* not by *muscle.* That is, stimulation of the motor cortex results not in a twitch of one muscle but in a smooth, synergistic movement of a group of muscles.

The Extrapyramidal System

The extrapyramidal system has its origin mainly in area 6, according to Brodmann's nomenclature. This area is rostral to area 4, the motor area, and is sometimes called the *premotor cortex.* Evidence, however, indicates that some of the fibers descending in the extrapyramidal tracts also originate with cell bodies in other areas, notably areas 8 and 5 and also in areas 3, 1, and 2, which are usually considered the sensory areas for somesthetic impulses.

The descending tracts that are composed of the axons from the neurons of the premotor cortex are considerably more complex. These fibers do not go directly to synapses with the lower motoneurons but by way of relay stations, which are called *motor nuclei.* The most important nuclei are *corpus striatum, substantia nigra,* and *red nucleus.* Some fibers also go by way of the pons to the cerebellum.

For the physical educator, the most important differences between the pyramidal and extrapyramidal systems are the functional differences. Whereas electrical stimulation of area 4 produces *specific movements,* stimulation of area 6 produces only large, general *movement patterns.* Consequently, it is believed that learning a new skill in which conscious attention must be devoted to the movements (as in learning a new dance step, where every movement is contemplated) involves area 4. As skill progresses, the origin of the movement is thought to shift to area 6 (dancers no longer concentrate on their feet but rather on very general patterns of movement, so that they can interpret the music better). However, area 4 still participates as a relay station, with fibers connecting area 6 to area 4.

The Proprioceptive-Cerebellar System

We have already dealt with some of the sensory functions of the proprioceptive-cerebellar system, namely, the kinesthesis and vestibular function in proprioception. In general, the pathway of vestibular proprioception leads to the cerebellum, either directly or by way of the vestibular nucleus in the medulla. Of the fibers that conduct kinesthetic information, some go to the thalamus and cortex to provide sensory knowledge of movement at the conscious level. Others go to the cerebellum. The confluence of sensory data on position, balance, and movement upon the cerebellum is indicative of the importance of this organ to movement.

The cerebellum rivals the cerebral cortex in complexity, but unfortunately it is not so well understood. Removing the cerebellum of experimental animals results in a loss of function that has three distinct components: 1) impairment of volitional movements, 2) disturbances of posture, and 3) impaired balance control. Consequently, its functions may be deduced. Without entering into anatomical detail we can say that the cerebellum receives constant sensory information from receptors in muscles, joints, tendons, and skin, and also from visual, auditory, and vestibular end organs.

Despite all this sensory reception, however, no conscious sensation is aroused in the cerebellum. This function is served by the sensory cortex of the cerebral hemispheres. The cerebellum is intimately connected with the motor centers, from the motor cortex all the way to the spinal cord, and may be considered to modify muscular activity from the beginning to the end of a movement pattern.

Posture, Balance, and Voluntary Movement

It is now appropriate to consider how all of the foregoing discussion relates to a better understanding of human muscular activity, which is the purpose of this text.

Posture

Human upright posture is mainly brought about through suprasegmental reflexes. The major part of these suprasegmental reflexes is the basic stretch, or myotatic reflex, which has been described. Let us therefore direct our attention to the postural mechanism that occurs about the knee joint. If the joint starts to collapse (flex), immediately as the muscle spindles of the quadriceps are stretched, an impulse is generated that is propagated over large afferents to the cord where synapse is made with a motoneuron, which innervates fibers in the quadriceps to contract and thus reextend the joint into its proper position. This reflex, however, occurs only in the presence of facilitation by the vestibular nucleus in the medulla, whose fibers in the cord tend to maintain a state of excitation of the motoneurons innervating the muscles, so that a relatively small afferent impulse can reach threshold value. Furthermore, postural reflexes also depend on effects of the extrapyramidal system and the autogenetic governor system to bring about smoothly coordinated contraction of the proper strength.

Balance

The balance aspect of muscular activity is best discussed by reference to the *righting reflex,* which illustrates the underlying principles rather well. If one drops a cat from a small height in supine position (upside down), one can observe the sequential events that invariably lead to its righting itself and landing on all four feet. The first reaction is a turning of the head toward the floor in the attempt to normalize the sensations coming from the otolith organs, which inform the cat it is not oriented in space as it would wish to be. This turning of the head innervates muscle spindles, tendon receptors, and other nerve endings in the neck muscles that initiate kinesthetic impulses and reflexly bring about the execution of a half twist, usually long before the cat hits the ground.

As the cat turns right side up, its visual receptors bring the necessary sensory data to the cerebellum for organization of muscle activity in the extensors to bring about a gradual acceptance of the force involved in landing. As the cat lands, the force that flexes the legs invokes the stretch reflex in the extensors. If the cat was an unwilling subject, the muscles of propulsion will already be underway. These principles apply equally well in diving, gymnastics, and all other activities in which balance is a factor.

Voluntary Movement

Let us now take a very simple voluntary movement and analyze the neural activity involved in bringing it about. Assume the right arm is at the side-horizontal position and the desired movement is to bring the right index fingertip to the end of the nose. Since this is not a usual movement, neural activity will probably originate in the arm section of area 4 of the motor cortex and proceed by way of the pyramidal tracts to synapse with the lower motoneuron in the cord and out to the appropriate muscles by way of the brachial plexus. At the same time, kinesthetic impulses traverse the afferent pathways to the cerebellum and bring about the proper control and coordination so that the shoulder muscles are activated to support the arm as it is moved through horizontal flexion adduction.

Furthermore, the same kinesthetic impulses act reflexly at the segmental level to relax the antagonists through reciprocal inhibition. The gamma efferent system is busy all the while innervating the muscle spindles so that constant measurements of the movement's progress can be fed back. As the movement accelerates, more and more motor units are innervated and the rate of impulse transmission to each motor unit increases, with each motor unit participating at the proper time in the sequential development of the movement (1). Finally, the movement has to be decelerated in reverse fashion.

Perception of Effort

Borg (2) developed a scale to rate an individual's perception of the level of exertion under conditions of work, play, or in diagnostic situations—exercise prescriptions and in epidemiological evaluation of daily exercise intensities. This scale, called the "Rating of Perceived Exertion" (RPE), is thought by some to be a valuable indicator of the degree of physical strain, because the RPE integrates various sources of information, including the many signals from the working muscles and joints, from the central cardiovascular and respiratory functions, and from the central nervous system (3).

One of the many interesting questions about perceived exertion is how the brain knows what the muscles are doing. It has been generally believed that kinesthetic information (discussed earlier at the reflex level only) such as joint angle, angular movement, and velocity and force is transmitted by one of the following three methods: 1) *feedforward:* a copy of the motor pattern initiated in the motor cortex is simultaneously transmitted to the sensory cortex; 2) *feedback:* afferent input to the sensory cortex from the peripheral receptors discussed earlier; or 3) a *combination of the feedforward + feedback,* which would allow comparing the movement as executed with the movement as planned and so increase precision of movement.

On the basis of his own interesting studies and the data available in the literature, Cafarelli (5) suggests that both feedforward and feedback elements are employed to evaluate the parameters of any contraction and that the numerical estimate of sensory intensity (RPE) obtained from subjects during running and cycling is also composed of both elements.

Use-Disuse Phenomena in the Nervous System

The effects of overload in bringing about hypertrophy and improved function in muscle is well known. Equally well recognized is the atrophy that accompanies disuse in muscle tissue. Unfortunately the evidence for similar responses in the nervous system has been neglected. As long ago as 1946, it was reported that the degree of activity of a particular neuron type has a great effect on its aging process (37). Destruction of nerve cells that normally stimulate other nerve cells causes premature aging of those cells that now receive fewer impulses. On the other hand the atrophy that accompanies aging is delayed not only by normal but also by such excessive activity (overload) of nerve cells as results in their hypertrophy. These conclusions of Vogt and Vogt are supported by more recent work on rats by Retzlaff and Fontaine (33).

Equally important data from the laboratory of the renowned neurophysiologist J. C. Eccles shows the importance of use and disuse in improving and decreasing synaptic transmission respectively (8). We may conclude that the "Use it or lose it" advice given with respect to muscle probably applies to nervous system function as well.

Does Viscerosomatic Motor Inhibition Limit Exercise?

Since 1967 Ginzel and Eldred have conducted a line of investigation describing a system of reflexes that originates in the heart, lung, and carotid region and when activated results in a generalized, somatic motor inhibition. Both alpha and gamma motoneurons are affected, with tonic motor activity and polysynaptic reflexes being more depressed than phasic activity. The existence of such an elaborate network of viscerosomatic reflexes exerting control over the entire somatic motor system prompted Ginzel and Eldred to propose that these reflexes may function to limit muscular exercise to protect the heart and lungs and other vital organs from excessive demands by an overly active musculature (9, 12).

Practical Considerations

Much of the discussion in this chapter has been technical. However, understanding the foregoing material can be of practical value in physical education and coaching. Examples will now be considered.

Effects of Hypnosis and Emotional Excitement on Performance

It is well known that emotional excitement can greatly increase muscular strength and endurance. Every coach and athlete is aware of the improvement of performance in the game situation from that in practice conditions. On occasion, however, a coach may also see examples of a decrease in performance due to a young, inexperienced athlete becoming overexcited.

Explanations of these phenomena rest upon a knowledge of the neural factors involved (as well as humoral factors, to be discussed later). Gellhorn (11) explains improved performance during emotional excitement in terms of an excitation of the hypothalamus that accompanies excitement. He cites studies that have shown that hypothalamic stimulation (which by itself does not elicit muscular movement) increases the intensity and complexity of a cortically induced movement. Furthermore, many muscles that were not activated by cortical stimulation alone became active, and activity even in other extremities was noted. Gellhorn attributes these effects to summation processes that take place at two sites:

1. In the spinal cord, as the result of the interaction of the subthreshold, extrapyramidal discharges from the hypothalamus, and the efferent discharges from the motor cortex.

2. In the motor cortex itself, due to the intensification of pyramidal discharges as the result of hypothalamic-cortical discharges (11).

This explains both the commonly seen improvement and the less commonly seen decrease in athletic performance, sometimes referred to as *tying up,* due to emotional excitement. The reason for improved performance is obvious from the above. An explanation for tying up, though less obvious, is also at hand. Nervous overflow to other muscles, and even to other extremities, could well be expected to result in innervation of synergistic muscles. In some cases antagonistic muscles will be innervated in a portion of the desired athletic movement. When the latter occurs, the level of performance declines.

Thus, to summarize the effect of emotional excitement on muscular performance, we can say that under normal conditions only some of the available motor units are activated but that this number can be augmented by activity of the hypothalamus due to emotional excitement. If the activity of the hypothalamus and humoral factors, such as an increased level of adrenaline in the muscle tissue, results in an activation of other muscles, some of which are antagonists, tying up and a decline in performance level may result.

Although great feats of strength and endurance have been claimed as the result of hypnotic trance states, demonstrations by competent investigators under controlled laboratory conditions have been less spectacular. Johnson and Kramer (25) were unable to demonstrate significant changes in the strength or power of ten athletes under hypnotic conditions, although muscular endurance improved enormously for one professional athlete.

Roush (34), in a study noted for its large number of subjects (twenty) and rigid criteria of the state of trance, found significant improvements in grip strength, arm strength, and muscular endurance, but Johnson and Kramer's (25) summary of the available research points out that the use of hypnosis to improve muscular strength or endurance is unreliable, even though great improvements have been found in a few persons. It is also Johnson and Kramer's opinion that the beneficial effects, when found, are the result of the neurophysiological mechanisms described in regard to emotional excitement. In any event, hypnosis is certainly not a practice to be indulged in by coaches and physical educators, unless it is supervised or directed by medical or other qualified personnel.

Proprioceptive Neuromuscular Facilitation (PNF)

This is a rationale for improving muscle compliance during stretching exercises by use of a maximal contraction of the muscle to be stretched immediately before the stretch is begun. As Hutton has pointed out (24), however, maximum or near maximum contraction prior to the onset of muscle stretch should exacerbate muscle stiffness rather than increase compliance. This is so because following a tetanic contraction both monosynaptic reflexes and muscle unit responses are potentiated (23), a phenomenon referred to as "post-tetanic-twitch potentiation" or PTP. The effectiveness of PNF for increasing flexibility is debatable and is discussed in detail in chapter 25.

The Dynamogenic Effect of Cocontractions

Hellebrandt, Houtz, and Kirkorian (16), after observing isometric contractions in the unexercised limb during cross-education experiments, postulated that the concurrent contraction of homologous (corresponding) parts (such as right and left arms) might function in augmenting the work output of a tiring or a weakened muscle. Their experiments, as well as the earlier experiments of Karpovich (26), demonstrated that this is indeed the case. When a limb was fatigued ergographically by rhythmic contractions, bringing the other unfatigued limb into synchronous movement resulted in a marked improvement of the work output of the fatigued limb. This phenomenon has much practical significance for corrective physical education and may prove of value in athletics as well.

Reaction Time and Movement Time

Of great interest and importance to all concerned with physical education and athletics is the speed with which an individual can react in a game situation. For example, this factor partly determines how successful a basketball player can be on defense. When the offensive player makes a move, the difference between a slow and a fast reaction by the defensive player (possibly 0.10 second) can result in the offensive player's getting a lead of several additional feet simply because the defensive player must react to the offensive move. In swimming races a difference in reaction to the pistol shot can result in several feet gained or lost. On such slim margins hang the fruits of victory in closely fought contests.

Reaction time is defined, for purposes of physical education, as the interval between presentation of the stimulus and the first sign of response. The measurement is easily made by electronic circuitry, which applies current to an electric timer (chronoscope) at the presentation of the stimulus and cuts the current when the subject's hand is removed from a push-button switch. The stimulus may be visual, audible, or tactile.

Movement time is defined as the interval between the start and the finish of a given movement. The movement may be terminated if it ends in striking an object, or it may be nonterminated if the chronoscope is stopped by interruption of a light beam or similar device that allows follow-through.

An interesting question here concerns the specificity versus the generality of these measures. In other words, if the reaction time is swift for removing a hand from a switch in response to a stimulus, can the motion be expected to be equally swift when performed by a leg on the same or the opposite side? Well-controlled studies by Henry and Rogers (19), Clarke and Glines (7), and Lotter (29) seem to indicate a relatively high degree of specificity by limb and movement. Thus an individual may be quick in reacting with an arm but slow when reacting with the legs.

In regard to gender, adequate data for the college-age group indicates that reaction and movement times are slower in women by approximately 14% and 30%, respectively (18, 19).

Effect of Fatigue

Kroll (28) has shown that total reflex and reflex motor times increase proportionately to the fatigue level assumed to be brought about by bench stepping. Such an effect may be related to the decrement in skilled motor performance known to accompany severe fatigue, such as occurs at the end of a marathon.

Motor Set versus Sensory Set

Set has been defined as the direction of the subject's attention preliminary to an anticipated movement. Thus *motor set* is obtained by directing the subject's attention to the movement response, as in thinking of the starting movement in track. *Sensory set* is the direction of attention to the stimulus, as in concentrating on the gunshot for the start.

It has been the accepted procedure in athletics to use the motor set on the assumption that it results in faster reaction. However, as a consequence of the *memory drum theory,* Henry and Rogers (19) hypothesized that attempts to institute conscious control of movement will interfere with the programming, thus increasing reaction time and resulting in a slower start. Their experiment on college age men and women indicated that both genders react approximately 2.6% slower and move 2.1% slower when using the motor set, compared with the sensory set. It should be pointed out, however, that they found 20% of the subjects had a natural preference for the motor set and that these subjects performed better with the motor set.

Although this phase of performance research cannot yet be considered closed, the evidence weighs in favor of the sensory set, contrary to widespread opinion. More recent research supports these findings (6).

Summary

1. The nervous system may be divided in two ways: (a) structurally, into *central* and *peripheral* components, and (b) functionally, into *somatic* and *autonomic* systems.

2. The basic structural unit of the nervous system is the nerve cell, called the *neuron.* The cell body has two types of processes: *dendrites,* which bring impulses to the cell body, and the *axon,* which conducts nerve impulses away.

3. The *reflex arc,* in its simplest form, is a discharge from a sensory receptor that is transmitted by an *afferent* pathway to a synapse in the spinal cord with a motor neuron, which conducts the *efferent* impulse to an *effector* organ (muscle or gland).

4. Reflexes may occur entirely at one level of the spinal cord (*segmental reflexes*), or they may traverse upward or downward in the cord (*intersegmental reflexes*), or they may be influenced by higher brain centers (*suprasegmental reflexes*).

5. Coordination of movement depends on feedback information of what the muscles are doing. This feedback is called *proprioception* and consists of two types of information: (a) *kinesthetic,* from receptors in the muscles, tendons, and joints, and (b) *vestibular,* from receptors of the nonauditory labyrinths of the inner ear.

6. Muscular control is mediated directly through the large *alpha motor nerve fibers* and indirectly through the smaller *gamma nerve fibers.* The alpha motor nerve fibers and their skeletal muscles, together with the gamma motor nerve fibers and their intrafusal fibers, form an interlocking servomechanism in which each reacts to the other's actions, thus bringing about very fine control of movement.

7. The *pyramidal system* is composed of area 4 of the motor cortex and the nerve fibers emanating therefrom, which descend through the pyramidal tracts to synapse directly or indirectly with the lower motoneuron in the cord. This system is involved mainly in conscious, specific, volitional movement.

8. The *extrapyramidal system* originates mainly in area 6 of the *premotor cortex.* Its descending fibers go to the cord indirectly, by way of various relay stations called *nuclei.* It is involved in general, diffuse motor patterns.

9. The *proprioceptive-cerebellar system,* although it arouses no conscious sensory sensation, is the clearinghouse for sensory data necessary for the coordination of movement patterns, which is mainly accomplished here.

10. *Upright posture* is maintained largely through the operation of *stretch reflexes,* also called *myotatic reflexes.* These reflexes make the minute adjustments in extensor tone that are necessary when extensor muscles start to slacken.

11. The perceived level of exertion as estimated from the Borg RPE is probably the result of both feedforward and feedback to the sensory cortex.

12. The "Use it or lose it" principle that is generally accepted with respect to muscle probably applies equally well to the nervous system.

13. Interesting research suggests the possibility of a negative feedback system in which reflexes from the heart, lung,

and carotid region result in generalized somatic motor inhibition, conceived as a factor that limits muscular exercise to protect the cardiovascular system from overstrain.

14. *Emotional excitement* or *hypnotic suggestion* can lead to an augmentation of the number of motor units participating in a given motor activity and thus improve performance. Both, however, can lead to a decrease in performance levels under certain conditions. For example, an overly emotional or inexperienced athlete can be *tied up* by overexcitement.

15. *Reaction time* and *movement time* appear to be unrelated, and neither is a general quality. That is, quick eye-hand reactions are not necessarily evidence that other reactions in the same individual will be similarly fast.

16. Tests of a hypothesized *memory drum theory* of neuromotor reaction have produced evidence that tends to overthrow older opinions of motor versus sensory set. Evidence indicates that, for most people, a sensory set results in quicker reactions.

References

1. Bigland, B., and Lippold, O. C. J. Motor unit activity in the voluntary contraction of human muscle. *J. Physiol.* 125: 322–35, 1954.

2. Borg, G. A. V. Perceived exertion as an indicator of somatic stress. *Scand. J. Rehab. Med.* 2:92–98, 1970.

3. ———. Psychophysical bases of perceived exertion. *Med. Sci. Sports Exer.* 14:377–81, 1982.

4. Bourne, G. A. *The Structure and Function of Muscle,* vol. 1. New York: Academic Press, 1960.

5. Cafarelli, E. Peripheral contributions to the perception of effort. *Med. Sci. Sports Exer.* 14:382–89, 1982.

6. Christina, R. W. Influence of enforced motor and sensory sets on reaction latency and movement speed. *Res. Q.* 44:483–87, 1973.

7. Clarke, H. H., and Glines, D. Relationships of reaction, movement and completion times to motor strength, anthropometric and maturity measures of thirteen-year-old boys. *Res. Q.* 33:194–201, 1962.

8. Eccles, J. C. *The Neurophysiological Basis of Mind,* pp. 193–216. London: Oxford University Press, 1953.

9. Eldred, E. Peripheral receptors: their excitation and relation to reflex patterns. *Am. J. Phys. Med.* 46:69–87, 1967.

10. Eldred, E., Granit, R., Holmgren, B., and Merton, P.A. Proprioceptive control of muscular contraction and the cerebellum. *J. Physiol.* 123:46–47, 1954.

11. Gellhorn, E. The physiology of the supraspinal mechanisms. *Science and Medicine of Exercise and Sports,* ed. W.R. Johnson, p. 737. New York: Harper & Row, 1960.

12. Ginzel, K. H. Interactions of somatic and autonomic functions in exercise. *Exercise and Sports Sciences Review,* vol. IV, ed. J. Keogh. Santa Barbara: Journal Publishing Affiliates, 1976.

13. Granit, R. Reflex self-regulation of muscle contraction and autogenetic inhibition. *J. Neurophysiol.* 13:351–72, 1950.

14. Granit, R., and Kaada, B. R. The influence of stimulation of central nervous structures in muscle spindles in the cat. *Acta Physiol. Scand.* 27: 130–60, 1952.

15. Hellebrandt, F. A. Cross education: ipsilateral and contralateral effects of unimanual training. *J. Appl. Physiol.* 4:136–44, 1951.

16. Hellebrandt, F. A., Houtz, S. J., and Kirkorian, A. M. Influence of bimanual exercise on unilateral work capacity. *J. Appl. Physiol.* 2:446–52, 1950.

17. Hellebrandt, F. A., Parrish, A. M., and Houtz, S. J. Cross education: the influence of unilateral exercise on the contralateral limb. *Arch. Phys. Med.* 28:76–84, 1947.

18. Henry, F. M. Influence of motor and sensory sets on reaction latency and speed of discrete movements. *Res. Q.* 31:459–68, 1960.

19. Henry, F. M., and Rogers, D. E. Increased response latency for complicated movements and "memory drum" theory of neuromotor reaction. *Res. Q.* 31:448–58, 1960.

20. Holmgren, B., and Merton, P.A. Local feedback control of motoneurons. *J. Physiol.* 123:47–48, 1954.

21. Houk, J., and Henneman, E. Responses of Golgi tendon organs to active contractions of soleus muscle of the cat. *J. Neurophysiol.* 30:466–81, 1967.

22. Hunt, C. C. The effect of stretch receptors from muscle on the discharge of motoneurons. *J. Physiol.* 117:359–79, 1952.

23. Hutton, R. S. Acute plasticity in spinal segmental pathways with use: Implications for training. Paper presented to Kyoto Satellite Symposium, July 26, 1981.

24. Hutton, R. S. Neuromuscular physiology. *Current Therapy in Sports Medicine,* eds. R. P. Welsh and R. J. Shephard, pp. 1–4. Toronto: B. C. Decker, Inc., 1985.

25. Johnson, W. R., and Kramer, G. F. Effects of stereotyped nonhypnotic, hypnotic, and post-hypnotic suggestions upon strength, power and endurance. *Res. Q.* 32:522–29, 1961.

26. Karpovich, P. V. Physiological and psychological dynamogenic factors in exercise. *Arbeitsphysiologie* 9:626, 1937.

27. Katz, B. Depolarization of sensory terminals and the initiation of impulses in the muscle spindle. *J. Physiol.* 111:261–82, 1950.

28. Kroll, W. Fractionated reaction and reflex time before and after fatiguing isotonic exercise. *Med. Sci. Sport.* 6:260–66, 1974.

29. Lotter, W. S. Interrelationships among reaction times and speeds of movement in different limbs. *Res. Q.* 31:147–55, 1960.

30. McCouch, G. P., Deering, I. D., and Stewart, W. B. Inhibition of knee jerk from tendon spindles of crureus. *J. Neurophysiol.* 13:343–50, 1950.

31. Moritani, T., and deVries, H. A. Neural factors vs. hypertrophy in the time course of muscle strength gain. *Am. J. Phys. Med.* 58:115–30, 1979.

32. Mountcastle, V. B. Reflex activity of the spinal cord. *Medical Physiology,* ed. Philip Bard. St. Louis: The C. V. Mosby Company, 1961.

33. Retzlaff, E., and Fontaine, J. Functional and structural changes in motor neurons with age. *Behavior, Aging, and the Nervous System,* eds. A. T. Welford and J. E. Birren. Springfield: Charles C Thomas, 1965.

34. Roush, E. S. Strength and endurance in the waking and hypnotic states. *J. Appl. Physiol.* 3:404–10, 1951.

35. Smith, J. L. Fusimotor loop properties and involvement during voluntary movement. *Exer. Sports Sci. Rev.* 4:297–333, 1977.

36. Taub, E. Movement in nonhuman primates deprived of somatosensory feedback. *Exer. Sports Sci. Rev.* 4:335–74, 1977.

37. Vogt, C., and Vogt, O. Aging of nerve cells. *Nature* 158:304, 1946.

38. Voss, H. Tabelle der absoluten und relativen muskelspindelzahlen der menschlichen skelettmuskulatur. *Anat. Anz.* 129:562–72, 1971.

39. Walters, C. E. The effect of overload on bilateral transfer of motor skill. *Phys. Ther. Rev.* 35:567–69, 1955.

6

The Heart and Exercise

Review of the Cardiac Cycle
Origin and Transmission of the Heartbeat
Pressure Relationships of the Cardiac Cycle

The Cardiac Output
Measurement of Cardiac Output
Control of Heart Rate
Control of Stroke Volume
Importance of the Venous Return

Coronary Circulation and Efficiency of the Heart
Coronary Circulation
Efficiency of the Heart

Factors Affecting the Heart Rate
Age
Gender
Size
Posture
Ingestion of Food
Emotion
Body Temperature
Environmental Factors
Smoking

The Heart Rate during and after Exercise
The Typical Heart Rate Response to Exercise
Response of the Heart Rate to Differences in Exercise

Effects of Athletic Training on the Heart
Heart Rate
Stroke Volume
Heart Size

Training Effects at the Cellular Level

The Cardiac Reserve Capacity

Heart Murmurs

It is the function of the heart and the circulatory system to provide the flow of blood necessary to maintain homeostasis of the various tissues of the body. *Homeostasis* can be defined as the sum total of regulatory functions that maintain a constant environment for the cells of the tissues. The *internal environment,* that is, the tissue fluid, must be held relatively constant in regard to nutrients and metabolites, oxygen and carbon dioxide, temperature and hormonal content. The blood must transport nutrients to the cells, wastes to the kidneys, and so on. The greatest concern in the physiology of exercise, however, is the transport of oxygen and carbon dioxide. During exercise, the supply of oxygen to the tissues is the most urgent tissue need. Oxygen cannot be stored, in any real sense, and its supply or lack of it is usually the critical factor in any endurance exercise. The removal of carbon dioxide is intimately related to the blood's transport of oxygen, as will be seen in a later discussion.

In other words, in the study of exercise physiology we are primarily interested in the heart as the pump in the *cardiorespiratory system* that maintains the proper pressure and flow of blood to active muscle tissues.

Review of the Cardiac Cycle

The salient anatomical features of the heart are reviewed in figure 6.1. Blood flows into the right atrium from the systemic circulation by way of the superior and inferior venae cavae. The thin-walled atrium acts as a combination storage basin and pump primer for blood flow through the tricuspid valve into the right ventricle. The right ventricle provides most of the energy for blood flow through the pulmonary valve and artery into the pulmonary circuit. Blood flows to and through the lungs and back to the heart through the pulmonary veins into the left atrium. Blood flow proceeds from the left atrium, through the mitral valve, and into the left ventricle. Contraction of the left ventricle provides the energy for blood flow through the aortic valve, through the aorta, and through the systemic arterial system to the capillary beds of the various tissues.

From the capillaries, the blood flow returns through veins of ever increasing size to the great veins: the superior and the inferior venae cavae. Thus the circulatory system is comprised of two loops, each with its own pump. The right heart and the pulmonary circuit form one loop, and the left heart and the systemic circuit form the other.

Origin and Transmission of the Heartbeat

The muscle tissue of the heart possesses *autorhythmicity*. It requires no innervation or stimuli from without to produce its regular contractions. Under normal conditions, the wave of excitation originates at the *sinoatrial* (SA) *node;* however, all cardiac tissue has the property of autorhythmicity. If, under abnormal conditions, the rate of emission from the SA node should slow unduly, any area of the myocardium that has a faster inherent rate may assume the role of pacemaker. This is what occurs in abnormal heart rhythms.

Figure 6.2 illustrates the transmission of the wave of excitation from the SA node, by way of the syncytium of muscle fibers in the atrium, to the atrioventricular (AV) node and then into the Purkinje system, which conducts the impulse throughout the ventricular myocardium.

Pressure Relationships of the Cardiac Cycle

Relating the events of the cardiac cycle to each other and placing them in time is best done by

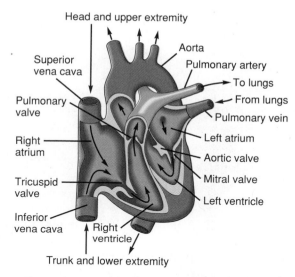

Head and upper extremity

Superior vena cava

Aorta

Pulmonary artery

To lungs

From lungs

Pulmonary valve

Pulmonary vein

Right atrium

Left atrium

Aortic valve

Mitral valve

Tricuspid valve

Left ventricle

Inferior vena cava

Right ventricle

Trunk and lower extremity

Figure 6.1 Details of the functional parts of the heart. (From Guyton, A. C. *Function of the Human Body.* © 1959 W. B. Saunders Company. Courtesy of W. B. Saunders Company, Philadelphia.)

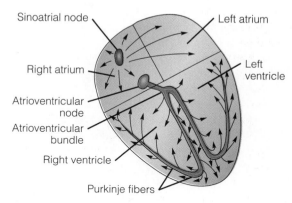

Sinoatrial node

Left atrium

Right atrium

Left ventricle

Atrioventricular node

Atrioventricular bundle

Right ventricle

Purkinje fibers

Figure 6.2 Transmission of the cardiac impulse from the sinoatrial (SA) node into the atria, then into the atrioventricular node, and finally through the Purkinje system to all parts of the ventricles. (From Guyton, A. C. *Function of the Human Body.* © 1959 W. B. Saunders Company. Courtesy of W. B. Saunders Company, Philadelphia.)

considering the *pressure relationships* that are basic to valve action in the heart. It is important to realize from the outset that all valve action is brought about by pressure differentials on the two sides of any given cardiac valve.

The pressure changes in figure 6.3 are recorded along with the events of the electrocardiogram, phonocardiogram (recording of heart sounds), and the heart volume curve. The vertical lines intersect these tracings to indicate events that occur simultaneously. The pressure curves depict the changes in the left heart, but the occurrences in the right heart are similar—though at a considerably lower pressure level.

Table 6.1 represents the events of an average cardiac cycle, under resting conditions, with a rate of seventy-four beats per minute. Under conditions of exercise, which necessitate higher heart rates, the relative durations of the phases of systole and diastole are altered somewhat. The most notable change and the change most important to the physiology of exercise is that the period of *diastasis* is the first to be shortened and may be eliminated completely as the heart rate increases. Because diastasis is the period during which the entire myocardium is at rest, a decrease in resting time at higher heart rates results in losses of efficiency.

The Cardiac Output

The cardiac output is the volume of blood ejected by the heart per unit of time and is usually expressed in liters per minute. At rest, in the average-size man, it is approximately 5 liters per minute, and it can be increased to over 40 liters per minute in a well-trained athlete. The amount of this increase in cardiac output is one important limiting factor in athletic performance. The output of the heart is determined by two factors: the heart rate and the stroke volume (the amount of blood ejected with each beat). Consequently, the cardiac output equals the heart rate times the stroke volume.

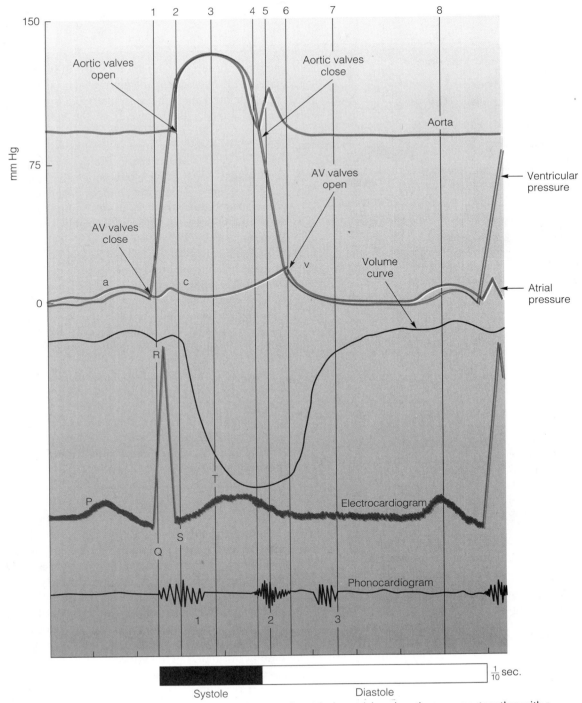

Figure 6.3 The cardiac cycle. Superimposed curves of ventricular, atrial, and aortic pressures, together with a ventricular volume curve, an electrocardiogram, and a phonocardiogram. (From Best, C. H., and Taylor, N. B. *The Physiological Basis of Medical Practice*, 3d ed., 1943. Courtesy of Williams & Wilkins Company, Baltimore.)

Table 6.1   Cardiac Cycle

Line	Nomenclature	Pressure Events	Valve Action	Average Duration
		Systole		
1		Ventricular pressure overcomes atrial pressure	AV valves close	
1–2	Period of isometric contraction (presphygmic)	Ventricular pressure increases	AV valves closed, aortic valve closed	0 05 sec
2		Ventricular pressure overcomes aortic pressure	Aortic valve opens	
2–3	Period of maximal ejection	Ventricular pressure continues to increase	Aortic valve open, AV valves closed	0.12
3–4	Period of reduced ejection	Ventricular pressure decreases	Aortic valve open, AV valves closed	0.14
			Systole Total	0.31 sec
		Diastole		
4–5	Protodiastolic phase	Ventricular pressure drops		0.04 sec
5		Ventricular pressure falls below aortic pressure	Aortic valve closes	
5–6	Isometric relaxation phase (postsphygmic)	Ventricular pressure continues to drop rapidly	Aortic valve closed, AV valves closed	0.08
6		Ventricular pressure falls below atrial pressure	AV valves open	
6–7	Period of rapid filling	Ventricular pressure falls to zero	Aortic valve closed, AV valves open	0.09
7–8	Diastasis—period of slower filling	Atrial and ventricular pressure both low	Aortic valve closed, AV valves open	0.19
8–1	Atrial systole	Increase in both atrial and ventricular pressure due to atrial contraction	Aortic valve closed, AV valves open	0.10
			Diastole Total	0.50 sec
			Total Cardiac Cycle	0.81 sec
			Heart Rate	74

Measurement of Cardiac Output

The most direct method of cardiac output measurement is based on the *Fick principle*. If we know how much O_2 an individual is consuming per unit time and if we also know the concentration of O_2 in the arterial and mixed venous blood, we can calculate the cardiac output as follows:

$$\text{Cardiac output in liters per minute} = \frac{O_2 \text{ consumption in milliliters per minute}}{\text{AV difference in } O_2 \text{ in milliliters per liter of blood}}$$

For example, in a resting subject we find an O_2 consumption of 250 ml/min. Arterial O_2 concentration is 20 volume percent, and mixed venous concentration is 15 volume percent. First we convert the volume percent, which means the volume in milliliters carried by 100 ml of blood, to milliliters per liter (1,000 ml). Thus each liter of arterial blood carries 200 ml of O_2, while the mixed venous blood returns only 150 ml to the heart and the lungs. Therefore we calculate the cardiac output:

$$\text{Cardiac output in liters per minute} = \frac{O_2 \text{ consumption (ml)}}{\text{AV difference in } O_2 \text{ (ml/liters)}}$$

$$= \frac{250}{50} = 5 \text{ liters.}$$

What we are really saying is that if we know the O_2 consumption is at a rate of 250 ml/min and the delivery of O_2 by the blood is such that it requires 1.0 liter blood to deliver 50 ml, then 250 ml requires the service of 5 liters of blood to deliver the 250 ml we know have been consumed. This is simple and direct, but unfortunately the calculation requires the value of O_2 in *mixed* venous blood, and a measure of truly mixed venous blood can only be obtained by catheterization of the right heart. This procedure involves inserting a tube into an arm vein and feeding it through the vein into the right ventricle or pulmonary artery. Although this is a standard hospital procedure for evaluating cardiac patients, it is not often used in exercise physiology.

Noninvasive techniques have been developed that involve the rebreathing of CO_2 and the estimation of mixed venous CO_2 from the rate at which CO_2 approaches a plateau. (The Fick principle is applied just as it was above, but CO_2 values are substituted for O_2 values.) This method is attractive in that no trauma is involved for the subject and it is feasible in the well-equipped exercise physiology laboratory. It is reasonably accurate and reproducible under exercise conditions, but deVries has found the reproducibility under resting conditions to be poor (4).

Control of Heart Rate

The rate of the heartbeat is determined by the frequency of impulse generation at the SA node. The activity of the SA node, in turn, is controlled by other factors, most important of which seems to be the effect of autonomic innervation upon the SA node. The autonomic nervous system supplies both parasympathetic and sympathetic fibers to the SA node. Parasympathetic fibers are supplied by the *vagus nerve* and sympathetic fibers by the *accelerator nerve*. In both cases the innervation arises in the cardioregulatory centers of the medulla.

It has long been known that severing the vagus fibers to the SA node results in an immediate quickening of the heart rate, and thus we know that these fibers are inhibitory and also that they exhibit *tone*—that is, they are chronically active. Further, the accelerator fibers also are constantly active, in the other direction. They have an accelerating effect called *accelerator tone*. Thus the heart rate is precisely adjusted by a balance of activity of the two divisions of the autonomic system.

For the adjustment of the heart rate to be meaningful and to serve the changing needs of the organism, it must reflect the demands of

**Sympathetic innervation
of the heart**

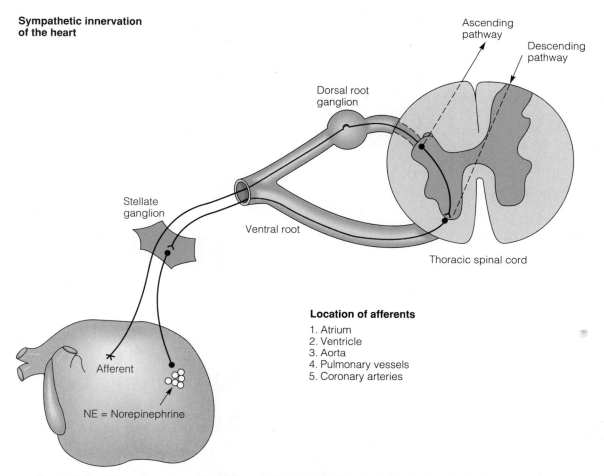

Figure 6.4   Schematic cross section of the spinal cord in the thoracic region showing the pathway taken for afferent and efferent sympathetic fibers. The known locations of sympathetic afferent nerve endings are listed in the figure. (From Stone, H. L., in *Medicine and Science in Sports* 9:253. Copyright © 1977 American College of Sports Medicine. Reprinted by permission.)

changing metabolic activity. To understand how this servomechanism works, we must know the origin of the afferent impulses that form the sensory side of the cardioregulatory reflexes, whose center lies in the medulla. These afferent nervous impulses come from a number of sources. The following impulses increase heart rate.

1. *Proprioceptive impulses* from the working muscles and joints

2. Impulses arising in the chemoreceptors of the *carotid body* and the *aortic body*

3. Impulses arising in the *cerebral cortex*

4. Impulses arising in the heart itself (fig. 6.4)

The sources of depressor afferent stimuli are mainly the *stretch receptors* of the *carotid sinus,* the *aortic arch,* and the heart itself (28) (fig. 6.5).

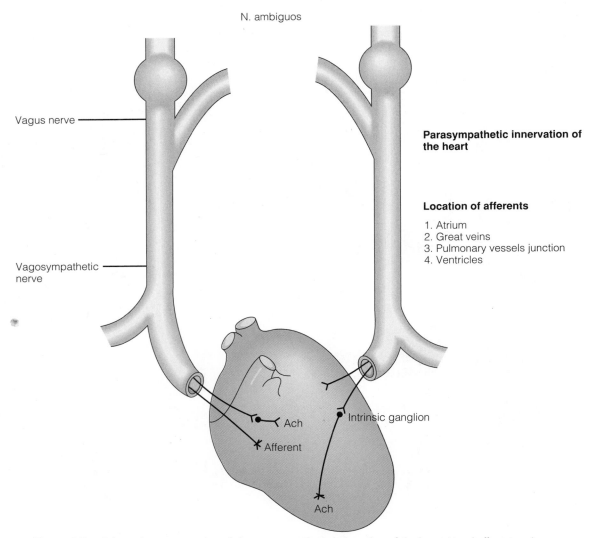

Figure 6.5 Schematic representation of the parasympathetic innervation of the heart. Vagal afferent and efferent fibers course in the vagosympathetic trunk in the cervical region. The cardiac branches leave the main nerve trunk near the heart. The locations of cardiac vagal afferent nerve endings are given in the figure. (From Stone, H. L., in *Medicine and Science in Sports* 9:253. Copyright © 1977 American College of Sports Medicine. Reprinted by permission.)

The effects of the autonomic nervous system in controlling the heart rate in an exercise bout may be summarized in three phases.

1. The anticipatory rise in heart rate, frequently seen before exercise begins, is undoubtedly the result of reflexes that arise in the cerebral cortex due to factors such as anxiety and excitement (1).

2. As exercise begins, stimuli from the working muscles influence the cardioregulatory centers (mainly, they inhibit the cardioinhibitory center), which results in a release from vagal inhibition and consequently produces an increased heart rate (7, 11).

3. As exercise continues beyond thirty or forty seconds, increases in heart rate—if the exercise is demanding—are mainly brought about by increases of tone in the accelerator nerve, and this through stimulation of the chemoreceptors in the carotid and aortic bodies by decreasing pH and increasing concentrations of carbon dioxide.

On the other hand, the frequency of the impulses in the pressure receptors of the carotid sinus and the aortic arch rises with increasing blood pressure and exerts a mitigating influence to prevent too high a rise in blood pressure. The receptors also function in bringing about an increase in heart rate (and blood pressure) when their discharge slows because of decreasing blood pressure, such as occurs in a change of posture from lying to standing.

In addition to the nervous control of the heart rate, at least two other factors are of considerable importance. An increase in adrenal activity also plays a large part in the increased heart rate of the third phase (described above). Both the nervous and the hormonal effects are superimposed, as it were, on the basic effects of body temperature on the heart rate. Increased body temperature results in increases in heart rate, and vice versa, in accordance with the reaction of all metabolic processes to temperature.

Control of Stroke Volume

Until relatively recently, the stroke volume of the heart had been considered a simple and direct function of the end diastolic volume of the ventricle, a conclusion based on the classic work of Frank and Starling. Starling's law of the heart states that the mechanical energy set free on passage from the resting to the contracted state depends on the length of the muscle fibers at the end of diastole. This is in agreement with the length-tension law of skeletal muscle discussed in chapter 4. However, X-ray motion pictures and X-ray kymograms have shown that the end diastolic volume of the heart is not larger in exercise than at rest and may even be smaller (9). Furthermore, whether the results of the Frank and Starling experiments on thoracotomized (open chest) dogs can be extrapolated to normal intact dogs—let alone to intact humans—is open to question (10). Because the classic work was done on heart-lung preparations in dogs, these limitations are serious challenges to its validity. Further research has shed more light on the mechanisms that control the stroke volume of the heart (2, 13, 19, 20).

First of all, there is no reason to challenge Starling's law as a determinant of stroke volume in a heart-lung preparation. Second, there is every reason to believe that a physiological law that can be as elegantly displayed as Starling's law of the heart must have some use for the intact organism. However, the weight of accumulating evidence indicates that although end diastolic volume may be a determining factor under certain conditions (postural changes and gravitational changes), several other factors are probably more important in the adjustments of stroke volume to the demands of exercise.

The stroke volume of the heart seems to be controlled by a physiological interplay of at least four factors:

1. Effective filling pressure
2. Distensibility of the ventricle in diastole
3. Contractility
4. Systemic arterial blood pressure

The first and second items are, in a sense, expressions of Starling's law. The third item needs elaboration. The *contractility* of the heart means its ability to produce force per unit of time or, in other words, power. Randall (19) has summarized the evidence that demonstrates increased contractility as the result of sympathetic stimulation. Under sympathetic stimulation, systolic pressures rise much faster and reach higher levels because of the development of augmented myocardial fiber tension. This means that, in addition to the obvious advantage of a more forceful beat, there is greater time for diastolic filling because systole is completed more rapidly within each cardiac cycle, resulting in even more advantage to the succeeding cycle due to the complete filling. Roskamm (21) has shown clearly that increases in heart rate and contractility are the important factors for humans during heavy exercise.

The importance of the fourth factor, systemic arterial blood pressure, is rather obvious in that the magnitude of this pressure is the resistance against which the blood must be ejected into the aorta. As this resistance grows, the stroke volume must inevitably decrease for any given force of contraction. However, this factor achieves importance only at relatively heavy exercise loads.

To summarize, Starling's law of the heart, while entirely valid in the experimentally controlled heart, is not nearly so important in the physiological control of stroke volume at exercise as was once believed. Furthermore, the law should probably be amended, as suggested by Rushmer (22): ". . . the energy released

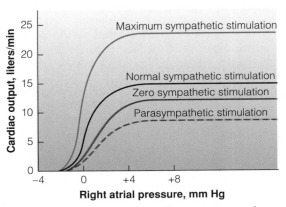

Figure 6.6   Effect on the cardiac output curve of different degrees of sympathetic and parasympathetic stimulation. (From Guyton, A. C. *Textbook of Medical Physiology.* © 1976 W. B. Saunders Company. Courtesy of W. B. Saunders Company, Philadelphia.)

during contraction is related to the initial length of the muscle fibers *under equal states of responsiveness.*"

Starling's law is probably quite important when the venous return is altered due to such changes as those in posture without concomitant changes in innervation or humoral content of the blood. During exercise, then, the most important changes in ventricular performance for providing the needed increase in cardiac output are 1) an accelerated heart rate and 2) an increased contractility due to increased sympathetic stimulation of the ventricular myocardium, which can result in a 100% increase in cardiac output (fig. 6.6).

Importance of the Venous Return

With the accumulating evidence against a greater end diastolic volume during exercise, the need for increased venous return during exercise may be forgotten. It is obvious that the heart cannot eject more blood than it receives. Therefore, although the increase in venous return can no longer be considered the single determining factor in increasing cardiac output, it is nevertheless an important limiting factor in cases where venous return may be curtailed in exercise, as in hot and humid environments. Furthermore, it is undoubtedly the major factor in increasing cardiac output when an erect person lies down; venous return is indeed temporarily increased due to the decreased effect of the force of gravity upon the circulatory system. The reduction of cardiac output in the change from the supine position to the standing position must be explained on a similar basis and will be discussed at greater length in chapter 7.

Coronary Circulation and Efficiency of the Heart

Cardiac output is one of the limiting factors that determines the level at which work output can be maintained because skeletal muscle tissues depend on a constant supply of oxygen from the blood to maintain their metabolic needs. As a consequence, we might suppose that the supply of blood to the heart muscle determines the upper limits of cardiac output and thus indirectly determines the maximum exercise load to be sustained by the skeletal muscles.

This, as it turns out, seems to be very sound reasoning. Arterial blood usually contains approximately 19 ml of oxygen per 100 ml of blood. In mixed venous blood, this may decrease to 12 to 14 ml per 100 ml of blood at rest, thus leaving some room for greater utilization in exercise. In the coronary veins under resting conditions, however, the oxygen content has already decreased to 4 to 6 ml per 100 ml of blood. Thus the oxygen extraction from blood in the coronary vessels is relatively high even at rest and consequently leaves little coronary venous oxygen reserve for the demands of exercise loads. For these reasons, the maximum sustained cardiac output is limited by two factors: the volume of the coronary blood

flow and the efficiency of the heart muscle in performing its work.

Coronary Circulation

Let us discuss first the control of the coronary blood flow and its adjustment to the demands of exercise. It is obvious that the blood flow through the heart is dependent on two factors: 1) the difference in pressure (pressure gradient) between the entering arterial blood and the venous outflow, and 2) the resistance to the flow, which in turn depends on the state of vasoconstriction or vasodilatation of the coronary vessels. The first factor, the pressure gradient, is determined largely by aortic pressure, since the coronary arteries derive from the aortic sinus. The resistance to flow is probably the more important factor of the two. Decreased oxygen tension has been shown to have a very strong dilatory effect upon the coronary vessels.

During exercise several factors tend to increase myocardial O_2 requirements and therefore operate to decrease coronary vascular resistance and thus increase coronary blood flow:

1. Heart rate (tachycardia)
2. Arterial pressure
3. Cardiac output
4. Left ventricular work
5. Myocardial contractility

Experiments on dogs have shown that about one-third of the increment in coronary flow and three-fourths of the decrease in coronary resistance during severe exercise can be accounted for by the tachycardia, unaffected by any other factor (30).

It seems, then, that increased coronary flow during exercise is brought about by at least two factors: 1) the increased arterial blood pressure provides a greater pressure gradient for driving blood through the myocardium, and 2) as the myocardial tissue increases its oxygen consumption, the lowering levels of oxygen result in dilatation of the coronary vessels.

Efficiency of the Heart

Before we enter a discussion of the efficiency of the heart, we must define some terms. *Efficiency,* in general, is the ratio of work production to energy input; thus, in this case:

$$\text{Efficiency} = \frac{\text{Work of the heart}}{\begin{array}{c}\text{Energy input}\\ \text{(in terms of } O_2 \text{ consumption)}\end{array}}$$

The *work of the heart* can be measured, as can any work done by fluid pressure:

$$\text{Work} = \text{Pressure} \times \text{Volume moved}$$

It should be noted here that pressure and volume moved (or flow rate) are independent of each other; that is, an increase in pressure may be associated with an increase, a decrease, or no change at all in flow rate.

A simple law of physics, the law of LaPlace, can also help us understand the cardiac function:

$$\begin{array}{c}\text{Tension (in the}\\ \text{cylinder wall)}\end{array} = \text{Pressure} \times \text{Radius of cylinder}$$

This formula tells us that the tension in the muscle fibers of the myocardium must be proportionately greater as the pressure rises. In other words, the tension required of the heart to move a given volume of blood increases as the arterial blood pressure rises. The formula also tells us that to move the same quantity of blood under equal pressures, the large heart (of greater radius) must exert greater tension than the small heart. Because the energy requirements of the heart are determined largely by the tension demanded of it, this means that a small heart is more efficient than the large heart in working against pressure, other things being equal.

The work of Sarnoff and his associates (23, 24) illustrates the conformance of practice to theory in this regard. Ingeniously devised experiments allowed measurement of the oxygen utilization of the myocardium of dogs when aortic pressure was increased and cardiac output and heart rate were held constant. In these *pressure runs* it was found that a 175% work increase was accompanied by a 178% increase in oxygen consumption. On the other hand, in *flow runs* where the work output was increased 696% through increasing the cardiac output while holding aortic pressure and heart rate constant, an oxygen consumption increase of only 53% was noted. Even this 53% seemed to be accounted for by an inadvertent increase in aortic pressure. Thus a striking difference in cardiac efficiency is seen when the work output of the heart is increased by pressure-load increases compared with volume-load increases.

Another very important observation in this series of experiments was that if the amount of work done by the heart is held constant by holding the cardiac output and the mean aortic pressure constant while increasing the heart rate, the oxygen consumption of the myocardium increases. Consequently, we may say that *high heart rates are less efficient than low rates,* other things being equal.

The researchers concluded that the principal, if not the sole, determinant of myocardial oxygen utilization is the *tension-time index* (mean systolic aortic pressure × duration of systole).

It has been shown that a reasonably valid estimate of the myocardial O_2 consumption (equivalent to work-load stress on the heart muscle) can be made even from the heart rate–blood pressure product using systolic pressure measured with a cuff (14, 15). This is important in any conditioning or testing program involving middle-aged or older adults, since the work of the heart is not always proportional to the work of the total body. Data from deVries's laboratory will be presented in chapter 19 to illustrate this point.

Some practical conclusions can be drawn from the preceding discussion that have large implications for exercise physiology. For any given set of conditions, 1) the heart of a subject with abnormally high blood pressure must work much harder than that of the normal subject; 2) the slower the heart rate for any given work load, the more efficiently the cardiac work is performed.

Factors Affecting the Heart Rate

The heart rate at rest varies widely from individual to individual and also within the same individual from one observation to another under similar circumstances. Therefore, it is almost meaningless to speak of a *normal* heart rate. We may, however, say that the *average* heart rate is 78 beats per minute without implying that a rate of 40 (observed in highly trained endurance athletes) or 100 is necessarily *abnormal*. Although heart rate during the stress of exercise or during the recovery period after exercise is a very valuable source of information for the exercise physiologist, the resting rate is affected by so many variables that it has very little meaning for the prediction of physical performance. Some of the factors that affect the resting rate will now be discussed.

Age

The heart rate at birth is approximately 130 beats per minute, and it slows down with each succeeding year until adolescence. The average rate in a resting adult male in standing position is approximately 78. The maximal attainable heart rate decreases with increasing age in the adult.

Gender

The resting heart rate in adult females averages 5 to 10 beats faster than in adult males under any given set of conditions.

Size

In the animal world in general, it seems to be a biological rule that the heart rate varies inversely with the size of the species. For example, the canary has a rate of approximately 1,000 beats per minute, whereas that of an elephant is about 25 beats per minute. However, no consistent relationship between size and heart rate in adult humans has been demonstrated.

Posture

Posture has a very definite effect upon heart rate. Although the results of different investigators show variances, the typical response to the change from recumbent to standing position seems to be an increase of 10 to 12 beats per minute.

Ingestion of Food

The resting heart rate is higher while digestive processes are in progress than in the postabsorptive state. This is also true in exercise. A given exercise load elicits a greater heart rate after a meal, one of many reasons that militate against heavy exercise immediately after a meal.

Emotion

Emotional stress brings about a cardiovascular response that is quite similar to the response to exercise. An increase in heart rate is the most notable factor and occurs in all but the most experienced athletes as an anticipatory reaction. Dill (5) found a mean increase of 19 beats per minute in the resting rate of teenage boys waiting to be tested in his laboratory. The effect of emotional excitement is most easily observed at rest, but it also occurs during exercise, where it tends to result in an excessive cardiovascular response (1). Under these conditions the response to a standard exercise load may be considerably greater, with the heart rate being elevated by the summation of the stimuli from exercise and from the emotional situation. The recovery period may also be unduly prolonged.

Body Temperature

With increases in body temperature above normal, the heart rate increases. Conversely, with decreases in temperature, the rate slows until a temperature of about 26°C is reached, at which temperature abnormal electrocardiograms are obtained that show danger of heart failure.

Environmental Factors

Ambient temperature is one of the most important factors affecting the heart rate and the total cardiovascular response to exercise. In moderate exercise, an increase of from 10 to 40 beats per minute may occur, depending upon the magnitude of the temperature rise. At rest, small increases in heart rate are seen as temperature increases. However, humidity and air movement also are factors. For any given temperature and work load, the rise in heart rate will be greater if the humidity is high and the air is motionless.

Smoking

It has been found that smoking even one cigarette significantly increases the resting heart rate, in either the sitting or the standing position (26).

The Heart Rate during and after Exercise

The ready availability of the pulse rate as a measure of what transpires internally has resulted in the accumulation of much interesting data that relate various exercise conditions and heart rate. We have pointed out that cardiac output is a determinant of how large an exercise load can be tolerated and that cardiac output is the result of two components: heart rate and stroke volume. Since heart rate is easily measured, it is indeed fortunate that research has shown heart rate to be the more important variable in response to the demands of exercise. The heart rate is more important for at least three reasons:

1. Stroke volume probably increases very little with an increase in metabolism until a level approximately eight times the resting level is reached.
2. Heart rate is proportional to the work load imposed.
3. Heart rate is proportional to the oxygen consumption during an exercise.

All three of these factors hold true only during the steady state, however, when the work is done aerobically.

It is obvious from preceding discussions that the slower the heart rate in response to a given exercise work load, the more efficient is the myocardium—again for at least three reasons:

1. The oxygen consumption of the heart increases with increasing heart rate, even though the work load is held constant (23).
2. As the heart rate increases, the filling time decreases.
3. Diastasis, the only resting period for the myocardium, is disproportionately shortened in faster rates and may disappear entirely at high rates.

All things considered, the rate of the heartbeat furnishes data that quite accurately reflects the degree of stress created by an exercise work load. Conversely, it provides insight into the adequacy of physiological responses to the exercise.

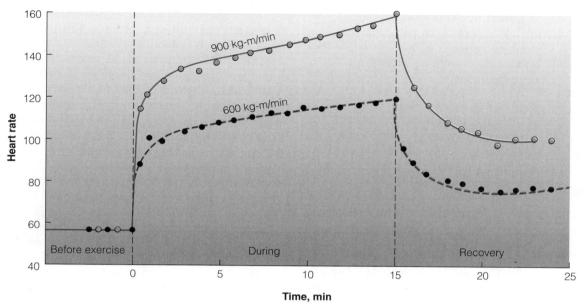

Figure 6.7   Heart rate changes in a moderately conditioned, middle-aged subject at work loads of 600 and 900 kg-m/min on a bicycle ergometer.

The Typical Heart Rate Response to Exercise

As exercise begins, the pulse rate elevates very rapidly. If the exercise is light or moderate, a plateau (leveling off) is seen in thirty to sixty seconds, and this pulse rate is relatively constant until cessation of the exercise. This rate is proportional to the work load of the exercise in any individual. If the work load is heavy (ten or more times the resting metabolic rate), the rate increases until exhaustion (fig. 6.7). For the first two to three minutes after the end of the exercise, the heart rate decreases almost as rapidly as it increased. After this initial decrease, the heart rate declines more slowly at a rate that is roughly related to the intensity and duration of the work.

Response of the Heart Rate to Differences in Exercise

Static versus Dynamic Exercise

In exercises that involve a held position or a straining of the musculature against a heavy load, as in weight lifting, only a very slight increase in heart rate is observed. At the other end of the continuum are exercises that involve rapid and vigorous alternating contractions, such as running and cycling, in which a large increase in heart rate occurs. This difference can be explained on two bases.

1. Venous return may be decreased in the straining exercise due to the increased intrathoracic pressure (chap. 7), and it may be increased in dynamic exercise due to the pumping action of the muscles.

2. The heart rate is proportional to the work load per unit of time, and slow, straining exercises seldom create a work load sufficient to bring about large responses in heart rate.

Intensity of the Exercise

Intensity is the number of foot-pounds (or kilogram-meters) of work per minute expended in an exercise. Since *Work = Force ×*
Distance, in a simple exercise such as bench-stepping the work load and thus the intensity may be increased by increasing the height of the bench, by increasing the rate of stepping, or by increasing both. Both factors would, of course, increase the distance per unit of time. The force could be increased by having the subject carry a weight on the back. Any and all of these factors increase the intensity of the exercise, which is the most important factor in determining the heart rate during exercise.

Duration of the Exercise

If a moderate work load is maintained over a considerable period of time, a secondary increase in heart rate can be observed after the plateau has been attained and held. This can best be explained in terms of fatigue of the skeletal musculature. Larger numbers of motor units are recruited, which results in a greater metabolic demand for the same level of exercise work load and thus an increase in the heart rate. This secondary increase is usually progressive, and continues until exhaustion ends the exercise.

Rest Periods in Discontinuous Exercise

Our discussion has centered on work or exercise that is done continuously. However, because of the advent of interval training methods in track, swimming, and many other sports, a discussion of the importance of rest periods and of their interaction with work load in influencing the stressfulness of the exercise or workout is in order.

For a light work load, a rest period of constant size can result in a return of the heart rate to the prework level after many work sessions. But if the intensity of the work session is increased beyond a certain point, recovery is no longer completed in each successive rest period unless the length of the rest periods is also progressively increased. On the other hand, if the rest interval is held constant and the intensity is increased, a progressively ascending heart rate will be observed during the work or exercise, and exhaustion will result if the work is carried on too long. A coach will, of course, end a workout after sufficient fatigue has occurred in bringing about the desired training effect and before exhaustion ensues.

In industry, on the other hand, where a six- to eight-hour day is involved, the rest periods must be adequate to prevent a progressive heart rate increase, or the intensity of the work must be decreased. In general, then, the stress of a day's work, or of an interval of a training and conditioning program, is the result of an interaction of two components: 1) total work done and 2) total amount of rest periods. The final recovery of the heart rate will be the result of these two components.

Heart Rate as a Measure of Stress

It is frequently desirable to evaluate the degree of stress imposed upon an individual's cardiovascular system by work loads in athletics and in industry. This is particularly important where the total load is increased by unfavorable environmental conditions, such as high ambient temperatures (chap. 28). Again, observation of the heart rate response to the work load provides the easiest and quickest evaluation.

Use of the cardiac cost concept provides reasonably valid information on the total stress an individual's cardiovascular system is subjected to under conditions in which the stress of exercise is complicated by the summation of the exercise stress and the stress imposed by the environment.

Cardiac cost = Total heartbeats during exercise minus resting rate for the same period of time

Recovery cost = Heartbeats between end of exercise and return to resting minus resting rate for the recovery period

Total cardiac cost = Cardiac cost during exercise plus cardiac cost during recovery

Effects of Athletic Training on the Heart

Heart Rate

As the result of training, the resting heart rate decreases as well as the heart rate for any given work load. Stated another way, other things being equal, the trained individual has a lower heart rate for any given work load. The slower resting heart rate appears to be the result of a reduction in intrinsic heart rate (the rate resulting when neural influences are blocked) (12), whereas the slower exercise rate is more likely due to a decreased sympathetic drive (8).

Stroke Volume

A preponderance of evidence indicates that the increased maximum cardiac output in athletes is due largely to an increase in stroke volume. This is not to say that the immediate adjustment to exercise, which was discussed earlier, is the result of an increased stroke volume. Rather, the stroke volume increase seems to be a long-term effect of training and is also manifest in the slower resting rate of the endurance-trained athlete. This greater stroke volume is the result of the greater contractility of the ventricle in the heart of the trained athlete (2, 21, 25, 29).

Heart Size

The effect of exercise on the heart in animals is well established. Many investigators have found that heavy exercise results in increases in the weight of the heart in different species. In recent years echocardiography (use of ultrasound to record the size, motion, and composition of cardiac structure) has provided information on the human heart. Investigators seem to agree that, in general, sports requiring dynamic endurance effort (such as running, skiing, swimming, and cycling) tend to produce left ventricular dilatation without marked left ventricular hypertrophy, whereas activities requiring heavy isometric effort (such as wrestling, weight lifting, and so on) increase left ventricular wall thickness and mass (3, 18, 31).

Training Effects at the Cellular Level

In chapter 3 we discussed the large and significant cellular adaptations that occur in skeletal muscle in response to endurance training. It would be reasonable to expect similar adaptations in the myocardium. While direct observations of cellular change in the skeletal muscles of humans have been made possible by the muscle biopsy technique, we must rely on extrapolation from animal experiments for information on myocardial adaptations.

Surprisingly, Oscai and coworkers have shown that in rats the heart does not appear to undergo any adaptive increase in cellular respiratory capacity in response to endurance exercise (16, 17). They found the levels of activity of various representative mitochondrial enzymes and the concentrations of cytochrome c and of mitochondrial protein to be unchanged in trained rats. More recent work on dogs has supported their work (27), so it appears unlikely that training adaptations in the human heart can be explained on this basis.

Since the heart muscle in the human, as in the animal preparations, shows large improvements in contractility with endurance training, we might expect some improvement in myofibrillar ATPase activity to accompany the training regimen, but three groups of investigators have shown that this is also not the case (6, 27, 29). At the present time the best available evidence suggests that the improved contractile function of the heart in response to endurance training lies in subtle changes in the mechanisms of calcium transport into and out of the sarcoplasmic reticulum (27, 29). See chapter 3 for the importance of calcium in initiating muscle contraction.

The Cardiac Reserve Capacity

Vigorous physical exercise provides the greatest challenge to the cardiovascular system. In the normal individual, only the increased metabolic demand of strenuous work loads can raise the output of the heart to its maximum values. Let us now consider the mechanisms available to the heart in its adjustment to supply the oxygen needs of exercised muscle tissue. It is convenient to think of these mechanisms, in total, as the *cardiac reserve*.

The first and probably the most important factor is the *reserve of heart rate*. In exercise, the rate can increase from its resting value of 70 to 80 beats per minute to a rate of 170 to 180 beats per minute. Although the heart rate can exceed these values, cardiac output will not be improved above approximately 180 because stroke volume will decrease as a result of the decreased diastolic filling times. Thus the cardiac output can be increased 2 to 2½ times by increases in heart rate.

The second factor is the *stroke volume reserve*. As was mentioned before, this factor probably comes into play only at a very high level of exertion. However, at very high levels of oxygen consumption, the heart has

two means by which stroke volume can be increased:

1. By reducing the blood volume remaining at the end of systole, a more complete ejection as the result of greater contractility.
2. By increasing the diastolic filling as the result of a greater effective filling pressure and possibly a more distensible ventricle.

The third factor is the possibility for *increased oxygen utilization* by the active muscle tissues. At rest, the arterial oxygen level supplied to the muscles is approximately 19 ml per 100 ml of blood, while the venous blood may have 13 to 14 ml per 100 ml of blood with a consequent utilization of 5 to 6 ml per 100 ml of blood supplied. However, when the muscle is exercising strenuously, 16 to 17 ml of oxygen per 100 ml of blood may be extracted, which results in a much larger arteriovenous oxygen difference—mainly at the expense of a lowered venous oxygen content in the blood flow from the active muscles.

Heart Murmurs

A heart murmur is the sound created by turbulent blood flow. The degree of turbulence necessary to create vibrations that can be heard is determined in the cardiovascular system by the velocity of blood flow and by the amount of eddy currents caused by obstructions, restrictions, and so on. Because the flow within the vascular system is normally streamlined (or laminar) and not turbulent, ordinarily no murmurs are heard. However, the velocity of flow in the roots of the aorta and in the pulmonary artery is sufficient to create murmurs during the rapid ejection phase of systole. These normal sounds, when they are heard or recorded, are termed *functional murmurs* and have no pathological significance.

On the other hand, cardiac valves are frequently damaged by disease, and the murmurs caused by regurgitation of blood through an insufficient valve or by the increased velocity due to a damaged valve (which creates a restriction in the orifice) are valuable diagnostic signs to the physician. The physical educator should at least understand the significance of these murmurs.

The significance of murmurs that result from valvular insufficiency is that in pumping a given volume of blood to the tissues to meet metabolic demands the heart must, in a sense, pump the blood that regurgitated twice. This results in a greater-than-normal *volume load* on the heart, and it responds by increasing its stroke volume through an increase in size (and probably by hypertrophy). In doing this, however, a portion of the cardiac reserve is lost because greater tension is required in the myocardial wall to maintain a given blood pressure in the systemic arteries, according to the law of LaPlace. As our discussion of the tension-time index indicated, oxygen consumption rises with tension. So it is apparent that the heart is now less efficient. This decreased efficiency may be so slight in some cases as to be a limiting factor only in very strenuous exercise, but in other cases it may severely limit the exercise tolerance.

In a murmur caused by a valvular restriction, the result is an increased *pressure load,* to which the heart responds by hypertrophy of the ventricular walls. Again, tension in the wall of the myocardium increases even more and efficiency consequently decreases. Obviously, individuals with heart murmurs who wish to participate in strenuous exercise or athletics should consult a physician. Present-day physicians and cardiologists recognize the advantages that accrue from exercise programs commensurate to the needs of individuals and their limitations. Both professions would be immeasurably helped in their efforts to attain a corrective physical education program if the physical educator and the physician were able to communicate, in quantitative terms, on exercise work loads. These terms might be kilogram meters per minute of work, liters of oxygen per minute, or the number of times the work load demand is greater than the resting metabolic demand. We will discuss this further in the second section of this text.

Summary

1. The heart and the vascular system maintain *homeostasis* of the various tissues of the body. Most important to the physical educator is an understanding of oxygen and carbon dioxide transport to and from the skeletal muscles.

2. Although the nervous impulse that stimulates the heart to beat originates within the myocardium, the rate is controlled to a large extent by a balance of the effects of the parasympathetic and sympathetic divisions of the autonomic system, acting through the *vagus* and *accelerator nerves,* respectively.

3. All cardiac valve action is the result of differences in pressure on the two sides of each valve. The cardiac cycle can best be understood in light of the pressure changes that occur in the heart.

4. One of the most important factors that limits human physical performance is the ability to increase cardiac output. Cardiac output = Heart rate × Stroke volume. Consequently, the cardiac output can be increased by an increase in rate, or stroke volume, or both.

5. The rise in heart rate with exercise seems to occur in three phases: (a) a preexercise, anticipatory rise due to cortical activity, (b) an early rise due largely to inhibition of vagal activity, and (c) a later rise that is probably the result of a combination of accelerator

nerve activity and increased adrenal activity.

6. Starling's law undoubtedly operates under all conditions, but it is the principal determinant of stroke volume only in changes of posture and other manifestations of gravitational changes. Under conditions of exercise, stroke volume is more likely determined by an interplay of the following factors: (a) effective filling pressure, (b) the distensibility of the ventricle in diastole, (c) contractility, and (d) the systemic arterial blood pressure.

7. Coronary blood flow is the limiting factor in cardiac output responses, and thus it indirectly sets the upper limit of exercise tolerance. Probably the most important factors that affect the increased coronary flow necessary for exercise conditions are (a) increased arterial blood pressure and (b) lowering levels of oxygen in the myocardium to bring about vasodilatation of the coronary vessels.

8. Many extrinsic factors affect the resting heart rate and, in many cases, the rate during exercise. All of the following factors must be considered in observing the effects of exercise upon heart rate: age, gender, size, posture, ingestion of food, emotion, body temperature, environmental factors, and smoking.

9. The heart rate responds to light or moderate exercise loads with a rapid increase to a plateau, at which the rate is proportional, in any individual, to the work load and to the oxygen consumption. In very heavy exercise, the rate continues to increase without leveling off until exhaustion ends the work bout. After exercise ends, the return to normal is very rapid for the first two to three minutes, then slows considerably to a rate of decrease that is roughly related to the intensity and duration of the exercise.

10. The heart rate responds differently to different types of exercise. In general, dynamic muscular activity brings about a much greater increase in heart rate than static, straining types of exercise. Increases in heart rate vary directly with the intensity and duration of the exercise and inversely with the number of rest periods in a long, continued work bout.

11. *Cardiac cost* has been proposed as a method for evaluating the stress imposed upon the cardiovascular system by a combination of exercise and environmental stress. Total cardiac cost includes the increase in heart rate during the work bout and the increase during recovery.

12. Athletic training brings about a complex of changes in heart rate, stroke volume, and other factors, all of which together interact to bring about a more effective and efficient adjustment of the organism to the increased metabolic demands of exercise. There seems to be no evidence that indicates a normal heart is harmed by the stress of exercise.

13. Although important training effects on the cellular respiratory capacity have been shown for skeletal muscle (chap. 3), this is not the case for heart muscle. The improved contractility of heart muscle in endurance training appears to be the result of better calcium transport in the sarcoplasmic reticulum.

14. The *cardiac reserve* for conditions of strenuous exercise is the result of three factors: (a) increase in heart rate, (b) increase in stroke volume, and (c) increased oxygen utilization of the active muscle tissues.

15. Heart murmurs are heart sounds that are brought about by increased turbulence in the blood flow through the heart or large vessels. This increased turbulence can be the result of increased velocity or of increased eddy currents in the blood flow. In some cases the velocity reaches the critical value without the existence of an abnormality, and the murmur is said to be *functional*. Heart murmurs are usually brought about by a valvular insufficiency that allows regurgitation of blood through a small opening at high velocity, or by restriction of a valvular orifice as a result of disease. Exercise or athletic participation under these conditions should be evaluated and controlled by the individual's physician.

References

1. Antel, J., and Cumming, G. R. Effect of emotional stimulation on exercise heart rate. *Res. Q.* 40:6–10, 1969.

2. Asmussen, E., and Nielsen, M. Cardiac output during muscular work and its regulation. *Physiol. Rev.* 35:778–800, 1955.

3. Cantwell, J. D. New concepts in sports medicine: A cardiologist's perspective. *Physician and Sportsmed.* 11 (June):162–63, 1983.

4. deVries, H. A. Physiological effects of an exercise training regimen upon men aged 52–88. *J. Geront.* 25:325–36, 1970.

5. Dill, D. B. Regulation of the heart rate. *Work and the Heart,* eds. F. F. Rosenbaum and E. L. Belknap. New York: Paul B. Hoeber, Inc., 1959.

6. Dowell, R. T., Stone, H. L., Sordahl, L. A., and Asimakis, G. K. Contractile function and myofibrillar ATPase activity in the exercise-trained dog heart. *J. Appl. Physiol.* 43:977–82, 1977.

7. Fagraeus, L., and Linnarsson, D. Autonomic origin of heart rate fluctuations at the onset of muscular exercise. *J. Appl. Physiol.* 40:679–82, 1976.

8. Frick, M. H., Elovainio, R. O., and Somer, T. The mechanism of bradycardia evoked by physical training. *Cardiologia* 51:46–54, 1967.

9. Gauer, O. H. Volume changes of the left ventricle during blood pooling and exercise in the intact animal: their effects on left ventricular performance. *Physiol. Rev.* 35:143–55, 1955.

10. Gregg, D. E., Sabiston, D. C., and Thielen, E. O. Performance of the heart: changes in left ventricular end-diastolic pressure and stroke work during infusion and following exercise. *Physiol. Rev.* 35:130–36, 1955.

11. Hollander, A. P., and Bouman, L. N. Cardiac acceleration in man elicited by a muscle-heart reflex. *J. Appl. Physiol.* 38:272–78, 1975.

12. Katona, P. G., McLean, M., Dighton, D. H., and Guz, A. Sympathetic and parasympathetic cardiac control in athletes and non-athletes at rest. *J. Appl. Physiol.* 52:1652–57, 1982.

13. Katz, L. N. Analysis of the several factors regulating the performance of the heart. *Physiol. Rev.* 35:91–106, 1955.

14. Kemp, G. L., Ellestad, M. H., Beland, A. J., and Allen, W. H. The maximal treadmill stress test for the evaluation of medical and surgical treatment of coronary insufficiency. *J. Thorac. Cardiovasc. Surg.* 57:708–13, 1969.

15. Kitamura, K., Jorgensen, C. R., Gobel, F. L., Taylor, H. L., and Wang, Y. Hemodynamic correlates of myocardial oxygen consumption during upright exercise. *J. Appl. Physiol.* 32:516–22, 1972.

16. Oscai, L. B., Mole, P. A., Brei, B., and Holloszy, J. O. Cardiac growth and respiratory enzyme levels in male rats subjected to a running program. *Am. J. Physiol.* 220:1238–41, 1971.

17. Oscai, L. B., Mole, P. A., and Holloszy, J. O. Effects of exercise on cardiac weight and mitochondria in male and female rats. *Am. J. Physiol.* 220: 1944–48, 1971.

18. Peronnet, F., Ferguson, R. J., Perrault, H., Ricci, G., and Lajoie, D. Echocardiography and the athlete's heart. *Physician and Sportsmed.* 9 (May):103–12, 1981.

19. Randall, W. C. Sympathetic control of the heart-peripheral mechanisms. *Cardiovascular Functions,* ed. A. A. Luisada. New York: McGraw-Hill Book Co., 1962.

20. Richards, D. Discussion of Starling's law of the heart. *Physiol. Rev.* 35: 156–60, 1955.

21. Roskamm, H. Myocardial contractility during exercise. *Limiting Factors of Human Performance,* ed. J. Keul. Stuttgart: Georg Thieme, 1973.

22. Rushmer, R. F. Applicability of Starling's law of the heart to intact, unanesthetized animals. *Physiol. Rev.* 35:138–42, 1955.

23. Sarnoff, S. J., and Braunwald, E. Hemodynamic determinants of myocardial oxygen consumption. *Cardiovascular Functions,* ed. A. A. Luisada. New York: McGraw-Hill Book Co., 1962.

24. Sarnoff, S. J., Braunwald, E., Welch, G. H., Stainsby, W. N., Case, R. B., and Macruz, R. Oxygen consumption of the heart, with special reference to the tension-time index. *Work and the Heart,* eds. F. F. Rosenbaum and E. L. Belknap. New York: Paul B. Hoeber, Inc., 1959.

25. Scheuer, J. The advantages and disadvantages of the isolated perfused working rat heart. *Med. Sci. Sports* 9:231–38, 1977.

26. Schilpp, R. W. A mathematical description of the heart rate curve of response to exercise, with some observations on the effects of smoking. *Res. Q.* 22:439–45, 1951.

27. Sordahl, L. A., Asimakis, G. K., Dowell, R. T., and Stone, H. L. Functions of selected biochemical systems from the exercise-trained dog heart. *J. Appl. Physiol.* 42:426–31, 1977.

28. Stone, H. L. The unanesthetized instrumented animal preparation. *Med. Sci. Sports* 9:253–61, 1977.

29. Tibbits, G., Koziol, B. J., Roberts, N. K., Baldwin, K. M., and Barnard, R. J. Adaptation of the rat myocardium to endurance training. *J. Appl. Physiol.* 44:85–89, 1978.

30. Vatner, S. F., Higgins, C. B., Franklin, D., and Braunwald, E. Role of tachycardia in mediating the coronary hemodynamic response to severe exercise. *J. Appl. Physiol.* 32:380–85, 1972.

31. Wolfe, L. A., Cunningham, D. A., Rechnitzer, P. A., and Nichol, P. M. Effects of endurance training on left ventricular dimensions in healthy men. *J. Appl. Physiol.* 47:207–12, 1979.

7

The Circulatory System and Exercise

Hemodynamics: Principles Governing
  Blood Flow
  Pressure Gradient
  Velocity of Blood Flow
  Resistance to Flow
  Poiseuille's Law
  Hydrostatic Pressure
The Microcirculation: Blood Flow
  through the Capillary Bed
Control of Blood Distribution
  Nervous Regulation
  Chemical Regulation
Blood Distribution in Rest and Exercise
Blood Pressure
  Measurement of Blood Pressure
  Maintenance of Arterial Blood
    Pressure
  Maintenance of Venous Return to the
    Heart

Arterial Blood Pressure during Exercise
  Type of Exercise
Blood Flow in Exercising Muscles
Blood and Fluid Changes during Exercise
  Hemoconcentration
  Erythrocyte Count
Blood and Fluid Changes from Training
  Blood Volume
  Hemoglobin
  Sports Anemia
  Alkaline Reserve
  Postural Effects on Circulation
  Cooling Down after Heavy Exercise

From the standpoint of exercise physiology, blood is primarily a tissue of respiration. Its importance lies in its ability to transport the respiratory gasses, oxygen and carbon dioxide, between the respiratory organs and the active tissues. Although blood serves many other very important general physiological functions, this transport of oxygen and carbon dioxide may become a limiting factor in physical performance and consequently assumes major importance.

It is tempting to liken the blood flow through the vascular system to the flow of water through a plumbing system. This is a very poor analogy, however, because the pipes in a plumbing system serve only *passively* as conduits for the transport of fluids, whereas the blood vessels are *active* participants in the adjustments made by the circulatory system for the demands of exercise. For example, a person can increase oxygen intake and energy output to twenty times the basal rate, but the increase of energy output by the *active muscles* can be as much as fifty times the resting rate. This difference, of course, is made possible by a redistribution of blood (and thus oxygen) by the vascular system through a vasoconstriction in inactive tissues and a vasodilatation of the active muscle tissues.

Hemodynamics: Principles Governing Blood Flow

Pressure Gradient

Blood flows through the vessels of the circulatory system because of differences in pressure. It flows from a point of high pressure to a point of lower pressure, and the difference in pressure between the two points is called a *pressure gradient*. In the systemic circulatory system, the point of highest pressure is within the left ventricle of the heart during systole. The pressure gradient between this point and the lowest pressure point, which is in the right atrium, is the driving force that brings about blood flow through the entire systemic circulation (although this is aided by the muscle pump, to be discussed below). An analogous situation exists in the pulmonary circulation.

Velocity of Blood Flow

The combination of systemic circulation and pulmonary circulation may be thought of as the two loops of a figure eight (fig. 7.1). The two loops are interconnected in series, and each has its own pressure gradient, provided by its side of the cardiac pump. It is apparent that this is a closed, single circuit—although possessed of two pressure gradients in series—and it follows that the *same volume* of blood must pass *each* and *any point* in the system per unit time (if we assume that no retention of blood occurs at any point). This being so, the *velocity of blood flow* past any point obviously depends on the total cross-sectional area of the vascular bed at that point. Where the area is smaller, the velocity must be higher, and vice versa (fig. 7.2).

The aorta has a cross-sectional area of approximately 2.5 to 5.0 cm^2. As the large arteries bifurcate, the combined area of the branches considerably exceeds the area of the parent vessel. As this branching of the arterial system progresses, the total cross-sectional area of the circulatory system constantly increases, and consequently the velocity of flow decreases proportionately. In the capillary bed, where each vessel is only 10μ (1/100 of a millimeter) in diameter, this multiplication has progressed to such an extent that the combined cross-sectional area of all capillaries is about 700 to 800 times the area of the aorta. This means that the flow rate or velocity has

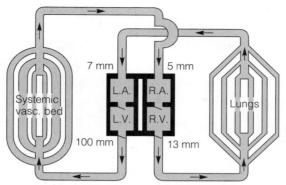

Figure 7.1   Interrelationships of systemic and pulmonary circulations and their pressure gradients.

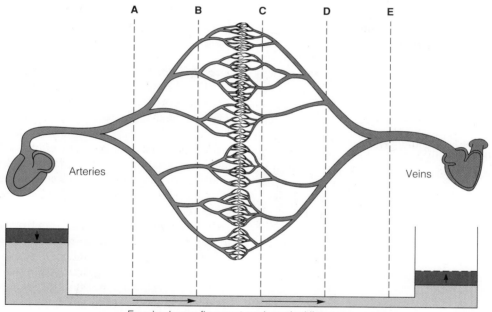

Equal volumes flow past each vertical line

Figure 7.2   Arborization of the systemic circulatory system is schematically represented with all vessels of the same caliber arranged vertically. This simplified illustration emphasizes the fact that the volume of fluid flowing past each vertical line in a unit of time must be equal to the quantity entering and leaving the system, just as in a single tube. (From Rushmer, R. F. *Cardiovascular Dynamics,* 2d ed. © 1961 W. B. Saunders Company. Courtesy of W. B. Saunders Company, Philadelphia.)

decreased in proportion. The result is a very slow flow of 0.5 to 1.0 mm/second through the capillaries, thus allowing adequate time for the exchange of respiratory gasses, nutrients, and so on.

Resistance to Flow

Resistance may be thought of as the sum of the forces opposing blood flow and may be illustrated by breathing through various sizes and lengths of glass tubing. It is readily seen that exhaling becomes progressively more difficult as the length of the tube is *increased;* it also becomes more difficult as the diameter of the tube is *decreased.* Another factor, the *viscosity* of the fluid, is also important. Other things being equal, the more viscous the fluid, the greater the resistance to its flow. For example, the flow of molasses is much slower than the flow of water.

Poiseuille's Law

If we make the simplifying assumption that the walls of the blood vessels are rigid, we can state the relationships discussed above as follows:

$$\text{Volume of blood flow} = \frac{\text{Pressure gradient}}{\text{Resistance}}$$

This can also be stated:

$$\text{Resistance} = \frac{\text{Pressure gradient}}{\text{Volume of blood flow}}$$

$$\text{Pressure gradient} = \text{Volume of blood flow} \times \text{Resistance}$$

A theoretically derived mathematical law that expresses all these relationships is frequently used by physiologists. This is Poiseuille's law (fig. 7.3), an approximation of which, in simplified form, can be stated as follows:

$$\text{Volume of blood flow} = \frac{\text{Pressure} \times (\text{Vessel radius})^4}{\text{Vessel length} \times \text{Viscosity}}$$

Hydrostatic Pressure

When one dives to the bottom of a swimming pool, one feels an increase in pressure on the ears. This increased pressure is *hydrostatic pressure,* and it increases with depth. It is also present in any vertical tube that contains a liquid because the weight of the liquid increases with increasing height (fig. 7.3). This principle is also applied when we *weigh* the atmospheric air by balancing it against a column of mercury to obtain barometric pressure. It is important to remember the effect of hydrostatic pressure in physiology because changes in body position alter the blood pressure in various parts of the body. Thus, when blood pressure is taken by a physician, it is taken at the level of the heart. Finding the blood pressure at any other level of the body requires correction for the hydrostatic pressure effect.

For example, in an individual whose mean blood pressure is 90 mm mercury (Hg) at heart level, we should expect to find a decrease of pressure of 30 cm of blood at the ear level. Converting 30 cm of blood to millimeters of mercury (1 mm Hg = 13.6 mm blood), we would expect a mean blood pressure at the ear of approximately 90 − 22 = 68 mm Hg. Conversely, at the ankle (in complete rest)—assuming a measurement of 125 cm from ankle to heart level in standing position (and neglecting such factors as frictional losses)—we should expect to find an increased pressure of some 125 × 10/13.6, or 90 + 92 = 182 mm Hg blood pressure at the ankle. These figures correspond closely to the pressures found experimentally (15).

The Microcirculation: Blood Flow through the Capillary Bed

The work of Zweifach (43, 44, 45) and Zweifach and Metz (46) has resulted in a better understanding of the capillary bed and allows

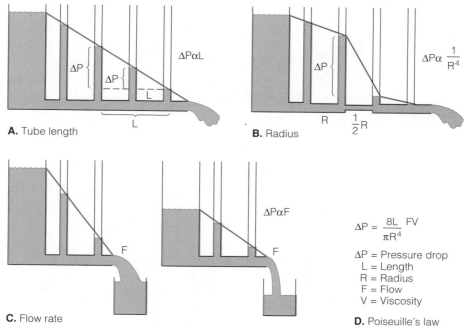

Figure 7.3   **A.** The drop in pressure (ΔP) during laminar flow of a homogeneous fluid through a rigid tube of constant caliber is directly proportional to the length of the tube. **B.** Under the same conditions, the pressure drop is also inversely proportional to the reciprocal of the radius to the fourth power ($1/R^4$) and directly proportional to the volume flow (F) through the tube and to the viscosity (V) of the fluid. (From Rushmer, R. F. *Cardiovascular Dynamics*, 2d ed. © 1961 W. B. Saunders Company. Courtesy of W. B. Saunders Company, Philadelphia.)

much better rationalization of the important circulatory changes that occur in muscle tissue during exercise.

The microcirculation is a well-organized network in which the arterioles give rise to *metarterioles* (fig. 7.4), which possess a gradually dispersing, thin muscular coat. These metarterioles constitute major thoroughfares, or *preferential channels,* through the tissue, and they remain open even during resting conditions. Eventually they join a collecting venule. The *true capillaries* are endothelial tubes, with no smooth muscle, which arise from the metarterioles by way of a *precapillary sphincter* that closes down the true capillaries during resting conditions and relaxes during muscle activity to allow the increased circulation demanded by the higher metabolic rate.

There is a third alternative route for blood flow through the microcirculation, by way of *arteriovenous anastomoses* (AVA) that form a short and direct connection between 1) small arteries and small veins, 2) arterioles and venules, and 3) metarterioles and adjacent venules. These AVA have a well-developed muscular coat and are under sympathetic nervous control. They seem to be most common in the extremities, and they function in bringing about greater losses of heat when environmental temperature rises or when heat is produced within, as during exercise. This loss of heat is brought about because the opening of the AVA causes a greater amount of blood to flow through the venous collection system, which is closer to the surface than the arteries

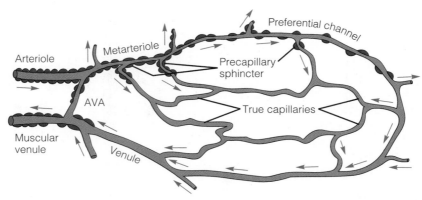

Figure 7.4   A schematic representation of the structural pattern of the capillary bed. The distribution of smooth muscle is indicated in the vessel wall. (From Zweifach, B. W. "Basic Mechanisms in Peripheral Vascular Homeostasis," in *Proceedings of Third Conference on Factors Regulating Blood Pressure,* 1950. Courtesy of Josiah Macy, Jr., Foundation, New York.)

and arterioles and thus provides greater heat losses.

We can think of the functions of the peripheral blood vessels as four-fold:

1. Maintenance of blood pressure by the arteries and arterioles.

2. Distribution of blood flow to the active tissues by the interaction of metarterioles and the precapillary sphincters in determining how much flow goes through the thoroughfare (preferential) channels and how much through the true capillaries.

3. Temperature control, largely by heat loss controlled through the AVA.

4. The return of blood to the heart, by way of the muscular venules to the small veins, and so on.

Various tissues have smaller or larger ranges of metabolic activity. Muscle tissue has the greatest range, from the resting state to forty or fifty times the resting level of energy metabolism. Apparently for this reason, the ratio of true capillaries to thoroughfare channels also varies considerably from tissue to tissue. Zweifach has estimated the ratio in skeletal muscle as eight or ten to one, whereas in tissues with less metabolic activity this ratio may be as low as two or three to one.

Control of Blood Distribution

Control of the flow of blood to the various tissues of the systemic circulation is brought about by changes in the diameter of the small arteries and arterioles. The effectiveness of change in the bore of these vessels is seen by referring to Poiseuille's law. If the diameter of a small vessel is doubled, the amount of blood flow will not be doubled, but will be increased sixteen times because the flow varies as the fourth power of vessel radius. These changes in diameter are brought about by two mechanisms: *nervous regulation* and *chemical regulation.* Since the main function of the small arteries and arterioles is to control by their degree of constriction the resistance to flow, they are properly referred to as the *resistance vessels.* The veins are thin-walled but nevertheless also have smooth muscle in their walls, and thus can also actively change their diameters. Changes in their wall tension do not have any great effect on resistance to flow, but they are very important in altering the *capacity* of the postcapillary system. Thus they are important in determining the rate of return flow to the heart and may be referred to as *capacity vessels*.

Nervous Regulation

So far as we know, all of the nervous regulation of blood flow to the skeletal muscles is brought about by the sympathetic system. However, this system supplies two types of fibers: 1) *adrenergic,* which bring about vasoconstriction, and 2) *cholinergic,* which cause active vasodilatation. The normal state of the resistance blood vessels that supply skeletal muscle tissue is one of vasoconstrictor tone. Greater blood supply to an active muscle can be brought about by release of its vasoconstrictor tone or by active vasodilatation. Release of vasoconstrictor tone in the active tissues, with concomitant vasoconstriction in less active tissues—particularly the skin and viscera—seems to be the more important factor. Vasodilatation of resistance vessels appears to function only in emotional reactions or in the expectation of an exercise bout. Furthermore, active vasodilatation probably does not contribute to the support of an increased metabolic rate because it does not result in an increased flow through the true capillaries but only through the AVA or thoroughfare channels discussed above (5).

Muscular exercise causes a reflex increase in the tension of the venous walls in both exercising and nonexercising limbs, which persists throughout the exercise and is proportional to the severity of the work (7). This closing down of the capacitance vessels along with the muscle pump and the abdominal-thoracic pump aids the venous return to the heart.

Chemical Regulation

Greater blood flow to active tissue is also brought about by the chemical results of metabolic activity. Lowered pH, increased CO_2 level, and other local changes in metabolites have such a potent effect on the microcirculation that these effects can override the more centrally mediated vasoconstrictor stimuli whether blood-borne or neurogenic in origin.

The overall picture in exercise appears to be one in which nervous regulation closes down, to a large extent, the circulation to inactive tissues, while it opens the precapillary sphincters of the microcirculation so that greater flow is provided through the true capillaries that serve the metabolic needs of the active muscle tissue. Simultaneously, or as soon as metabolic products of the activity accumulate, chemical regulation augments the blood flow by further local vasodilatation.

Blood Distribution in Rest and Exercise

As we described earlier, the volume of blood flow to a particular tissue depends on the resistance it offers in relation to the pressure gradient of its blood flow. Thus the resistance to flow is frequently described in R units, where:

$$R = \frac{\text{Pressure gradient in millimeters mercury}}{\text{Flow rate in milliliters per second}}$$

This is a very convenient method. If we assume an average human at rest has a cardiac output of 5,400 ml/min, then with the usually accepted average resting mean arterial blood pressure of 90 mm Hg (diastolic + ⅓ pulse pressure), the resistance for the total circulatory system—with essentially zero central venous pressure—becomes:

$$R = \frac{90 - 0}{5,400/60} = \frac{90}{90} = 1$$

This resistance of one R unit can be broken down into its component parts according to the part of the circulatory system that interests us. Thus the resistance of the arterial system can be compared with that of the venous system under resting conditions as follows:

Flow rate = 90 ml/sec

Central venous pressure = 0.0

Mean arterial pressure = 90 mm Hg

Mean pressure in middle of capillary = 25 mm Hg

Arterial resistance equals: $\dfrac{90 - 25}{90} = 0.72\ R$

and venous resistance equals: $\dfrac{25 - 0.0}{90} = 0.28\ R$

Total = 1.00 R

Under a moderate exercise load, the same average human will increase cardiac output some three times, to 16,200 ml/min. Let us examine some typical figures and determine the resistance changes.

Flow rate = 16,200 ml/min = 270 ml/sec

Central venous pressure = 0.0

Mean arterial pressure = 120 mm Hg

Mean capillary pressure = 25 mm Hg

Arterial resistance equals: $\dfrac{120 - 25}{270} = 0.35\ R$

and venous resistance equals: $\dfrac{25 - 0}{270} = 0.09\ R$

Total = 0.44 R

These figures, which are quite realistic, illustrate what happens in the circulatory system during exercise. First, the total peripheral resistance is greatly reduced because the blood pressure gradients do not rise nearly as much as the flow rate. This, of course, is the result of vasodilatation in the active skeletal muscles, which far outweighs the accompanying vasoconstriction in less active tissues. Second, the decrease in resistance is even greater in the venous than in the arterial system. The decrease in the arterial system is the result of vasodilatation of the arterioles, while the decrease in the venous system results from the assistance to blood flow given by the muscle pump. Overall, it is this decreased total peripheral resistance that allows the heart to function at a greatly elevated output without strain.

It is also of interest to know where and to what extent compensatory vasoconstriction occurs to support the increased blood flow to the active muscles in exercise. It has been estimated that the resistance to flow in the muscles is reduced from 3.1 R units to 0.37 R during exercise, while the resistance in the portal arteries increases from 2.6 R to 12.0 R, and the portal venous and liver resistance increases from 1.0 R to 3.0 R (6).

Blood Pressure

The importance of blood pressure as the driving force for the circulatory system has been emphasized. Equally worth emphasizing is the importance of hypertension (higher than normal levels of blood pressure) as a determinant of the hazard and incidence of such serious health problems as heart attacks, strokes, and kidney disease. Now let us consider the practical problem of measurement and how observed measurements can change under varying conditions.

Measurement of Blood Pressure

The common indirect method of measuring blood pressure involves using a pressure cuff whose pressure is read from a mercury or aneroid manometer. This device is called a *sphygmomanometer*. The sphygmomanometer's cuff is applied to the upper arm, as the subject sits comfortably, so that the cuff is approximately at heart level. The pressure required to occlude the brachial artery is noted by listening to the flow of blood below the cuff. This is read as *systolic blood pressure. Diastolic blood pressure* is recorded as the pressure at which the sounds resulting from occlusion become muffled, or disappear, as the cuff pressure is reduced. The systolic-diastolic difference is *pulse pressure.*

Blood pressure measurements made by the indirect method during exercise must be viewed with caution. Comparisons between indirect (sphygmomanometer) and direct (catheter) methods showed that systolic pressure was underestimated by mean values of 8 to 15 mm Hg by the indirect method and overestimated during recovery by 16 to 38 mm Hg (17). Other investigators (30) have found that the indirect method provides satisfactory data on systolic but not diastolic pressure. Some sources of variability in blood pressure follow.

Age

Figure 7.5 illustrates the increase of systolic and diastolic pressures with age. It also shows the more enlightened approach to the problem of *normality*, in which ranges are given instead of single figures. It is of interest that not all cultures show this increase in blood pressure with age. Henry and Cassel (16) have furnished impressive evidence for a psychosocial effect in which dissonance between the social milieu in later life and expectations based on early experiences brings about the often observed increase in blood pressure with age.

Gender

The blood pressure in women prior to menopause tends to be slightly lower—and after menopause somewhat higher—than it is in men of the same age.

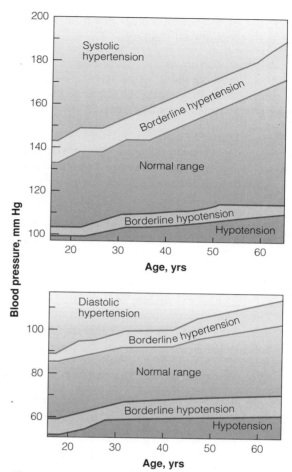

Figure 7.5   Range of systemic arterial blood pressure as a function of age. (From Rushmer, R. F. *Cardiovascular Dynamics*, 2d ed. © 1961 W. B. Saunders Company. Courtesy of W. B. Saunders Company, Philadelphia.)

Emotion

The problem of measuring blood pressure is greatly complicated by the fact that the slightest emotional involvement is reflected by significant rises in blood pressure. This fact is used to advantage in the *polygraph* or lie detector because the act of lying creates emotional conflict that is sensed and recorded, along with other physiological variables that react to emotional changes.

Diurnal Variation

Blood pressure tends to rise from a low point during sleep to a high point (15 to 20 mm Hg higher) after the evening meal.

Ingestion of Food

After a large meal, there is normally a considerable rise in systolic pressure and sometimes a fall in diastolic pressure.

Posture

In changing from supine to erect posture, the hydrostatic pressure increase requires greater arterial pressure, and the response by the cardiovascular system usually overshoots the mark so that systolic and diastolic pressures usually show an increase of 5 to 10 mm Hg. The pulse pressure usually shows a decrease due to the relatively greater increase in diastolic pressure.

Maintenance of Arterial Blood Pressure

The formula

$$\text{Pressure gradient} = \text{Volume of blood flow} \times \text{Resistance}$$

shows clearly that blood pressure is maintained by the interaction of two factors: volume of blood flow and resistance. The volume of blood flow is in turn dependent on 1) heart rate and 2) stroke volume. The resistance is largely determined by the vasoconstrictor tone of the arterioles.

Maintenance of Venous Return to the Heart

The venous blood pressure at the ankle in the standing posture (under conditions of no muscular activity) is roughly equivalent to the hydrostatic pressure 92 mm Hg if we assume a vertical distance from ankle to right atrium of 125 cm. However, such a pressure, if maintained for any length of time, results in filtration of fluids from the vascular system into the tissue spaces, which results in considerable *edema* (swelling). This happens when a person is forced to stand motionless for a protracted period of time, but it does not occur if the muscles of the leg are active. If the venous pressure is measured in a leg whose muscles are active—as in walking—the pressure is greatly reduced (to 20 or 25 mm Hg) because of one-way valves in the veins that serve the musculature. Thus the contraction of muscle drives blood toward the heart, and during the relaxation phase these valves prevent a backward flow. This is the first of three major factors that maintain venous return: *the pumping action of contracting muscles*. The importance of this muscle pump, sometimes called a peripheral heart, is shown by the fact that it has been calculated to provide more than 30% of the energy required to circulate the blood during running (41).

A second factor is the *abdominothoracic pump*. The descent of the diaphragm in inspiration creates an increase in intra-abdominal pressure while simultaneously lowering intrathoracic pressure. This increased pressure gradient, from abdomen to right atrium, aids the venous return. During expiration, the backward flow is prevented by the valves in the veins of the muscles of the legs.

A third factor is the *shortening of the inferior vena cava* during the descent of the diaphragm, which results in its having smaller volume, which in turn aids the flow from abdomen to thorax. The lengthening inferior vena cava during expiration lowers pressure within its walls and allows a better pressure gradient for its filling, preparatory to the next descent of the diaphragm.

Arterial Blood Pressure during Exercise

The effects of exercise upon arterial blood pressure can best be described as the end result of the balance struck between the increased blood flow due to the increased cardiac output and the decreased peripheral resistance caused by the vasodilatation of the microcirculation. Consequently, the end result is considerably influenced by the *type* and *intensity* of the exercise and by the physical condition of the subject.

Type of Exercise

In rhythmic exercise that involves moderate to strenuous work loads, the typical response is an elevation of systolic pressure with little, if any, elevation in diastolic pressure. Figure 7.6 shows a typical response for a young male. The mean arterial pressure is usually calculated at one-third of the way between diastolic and systolic pressures because of the shape of the arterial pressure wave form. Therefore, the mean pressure is much less affected by exercise.

In static or isometric exercise, where an expiratory effort is made against a closed glottis, the situation is quite different. The intrathoracic pressure is raised from 80 to 200 mm Hg or more, and this increased pressure is transmitted through the thin walls of the great veins. Venous return to the right atrium is thus severely decreased, resulting in the following sequence of events.

1. There is a sharp increase in pressure, both systolic and diastolic, which reflects the increase in intrathoracic pressure.
2. After a period of several seconds, during which blood in the lungs furnishes the venous return, the decreased venous

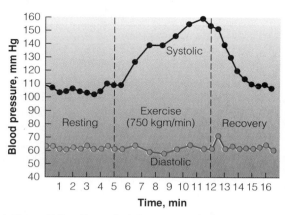

Figure 7.6   The typical time course of the arterial blood pressure response to rest-exercise-recovery in a healthy young man.

return brings about a decreased pulse pressure.
3. After release of the straining activity, there is an increase in both mean pressure and pulse pressure due to the improved venous return of blood, which had been blocked.

This sequence of events is called the *Valsalva effect*.

Although exercise physiologists have often cautioned against strength exercises with a large static component because of possibly harmful effects of the increased pressure on the heart and large blood vessels, the work of Hamilton and others (14) shows that no increased difference in pressure across the walls of the heart and great vessels can exist. As the pressure increases within these walls, it increases proportionately outside them. In fact, the pressure difference decreases.

The vessels of the cerebral circulation are similarly protected in that the increased intrathoracic pressure is also transmitted to the cerebrospinal fluid. The only possible danger, then, is in peripheral vessels. But the peripheral vessels are small in diameter, and the laws of physics tell us they are consequently better able to withstand pressure.

However, it must be recalled from the earlier discussion that the work of the heart is determined to a great extent by the arterial pressure against which it is working. It will also be recalled that during exercise the redistribution of blood flow is accomplished by increased sympathetic adrenergic vasomotor tone in the inactive areas, while this tone is overridden in the active muscles by local effects to increase the blood flow to the active muscles.

Considerable evidence has suggested that the systemic level of arterial blood pressure is set by the perfusion pressure required to get through that muscle tissue that is contracting most strongly (2, 3, 10, 13, 28). More recent evidence suggests that the amount of total muscle mass involved is at least equally important both in dynamic exercise (27) and in isometric contraction (39). At a given relative work intensity, cardiac output and heart rate increase in proportion to O_2 uptake and therefore rise to a greater extent in large muscle work. On the other hand, in small muscle exercise the local vasodilator effect of lowering pH, increasing CO_2, and other metabolites as discussed earlier, has only a small effect on the total systemic resistance in spite of the strong local effect. In large muscle exercise, the much more extensive metabolic vasodilatation markedly reduces total peripheral resistance and results in a relatively small rise in mean arterial pressure in spite of the much greater increases in heart rate and cardiac output.

Thus, to summarize, in exercise involving large muscle mass, the forces that drive blood pressure up—that is, heart rate and cardiac output—are high but are more than offset by the large decrease in total peripheral resistance. With small muscle mass exercise, the heart rate and cardiac output provide less drive to raise blood pressure. But the vasodilator effect is virtually negligible with respect to the total muscle mass, so that systolic and mean blood pressure rise to a greater extent in small muscle work.

There is also evidence from animal experiments to suggest that, at least in isometric contraction, a contraction of slow twitch muscle causes a much smaller rise in arterial pressure than contraction in muscle of mixed FT and ST fibers (33).

Lind and McNicol (28) performed an experiment in which their subjects walked on a treadmill at three miles per hour against a grade of 22%, which required an O_2 uptake of 2.8 liters/min. In spite of this very heavy work load sustained by the entire body musculature, when they then performed an isometric contraction, while walking, of 50% maximum on a handgrip dynamometer for one minute, their systolic pressure rose by 45 mm Hg and diastolic by 40 mm Hg. This illustrates clearly the need to avoid isometric contractions and also high loadings of small muscles in any exercise situation where high cardiac work loads are undesirable, as in cardiac rehabilitation exercise or in conditioning programs for older adults.

Blood Flow in Exercising Muscles

As soon as exercise begins, the metabolic demands of the active muscle tissue increase (by as much as fiftyfold in all-out activity). Many physiological mechanisms cooperate to supply the demand. In addition to the increased cardiac output and redistribution of blood from inactive to active tissues, changes in blood flow occur within the active tissues. In an interesting experiment in 1932—in which India ink was injected into dogs' muscles—Martin and others (29) showed that in the active gracilis muscle there were 2,010 open capillaries per square millimeter, compared with 1,050 in the same muscle when resting.

Concurrently with the increased flow rate through the tissue, the rate of O_2 consumption per cell (muscle fiber) increases rapidly, and this results in a fall in the partial pressure of O_2 within the cell. The partial pressure of O_2 in the tissue fluid bathing the cells, on the other hand, falls very little. Thus a much higher pressure gradient exists to move O_2 from the capillary through the tissue fluid and into the muscle fiber. Better O_2 extraction per volume of circulating blood helps supply the increased metabolic demand. The presence of greater concentrations of CO_2 in the cell further aid the gas exchange (this factor is discussed in chap. 9).

According to the work of Reeves and others (34, 35), it seems that the increased O_2 extraction plays the greater part in making the adjustment to mild exercise (two to three times the resting level), but that in moderate to heavy exercise the increase in cardiac output and the improved flow through tissues is more important. In general, the blood flow through muscle increases in proportion to the metabolic demand.

The type of activity is an important factor not only in the circulation through large vessels but also in the blood flow within the muscle itself. The classic early work of Barcroft and Millen (4) on the plantar flexors of the foot demonstrated an increased flow (hyperemia) when muscular contractions were 0.1 maximum or less but a cessation of flow when the contractions were above 0.3 maximum. Other work (38, 40) has shown that isometric contraction of the forearm muscles and elbow flexors occludes the blood flow in these muscles also but requires 0.6 maximal contraction strength. Thus it would seem that muscles held unnecessarily in tension during athletic activity may suffer the effects of ischemia with its accompanying pain and loss of endurance.

According to Folkow and coworkers (12), the optimal rhythm for maximizing muscle blood flow is one contraction of about 0.3

second duration per second, a rhythm which is often spontaneously chosen by human subjects during bicycling, running, and swimming. The advantage from this activity pattern seems to be that it enables the muscle pump to keep the local mean venous pressure at a minimum during the relaxation phase, thus increasing the effective perfusion pressure.

There are also interesting differences in hemodynamics from sport to sport. For example, in comparing the responses to swimming and running, it was found that arterial blood pressure was higher in swimming than running by 20% at submaximal work loads and 16% at maximal, although cardiac output was lower in swimming as the result of lower heart rates (19).

As would be expected, training and conditioning have an effect on the level of blood flow through the muscles involved. Rohter and others (37) demonstrated an increase of almost 60% in blood flow through the forearm flexors in swimmers after five weeks of training, compared with controls. This work was confirmed by Rochelle and associates (36) (fig. 7.7). It has also been shown that isometric training can increase exercise blood flow, at least when measured with a contraction of not over 50% of maximal (8).

It is tempting to explain this improved blood flow that results from training on the basis of the older and often cited work that showed capillarization to increase as a result of training in animals (32). However, this work depended on staining the red blood cells, and accurate counts probably cannot be made in this fashion. More recent work has shown that 30 minutes of endurance training three times per week for eight weeks resulted in a 20% increase in the number of capillaries per mm^2 and in the number of capillaries per fiber (25). Detraining for eight weeks resulted in a loss of the capillaries per fiber improvement, but when expressed as capillaries/mm^2 the improvement was unchanged after detraining and

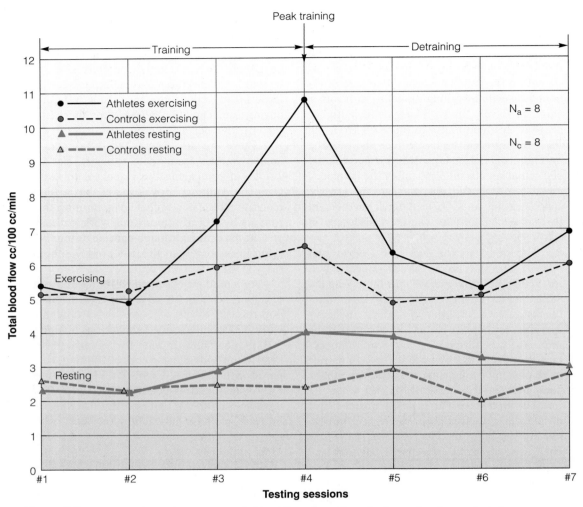

Figure 7.7   Mean resting and exercise muscle blood flows for athletes (swimmers) and controls during a twenty-week training and detraining program. Testing sessions 1, 2, 3, 4, 5, 6, and 7 correspond to the 1st, 4th, 7th, and 10th weeks of training and 4th, 7th, and 10th weeks of detraining, respectively. (From Rochelle, R. H. et al., in *Medicine and Science in Sports* 3:122–129. © 1971 American College of Sports Medicine. Reprinted by permission.)

probably represents a favorable long-term effect.

Retrospective comparisons of endurance-trained persons with untrained men (20) and women (21) have shown even larger advantages with respect to capillarization, and this existed in all three muscle fiber types (20).

Recent data suggests that heavy resistance training in contrast to endurance training does not result in increased capillary density (42). In fact, because of muscle fiber hypertrophy induced by the muscle overloads, the ratio of capillary to cross-sectional muscle area may decrease somewhat.

In general, the immediate short-term effects of exercise are an increase of blood flow through muscles that are active in light, rhythmic activity and a decrease during heavy, sustained contraction, which is followed by a period of increased flow called *reactive hyperemia*. The long-term effect of exercise includes almost certainly improved perfusion of the active tissues.

Blood and Fluid Changes during Exercise

The total body fluid is composed of four components:

1. Blood plasma
2. Interstitial fluid
3. Intracellular fluid
4. Miscellaneous components

Only the first three are important to exercise physiology. Because the capillary wall is freely permeable to most of the substances in the plasma (except the plasma protein), the plasma and interstitial fluid constantly mix and are very similar in makeup. Therefore the two together are referred to as extracellular fluid.

To maintain normal osmotic pressures in intracellular and extracellular fluids, water diffuses in the direction needed through the cell membrane. Thus in excessive sweating as in heavy exercise, water that is lost in sweat comes directly from an extracellular component. This raises the concentration of nondiffusible substances of the interstitial fluid, which results in transfer of water across the cell membranes of the various tissue cells from intracellular to extracellular components, thus dehydrating the tissues as well. Obviously, ingestion of water causes a reverse reaction in which tissue hydration is restored to normal.

Hemoconcentration

Moderate to heavy exercise bouts result in a shift of fluid from the plasma to the interstitial fluid. This, in turn, results in higher hemoglobin and serum protein concentrations and in a higher proportion of cellular elements in the plasma. If the exercise bouts involve heavy work in a hot environment, dehydration contributes to exaggerate this phenomenon. Weight loss in wrestlers by dehydration has been reported as high as 8.8 lb, and in marathon runners it may be as high as 7% of body weight. A dehydration of 2% may cause deterioration of performance in some persons (1).

Erythrocyte Count

The hemoconcentration discussed above results in a considerable rise in the cell count per cubic millimeter. In the normal male, the count is ordinarily 5.5 million per cubic millimeter (female, 4.8 million per cubic millimeter). These values can be raised by as much as 20% to 25% in vigorous exercise. Whether this rise is due entirely to hemoconcentration, or in part to release of stored cells, is still unclear. In some animals the spleen releases erythrocytes to the general circulation during exercise, but this does not seem to be the case in humans.

Blood and Fluid Changes from Training

Blood Volume

Evidence indicates that blood volume first falls, then rises above normal during a four- to nine-week training period in dogs (9). The increased blood volume persisted about four weeks after cessation of training. Kjellberg and others (24) found similar results with men and women: blood volumes were found to be 10% to 19% higher after training than before. They also found blood volume was as much as 41%

to 44% higher in an athletically trained group than in a comparable untrained group.

Changes in the opposite direction occur with prolonged bed rest. Thus it would seem that blood volume varies proportionately with the amount of physical activity. Increased blood volume is a considerable advantage in heavy exercise because a circulatory demand may exist for purposes of heat dissipation at the same time that active muscle tissues also demand a greatly increased blood volume. Under these conditions, increased blood volume helps ensure an adequate venous return to the heart.

Hemoglobin

Increases of *total hemoglobin* have been found in dogs and in humans as the result of physical conditioning (9, 25). These increases seem to parallel the increased blood volume, so that no increase in *hemoglobin concentration* (hemoglobin per unit blood volume) seems to occur. Indeed Dill and associates (11) found hemoglobin concentration to be 4% *lower* in highly trained runners than in controls. They concluded that endurance athletes have thin blood but so much of it that their total hemoglobin exceeds that of nonathletes. Recent work supports this conclusion by showing that the total amount of hemoglobin rather than its concentration in the blood is the determining factor for reaching a maximal VO_2 (23).

Sports Anemia

While the above discussion deals with a lowered hemoconcentration in athletes that may be only apparent due to an increasing blood volume, there may also be cause for concern about real "sports anemia." Pate has provided an excellent review of this literature (31) and points out that its causes (other than the aforementioned plasma volume expansion) may include: 1) reduced hemoglobin synthesis, 2) reduced erythropoiesis, and 3) increased destruction of red blood cells. Physicians should screen athletes, especially female endurance athletes, for: 1) a diet that is low in iron, protein, vitamin C, vitamin B_{12}, or folic acid, 2) high rates of iron loss, and 3) too intensive a training regimen, especially at the outset of the training season.

Alkaline Reserve

Alkaline reserve may be defined as the buffering capacity of the blood. Many investigators have shown that there is an increased ability to tolerate acid metabolites (mainly lactic acid) after a period of training. Thus it seems a likely hypothesis that this increased tolerance is due to an increase in buffering ability of the blood. It has been shown that an induced alkalosis does indeed improve power output (22) (chap. 30).

Postural Effects on Circulation

Posture during physical activity varies from the usual, upright position, to sitting while rowing, to the prone or supine position in swimming, to the head-down position in gymnastics. Changes in posture might be expected to exert effects upon the circulation, and these effects have been demonstrated.

The responses to exercise in supine and sitting positions (bicycle ergometer) and standing (treadmill) positions have been studied by many investigators. In general, the cardiac output is about 2 liters/min greater in supine position than in the upright positions. This is due to the greater stroke volume while supine. A higher arteriovenous O_2 difference in the upright position compensates for the lower cardiac output and stroke volume (7).

Tilttable changes of a subject's position, from standing upright to the head-down position, produced a *vagal rebound phenomenon* (26) in which the subjects' heart rates slowed by an average of fifteen beats per minute (fig. 7.8). This can be explained by the fact that in upright posture the peripheral resistance is maintained by sympathetic nervous activity that reflexly maintains a state of vasoconstriction in the arterioles of the lower extremities. When the body is tilted head downward, the redistribution of blood due to the changed direction of the force of gravity brings about greater stimulation of the carotid sinus and central nervous system receptors, which induces vagal efferent stimulation with cardioinhibitory responses. Surprisingly, no relationship was found between the reaction to head-down tilting and physical fitness (measured by endurance in treadmill walking).

The circulatory reserves that can be called upon also seem to vary with body position. As soon as one assumes the standing position, one's O_2 extraction (as measured by the difference between arterial and venous oxygen levels of the working muscle) has already greatly increased. One's circulatory reserve therefore depends largely on the factors that can increase the flow rate. In the supine position, mild demands of exercise can be satisfied by increased O_2 extraction before any increase in blood flow is demanded.

Cooling Down after Heavy Exercise

It has been the common practice in athletic events that involve large circulatory adjustments (such as distance running) to *cool down* at the end of the competitive effort by jogging for a few minutes. This procedure rests on sound physiological principles and should be encouraged. If this cooling down is not done, venous return to the heart—which has been largely supported by the muscle pump—drops too abruptly, and blood pooling may occur in the extremities. This, in turn, may result in shock, or at least in hyperventilation, which causes lower levels of CO_2 and muscle cramps.

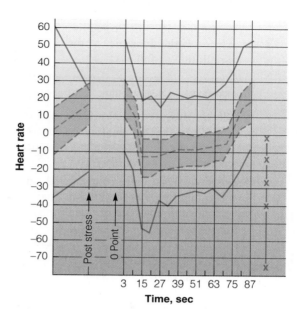

Figure 7.8   The mean change in heart rate from the baseline level for 215 subjects is plotted against time. The 0 point is a six-second period just prior to the head-down tilt. Heart rate is plotted for each six-second interval thereafter. The increase in heart rate after the sixty-second period is following rotation to the feet-down position. The shaded area is the standard deviation of the mean. The upper and lower graphs represent the extremes, the high and low values for the group. (From Lamb, L. E., and Roman, J. "The Head-Down Tilt and Adaptability for Aerospace Flight," in *Aerospace Medicine* 32:473, 1961. Reprinted by permission.)

Summary

1. Blood flow is the result of a difference in pressure between two points in the circulation. This difference in pressure is called a *pressure gradient*.

   a. Other things being equal, the velocity of blood flow through any given type of blood vessel varies inversely with the cross-sectional area of the total vessels of that type.

b. A simplification of Poiseuille's law expresses the dynamics of the circulation as follows:

$$\frac{\text{Volume of}}{\text{blood flow}} = \frac{\text{Pressure} \times (\text{Vessel radius})^4}{\text{Vessel length} \times \text{Viscosity}}$$

c. Blood pressure must always be referred to a specific point in the body to account for the effects of hydrostatic pressure.

2. There are at least three routes for blood flow through the microcirculation that serve differing physiological conditions: (a) *thoroughfare* or *preferential channels* that serve the metabolic needs of resting tissue; (b) *true capillaries,* which open to serve the needs of an increased metabolic activity; and (c) *arteriovenous anastomoses* that probably dissipate heat.

3. Control of blood distribution is mediated by the sympathetic nervous system and chemical regulation. *Adrenergic fibers* of the sympathetic system bring about vasoconstriction of inactive tissues, and *cholinergic fibers* of the same system cause vasodilatation of the active tissue, which is augmented by chemical activity of the metabolites after exercise is well under way.

4. Approximately 72% of the resistance of the circulatory system at rest arises in the arterial system (largely in the arterioles) and only 28% in the venous system. In exercise, the total resistance may be reduced by at least 50%.

5. Blood pressure is subject to the effects of many variables, such as age, gender, emotional state, time of day, nutritional state, and posture.

6. Blood pressure usually shows a rise during exercise in systolic and mean values but no change or a very small rise in diastolic pressure. The effects vary with the type of exercise.

7. The systemic arterial pressure is set both by the general level of the work load sustained by the total body and by the pressure required to perfuse that muscle or muscle group that is working under greatest tension.

8. During exercise, the number of open capillaries is approximately double the number observed during rest.

9. The training and conditioning of athletes has been shown to bring improved blood flow to the active muscles at the peak of training. These changes are reversible and show a detraining effect within three weeks of the end of training.

10. Exercise that results in heavy sweating causes a loss of intracellular as well as extracellular fluid, which must be replaced during or after the workout to maintain normal tissue hydration and electrolyte balance.

11. Total blood volume responds to training with significant increases and declines in persons confined to the inactivity of bed rest.

12. The response of the circulatory system to exercise varies with posture. Even at rest, changes in posture are reflected in predictable and typical circulatory response patterns.

13. *Cooling down* after heavy exercise is necessary to prevent blood pooling, which may result in muscle cramps or even shock.

References

1. Ahlman, K., and Karvonen, M. J. Weight reduction by sweating in wrestlers and its effect on physical fitness. *J. Sports Med. Phys. Fitness* 1:58–62, 1962.

2. Astrand, P. O., Ekblom, B., Messin, R., Saltin, B., and Stenberg, J. Intraarterial blood pressure during exercise with different muscle groups. *J. Appl. Physiol.* 20:253–56, 1965.

3. Astrand, I., Guharay, A., and Wahren, J. Circulatory responses to arm exercise with different arm positions. *J. Appl. Physiol.* 25:528–32, 1968.

4. Barcroft, H., and Millen, J. L. E. The blood flow through muscle during sustained contraction. *J. Physiol.* 97:17–31, 1939.

5. Barcroft, H., and Swan, H. J. C. *Sympathetic Control of Human Blood Vessels.* London: E. Arnold, 1953.

6. Bazett, H. C. A consideration of the venous circulation. *Factors Regulating Blood Pressure,* eds. B. W. Zweifach and E. Shorr. New York: Josiah Macy, Jr., Foundation, 1949.

7. Bevegard, B. S., and Shepherd, J. T. Regulation of the circulation during exercise in man. *Physiol. Rev.* 47: 178–213, 1967.

8. Byrd, R. J., and Hills, W. L. Strength, endurance and blood flow responses to isometric training. *Res. Q.* 42:357–61, 1971.

9. Davis, J. E., and Brewer, N. Effect of physical training on blood volume, hemoglobin, alkali reserve, and osmotic resistance of erythrocytes. *Am. J. Physiol.* 113:586–91, 1935.

10. deVries, H. A., and Adams, G. M. Total muscle mass activation versus relative loading of individual muscles as determinants of exercise response in older men. *Med. Sci. Sports* 4:146–54, 1972.

11. Dill, D. B., Braithwaite, K., Adams, W. C., and Bernauer, E. M. Blood volume of middle distance runners; effect of 2300 m altitude and comparison with nonathletes. *Med. Sci. Sports* 6:1–7, 1974.

12. Folkow B., Gaskell P., and Waaler B. A. Blood flow through limb muscles during heavy rhythmic exercise. *Acta Physiol. Scand.* 80:61–72, 1970.

13. Freyschuss, V., and Strandell, T. Circulatory adaptation to one- and two-leg exercise in supine position. *J. Appl. Physiol.* 25:511–15, 1968.

14. Hamilton, W. F., Woodbury, R. A., and Harper, Jr., H. T. Arterial, cerebrospinal and venous pressures in man during cough and strain. *Am. J. Physiol.* 141:42–50, 1944.

15. Hargens, A. R. Fluid shifts in vascular and extra-vascular spaces during and after simulated weightlessness. *Med. Sci. Sports Exer.* 15:421–27, 1983.

16. Henry, J. P., and Cassel, J. C. Psychosocial factors in essential hypertension. *Am. J. Epidemiol.* 90:171–200, 1969.

17. Henschel, A., De la Vega, F., and Taylor, H. L. Simultaneous direct and indirect blood pressure measurements in man at rest and work. *J. Appl. Physiol.* 6:506–12, 1954.

18. Hermansen, L., and Wachtlova, M. Capillary density of skeletal muscle in well-trained and untrained men. *J. Appl. Physiol.* 30:860–63, 1971.

19. Holmer, I., Stein, E. M., Saltin, B., Ekblom, B., and Astrand, P. O. Hemodynamics and respiratory responses compared in swimming and running. *J. Appl. Physiol.* 37:49–54, 1974.

20. Ingjer, F. Capillary supply and mitochondrial content of different muscle fiber types in untrained and endurance trained men. *Eur. J. Appl. Physiol.* 40:197–209, 1979.

21. Ingjer, F., and Brodal, P. Capillary supply of skeletal muscle fibers in untrained and endurance trained women. *Eur. J. Appl. Physiol.* 38:291–99, 1978.

22. Jones, N. L., Sutton, J. R., Taylor, R., Toews, C. J. Effect of pH on cardiorespiratory and metabolic responses to exercise. *J. Appl. Physiol.* 43:959–64, 1977.

23. Kanstrup, I-L., and Ekblom, B. Blood volume and hemoglobin concentration as determinants of maximal aerobic power. *Med. Sci. Sports Exer.* 16:256–62, 1984.

24. Kjellberg, S. R., Rudhe, V., and Sjostrand, T. Increase of the amount of hemoglobin and blood volume in connection with physical training. *Acta Physiol. Scand.* 19:146–51, 1949.

25. Klausen, K., Anderson, L. B., and Pelle, I. Adaptive changes in work capacity, skeletal muscle capillarization and enzyme levels during training and detraining. *Acta Physiol. Scand.* 113:9–16, 1981.

26. Lamb, L. E., and Roman J. The head-down tilt and adaptability for aerospace flight. *Aerospace Med.* 32:473–86, 1961.

27. Lewis, S. F., Taylor, W. F., Graham, R. M., Pettinger, W. A., Schutte, J. E., and Blomgrist, C. G. Cardiovascular responses to exercise as functions of absolute and relative workloads. *J. Appl. Physiol.* 54:1314–23, 1983.

28. Lind, A. R., and McNicol, G. W. Muscular factors which determine the cardiovascular responses to sustained and rhythmic exercise. *Can. Med. Assoc. J.* 96:706–13, 1967.

29. Martin, E. G., Wooley, E. C., and Miller, M. Capillary counts in resting and active muscle. *Am. J. Physiol.* 100:407–16, 1932.

30. Nagle, F. J., Naughton, J., and Balke, B. Comparison of direct and indirect blood pressure with pressure-flow dynamics during exercise. *J. Appl. Physiol.* 21:317–20, 1966.

31. Pate, R. Sports anemia: A review of the current research literature. *Physician and Sportsmed.* 11 (Feb.):115–26, 1983.

32. Petren, T., Sjostrand, T., and Sylven, B. Der Einfluss des Trainings auf die Häufigkeit der Capillaren in Herz und Skeletmuskulatur. *Arbeitsphysiologie* 9:376–86, 1936.

33. Petrofsky, J. C., Phillips, C. A., Sawka, M. N., Hanpeter, P., Lind, A. R., and Stafford, D. Muscle fiber recruitment and blood pressure response to isometric exercise. *J. Appl. Physiol.* 50:32–37, 1981.

34. Reeves, J. T., Grover, R. F., Filley, G. F., and Blount, S. G. Circulatory changes in man during mild supine exercise. *J. Appl. Physiol.* 16:279–82, 1961.

35. ———. Cardiac output response to standing and treadmill walking. *J. Appl. Physiol.* 16:283–88, 1961.

36. Rochelle, R. H., Stumpner, R. L., Robinson, S., Dill, D. B., and Horvath, S. M. Peripheral blood flow response to exercise consequent to physical training. *Med. Sci. Sports* 3:122–29, 1971.

37. Rohter, F. D., Rochelle, R. H., and Hyman, C. Exercise blood flow changes in the human forearm during physical training. *J. Appl. Physiol.* 18:789–93, 1963.

38. Royce, J. Isometric fatigue curves in human muscle with normal and occluded circulation. *Res. Q.* 29:204–12, 1958.

39. Seals, D. R., Washburn, R. A., Hanson, P. G., Painter, P. L., and Nagle, F. J. Increased cardiovascular responses to static contraction of larger muscle groups. *J. Appl. Physiol.* 54:434–37, 1983.

40. Start, K. B., and Holmes, R. Local muscle endurance with open and occluded intramuscular circulation. *J. Appl. Physiol.* 18:804–7, 1963.

41. Stegall, H. F. Muscle pumping in the dependent leg. *Circ. Res.* 19:180–90, 1966.

42. Tesch, P. A., Thorsson, A., and Kaiser, P. Muscle capillary supply and fiber type characteristics in weight and power lifters. *J. Appl. Physiol.* 56:35–38, 1984.

43. Zweifach, B. W. Basic mechanisms in peripheral vascular homeostasis. *Proceedings of Third Conference on Factors Regulating Blood Pressure.* New York: Josiah Macy, Jr., Foundation, 1949.

44. ————. General principles governing the behavior of the microcirculation. *Am. J. Med.* 23:684–96, 1957.

45. ————. Structural and functional aspects of the microcirculation in the skin. *The Microcirculation,* eds. S. R. M. Reynolds and B. W. Zweifach, pp. 144–52. Urbana: The University of Illinois Press, 1959.

46. Zweifach, B. W., and Metz, D. B. Selective distribution of blood through the terminal vascular bed of mesenteric structures and skeletal muscle. *Angiology* 6:282–90, 1955.

8

The Lungs and External Respiration

Anatomy of External Respiration

Mechanics of Lung Ventilation

Nomenclature for the Lung Volumes and Capacities

Respiratory Control
Carbon Dioxide and Subsequent pH Changes
Oxygen (Anoxia)
Proprioceptive Reflexes from Joints and Muscles
Temperature
Cerebral Factors

Importance of Breathing Pattern
Rate versus Depth
Effect of Type of Exercise on Breathing Pattern
Diaphragmatic versus Costal Breathing
Oral versus Nasal Breathing

Efficiency of Breathing
Lung Ventilation versus O_2 Consumption in Exercise
Oxygen Cost of Breathing

Improving Performance by Better Breathing

Training Effects on Pulmonary Function
Genetic Effects on Respiratory Responses to Endurance Exercise

Respiratory Phenomena
Stitch in the Side
Second Wind
Exercise-Induced Asthma (EIA)

Unusual Respiratory Maneuvers
Hypoventilation
Hyperventilation
Breath-Holding
Valsalva Maneuver

Effects of Air Pollution on Respiration
Effect on Performance
Toxicity

Smoking—Self-Induced Air Pollution

Each cell of every tissue in the human body depends on oxidative reactions to provide the energy for its metabolism. In very simple biological organisms, each cell is in contact with the external environment and thus derives its supply of oxygen directly. In the human organism, the vast majority of tissues are not in direct contact with the external environment, and for this reason a specialized respiratory system is necessary to provide the oxygen for their metabolic demands.

The respiratory process can be broken down into three component functions:

1. Gas exchange in the lungs, in which the lung capillaries take up oxygen and give up much of their carbon dioxide.
2. Gas transport and distribution from the lungs to the various tissues by the blood.
3. Gas exchange between the blood and the tissue fluids bathing the ultimate consumers, the cells.

The first process is also referred to as *external respiration* or *pulmonary ventilation;* the third process is referred to as *internal* or *tissue respiration;* and the second process, *gas transport,* is the function of the cardiovascular system. This chapter is concerned with the first process, external respiration. The respiratory function of the cardiovascular system and internal respiration are discussed in chapter 9.

Anatomy of External Respiration

It will be recalled from elementary physiology and anatomy that the flow of air proceeds through the nose (or mouth) into the nasal cavity, where it is warmed, humidified, and agitated by striking the *turbinates.* From the nasopharynx, air is conducted past the *glottis,* where the pharynx separates into the *trachea* for air conduction and the *esophagus* for the passage of food. The trachea splits into the two chief *bronchi,* one going to the left lung and the other to the right lung (fig. 8.1).

The lungs can be considered a system of branching tubes that perform two major functions: conduction of air and respiration. The conductive portion of the system proceeds from the chief bronchi that branch in the lung root. Subsequent branching of the conductive pathway occurs within the lungs and results in smaller bronchi, which in turn branch into smaller tubes called *bronchioles.* Throughout the repeated branchings, each branching results in a larger total cross-sectional area, as is also the case in the circulatory system. The bronchioles eventually branch into the *terminal bronchioles,* the last units of the conductive system, which are from 0.5 to 1.0 mm in diameter.

Each terminal bronchiole divides into two *respiratory bronchioles,* which in turn may divide once more (or even twice), with these divisions forming *alveolar ducts.* The alveolar ducts may or may not branch, but they eventually terminate in thin-walled sacs called *alveoli* (singular: *alveolus*). These alveoli, with their supporting structures, are highly vascularized. Thus the *lung unit* is considered to consist of the alveolar duct and its subdivisions (alveoli), together with the blood and lymph vessels and the nerve supply. Within the lung unit, only two very thin endothelial layers separate the air in the system from the blood in the capillaries, thus allowing for very efficient diffusion of gasses. Furthermore, the total cross-sectional area available for diffusion has been estimated to be between 500 and 1,000 sq ft.

Mechanics of Lung Ventilation

The laws governing fluid flow also apply to gasses. It has been pointed out that the flow of

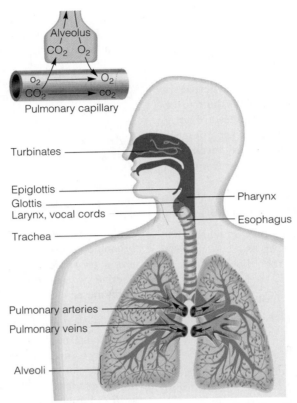

Figure 8.1   The respiratory system, showing the respiratory passages and the function of the alveolus to oxygenate the blood and to remove carbon dioxide. (From Guyton, A. C. *Function of the Human Body*, 1959. Courtesy of W. B. Saunders Company, Philadelphia.)

blood in the vascular system is brought about through differences in pressure, called a pressure gradient. The flow of respiratory gas similarly depends on a pressure gradient between the air in the lungs and the ambient (outside) air. For air to flow into the lungs, the pressure within must be lower than atmospheric pressure. This lowering of pressure in the lungs is brought about by the descent of the diaphragm (contraction of the muscle fibers) and the action of the external and anterior internal intercostal muscles in raising the ribs. Campbell (9) has shown by X-ray technique that the diaphragm descends approximately 1.5 cm in

normal, quiet respiration and as much as 6 to 10 cm during maximal breathing. Thus the volume of the lungs is considerably increased during inspiration, largely by virtue of elongation. This increase in volume results in a temporary lowering of pressure within the lungs so that a pressure gradient exists, with the ambient air having the higher pressure and thus moving into the lungs during inspiration.

In the respiratory cycle, the inspiration phase is the active phase and is brought about by the active contraction of the ordinary muscles of respiration, the diaphragm and the intercostals. The expiration phase under resting conditions is largely due to the elastic recoil of these muscles and associated structures as they snap back to their resting length. Thus the elastic recoil creates a higher-than-atmospheric pressure within the lung, which results in the necessary pressure gradient for moving the air out in expiration.

Ventilation of the alveoli, where the greatest part of the diffusion process occurs, has been attributed to the enlargement of the alveolar ducts in length and width without a concomitant enlargement of the alveoli themselves. However, it appears more likely that the alveoli participate proportionately in the overall enlargement during inspiration, this enlargement being about twofold for the alveolar duct and the alveolus. This twofold increase in volume was calculated to result in a 70% increase in alveolar area for diffusion.

The description so far holds only for normal resting breathing conditions. During exercise, metabolic demands are greater, and rate and depth of breathing are increased. The increased depth of respiration is brought about by the *accessory muscles* of breathing. In inspiration, greater volume is obtained by activity of the *scalene* and the *sternocleidomastoid* muscles, which help lift the ribs. In the expiratory phase of heavy exercise, the passive elastic recoil of the ordinary muscles of breathing is greatly aided by the active contraction of the abdominal muscles. The abdominal muscles serve two important mechanical functions: 1) raising the intraabdominal pressure, which results in greater intrathoracic pressure to aid in expiration, and 2) drawing the lower ribs downward and medially. The lateral muscles (oblique and transverse) are more important than the rectus abdominis (9).

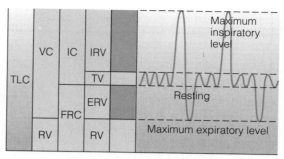

Lung volumes

Figure 8.2   Lung volumes. (From *The Lung,* 2nd edition, by Julius H. Comroe, Jr., et al. Copyright © 1962, Year Book Medical Publishers, Inc. Used by permission of Year Book Medical Publishers, Inc.)

Nomenclature for the Lung Volumes and Capacities

Because respiratory physiology had been plagued by an ambiguity of terms, a group of American physiologists agreed in 1950 to standardize terms and definitions. The result of this agreement is given in table 8.1 and is illustrated in figure 8.2. Table 8.2 provides illustrative values for the lung volumes in healthy, recumbent subjects.

Respiratory Control

The question of how pulmonary ventilation is controlled has been the subject of much physiological research. It is obvious that the rate and depth of respiration must be so controlled as to maintain homeostasis in the face of varying metabolic demands, ranging from rest to the very vigorous exercise of competitive athletics. However, the physiological mechanisms by which this homeostasis is brought about are, as yet, not so obvious.

Table 8.1	Lung Volumes and Capacities

A. Volumes. There are four primary volumes, which do not overlap.

1. Tidal volume, or the depth of breathing, is the volume of gas inspired or expired during each respiratory cycle.
2. Inspiratory reserve volume is the maximal amount of gas that can be inspired from the end inspiratory position.
3. Expiratory reserve volume is the maximal volume of gas that can be expired from the end expiratory level.
4. Residual volume is the volume of gas remaining in the lungs at the end of a maximal expiration.

B. Capacities. There are four capacities, each of which includes two or more of the primary volumes.

1. Total lung capacity is the amount of gas contained in the lung at the end of a maximal inspiration.
2. Vital capacity is the maximal volume of gas that can be expelled from the lungs by forceful effort following a maximal inspiration.
3. Inspiratory capacity is the maximal volume of gas that can be inspired from the resting expiratory level.
4. Functional residual capacity is the volume of gas remaining in the lungs at the resting expiratory level. The resting end expiratory position is used here as a baseline because it varies less than the end inspiratory position.

(From *The Lung*, 2d ed., by Julius H. Comroe, Jr., et al. Copyright © 1962, Year Book Medical Publishers, Inc. Used by permission of Year Book Medical Publishers, Inc.)

Table 8.2	Lung Volumes in Healthy Recumbent Subjects (Approximate values in milliliters)

	Male Aged 20–30 1.7 M²	Male Aged 50–60 1.7 M²	Female Aged 20–30 1.6 M²
Inspired capacity	3600	2600	2400
Expiratory reserve volume	1200	1000	800
Vital capacity	4800	3600	3200
Residual volume (RV)	1200	2400	1000
Functional residual capacity	2400	3400	1800
Total lung capacity (TLC)	6000	6000	4200
RV/TLC × 100	20%	40%	24%

(From *The Lung*, 2d ed., by Julius H. Comroe, Jr., et al. Copyright © 1962, Year Book Medical Publishers, Inc. Used by permission of Year Book Medical Publishers, Inc.)

The nerve cells responsible for the automatic and rhythmic innervation of the muscles of respiration lie in the reticular formation of the medulla. As a group, these nerve cells are referred to as the respiratory center.* The best available evidence seems to indicate that this center possesses automatic rhythmicity, which would account for the phases of inspiration and expiration, with expiration being the result of inactivity of the respiratory center.

The breathing frequency (f) and depth (tidal volume or V_T) are adjusted to metabolic demands for oxygen by a complex of factors, some of which act directly upon the nerve cells of the respiratory center (chemosensitive cells of the medulla), and some of which operate reflexly through the aortic and carotid bodies, which are sensitive chemoreceptors. The most important factors are as follows.

Carbon Dioxide and Subsequent pH Changes

In resting humans, rises in arterial carbon dioxide tensions have been shown to be a very potent stimulant for the respiratory processes. Lambertsen and others (33) have shown that approximately 45% of this respiratory drive is due to the lowered pH brought about by the increased CO_2. The other 55% of respiratory drive may be caused by extravascular pH changes due to CO_2, or by direct action of the CO_2 itself. The effect of the CO_2 and pH factors seems to be mediated directly through chemosensitive receptors in the medulla.

---

*Evidence is accumulating that the respiratory center is probably not as discrete an entity as had been thought. However, for the purposes of this text, the term is useful and will be retained to eliminate unnecessary discussions of neurological concepts that are not yet completely elucidated.

Oxygen (Anoxia)

A low arterial level of oxygen has also been demonstrated to bring about greater ventilatory activity. However, it had been thought that the level of O_2 had to drop from a normal arterial partial pressure (PaO_2) of 100 mm Hg to about 60 mm Hg to have any effect. Hornbein and others (29) have shown that very small changes of 6 to 7 mm Hg are effective if they are sudden changes and also that, during exercise, responses are elicited by a drop in PaO_2 of 6 to 7 mm Hg. They suggest that this difference in response between the resting and exercise states may be due to increased sympathetic activity during exercise that decreases blood flow to the chemoreceptors of the carotid and aortic bodies where this reflex arises.

Proprioceptive Reflexes from Joints and Muscles

Considerable evidence exists that movement per se, independent of any other change, can have a reasonably large effect in bringing about the increased ventilation that occurs during exercise. This effect has been best demonstrated for the knee joint, but it undoubtedly is also operative at other joints and arises from receptors in the joints and muscle tissues. It has been shown (31) that not only can the afferents from stretch receptors elicit a ventilatory response but that even the nonmedullated C fibers can do so. However, the importance of neurogenic factors in general has been challenged by the work of Beaver and Wasserman (4), who have shown that the rise and fall of ventilation is not generally so precipitous as had been believed. Consequently, the neurogenic factor is no longer necessary to explain a response that was thought to be too rapid for other than a reflex mechanism. Further work in their laboratory (10) has shown that variation in bicycle pedaling rate produces no change in ventilatory response. This finding is, of course, inconsistent with any appreciable role for proprioceptive reflexes in the control of breathing during exercise.

Temperature

As body temperature goes up, the ventilation rate goes up in direct proportion. Since the body temperature rises from 1° to 5° F during exercise, this is one of the factors involved. However, it cannot be responsible for the early and large ventilatory response to exercise because the temperature rise requires too much time (twenty to thirty minutes for any appreciable increase). It may be noted, in passing, that respiration also drops in direct proportion to temperatures lower than normal, until death ensues from respiratory failure.

Cerebral Factors

An increase in the ventilation rate is frequently observed in anticipation of exercise before any of the aforementioned factors can have an effect. This increase is attributed to cerebral innervation aroused psychically in the forebrain.

Note that all of the above factors except cerebral activity are feedback mechanisms. It has also been shown that a *feedforward* mechanism can bring about a proportional driving of locomotion and respiration during exercise through stimulated activity in the "locomotor" region of the hypothalamus in cats (19). Most importantly, it was also shown that this mechanism operated when the animals were paralyzed, when no *feedback* mechanisms should have been in effect. While this system *could* bring about the necessary exercise hyperpnea, it seems likely that the feedback systems also contribute.

Control of respiratory activity is undoubtedly brought about by a combination of the above factors in complex interactions that have not yet been completely elucidated. An excellent review of this literature is available (15).

Obviously, the muscular movements of breathing are also under voluntary control. Rate and depth can be changed at will, and the breath can be held for varying periods of time.

It is also interesting to note that vibration of the human body—as occurs on trucks, tractors, and high-speed, low-flying aircraft—results in hyperventilation (increase over normal ventilation). Exactly how this hyperventilation is brought about is not yet known.

Importance of Breathing Pattern

Rate versus Depth

Lung ventilation rate (minute volume of breathing) is the result of two variable factors: *rate* and *depth,* or tidal volume (V_T). There are also two types of resistance to be overcome for the respiratory muscles: the *elastic resistance,* met in stretching the lungs and muscular and connective tissues of the thorax, and *airway resistance,* met by the movement of air flowing in through the small tubes of the lungs. The elastic resistance increases with increasing tidal volume for any given lung ventilation rate because the elastic tissues are stretched farther in deeper breathing. On the other hand, the airway resistance does not increase with rate or with depth if the minute volume of breathing is held constant. On the face of it then, it would seem to be more efficient to breathe at a high rate and shallow depth. However, this is not so because of the *anatomical dead space,* which is defined most simply as the volume of the conducting portion of the airways of the lung where no gas exchange occurs.

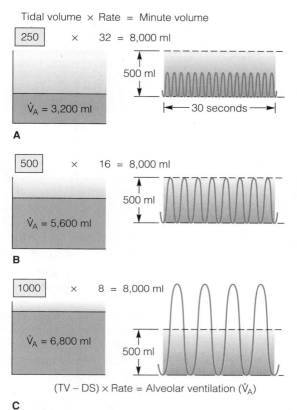

Figure 8.3   Area of each small block represents tidal volume (250, 500, or 1,000 ml). Total area of each large block (shaded and unshaded areas) = minute volume of ventilation; in each case it is 8,000 ml. Shaded area of each block represents volume of alveolar ventilation per minute; this varies in each case since Alveolar ventilation/ min = (Tidal volume − Dead space) × Frequency. A dead space of 150 ml is assumed in each case, although actually the dead space would increase somewhat with increasing tidal volume. *Right*, spirographic tracings. (From *The Lung*, 2nd edition, by Julius H. Comroe, Jr., et al. Copyright © 1962, Year Book Medical Publishers, Inc. Used by permission of Year Book Medical Publishers, Inc.)

Figure 8.3 illustrates how the anatomical dead space helps determine the optimum rate and tidal volume of breathing. It shows that although the minute volume is the same 8,000 ml and the dead space is 150 ml in all three cases, if the tidal volume is small and the rate is high (A), the dead-space air represents 4,800/8,000 of the total minute volume. In C, where the rate is low and the tidal volume is high, the dead-space air represents only 1,200/ 8,000 of the total minute volume.

The importance of the dead-space air is perhaps more evident if we consider the extreme case: where the dead-space air is 150 ml, the rate is increased and the depth decreased until the tidal volume is also 150 ml. In this case, of course, no real alveolar ventilation can occur because the dead-space air would simply be moved back and forth between conductive airways and the alveoli.

Thus it might be predicted that for each individual, with varying degrees of elastic resistance, airway resistance, and volume of dead space, an optimum rate and depth of breathing exists, and this has proven essentially true. In near maximal exercise the rate commonly adopted by the athlete (30 to 35 breaths per minute) is marginally more efficient than either slower or faster rates (46). This relatively slow breathing pattern probably minimizes the O_2 consumption of the chest muscles and is also most effective in terms of gas exchange. There is a close relationship between the maximum V_T in exercise and VC in healthy adults, as expressed in the following equation (30):

$$V_T \, max = 0.74 \, VC - 1.11$$

Under resting conditions, the rate of breathing varies considerably, from six or seven to twenty respirations per minute; during vigorous exercise, it may go as high as fifty to sixty per minute. The tidal volume is roughly 500 ml for an average man and may increase to approximately 2,500 ml in high-intensity, short-duration (two to three minutes) exercise. The total lung ventilation averages about 7.0 liters/min for healthy male adults at rest and may go up to 150 liters/min or more in heavy exercise.

Effect of Type of Exercise on Breathing Pattern

The fact that various sports activities result in considerably different respiratory responses is not surprising. To begin with, the rhythm of exercise is likely to affect the rhythm of breathing, even in such sports as running and cycling (5). In some sports such as swimming (crawl stroke), the rate of breathing is totally dictated by the stroke rhythm, and even tidal volume is probably constrained to some extent. In a comparison of running and swimming it has been shown that, at maximum effort, swimming resulted in a minute ventilation of 111 liters/min compared with 154 liters for maximal running. Since arterial O_2 saturation remained similar, better O_2 extraction must have compensated for the low ventilation in swimming (28).

Diaphragmatic versus Costal Breathing

At rest, there are apparently no major differences with respect to either gender or age in the relative contribution of the diaphragm and the intercostal muscles to the movement of the tidal volume (45). Most normal subjects are abdominal breathers when supine and thoracic when upright (18).

In moderate and heavy exercise tidal volume increases both in inspiratory and expiratory directions. Virtually all of the inspiratory increase is produced by the rib cage and most of the expiratory increase by the abdomen (diaphragm) (25). Physical education and singing instructors have often advised modification of costal breathing (chest) to abdominal breathing (greater use of the diaphragm). Campbell (9), after electromyographic research into the muscular activity of breathing, concluded that the activity pattern of the normal muscles of breathing (diaphragm and intercostals) is probably not changed by any of the breathing exercises advocated, even though externally observed movements of the thorax and abdomen may seem different. He feels, however, that the accessory muscles of breathing (abdominals and elevators of ribs) can be trained through breathing exercises but that their activity probably does not become an unconscious habit pattern. Thus a change in the breathing pattern would require constant voluntary control and attention.

Oral versus Nasal Breathing

It is surprising that such an obvious difference in breathing pattern as oral versus nasal breathing has received no attention until recently. As might be expected there is considerable variation among persons in breathing pattern, with most normal adults bringing about the oro-nasal-breathing-shift (ONBS) at 35 to 40 liters of ventilation (39, 42), while 13% to 16% breathed only through the mouth and 8% to 16% breathed only through the nose. The pattern did not appear to be related to either gender or nasal resistance (42), but was best related to the perceived exertion and to the nasal work of breathing (39). Further investigation is needed to determine the effect of breathing pattern on endurance.

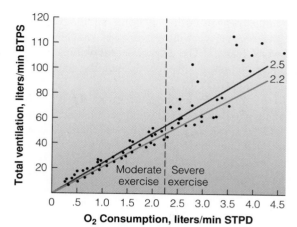

Figure 8.4   Ventilation as a function of O_2 consumption in physical exercise (walking, running, bicycling). The experimental points represent the means of 611 determinations in eighty-six subjects reported by eleven different authors. The straight lines correspond to ventilation equivalents for O_2 of 2.2 and 2.5 liters/min STPD. (From Gray, J. S. *Pulmonary Ventilation and Its Physiological Regulation*, 1950. Courtesy of Charles C. Thomas, Publisher, Springfield, Ill.)

Efficiency of Breathing

Lung Ventilation versus O_2 Consumption in Exercise

Between the resting state and a moderate level of exercise (approximately 2.0 liters of O_2 consumption), a very constant ratio of ventilation rate to O_2 consumption is maintained. This ratio is usually termed the *ventilation equivalent* and is defined as the number of liters of air breathed for every 100 ml of oxygen consumed. Thus at rest the ventilation equivalent (VE) is

$$\frac{7.0 \text{ liters air breathed/min}}{275 \text{ ml } O_2 \text{ uptake/min}} \text{ or}$$

$$\frac{7.0}{2.75 \text{ (hundred ml)}} = 2.54$$

This ratio also indicates that 25.4 liters of air must be respired to achieve an O_2 uptake of 1 liter:

$$\frac{7.0 \text{ liters}}{.275 \text{ liters}} = 25.4 \text{ liters.}$$

This ratio holds until the work load demands more than 2 liters of O_2 per minute, at which point the ratio grows higher. This relationship is shown in figure 8.4. The reason for the higher ventilation equivalent at the higher work loads is that the steady state is no longer maintained, and lactic acid accumulates that acts on the respiratory center through lowering the pH.

Oxygen Cost of Breathing

Under resting conditions, the muscular work done in breathing is relatively small. Probably not much more than 1% of the resting metabolism is devoted to this function. As exercise becomes vigorous, however, the oxygen cost of breathing increases disproportionately. Probably at a point between 150 and 250 liters of ventilation, the cost of moving the air takes all of the additional O_2 provided. However, this range of ventilation is seldom achieved in the normal ventilation of even the heaviest work loads. (The experimental values have been achieved through artificially contrived hyperventilation.)

One of the important factors in the physiology of athletic training is the increased efficiency of the breathing mechanics. The ventilation equivalent discussed above is smaller in conditioned athletes, meaning that less breathing work is required to maintain a given O_2 supply. It is quite likely that high efficiency of breathing (as measured by the VE) is a very important factor in such feats as the four-minute mile.

Improving Performance by Better Breathing

It is of practical interest that efficiency of lung ventilation apparently could be improved on theoretical bases (51) by changing the breathing pattern from the normal, which approximates a sine wave, to that approaching a square wave involving an end inspiratory pause. It has been shown in experiments on dogs that such a change in breathing pattern results in an increase in the arterial O_2 pressure of 9.5%, a decrease in arterial CO_2 of 8.2%, and 20.3% better alveolar ventilation (32). The only experimental evidence available on human subjects suggests that spontaneously chosen breathing patterns result in the most effective combination of O_2 transport and ventilation cost (19). However, this study included only the very lightest of exercise loads. This is an interesting area for further experimentation by scientifically inclined coaches. Acquiring such new breathing patterns would not be a simple matter, however.

Training Effects on Pulmonary Function

In a review of pulmonary adaptations to acute and chronic exercise (training), Dempsey and others (17) pointed out that neither they nor other investigators had been able to demonstrate a training effect on the lung tissue itself in terms of improved diffusion capacity.

However, it has long been known that the VE for O_2 under exercise conditions decreases as the result of training. But this improved efficiency in breathing is not the result of improvement in the lung tissue per se but rather of a reduced metabolic acidosis and thus a lower drive to increase ventilation.

Endurance training does appear to bring about important changes in the lung volumes and capacities. Bachman and Horvath (3) found significant decreases in functional residual capacity, residual volume, and the ratio of residual volume/total lung capacity in swimmers after four months of training. Controls and a similar group of wrestlers showed no significant changes. The swimmers also showed significantly increased vital capacity, which was the result of an increased inspiratory capacity. All of these changes would result in better alveolar ventilation and consequently should weigh in favor of improved athletic performance.

We now have evidence that respiratory muscle fatigue can lead to exercise limitations even in normal young subjects (41), but we also have evidence that the diaphragm and other respiratory muscles are trainable like other skeletal muscles (6, 34). Aerobic training or training directed to the diaphragm itself improves contractility and endurance (20), apparently the result of increasing the percentage of FT fatigue-resistant fibers and decreasing the percentage of FT fatiguable fibers. All fibers displayed increased mitochondrial density and oxidative capacity (21).

Genetic Effects on Respiratory Responses to Endurance Exercise

Endurance athletes compared to nonathletes have a decreased ventilatory response to hypoxia (low blood O_2 level) and to hypercapnia (high blood CO_2 level). Interestingly, the former is a genetic effect, but the latter is probably not (1, 44). In any event, the lesser sensitivity to the buildup of CO_2 acting in concert with the smaller amount of CO_2 produced in the muscle tissue (chap. 3) results in the significantly lower VE discussed above.

Respiratory Phenomena

Stitch in the Side

Frequently, in the course of making the respiratory adjustment to a heavy exercise load such as distance running, athletes experience a rather severe, sharp pain on the lower, lateral aspects of the thoracic wall. This pain has been called a "stitch in the side." No scientific evidence is available to explain its cause. Because it usually occurs during adjustment to new metabolic demands, it seems reasonable to postulate that ischemia of either the diaphragm or intercostal muscles is the cause. Ischemia of any skeletal muscle brings the sensation of pain.

Second Wind

"Second wind," familiar to most endurance athletes, is typified by the feeling of relief upon making the necessary metabolic adjustments to a heavy endurance load. Although it is not entirely, and probably not even mainly, a respiratory adjustment, it is treated under respiratory phenomena because the major manifestation to the athlete is the changeover from dyspnea (labored breathing, shortness of breath) to eupnea (normal breathing).

Again, very little scientific evidence can be brought to bear on this phenomenon. Close observation seems to indicate a discontinuity between the time of occurrence and cardiovascular adjustments. Furthermore, the respiratory adjustment is probably only a reflection (an effect rather than a cause) of metabolic adjustment to the exercise load. The most likely explanation seems to be one that invokes a change in skeletal muscular efficiency such as might be brought about by increasing muscle temperature.

Scharf and colleagues (43) measured the EMG response of the diaphragm to breathing against measured resistance. They found that at the point of second wind the EMG was reduced. They concluded this was the result of increased contractility of the diaphragm, which resulted in a lower neural drive (lower EMG) necessary to maintain the target breathing pattern. In any event they have provided evidence that this phenomenon is subject to experimental verification, and their method should lead to further research.

Exercise-Induced Asthma (EIA)

It is now a well-established fact that exercise can induce bronchoconstriction (asthma attack, or EIA) in asthmatics (24). There is probably also a significant number of people who have never experienced classic asthma but have some form of bronchospasm with exercise (8). However, physical educators and coaches should realize that the asthmatic, like the nonasthmatic, will benefit from regular aerobic exercise by improvements in cardiovascular-respiratory function, body composition, and in the size, number, and oxidative capacity of the mitochondria (35). The American Academy of Pediatrics has issued a position statement recommending that a child with asthma be advised to participate in school and recreational physical activity and sports programs with minimal restrictions.

The nature of the exercise programs appears to be of critical importance in reducing the frequency and severity of EIA. Swimming seems to be the best tolerated aerobic activity. This may be due to the usually higher ambient temperature and humidity (7), but not all investigators agree on this point (3). Considerable evidence suggests that intermittent exercise is much preferable to continuous, and continuous running may be the activity most likely to cause EIA (36). For the reader interested in asthma, an excellent review of the pertinent literature is available (35).

Unusual Respiratory Maneuvers

Hypoventilation

If lung ventilation is decreased, either voluntarily or involuntarily, without a corresponding decrease in metabolic rate, the reduction is called *hypoventilation.* It occurs only in abnormal situations, such as those involving airway obstruction. Because metabolism continues at a faster rate than lung ventilation, CO_2 accumulates and the arterial CO_2 must rise (hypercapnia).

Hyperventilation

The converse of hypoventilation is *hyperventilation,* in which the lung ventilation rate is greater than is needed for the existing metabolic rate. In this case, CO_2 is *blown off* faster than it is produced. Thus hyperventilation or forced breathing results in decreasing quantities of CO_2 in the circulorespiratory system. This lowering of blood CO_2 is called *hypocapnia.* Hyperventilation and hypocapnia are very interesting since they occur accidentally as the result of emotional excitement, particularly in the inexperienced athlete, or are brought about intentionally to increase breath-holding ability. It should be pointed out here that hyperventilation has no appreciable effect on O_2 values in the blood since blood is virtually saturated with O_2 when it leaves the lungs anyway.

That hyperventilation increases breath-holding time is shown by table 8.3, which illustrates an experiment by deVries on sixteen college men and women. One minute of hyperventilation more than doubled the mean breath-holding time. In light of the earlier discussion on the significance of the dead space, one can readily understand why hyperventilation is best performed by increasing the depth rather than the rate of breathing.

There is no doubt that hyperventilation can provide a significant advantage in competitive athletics wherever breath-holding time is a factor in overall performance. In swimming the crawl stroke, for example, turning the head away from the midline to breathe slows the sprint swimmer's time. Hyperventilation immediately before an event allows the swimmer to go farther before breathing becomes necessary.

A physical educator or coach will occasionally see an inexperienced person pass out immediately after completing a sprint run. If the subject's fingernails show cyanosis (blue color) and there is evidence of tetany (such as involuntary flexing of the fingers or toes), the faint may well have been caused by prolonged, unintentional hyperventilation brought on by emotional factors associated with the run (such as testing for grading purposes). In any event, the situation calls for medical attention to determine if the causes are more serious.

Individual variations in reaction to hyperventilation are illustrated by the symptoms listed in table 8.3. If overbreathing is done at a lesser depth, it can be continued for a longer period before symptoms become evident.

Breath-Holding

Many athletic events are performed with the breath held, notably swimming and track

Table 8.3   Seconds of Breath-holding with and without
             Hyperventilation* (Sitting at Rest)

Subject	Without Hyperventilation	10 Times in 30 Sec	20 Times in 60 Sec	Dizziness at	Other Symptoms
1	35	95	110	20 breaths	none
2	63	83	93	10	cyanosis of fingers
3	80	122	183	20	cyanosis of fingers
4	40	70	152	20	none
5	45	63	105	10	tension in fingers
6	65	125	160	10	cyanosis of fingers
7	45	80	120	20	none
8	63	108	153	20	none
9	90	135	120		none
10	80	180	140		none
11	35	55	80	10	none
12	55	95	120		cyanosis of fingers
13	55	105	145	20	cyanosis of fingers
14	105	150	195	20	tension, headache
15	120	150	160		finger perspiration
16	30	60	75		tension in gastrocnemius
mean	62.9	104.8	131.9		

*Hyperventilation achieved through increasing depth by using both inspiratory and expiratory reserve volumes.

sprints. The physiology of breath-holding involves respiratory, circulatory, and cardiac changes, all of which are important in the light of recent research. The most obvious changes when the breath is held are the increasing level of CO_2 and the decreasing level of O_2 in the alveolar air. These changes, of course, reflect the changes in the level of the respiratory gasses in the blood, the result of the continuing metabolism. You will recall that O_2 and CO_2 levels are involved in respiratory control, but the rising CO_2 level is more important in determining the length of time the breath can be held.

The maximum duration of a voluntary breath-hold is longer at high lung volumes than at low volumes. This is probably due to the inhibitory effect of lung inflation on respiratory motor neuron activity (48). The longest breath-hold is probably found at volumes close to TLC.

It has been shown by Craig and his associates (11, 13, 14) that when the partial pressure of CO_2 in the alveolar air exceeds approximately 50 mm Hg, the stimulus to breathe is so strong that the breath can no longer be held. This is called the *break point*, at which breathing recommences. It has, however, become common practice to hyperventilate in preparation for any event that requires breath-holding, and this procedure, since it allows athletes to start with a lower level of CO_2, also enables them to continue the breath-hold longer (table 8.3). As the breath-hold continues, lower levels of alveolar O_2 are reached because of the continuing consumption for metabolic needs. When the partial pressure of O_2 in the alveolar air has been reduced from its normal value (approximately 100 mm Hg) to 25 or 30 mm Hg, cerebral function is affected and consciousness is lost. Craig's work (11) indicates this may happen in underwater swimming at distances of 114 to 185 feet. Thus the combination of hyperventilation and subsequent underwater swimming constitutes a hazardous situation.

Craig has recently summarized fifty-eight cases of loss of consciousness during underwater swimming and diving in which twenty-three athletes died (12). His breath-holding experiments indicated that the time between loss of consciousness and death may be no longer than 2.5 minutes. Those responsible for aquatic safety must watch for swimmers who are practicing hyperventilation and underwater swimming in competition with themselves or with others.

Valsalva Maneuver

The Valsalva maneuver involves a deep inspiration that is followed by attempted expiration against a closed glottis. Its physiology was described in chapter 7.

Effects of Air Pollution on Respiration

Many different chemical entities pollute our urban environments. The major contaminants are 1) *particulate matter* (dusts, fumes, and mists of solid particles); 2) *carbon monoxide,* or CO, the result of incomplete combustion of hydrocarbons such as gasoline; 3) *hydrocarbons* from industrial plants, and so on; 4) *sulfur oxides,* which result from burning of fossil fuels such as coal; 5) *nitrogen oxides,* which are formed when most combustibles are burned because of the large fraction of nitrogen in air; 6) *ozone,* which is the result of the sun's action on nitrogen dioxide and certain hydrocarbons. Many other contaminants become important under certain specified and unusual circumstances.

Of greatest importance to us is ozone, because it is such a common and typical constituent of the upper atmosphere and because it is a toxic contaminant predominant in the smog of numerous urban areas. It is one of the most potent oxidizing agents in our atmosphere and can seriously disrupt biochemical and physiological functions through direct oxidative lesions in the respiratory tissues and blood.

Until recently, most experimentation with air pollutants had been carried out with exposure to varying levels of contaminant only at rest or light exercise. But the total exposure to ozone (O_3), for example, is related not only to its concentration in the air breathed but also to ventilation, which may increase by twenty times in heavy work or exercise. Thus the important question for us is, What is the effect of smog as measured by O_3 concentration on the exercising human?

Effect on Performance

One of the earlier studies on this problem showed that the performance of high school cross-country runners decreased with increasing concentrations of photochemical oxidants (smog) (50). The basis for these losses in endurance performance is probably a loss of aerobic capacity. It has been shown that exposure to ozone concentrations approximating peak ambient levels resulted in significant reductions of 10% in aerobic capacity accompanied by a 16% loss in maximum ventilation (22).

Toxicity

At rest, the short-term effects (less than twenty-four hours exposure) of the nitrogen oxides are mainly a loss in visual dark adaptation and increases in airway resistance. The effects of chronic exposure are more serious and include a lowered resistance to infection in the respiratory system, ciliary loss, alveolar cell disruption, and obstruction of respiratory bronchioles, at least in animal studies and quite probably in humans as well (38).

At an exercise in which normal young males were exposed to ozone concentrations below current smog-alert levels, all subjects clearly demonstrated some signs of toxicity while working at 45% to 65% of maximum $\dot{V}O_2$. The major ventilatory effects were a trend toward shallower breathing, leading to a 25% increase in breathing frequency and a 30% decrease in mean tidal volume. DeLucia and Adams (16) also showed distinct differences in individual sensitivity to ozone. Their two most sensitive subjects were unable to complete one hour at 65% maximum exercise.

Silverman and colleagues (47) have shown that ozone exposure at concentrations that may be encountered in some North American cities is associated with significant decrements in breathing function and that the addition of even light exercise increased these losses of function. They concluded that currently encountered ambient levels are too high and may provoke physiological responses even in healthy, normal individuals.

On the other hand, Hackney and his colleagues (26) have found that some human subjects seem to adapt to severe ambient ozone exposure, at least to the extent that obvious acute respiratory effects are prevented. Whether this is also true for the chronic effects of smog exposure is not yet known.

In any event, the only dose-response data available at the present time suggest that for subjects engaged in vigorous exercise, 0.30 ppm of ozone is an unacceptably high level of exposure (22). On the basis of these data, it appears that physical educators, coaches, and school administrators in urban areas exposed to smog would be well advised to set standards along these lines, followed by day-to-day monitoring of ozone level. Classes and team exercises involving vigorous activity should be discontinued, or activities should be made less vigorous, when ozone levels approach 0.30 ppm.

Smoking— Self-Induced Air Pollution

Although smoking has long been indicted as a cause of respiratory problems in athletes and has customarily been forbidden for members of athletic teams, the scientific evidence has been meager. Nadel and Comroe (37), in a well-controlled study, demonstrated that fifteen puffs of cigarette smoke in five minutes caused an average decrease in airway conductance of 31% in thirty-six normal subjects. This finding was highly significant and was found in both smokers and nonsmokers. Changes occurred as early as one minute after smoking began and lasted from ten to eighty minutes (mean was equal to thirty-five minutes). These investigators attributed the changes to inhalation of submicronic particles rather than nicotine or oxides of nitrogen.

In light of the earlier discussion on the cost and efficiency of breathing, it is readily seen that smoking, which can increase airway resistance by 31% under resting conditions, can be a very great detriment under conditions of maximum ventilation to an athlete.

Indeed, this increased resistance to breathing may usurp as much as 5% to 10% of the total O_2 supply at heavy exercise work loads such as those encountered in endurance-type athletic activities (40). This is one form of air pollution we can and should remove immediately. While other forms of air pollution are difficult to control, this self-induced air pollution is completely within our control.

Summary

1. The total respiratory process consists of three component functions: (a) gas exchange in the lungs, (b) gas transport to the tissues by the blood, and (c) gas exchange between the blood and the tissue fluids bathing the cells.

2. The lungs consist of two systems: (a) a conductive system, whose smallest components are the *terminal bronchioles,* and (b) a respiratory system, whose function is performed largely by the *alveoli.*

3. Air flow into and out of the lungs depends on differences of pressure between the ambient air and the air within the lung. This pressure gradient is brought about by the muscular activity of the diaphragm and intercostals in normal resting breathing.

4. Respiration during vigorous exercise brings accessory muscles into play. Inspiration is aided by action of the *sternomastoids* and *scalenes.* Expiration is aided by the abdominal group.

5. Respiratory control is brought about by the interaction of several factors, acting either directly or reflexly on the respiratory center in the medulla: (a) CO_2 rise and consequent pH depression; (b) anoxia; (c) proprioceptive reflexes from the joints and muscles; (d) body temperature rise; (e) cerebral factors; (f) Hering-Breuer reflexes.

6. Every individual has an optimal combination of rate and depth of breathing for greatest efficiency. In normal individuals, increases in depth are more effective because of the decreasing effect of the anatomical dead space as depth is increased.

7. Various types of athletic activity require considerably different breathing patterns. Where minute ventilation is restricted by the nature of the movement, as in swimming, better O_2 extraction appears to compensate.

8. Under steady-state conditions, approximately twenty-five liters of air are required to furnish one liter of O_2 to the tissues. The ratio goes even higher during overload conditions.

9. The work of breathing is relatively small at rest. Under vigorous exercise conditions, however, a point is reached at which all of the extra O_2 made available by increased breathing is necessary to supply the needs of the respiratory muscles.

10. Theoretical considerations suggest performance can be improved by optimizing the mechanics of breathing, but presently available evidence relating to application is meager.

11. Training results in more efficient breathing in that less ventilation is required per liter O_2 consumption. This appears to be more a matter of improving various lung volumes and capacities than of bringing about changes in the lung tissue per se.

12. Exercise commonly results in asthmatic attacks in asthmatics and on occasion in those who have no history of chronic asthma. In spite of this, the available evidence suggests that the benefits of physical fitness gained through appropriate exercise far outweigh the disadvantages.

13. *Hyperventilation* has important physiological advantages in increasing breath-holding time. On the other hand, every physical educator, coach, and athlete should be aware of its hazards.

14. The effects of air pollution upon respiration are well documented. Pollution significantly affects performance as well as health.

15. Scientific evidence indicates that smoking has a deleterious effect not only on the circulatory system but also on the respiratory system, and on performance as well as health.

References

1. Arkinstall, W. W., Nirmel, K., Klissouras, V., and Milic-Emili, J. Genetic differences in the ventilatory response to inhaled CO_2. *J. Appl. Physiol.* 36:6–11, 1974.

2. Bachman, J. C., and Horvath, S. M. Pulmonary function changes which accompany athletic conditioning programs. *Res. Q.* 39:235–39, 1968.

3. Bar-Yishay, E., Gur, I., Inbar, O., et al. Differences between swimming and running as stimuli for exercised induced asthma. *Eur. J. Appl. Physiol.* 48:387–97, 1982.

4. Beaver, W. L., and Wasserman, K. Transients in ventilation at start and end of exercise. *J. Appl. Physiol.* 25:390–99, 1968.

5. Bechbache, V., Bechbache, R. R., and Duffin, J. The entrainment of breathing frequency by exercise rhythm. *J. Physiol.* 272:553–61, 1977.

6. Bradley, M. E., and Leith, D. E. Ventilatory muscle training and the oxygen cost of sustained hyperpnea. *J. Appl. Physiol.* 45:885–92, 1978.

7. Bundgaard, A., Schmidt, A., Ingemann-Hansen, T., et al. Exercise induced asthma after swimming and bicycle exercise. *Eur. J. Respir. Dis.* 63:245–48, 1982.

8. Burton, R. M. Exercise-induced asthma in cold weather. *Physician and Sportmed.* Sept. 1981, pp. 131–32.

9. Campbell, E. J. M. *The Respiratory Muscles and the Mechanics of Breathing*. Chicago: Year Book Medical Publishers, 1958.

10. Casaburi, R., Whipp, B. J., Wasserman, K., and Koyal, S. N. Ventilatory and gas exchange responses to cycling with sinusoidally varying pedal rate. *J. Appl. Physiol.* 44:97–103, 1978.

11. Craig, A. B., Jr. Causes of loss of consciousness during underwater swimming. *J. Appl. Physiol.* 16:583–86, 1961.

12. ———. Summary of 58 cases of loss of consciousness during underwater swimming and diving. *Med. Sci. Sports* 8:171–75, 1976.

13. Craig, A. B., Jr., and Babcock, S. A. Alveolar CO_2 during breath-holding and exercise. *J. Appl. Physiol.* 17:874–76, 1962.

14. Craig, A. B., Jr., Halstead, L. S., Schmidt, G. H., and Schnier, B. R. Influences of exercise and oxygen on breath-holding. *J. Appl. Physiol.* 17:225–27, 1962.

15. Davis, J. A. Symposium on ventilatory control during exercise. *Med. Sci. Sports* 11:190, 1979.

16. DeLucia, A. J., and Adams, W. C. Effects of O_3 inhalation during exercise on pulmonary function and blood biochemistry. *J. Appl. Physiol.* 43:75–81, 1977.

17. Dempsey, J. A., Gledhill, N., Reddan, W. G., Forster, H. V., Hanson, P. G., and Claremont, A. D. Pulmonary adaptation to exercise: Effects of exercise type and duration, chronic hypoxia and physical training. *Ann. N.Y. Acad. Sci.* 301:243–61, 1977.

18. Druz, W. S., and Sharp, J. T. Activity of respiratory muscles in upright and recumbent humans. *J. Appl. Physiol.* 51:1552–61, 1981.

19. Eldridge, F. L., Millhorn, D. E., and Waldrop, T. G. Exercise hyperpnea and locomotion: Parallel activation from the hypothalamus. *Science* 211:844–46, 1981.

20. Farrell, P. A. Maximum expiratory flow-volume relationship before and after eight weeks of endurance testing. *J. Sports Med. Phys. Fit.* 21:145–49, 1981.

21. Faulkner, J. A., Maxwell, L. C., Ruff, G. L., and White, T. P. The diaphragm as a muscle. *Am. Rev. Resp. Dis.* 119:89–92, 1979.

22. Folinsbee, L. J., Drinkwater, B. L., Bedi, J. F., and Horvath, S. M. The influence of exercise on the pulmonary function changes due to exposure to low concentrations of ozone. *Environmental Stress: Individual Human Adaptations,* eds. L.J. Folinsbee et al. New York: Academic Press, 1978.

23. Folinsbee, L. J., Silverman, F., and Shephard, R. J. Decrease of maximum work performance following ozone exposure. *J. Appl. Physiol.* 42:531–36, 1977.

24. Freedman, S., Tattersfield, A. E., and Pride, N. B. Changes in lung mechanics during asthma induced by exercise. *J. Appl. Physiol.* 38:974–82, 1975.

25. Grimby, G., Bunn, J., and Mead, J. Relative contributions of rib cage and abdomen to ventilation during exercise. *J. Appl. Physiol.* 24:159–66, 1968.

26. Hackney, J. D., Linn, W. S., Mohler, J. G., and Collier, C. R. Adaptation to short-term respiratory effects of ozone in men exposed repeatedly. *J. Appl. Physiol.* 43:82–85, 1977.

27. Hanson, P. G., Lin, K. H., and McIlroy, M. B. Influence of breathing pattern on oxygen exchange during hypoxia and exercise. *J. Appl. Physiol.* 38:1062–66, 1975.

28. Holmer, I., Stein, E. M., Saltin, B., Ekblom, B., and Astrand, P-O. Hemodynamic and respiratory responses compared in swimming and running. *J. Appl. Physiol.* 37:49–54, 1974.

29. Hornbein, T. F., Roos, A., and Griffo, Z. J. Transient effect of sudden mild hypoxia on respiration. *J. Appl. Physiol.* 16:11–14, 1961.

30. Jones, N. L. Dyspnea in exercise. *Med. Sci. Sports Exer.* 16:14–19, 1984.

31. Kalia, M., Senapati, J. M., Parida, B., and Panda, A. Reflex increase in ventilation by muscle receptors with nonmedullated fibers (C fibers). *J. Appl. Physiol.* 32:189–93, 1972.

32. Knelson, J. H., Howatt, W. F., and DeMuth, G. R. Effect of respiratory pattern on alveolar gas exchange. *J. Appl. Physiol.* 29:328–31, 1970.

33. Lambertsen, C. J., Semple, S. J. G., Smyth, M. G., and Gelfand, R. H+ and pCO_2 as chemical factors in respiratory and cerebral circulatory control. *J. Appl. Physiol.* 16:473–84, 1961.

34. Leith, D. E., and Bradley, M. Ventilatory muscle strength and endurance training. *J. Appl. Physiol.* 41:508–16, 1976.

35. Morton, A. R., Fitch, K. D., and Hahn, A. G. Physical activity and the asthmatic. *Physician and Sportsmed.* 9:51–64, 1981.

36. Morton, A. R., Hahn, A. G., and Fitch, K. D. Continuous and intermittent running in the provocation of asthma. *Ann. Allergy* 48:123–29, 1982.

37. Nadel, J. A., and Comroe, J. H., Jr. Acute effects of inhalation of cigaret smoke on airway conductance. *J. Appl. Physiol.* 16:713–16, 1961.

38. National Academy of Sciences. *Medical and Biological Effects of Environmental Pollutants: Nitrogen Oxides.* Washington D.C.: The Academy, 1977.

39. Niinimaa, V., Cole, P., Mihitz, S., and Shephard, R. J. The switching point from nasal to oronasal breathing. *Respir. Physiol.* 42:61–71, 1980.

40. Rode, A., and Shephard, R. J. The influence of cigarette smoking upon the oxygen cost of breathing in near maximal exercise. *Med. Sci. Sports* 3:51–55, 1971.

41. Roussos, C. S., and Macklem, P. T. Diaphragmatic fatigue in man. *J. Appl. Physiol.* 43:189–97, 1977.

42. Saibene, F., Mognoni, C. L., LaFortuna, L., and Mostardi, R. Oronasal breathing during exercise. *Pfluegers Arch.* 378:65–69, 1978.

43. Scharf, S. M., Bark, H., Heimer, D., Cohen, A., and Macklem, P. T. "Second wind" during inspiratory loading. *Med. Sci. Sports Exer.* 16:87–91, 1984.

44. Scoggin, C. H., Doekel, R. D., Kryger, M. H., Zwillich, C. W., and Weil, J. V. Familial aspects of decreased hypoxic drive in endurance athletes. *J. Appl. Physiol.* 44:464–68, 1978.

45. Sharp, J. T., Goldberg, N. B., Druz, W. S., and Danon, J. Relative contributions of rib cage and abdomen to breathing in normal subjects. *J. Appl. Physiol.* 39:608–18, 1975.

46. Shephard, R. J., and Bar-Or, O. Alveolar ventilation in near-maximum exercise. *Med. Sci. Sports* 2:83–92, 1970.

47. Silverman, F., Folinsbee, L. J., Barnard, J., and Shephard, R. J. Pulmonary function changes in ozone-interaction of concentration and ventilation. *J. Appl. Physiol.* 41:859–64, 1976.

48. Stanley, N. N., Altose, M. D., Kelsen, S. G., Ward, C. F., and Cherniak, N. S. Changing effect of lung volume on respiratory drive in man. *J. Appl. Physiol.* 38:768–73, 1975.

49. Sutton, J. R., and Jones, N. L. Control of pulmonary ventilation during exercise and mediators in the blood: CO_2 and hydrogen ion. *Med. Sci. Sports* 11:198–203, 1979.

50. Wayne, W. S., and Wehrle, P. F. Oxidant air pollution and school absenteeism. *Arch. Environ. Health* 19:315–22, 1969.

51. Yamashiro, S. M., and Grodins, F. S. Optimal regulation of respiratory airflow. *J. Appl. Physiol.* 30:597–602, 1971.

9

Gas Transport and Internal Respiration

Properties of Gasses and Liquids
    Composition of Respiratory Gasses
    Acids, Bases, and pH
Gas Transport by the Blood
    Oxygen
    Carbon Dioxide
Internal Respiration
    O_2 Dissociation Curve
    Coefficient of O_2 Utilization
Regulation of Acid-Base Balance
    Buffer Systems
    Physiological Regulation of Acid-
    Base Balance

Acid-Base Balance as a Factor Limiting
    Performance
Changes in Lung Diffusion in Exercise
Use of Oxygen to Improve Performance
    O_2 before Exercise
    O_2 during Exercise
    O_2 during Recovery
What Sets the Limits of Aerobic Power?

Thus far we have discussed the mechanical factors involved in breathing and their physiological controls. We will now consider the processes that are necessary for bringing about the ultimate goal of tissue respiration. Three processes intervene between lung ventilation and actual tissue respiration: 1) diffusion of O_2 across two very thin membranes—the wall of the alveolus and the wall of the capillary; 2) transport of O_2 via the blood to the capillary bed of the active tissues; 3) diffusion of O_2 across the capillary wall to the tissue fluids that bathe the actual consumers, the metabolizing cells. As O_2 is unloaded from the blood, CO_2 is being taken on for the return trip to the right heart and back to the lungs.

At this point we must consider the nature of the diffusion process and some of the laws that govern it. Recall that fluids flow from point to point only because of differences in pressure called *pressure gradients*. This is equally true for gasses. For this reason physiologists usually refer to respiratory gasses in terms of pressure rather than in terms of concentration (percentage, and so on).

Table 9.1 gives percentages and approximate pressures of O_2 exerted in a standard atmosphere. Note that the percentage concentration of O_2 is the same at 40,000 feet as it is at sea level. However, since one becomes unconscious in a matter of seconds at 40,000 feet altitude due to lack of O_2, it is obvious that percentage has little meaning in this situation. The atmospheric pressure of O_2, on the other hand, tells the story rather well.

Properties of Gasses and Liquids

Basic to all gas laws is the molecular theory that all gasses are composed of molecules that are constantly in motion at very high velocities. A gas has no definite shape or volume and conforms to the shape and volume of its container. Its pressure is the result of the constant impact of its many molecules upon the walls of the container. Obviously, the pressure of a gas is increased by confining it in a smaller volume or by increasing the activity of each molecule. Because a rise in temperature increases the velocity of molecular movement, heat increases pressure.

Liquids, on the other hand, are composed of molecules that are much closer together. This closeness results in their having a definite, independent volume that varies little with temperature or with the size and shape of the container.

For the student to understand respiratory physiology (a very important part of exercise physiology), knowledge of the laws that govern behavior of gasses is essential.

Boyle's Law
Boyle's law states that if temperature remains constant, the pressure of a gas varies inversely with its volume. If, for example, we decrease the volume by one-half, the pressure will be doubled.

Gay-Lussac's Law
Gay-Lussac's law states that if its volume remains constant, the pressure of a gas increases directly in proportion to its (absolute) temperature.

Law of Partial Pressures
According to the law of partial pressures, in a mixture of gasses, each gas exerts a *partial pressure* proportional to its concentration. Thus in atmospheric air with a total pressure of 760 mm Hg, O_2—which makes up 20.93%—has a partial pressure of 159 mm Hg: $20.93/100 \times 760$ mm Hg $= 159$ mm Hg.

Table 9.1	Percentage and Partial Pressures of O_2 by Altitude		
Altitude	Atmospheric Pressure (mm Hg)	Percent O_2	Approximate Pressure Exerted by O_2 in the Atmosphere (mm Hg)
Sea level	760	20.93	159
10,000	523	20.93	109
20,000	349	20.93	73
30,000	226	20.93	47
40,000	141	20.93	29

Henry's Law

Henry's law states that the quantity of a gas that will dissolve in a liquid is directly proportional to its partial pressure, if temperature remains constant.

Composition of Respiratory Gasses

The atmospheric air is composed mainly of nitrogen (N_2), oxygen (O_2), and carbon dioxide (CO_2). There are also rare gasses (such as argon and krypton), but these are ordinarily lumped together and included with the nitrogen fraction.

Table 9.2 illustrates the salient features of the respiratory gas exchange. It will be noted that the partial pressures of dry atmospheric air are proportional to the percentages as per the law of partial pressures. However, the alveolar air is saturated with water vapor, which contributes a partial pressure of 47 mm Hg at body temperature. The partial pressure of O_2 in the lungs, then, would be 20.93% of 713 $(760 - 47)$ mm, or approximately 149 mm Hg—if we could completely exchange the air in the lungs. This, of course, is impossible because alveolar air in the lungs is a mixture of atmospheric air with air that has already participated in the respiratory exchange. For this reason, note in table 9.2 that the actual partial

pressure of O_2 in the alveolar air is 100 mm instead of the 149 mm that would be present if there were no dead space and if the lung collapsed to empty itself completely at each breath.

The importance of all this lies in the *diffusion gradients* for O_2 and CO_2 that, after all, ultimately determine the amount of gaseous exchange taking place. The diffusion gradient for O_2 is some 60 mm Hg, for CO_2 only 5 to 6 mm Hg. Since these figures are based on normal, healthy individuals, the diffusion gradient for CO_2 is obviously sufficient to maintain the necessary homeostatic relations for CO_2 levels. This can be explained by the fact that diffusion of gasses across a membrane depends not only on the gradient but also on the ease with which a particular gas can penetrate the membrane. This, in turn, depends on the solubility of the gas in the membrane (largely water). The fact that the solubility of CO_2 in water is some twenty or more times that of O_2 explains the need for a greater diffusion gradient for O_2.

Acids, Bases, and pH

Acids can be defined as compounds that yield positively charged hydrogen ions (H^+) in solution. Conversely, bases can be defined as compounds that yield negatively charged hydroxyl ions (OH^-) in solution. pH, which is the

Gas	Percent in Dry Atmosphere	Partial Pressure in Dry Atmosphere	Partial Pressure in Alveolar Air	Partial Pressure in Mixed Venous Blood	Diffusion Gradient
Total	100	760	760	705	
H_2O	0	0	47	47	
O_2	20.93	159	100	40	60
CO_2	0.03	0.2	40	45	5
N_2	79.04	600.8	573	573	

Table 9.2   Composition of Atmospheric Air and the Consequent Partial Pressures of Respiratory Gasses

negative logarithm of the hydrogen ion concentration in gram molecular weight, is a very convenient yardstick for measuring and describing degrees of acidity or alkalinity. This may be visualized as follows:

Strongest Acid   Strongest Base

← Increasing Acidity   Neutrality   Increasing Alkalinity →

pH = 1   2   3   4   5   6   7   8   9   10   11   12   13   14

Since this is a logarithmic scale, a very small change of pH makes a considerable change in acidity or alkalinity. Therefore pH is given to at least one and usually two decimal places. For example, the extreme fluctuations of the pH of normal blood lie within pH values of 7.30 to 7.50. The extreme values in illness have been known to go as low as 6.95 and as high as 7.80. However, in healthy subjects, recent work has shown (12) that surprisingly low values (down to 6.80) can result from heavy anaerobic exercise. Such *short-term* pH changes appeared to be well tolerated in *healthy subjects*. For a more complete treatment of pH and acid-base balance, the student is referred to a text in physiological chemistry.

Gas Transport by the Blood

Oxygen

Although chemical analyses have demonstrated that blood is capable of carrying only about 0.2 volume percent of O_2 (0.2 ml of O_2 per 100 ml of blood) in solution at normal atmospheric pressures, it actually transports 20 volume percent of O_2, 100 times as much as will dissolve in physical solution.

The reason for this great discrepancy is the presence of hemoglobin in the erythrocytes. Hemoglobin is an iron-bearing pigment, consisting of *heme* (which contains iron) and *globin* (which is a protein). Hemoglobin has the unique characteristic of combining with O_2 quickly and reversibly and without requiring help from enzyme reactions. This is not true of typical oxidation reactions in which the O_2, once combined, is separated only with difficulty. Therefore the term *oxygenation,* rather than *oxidation,* is used for the process and the reaction can be described thus:

Hemoglobin + Oxygen $\rightleftharpoons$ Oxyhemoglobin
Hb   + O_2 $\rightleftharpoons$ HbO_2

As is the case with all reversible reactions, if the end product on the right, HbO_2, is constantly removed, as in the lungs where oxygenated blood moves off to the tissues, the reaction continues to proceed from left to right. On the other hand, in the tissue exchange the O_2 is carried off by tissue fluids to the cells, and the reaction proceeds to the left.

If the organism depended on dissolved O_2, an all-out effort by the cardiovascular and respiratory systems could not meet the O_2 needs of the resting metabolism, let alone the metabolism of exercise.

Carbon Dioxide

CO_2, which is the constant end product of metabolism in the cell, diffuses across the cell membrane into the tissue fluid, thence across the capillary wall into the blood plasma where a small portion of it is transported. The larger proportion, probably 90% to 95%, diffuses from the plasma into the erythrocytes. It is transported by the erythrocyte in three forms: 1) in combination with hemoglobin as carbaminohemoglobin; 2) as bicarbonate, HCO_3; and 3) as dissolved CO_2, a portion of which ionizes into carbonic acid, H_2CO_3.

The exchange of CO_2, at the lungs and at the tissues, involves the following reversible reaction.

$$\text{In the Lungs} \rightarrow$$
$$HCO_3^- + H^+ \rightleftharpoons H_2CO_3 \rightleftharpoons H_2O + CO_2$$
$$\leftarrow \text{In the Tissues}$$

This is ordinarily a slow reaction. However, an enzyme, *carbonic anhydrase,* catalyzes these reactions so that they can go to completion before the blood leaves the lung or tissue capillaries.

Internal Respiration

Much of the story concerning internal respiration, or gas exchange in the tissues, has already been told. Two other factors, however, are basic to an understanding of the respiratory exchange.

O_2 Dissociation Curve

It is an interesting biochemical fact that the loading of CO_2 into the blood at the tissues considerably aids the unloading of O_2 from blood to tissues. The reverse is also true in the lungs: the unloading of CO_2 in the lungs aids the loading of O_2 into the blood.

These facts are best illustrated by the O_2 dissociation curve (fig. 9.1). If one places a straightedge vertically along the line representing a partial pressure of O_2 of 30 mm Hg (that of the tissues), the difference in hemoglobin saturation level between the points where the 40 mm CO_2 curve (blood CO_2 level) and the 80 mm CO_2 curve (active tissue level) cross this vertical line represents the difference of O_2 that the hemoglobin can hold.

This amount of O_2—in this case from approximately 58% to approximately 42% (16%)—is driven off by changing CO_2 levels in the tissues. In other words, increasing the CO_2 level of the blood from its arterialized level of 40 mm Hg to 80 mm Hg, which probably represents the temporary local changes in blood level at the tissues, results in driving off 16% of the total O_2 load.

Another point regarding the O_2 dissociation curve is of very practical interest in regard to the effect of altitude on human respiration.

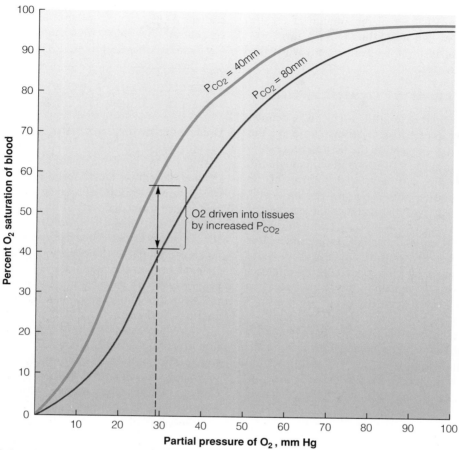

Figure 9.1   The oxygen dissociation curve for human blood. (Drawn from the data of J. W. Severinghaus, in *Journal of Applied Physiology* 21:1108, 1966; and R. M. Winslow et al., *Journal of Applied Physiology* 45:289, 1978.)

Note that the curve for 40 mm of CO_2, which represents the mixed venous blood (typical of the body as a whole but not of any localized tissue site), is not very steep from 100 mm to approximately 60 mm of O_2 partial pressure. The upper figure is typical of alveolar O_2 tension at sea level. The lower figure represents alveolar O_2 tension at about 15,000 to 16,000 feet above sea level, the level at which resting humans (pilots and others) begin showing serious symptoms due to the lack of O_2. (Military regulations require the use of oxygen above 10,000 feet to provide a safety margin that allows for individual variance.) If this O_2 dissociation curve were a straight diagonal line, physical impairment would probably commence at about 90 mm of O_2 tension instead of at 60 mm, or at an altitude of about 6,000 feet.

Another salient feature of the O_2 dissociation curve is that it is steep (close to vertical) when the partial pressures of O_2 are low. This means, of course, that small changes in partial pressure of O_2 on this part of the curve make large changes in the amount of O_2 the hemoglobin can hold, thus making large exchanges of respiratory gas efficient when the need is greatest.

Coefficient of O_2 Utilization

The coefficient of O_2 utilization can be defined as the proportion of O_2 transported by the blood that is given off to the tissues. Since 99% of the transported O_2 is bound to hemoglobin, this story also can be related in terms of the O_2 dissociation curve. During resting conditions at sea level, the hemoglobin leaving the lungs is at least 95% saturated with O_2. After leaving the capillary bed of resting tissue, it is still at least 70% saturated. (In figure 9.1, use the 40 mm CO_2 curve and note its intersections at the 100 mm and the 40 mm O_2 tension lines.) Thus the hemoglobin has given off 23/98 of its O_2, or 23%, in resting conditions.

In exercise, this situation becomes much more favorable. The hemoglobin leaving the lungs is still approximately 95% saturated, but after leaving active muscle tissue it may approach zero saturation. Thus the coefficient of oxygen utilization may increase from three to four times in exercise. It should be repeated that this increase is facilitated by the steepness of the O_2 dissociation curve at the lower O_2 tensions (as was mentioned before).

At this point it may be well to note the combination of factors that contribute to supplying the increased oxygen demands of exercising muscle tissue. First, recall that cardiac output can increase about six times its resting value. Second, in combination with an increased utilization coefficient of three to four times, this means a possible increase of at least eighteen times the resting value. Third, in respect to the local situation at any given active muscle, this may be multiplied by another factor of two, due to the approximate doubling of the number of open capillaries (discussed

earlier). Thus a total increase of at least thirty-six times the resting oxygen supply is possible at any active muscle group.

Regulation of Acid-Base Balance

Even under resting conditions, the acid-base equilibrium of the body fluids is constantly challenged by the formation of CO_2 as the end product of cellular metabolism. Furthermore, when exercise work loads become severe, lactic acid is also formed, constituting an additional influence that tends to drive pH downward. Illness brings about other acidifying or alkalinizing influences. Because long-term pH changes beyond the range of 7.30 to 7.50 are inconsistent with good health, it is obvious that the human organism must be able to control acid-base balance.

Two processes are involved in this. The first line of defense against pH changes is the combination of three *buffer systems* that serve to absorb the shock, as it were, of sudden changes. Ultimately, however, *physiological changes* have to be brought about to maintain the organism in homeostasis over the longer period of time, and these physiological changes mainly involve the lungs and the kidneys.

Buffer Systems

A buffer system consists of a weak acid and a salt of that acid. The system functions as follows.

HL	$NaHCO_3$		NaL	H_2CO_3
Lactic +	Sodium	→	Sodium +	Carbonic
acid	bicarbonate		lactate	acid

In this schema, lactic acid (a relatively strong acid) combines with sodium bicarbonate (salt of a weak acid) to form sodium lactate (which no longer has acid tendencies) and carbonic acid (which is a very weak acid). Thus a strong

Table 9.3	Effect of Buffering in Combating Acidifying Effect of Adding Hydrochloric Acid to a Solution			
HCl (gm) Added	Buffer Ratio $H_2CO_3/$ $NaHCO_3$	H^+ Concentration	pH	Relative Acidity
0	2.27:11.9	0.000000057N	7.24	.57
10	2.27:11.5	0.000000059	7.23	.59
50	2.27:10.0	0.000000068	7.13	.68
100	2.27: 8.2	0.000000083	7.08	.83
150	2.27: 6.3	0.000000108	6.97	1.08
200	2.27: 4.4	0.000000154	6.81	1.54
250	2.27: 2.6	0.000000260	6.59	2.60
300	2.27:0.68	0.000001000	6.00	10.
310	2.27:0.31	0.000002200	5.66	22.
318		0.000260000	3.59	260.
320		0.000450000	3.35	450.
330		0.002700000	2.57	2,700.

Based on data from L. J. Henderson in C. H. Best and N. B. Taylor, *The Physiological Basis of Medical Practice,* 1943, p. 170. Courtesy of Williams & Wilkins Company, Baltimore.

acid has been exchanged for a weak acid, and the tendency for the lactic acid to lower the pH of the blood has been greatly lessened by the buffering action of the carbonic acid bicarbonate system.

Table 9.3 illustrates what happens when a strong acid, HCl, is added to a water solution that contains the bicarbonate buffer system. Note that when the ratio of H_2CO_3 and $NaHCO_3$ is favorable (about 1:5), the addition of the first 10 gm of acid brings about almost no change in relative acidity or pH. When the buffer ratio becomes less favorable, however, the addition of the same quantity of acid (300–310 gm) more than doubles the relative acidity, and the pH changes from 6.00 downward to 5.66. When the bicarbonate is used up, there is no longer any buffering, and the addition of 10 gm of HCl (bringing the HCl from 320 to 330 gm) brings about a *sixfold* increase in relative acidity and, of course, a much larger drop in pH. The effectiveness of the buffer system depends on the ratio of the acid to the salt.

Blood must now be considered as two fluids that need buffering: the plasma and the fluid within the erythrocytes. In the plasma, the acids to be buffered are largely *fixed acids,* so called because they are not subject to rapid excretion. They are, in general, stronger acids, such as hydrochloric, phosphoric, sulfuric, and lactic acids (the stronger acids occur in very small quantities). The most important buffers in the plasma are

$$\frac{H_2CO_3}{NaHCO_3} \quad \text{and} \quad \frac{H \text{ protein}}{Na \text{ proteinate}}$$

The blood proteins can act as buffer systems because, at the pH of blood, they behave as weak acids and react with the base to form a salt. In the intracellular fluids of the erythrocytes, on the other hand, the major acid to be buffered is the carbonic acid that results from the respiratory exchange. The buffer systems mainly responsible for this are hemoglobin and oxyhemoglobin, each of which can act as a weak acid or as a potassium salt as follows:

$$\frac{H\ Hb\ O_2}{K\ Hb\ O_2} \quad \text{and} \quad \frac{H\ Hb}{K\ Hb}$$

Oxyhemoglobin   Hemoglobin
system   system

There are also other, less important buffer systems in both plasma and cells, such as the acid and basic sodium and potassium phosphates.

Physiological Regulation of Acid-Base Balance

Although the buffering systems can resist fast changes in pH, a change does occur with the addition of an acid (or base) to the body fluids (table 9.3). These changes are corrected by two physiological mechanisms for excretion of the acid (or base): changes in respiratory function and changes in kidney function.

The function of the lungs in regulating acid-base balance is another example of the body's servomechanisms. For example, if the breath is held, the CO_2 resulting from metabolism accumulates. This has the effect of pouring acid into the tissue fluids and blood: $CO_2 + H_2O \rightarrow H_2CO_3$. This decrease in pH is interpreted as the *error signal* by the respiratory center in the medulla, which corrects the situation by increasing the rate and depth of ventilation (if possible). When the breath is held, the error signal simply grows larger and larger, until the urge to breathe overcomes the willpower to hold the breath. The rate and depth will then be greater than normal until equilibrium has been reestablished by *blowing off* more CO_2 than is being formed: $H_2CO_3 \rightarrow CO_2 + H_2O$.

Thus the importance of the respiratory function in acid-base regulation lies in the fact that the decomposition products of carbonic acid are volatile and can be readily blown off by the lungs.

In hyperventilation, on the other hand, more CO_2 is blown off than is formed, bringing about a change in the ratio of H_2CO_3 to $NaHCO_3$. The normal ratio is 1:20. If H_2CO_3 and $NaHCO_3$ are increased or decreased proportionately, the ratio does not change and consequently there is no change in pH. In the case of hyperventilation, however, the H_2CO_3 decreases disproportionately because the $NaHCO_3$ remains the same. Thus a relative increase in the base occurs with a rise in pH.

If the hyperventilation is of short duration—as in preparing for an athletic event—the increased production of CO_2 during the event corrects the situation. But if hyperventilation is long-term (one hour or more), as in fever, a secondary adjustment must be made to excrete some of the bicarbonate to keep the ratio close to 1:20. This excretion of bicarbonate is done through the kidney.

The last line of defense and the one concerned with long-term changes in acid-base equilibrium is the excretion of abnormal amounts of acid or base by the kidney to maintain all the buffer systems at the proper acid-salt ratio for maintaining normal pH. When it is no longer possible to maintain these ratios, acidosis or alkalosis ensues. In severe acidosis, death ensues as a result of coma. In severe alkalosis, death may be brought about by tetany and the resulting muscle spasm of respiratory muscles.

Acid-Base Balance as a Factor Limiting Performance

The preceding discussion makes it obvious that metabolism in general provides a constant acidifying influence. When the metabolic rate is raised to seven or eight times that of the resting level, the increase in CO_2 is proportional, but ventilation can usually keep pace to maintain acid-base equilibrium. However, when the work load goes beyond aerobic capacity, lactic acid becomes the end product of metabolism, instead of CO_2. This is a much stronger acid, and it cannot be excreted quickly by respiration as can the CO_2. It has already been pointed out that under conditions of heavy anaerobic exercise the pH can drop as low as 6.80 (14).

This line of reasoning seems to indicate that the body's ability to buffer fixed acids (such as lactic acid) plays a large part in determining the end point of anaerobic activity. There is evidence that this is indeed the case (7). See chapter 30 for further discussion. Because these fixed acids are largely buffered by the bicarbonate system, the combining power of the plasma bicarbonate has been referred to as the *alkaline reserve*. Although this concept rests on a reasonably sound rationale, it is an oversimplification of the complex biochemical interactions involved in acid-base regulation.

Changes in Lung Diffusion in Exercise

The diffusion of oxygen from the alveoli to the pulmonary capillaries increases in virtually direct proportion to the effort involved in the exercise, as measured by O_2 consumption. This relationship has been demonstrated to a level at least seven or eight times that of the resting metabolism (21). In the absence of disease processes, it is very unlikely that pulmonary diffusing capacity for O_2 is a limiting factor in exercise.

The reasons for increased pulmonary diffusion are not yet completely understood, but the increased ventilation of exercise does not seem to be a necessary factor. It has been shown that similar increases in pulmonary diffusion can occur during exercise when the ventilation is voluntarily held to resting levels (16). It seems most likely that the increase in pulmonary diffusion is the result of increased pulmonary capillary blood volume during exercise brought about by the opening of previously unopened capillaries—as discussed in the chapter on circulation (chap. 7).

There is evidence that highly trained athletes demonstrate better pulmonary diffusion under maximal (13) and submaximal work rates (2) than do nonathletes. This effect may be an innate, inherited characteristic of champion athletes, but it can also be brought about by the effects of a rigorous training program (13).

The work of Mostyn and others (12) seems to indicate that championship-level swimmers have an unusually high pulmonary diffusing capacity. Their experiments indicate this is due to a larger-than-normal pulmonary capillary blood volume. However, a change in breathing pattern can bring about significant increases in normal nonswimmers. When subjects breathed during exercise with a *held inspiration* maneuver in which they took a fast inspiration to full capacity (one second), held the breath at full inspiration for about seven seconds, then exhaled as fast as possible, they showed a significant improvement in pulmonary diffusion. Obviously, this type of breathing is very similar to that imposed upon competitive swimmers by their environment.

Thus it would seem that in activities in which the respiratory exchange is made under unfavorable conditions such as swimming or mountain climbing, or during other activities in which the ambient atmospheric pressure of O_2 is low, the held inspiration type of breathing might provide an advantage in increasing pulmonary diffusing capacity. This procedure might be of practical use to athletes who must compete at higher-than-normal elevations.

Use of Oxygen to Improve Performance

It is not uncommon to see a coach administer O_2 to his athletes. This has been done by track and swimming coaches immediately before the event and by many other coaches to hasten the recovery process—for example, between halves of a football or basketball game. Let us consider first the theoretical aspects of this procedure to determine its likely validity and then take note of the applied research.

We must remember that the arterial blood that leaves the lungs is saturated to the extent of 95% to 98%. This degree of saturation does not seem to change in vigorous exercise in a normal subject at sea level. (All of this discussion will apply only to sea-level atmosphere.) If alveolar air increases its partial pressure of O_2 by a factor of three (not unreasonable in 70% to 100% mixtures), O_2 transport is conceivably enhanced by two factors.

1. Hemoglobin saturation increases to a maximum of 95% to 100%. Because blood normally carries twenty volume percent O_2 or 20 ml of O_2 in 100 ml of blood (in round figures), it increases by 5% (0.05×20), for an increase of 1 ml/100 ml of blood.

2. The O_2 in solution increases in proportion to the increased partial pressure of O_2 (Henry's law). The amount in solution is ordinarily about 0.2 ml/100 ml of blood. This, then, becomes about 0.6 ml/100 ml of blood, or an increase of 0.4 ml. The total potential advantage accruing in O_2 transport is therefore something like 1.4 ml, or 1.4/20, or about 7%.

It must be realized, however, that this discussion is predicated upon the breathing of O_2 *during* the athletic performance. If it is breathed before the performance, the O_2 would have to be stored to benefit the performance, unless subjects were able to use O_2 right up to the start of the performance and then hold their breath during the performance. In this unlikely event, storage of O_2 might be thought to occur in the sense of a higher partial pressure of O_2 in the lungs at the start of the event.

Now let us review the research in this area under three categories: O_2 before exercise, O_2 during exercise, and O_2 during recovery.

O_2 before Exercise

In a well-controlled study by Miller (11) in which he administered O_2 before, during, and after a treadmill exercise, no changes in heart rate, blood pressure, blood lactate, or endurance were found when the O_2 was administered before exercise or during recovery from the exercise. He was able to show a psychological effect from breathing air that had been marked *oxygen*. This very likely is also the explanation for earlier studies that had shown improved performance after O_2 breathing.

O_2 during Exercise

Available research seems to agree upon the value of O_2 administration during exercise. Miller found a significant decrease in blood lactate and an increase in running time to exhaustion when O_2 was administered during the treadmill run. Elbel and others (4) found significantly slower heart rates when O_2 was administered during exercise. Bannister and Cunningham (3) set exercise loads on a treadmill so that their four subjects would run to exhaustion in seven to ten minutes while breathing air. While breathing 66% O_2, all subjects were able to maintain these work loads for longer periods, and three of the four subjects went beyond twenty-three minutes. They also compared the effects of 21%, 33%, 66%, and 100% O_2. Interestingly, the best results were obtained with 66%. Subjective reports of euphoria were gotten only from the 66% mixture.

A recent review of the literature (22) in this area suggests considerable doubt as to whether O_2 delivery to the tissues is actually improved during O_2 breathing.

O_2 during Recovery

Miller found no improvement in recovery for any of the measurements made as the result of breathing O_2 during recovery. Elbel and colleagues (4) found no significant changes in O_2 debt repayment as the result of breathing O_2 during recovery, but they found significantly slower heart rates. Their heart rate findings could be construed as a hastening of the recovery process, but the differences were very small, one to five beats per minute.

To summarize the case for breathing O_2 to improve performance, it seems unlikely that any *physiological* changes are brought about by breathing it before the event and (at best) only very small improvements in the recovery rate. Improved performance undoubtedly can result if O_2 is breathed *during* the event, but this can have no practical importance in athletics.

On the other hand, *psychological* improvement in performance can be brought about through suggestion (in the use of oxygen). Also, if an athlete is conditioned to the use of O_2, accidental deprivation at an important meet or game could result in a calamitous decrement in performance.

What Sets the Limits of Aerobic Power?

Aerobic power—the maximum O_2 consumption—depends on the transport of O_2 from the atmosphere to the mitochondria of the muscle cells. This transit involves basically four processes: 1) lung ventilation, or more precisely, alveolar ventilation; 2) the interaction between pulmonary diffusion and blood transport; 3) blood transport; and 4) the interaction between tissue diffusion and blood transport.

R.J. Shephard (18) has suggested using the *O_2 conductance equation* to estimate where the bottleneck to O_2 transport may lie on theoretical bases. In this approach each of the four links in the O_2 transport chain is treated as a conductance. Conductances can be added as reciprocals to give the sum of series conductances, so that the total conductance, which is equivalent to aerobic power or maximal O_2 consumption, can be predicted in simplified form as follows:

$$\frac{1}{Uo_2} = \frac{1}{A} + \frac{1}{B} + \frac{1}{C} + \frac{1}{D}$$

where Uo_2 is the total conductance and A, B, C, D represent the four phases in gas transport.

When realistic estimates for maximal conductance are substituted for each of the four links in the chain, the equation looks like this:

$$\frac{1}{Uo_2} = \frac{1}{90} + \frac{1}{176} + \frac{1}{30} + \frac{1}{681}$$

It can readily be seen that the term C, which represents blood transport, has the greatest effect in setting the limit for maximal aerobic capacity. All of these data apply only to normal young subjects at sea level. Thus the theoretical application of the O_2 conductance equation suggests that the most important determinants of aerobic power are the interaction of cardiac output and hemoglobin level, which together determine the level of blood transport. However, subsequent work (10) that shows the O_2 consumption of the ventilatory muscles to be considerably higher than had been previously estimated suggests that the first factor—lung ventilation—may play a larger role.

Furthermore, in the last few years during which muscle energetics at the cellular level have come under closer investigation, it no longer appears so certain that human endurance performance (as measured by aerobic power, $\dot{V}O_2$ max) is limited by O_2 transport. Considerable evidence now suggests that endurance performance may be limited by the ability of active muscle tissue to utilize O_2 rather than by the delivery of O_2 to it.

Two lines of research have been most popular in attempts to resolve this rather basic question. The first research paradigm is based on the concept that adding more active muscle mass should increase the $\dot{V}O_2$ max, if the limits are set by O_2 utilization. On the other hand, if aerobic capacity is limited by O_2 transport, there should be no increase by adding muscle mass. In such studies where arm work has been added to leg work on the bicycle ergometer, some investigators have found that arm plus leg work elicited greater $\dot{V}O_2$ max than leg work alone (5, 6, 17, 20). Other investigators have been unable to demonstrate any difference between arm plus leg work and leg work only (1, 19).

Evidence suggests that the divergent results can be explained on the basis of interindividual difference. Those subjects having high fitness levels for leg work show no increase by adding muscle mass because the high O_2 utilization of well-trained legs may reach the capacity for O_2 delivery. Less well-conditioned subjects can increase $\dot{V}O_2$ max because the capacity of the O_2 transport system exceeds the demand of the poorly trained leg muscles (15). This is an attractive hypothesis to explain the divergent research findings, but unfortunately it rests on findings from only three subjects.

The second research paradigm is based on the response of $\dot{V}O_2$ max when subjects breathe greater than normal values of O_2 (hyperoxia), either by breathing gasses with a greater than normal percentage of O_2 (20.93) or by breathing air at greater than sea-level pressure. Again, there is disagreement in the experimental results. Some investigators have found an increased $\dot{V}O_2$ max or improved performance resulting from hyperoxia (1, 9, 22, 24, 25), which suggests that the limit is set by O_2 transport. If increasing the O_2 offered to the tissues increases O_2 consumption, then obviously O_2 utilization could not have been limiting. But other investigators have found no increase in $\dot{V}O_2$ max as a result of hyperoxia (8, 11).

In any event, the hyperoxic paradigm is not very convincing even when an increased $\dot{V}O_2$ max is found, because the CO_2 produced does not increase under these conditions, and therefore it is unlikely to represent a real increase in metabolic activity (chap. 3). Furthermore, Welch and associates (23) have recently shown that during exercise under hyperoxic conditions, leg muscle blood flow is reduced, and therefore the O_2 available to the active leg muscles is not really increased.

While this question of where the limits are set is not finally resolved, the available evidence suggests that in activities involving large muscle masses (such as running), aerobic power is probably limited by cardiac output. In activities involving smaller muscle masses, as in sports in which only arms or only legs are used, peripheral factors such as muscle blood flow and muscle O_2 utilization probably set the limit. It is also likely that interindividual differences in cardiovascular dimensions and the functional capacities of the various systems involved determine the limits for any given individual.

Summary

1. The important factor governing the diffusion of respiratory gasses is the difference in pressure between two points, called a *diffusion gradient*.

2. If atmospheric pressure is much below sea-level pressure, the percentage concentration of a gas such as O_2 is meaningless, because its partial pressure may be insufficient to bring about sufficient diffusion.

3. At sea level, the partial pressures of O_2 are approximately 100 and 40 mm Hg in the alveoli and venous blood, respectively, yielding a diffusion gradient of 60 mm Hg. For CO_2, the corresponding figures are 45 and 40 mm in venous blood and alveoli, respectively, with a diffusion gradient of 5 mm Hg.

4. CO_2 requires a smaller diffusion gradient than O_2 because of its greater solubility in water and hence its greater solubility in the alveolar and endothelial tissues.

5. Acidity and alkalinity are expressed in pH units: 7.00 represents neutrality, higher values represent alkalinity, and lower values represent acidity.

6. Ninety-nine percent of the oxygen transport of the blood is accomplished by combination with hemoglobin; about 1% is carried in physical solution.

7. Carbon dioxide transport is accomplished largely within the erythrocytes and in three forms: (a) carbamino-hemoglobin, (b) bicarbonate, and (c) dissolved CO_2.

8. The shape of the O_2 dissociation curve is such that gaseous exchange is greatly expedited at the lungs and at the tissues.

9. At rest, hemoglobin enters the tissues about 95% saturated and leaves about 70% saturated. This difference is called the *coefficient of O_2 utilization*. In exercise, comparable percentages may be 95% and close to 0%, thus effecting a great increase in O_2 utilization.

10. Acid-base balance is maintained throughout the body by buffer systems. Each is composed of a weak acid and a salt of the acid and functions by converting strong acids to weak acids and neutral salts.

11. When the capacity for buffering is stressed, acids and bases are excreted by the lungs and kidneys as a secondary line of defense against pH changes that may be inconsistent with the welfare of the organism.

12. As the rate of metabolism increases in exercise, the rate of diffusion for O_2 increases proportionately. This is probably brought about by the better perfusion of the lung capillaries with blood.

13. Use of O_2 to improve performance rests on sound scientific evidence only when it is used during the exercise period. A small improvement in rate of recovery seems to be possible, but this awaits corroborative evidence.

14. Both theoretical and experimental data suggest that the limits for maximal O_2 transport (*aerobic power*) for healthy young subjects exercising at sea level are set by the interaction of cardiac output and hemoglobin level when large muscle masses are involved. In exercise involving small muscle masses, muscle O_2 utilization and muscle blood flow may become critical. Recent research also suggests that lung ventilation can become a limiting factor under certain conditions.

References

1. Astrand, P-O., and Saltin, B. Maximal oxygen uptake and heart rate in various types of muscular activity. *J. Appl. Physiol.* 16:977–81, 1961.

2. Bannister, R. G., Cotes, J. E., Jones, R. S., and Meade, F. Pulmonary diffusing capacity on exercise in athletes and nonathletic subjects. *J. Physiol.* 152:66–67, 1960.

3. Bannister, R. G., and Cunningham, D. J. The effects on the respiration and performance during exercise of adding oxygen to the inspired air. *J. Physiol.* 125:118, 1954.

4. Elbel, E. R., Ormond, D., and Close, D. Some effects of breathing O_2 before and after exercise. *J. Appl. Physiol.* 16:48–52, 1961.

5. Gleser, M. A., Horstman, D. H., and Mello, R. P. The effect on $\dot{V}O_2$ max of adding arm work to maximal leg work. *Med. Sci. Sports* 6:104–7, 1974.

6. Hermansen, L. Oxygen transport during exercise in human subjects. *Acta Physiol. Scand.* [Suppl.]: 399, 1973.

7. Jones, N. L., Sutton, J. R., Taylor, R., and Toews, C. J. Effect of pH on cardiorespiratory and metabolic responses to exercise. *J. Appl. Physiol.* 43:959–64, 1977.

8. Kaijser, L. Oxygen supply as a limiting factor in physical performance. *Limiting Factors of Human Performance,* ed. J. Keul. Stuttgart: Georg Thieme, 1973.

9. Margaria, R., Camporesi, E., Aghemo, P., and Sassi, G. The effect of O_2 breathing on maximal aerobic power. *Pfluegers Arch.* 336:225–35, 1972.

10. Martin, B. J., and Steger, J. M. Ventilatory endurance in athletes and non-athletes. *Med. Sci. Sports Exer.* 13:21–26, 1981.

11. Miller, A. T., Jr. Influence of oxygen administration on cardiovascular function during exercise and recovery. *J. Appl. Physiol.* 5:165–68, 1952.

12. Mostyn, E. M., Helle, S., Gee, J. B. L., Bentivoglio, L. G., and Bates, D. V. Pulmonary diffusing capacity of athletes. *J. Appl. Physiol.* 18:687–95, 1963.

13. Newman, F., Smalley, B. F., and Thomson, M. L. Effect of exercise, body and lung size on CO diffusion in athletes and nonathletes. *J. Appl. Physiol.* 17:649–55, 1962.

14. Osnes, J. B., and Hermansen, L. Acid-base balance after maximal exercise of short duration. *J. Appl. Physiol.* 32:59–63, 1971.

15. Reybrouck, T., Heigenhauser, G. F., and Faulkner, J. A. Limitations to maximum oxygen uptake in arm, leg and combined arm-leg ergometry. *J. Appl. Physiol.* 38:774–79, 1975.

16. Ross, J. C., Reinhart, R. W., Boxell, J. F., and King, L. H., Jr. Relationship of increased breath-holding diffusing capacity to ventilation in exercise. *J. Appl. Physiol.* 18:794–97, 1963.

17. Secher, N. H., Ruberg-Larson, N., Binkhorst, R. A., and Bonde-Peterson, F. Maximal oxygen uptake during arm cranking and combined arm plus leg exercise. *J. Appl. Physiol.* 36:515–18, 1974.

18. Shephard, R. J. The validity of the oxygen conductance equation. *Int. Z. Angew. Physiol.* 28:61–75, 1969.

19. Stenberg, J., Astrand, P-O., Ekblom, B., Royce, J., and Saltin, B. Hemodynamic response to work with different muscle groups, sitting and supine. *J. Appl. Physiol.* 22:61–70, 1967.

20. Taylor, H. L., Buskirk, E., and Henschel, A. Maximal oxygen uptake as an objective measure of cardio-respiratory performance. *J. Appl. Physiol.* 8:73–80, 1955.

21. Turino, G. M., Bergofsky, E. H., Goldring, R., and Fishman, A. P. Effect of exercise on pulmonary diffusing capacity. *J. Appl. Physiol.* 18:447–56, 1963.

22. Welch, H. G. Hyperoxia and human performance: A brief review. *Med. Sci. Sports Exer.* 14:253–62, 1982.

23. Welch, H. G., Bonde-Petersen, F., Graham, T., Klausen, K., and Secher, N. Effects of hyperoxia on leg blood flow and metabolism during exercise. *J. Appl. Physiol.* 42:385–90, 1977.

24. Wilson, B. A., Welch, H. G., and Liles, J. N. Effects of hyperoxic gas mixtures on energy metabolism during prolonged work. *J. Appl. Physiol.* 39:267–71, 1975.

25. Wilson, G. D., and Welch, H. G. Effects of hyperoxic gas mixtures on exercise tolerance in man. *Med. Sci. Sports* 7:48–52, 1975.

10

The Endocrine System and Exercise

Nature of Hormones

Importance of Hormones in Exercise and Sports

Endocrine Effects on Performance-Related Parameters
Control of Energy Substrates by Pancreatic Hormones
Catecholamine Effects on Muscle Contraction
Circulatory Effects of Norepinephrine
Effect of Gonadal Hormones on Muscle
Thyroid Hormones and Metabolic Rate

Pituitary-Adrenocortical Axis and Stress Theory
The Selye Theory of Stress
Implications of the Selye Theory for Health and Physical Education
Exercise and Stress
Function of the Adrenal Cortex in Training and Conditioning

Effect of Exercise on Endocrine Function
Hypothalamus-Pituitary-Adrenal Axis
Adrenal Medulla (Catecholamine Effects)
Pancreatic Hormones
Thyroid Function
Parathyroid Hormone
Gonadal Hormones

For the human organism to meet the demands of exercise that may increase the metabolic rate by as much as twentyfold requires coordination of many physiological systems. It would be futile for the lungs to operate at maximum capacity if the heart did not cooperate by pumping blood at a commensurate rate to move the necessary blood gasses and nutrients needed by the muscle tissues involved. In fact, most of the systems of the body become involved in the adjustments necessary to support all-out athletic efforts. Obviously, the various physiological systems must be properly coordinated to bring about the appropriate response to the imposed demand.

There are essentially two systems for coordinating the physiological functions of the human organism: the nervous system provides the mechanism for bringing about quick homeostatic responses, and the endocrine system provides the long-term (slower) control of the systems involved. The functions of the two systems are also highly interrelated. Each affects the function of the other.

The term *endocrine* describes the system of ductless glands that secrete their products called *hormones* into the blood, which carries them to "target" organs or systems where they have their effects. The organs or systems may be quite distant. This is in distinction to *exocrine* glands (such as sweat glands), which secrete their products through ducts to the exterior. Figure 10.1 shows the location of the major endocrine glands.

Nature of Hormones

Hormone is the term for the chemical entity secreted by an endocrine gland. Hormones are chemically either steroid, as in the case of the sex glands and some of the hormones of the adrenal cortex, protein, as in the case of some of the pituitary hormones, or amine derivatives of proteins (or amino acids), such as the catecholamines, epinephrine and norepinephrine, which are produced in the adrenal medulla. The latter two hormones are also known as adrenaline and noradrenaline, respectively.

The action of a hormone on its target cell or tissue is usually a control function that results in accelerating or decelerating normal cellular processes. Figure 10.2 illustrates the process by which steroid-type hormones gain entry to the cells' internal machinery. Since both the steroid hormone and the cell membrane are lipids, the steroid hormones easily enter the cell through the membrane. Once inside they combine with specific protein molecules called *receptors*. The hormone and its receptor are analogous to a key and lock in that both hormone and receptor are specific for each other. This steroid protein complex enters the nucleus and activates the synthesis of messenger RNA, which then proceeds to the ribosome to provide a template for the manufacture of new protein molecules.

On the other hand, protein hormones such as insulin need a mechanism for getting through the cell membrane. Figure 10.3 shows how this is accomplished. The hormone and receptor combine on the membrane of the target cell (instead of internally), resulting in the formation of adenylcyclase, which acts as an enzyme to allow conversion of some of the cell's ATP into cyclic AMP (cAMP). The cAMP then initiates any number of cellular functions before it is destroyed. Such functions may include: 1) increasing the number of enzymes in the cell, 2) altering cell permeability, or 3) initiating synthesis of specific biochemical entities. The effects within the cell are of course determined by the nature of the cell itself. Such stimulation of cells in the adrenal medulla result in the formation of catecholamines, while similar stimulation in the adrenal cortex cells results in the production of adrenocortical hormones.

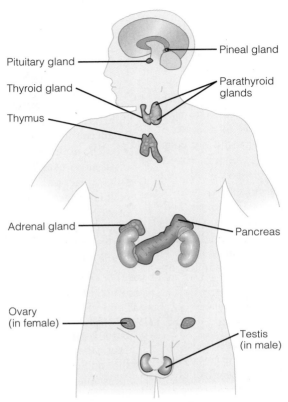

Figure 10.1   Locations of major endocrine glands. (From J. W. Hole, Jr. *Human Anatomy and Physiology,* 3d ed. Copyright © 1984 Wm. C. Brown Communications, Inc., Dubuque, Iowa. All rights reserved. Reprinted by permission.)

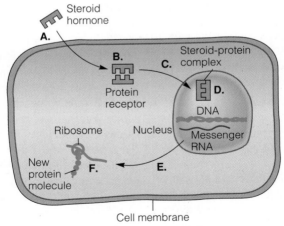

Figure 10.2   (a) A steroid hormone passes through a cell membrane and (b) combines with a receptor protein in the cytoplasm. (c) The steroid-protein complex enters the nucleus and (d) activates the synthesis of messenger RNA. (e) The messenger RNA leaves the nucleus and (f) functions in the manufacture of protein molecules. (From J. W. Hole, Jr. *Human Anatomy and Physiology,* 3d ed. Copyright © 1984 Wm. C. Brown Communications, Inc., Dubuque, Iowa. All rights reserved. Reprinted by permission.)

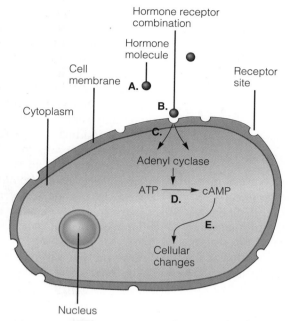

Figure 10.3   (a) Hormone molecules first reach target cells by means of body fluids and (b) combine with receptor sites on the cell membrane. (c) As a result, molecules of adenylate cyclase are activated and (d) cause the change of ATP into cyclic AMP. (e) Cyclic AMP brings about various cellular changes. (From J. W. Hole, Jr. *Human Anatomy and Physiology,* 3d ed. Copyright © 1984 Wm. C. Brown Communications, Inc., Dubuque, Iowa. All rights reserved. Reprinted by permission.)

Importance of Hormones in Exercise and Sports

Our knowledge of the hormonal response to exercise and conversely the effects of the level of secretion of various hormones on health and performance is still far from complete. Only in recent years have methods become available for measuring many of the hormones in blood *during* exercise. Previously, many of the important hormones such as those produced by the adrenal cortex had to be estimated from breakdown products that appear in the urine after completion of the exercise bout. Obviously, urinalyses could not provide a very accurate time relation between physical exercise and the hormonal response elicited.

During the last twenty years, as the result of newer methods such as radio enzymatic techniques, investigators have made measurements of much improved sensitivity, specificity, and precision and accuracy. While our body of knowledge is still fragmentary, the emerging evidence indicates that endocrine effects on exercise performance are of considerable importance and likewise that the effects of exercise on endocrine function are considerable, with all that implies for the health sciences in general.

Endocrine Effects on Performance-Related Parameters

Control of Energy Substrates by Pancreatic Hormones

The pancreas contains two types of glandular tissue, one of which (exocrine glands) secretes digestive juices, the other of which (endocrine glands) consists of the islets of Langerhans in which there are two types of secretory cells, the alpha and beta cells. The alpha cells secrete glucagon, the beta cells insulin. These hormones are important in carbohydrate and fat metabolism.

Insulin is necessary for the transport of glucose through the cell membrane in muscle tissue. In diabetes, an insufficient secretion of insulin causes blood glucose levels to rise to intolerable values. Heavy exercise may also cause decreasing blood levels of insulin but not to the same extent. This exercise *hypoinsulinemia* (low blood level of insulin) facilitates glucose production and release of glucose by the liver. There is in fact an inverse relationship between glucose output and plasma insulin level during exercise (41).

A low blood level of insulin is also probably a determinant in promoting an increase in lipolysis (breakdown of fat tissue) and the consequent rise in the blood level of free fatty acids (FFA) and glycerol (42).

Glucagon, the hormone produced by the alpha cells of the pancreas, mainly acts to raise blood glucose levels by promoting release of glucose from the liver. In a sense, glucagon is antagonistic to insulin in that it tends to raise blood glucose level while insulin depresses it. It has been shown that exercise is a powerful stimulus for glucagon secretion (24). Thus it appears that the pancreatic hormones are important in increasing the mobilization of fuels necessary during prolonged work. Available data suggest that hepatic glucose production increases within a few minutes after start of exercise and varies proportionately with increasing work load (79).

In addition to the effect of the pancreatic hormones, the catecholamines epinephrine (E) (produced in the adrenal medulla) and norepinephrine (NE) (mainly from the sympathetic adrenergic nerve endings) also serve to increase the availability of fuel to the active muscles (78).

Catecholamine Effects on Muscle Contraction

Studies of incubated skeletal muscle have shown that stimulation by the catecholamines results in increased tension and duration of twitches in FT muscle (59), while ST muscle may respond with reduced tension and duration of twitches (81).

Catecholamine stimulation of heart muscle also exerts positive inotropic effects (a more forceful contraction) (10).

Circulatory Effects of Norepinephrine

We have already discussed the control of blood distribution (chap. 7). You will recall that resting blood pressure as well as exercise blood pressure is maintained by vasoconstrictor tone. To a large extent this is brought about by the release of NE from the sympathetic adrenergic nerve fibers.

Effect of Gonadal Hormones on Muscle

Of the several androgenic hormones (having a masculinizing effect), testosterone seems to be the only one of importance in exercise physiology. It is a naturally produced circulating hormone in both male and female adults but occurs at some fifty times greater concentration in the male. As Lamb has pointed out (51), perhaps the best evidence that androgens are involved in athletic performance is that boys become more athletically proficient than girls at puberty, the time of the greatest changes in blood testosterone.

The available evidence suggests that only minimal amounts of androgen are necessary to bring about the normal male-female differences in secondary sex characteristics. Animal experiments in Russia, using synthetically developed analogs of testosterone (anabolic steroids—chap. 30), suggest that the increases in protein synthesis and lean body mass long associated with testosterone are the result of better transcription of ribosomal RNA in skeletal muscle, which brings about an increased synthesis of myofibrillar and sarcoplasmic protein (63, 64).

Thyroid Hormones and Metabolic Rate

The thyroid gland produces several hormones that have important effects on the metabolic rates of most body cells, the most important of which are *thyroxine* and *triiodothyronine,* which act to increase the rate of energy release from carbohydrates and the rate of protein synthesis. Indeed until recent years the physician's standard test for thyroid function was to measure basal metabolic rate (BMR). Too low a BMR indicated hypothyroidism, while too high indicated hyperthyroidism. The release of these hormones is controlled by the hypothalamus and pituitary gland. These hormones also have marked effects on the activation level of the nervous system and accelerate growth in young persons.

Because of the factors discussed previously, even brief treatment with thyroid hormones increases the temperature response to exercise in dogs. Similarly, during exercise in humans, core temperature is higher in hyperthyroid patients than in controls. These findings indicate that the thyroid status is important for the setting of the thermoregulatory centers in exercise.

In general, work tolerance is typically poor in both hypo- and hyperthyroidism (74).

Pituitary-Adrenocortical Axis and Stress Theory

The Selye Theory of Stress

It has long been known that stressful situations call forth various physiological responses. However, Hans Selye, a Canadian endocrinologist, was the first to observe and report the fact that regardless of the form the stressor might take the response was always the same: a stress *syndrome* (concurrent symptoms that characterize a disease) consisting of 1) adrenal enlargement, 2) thymus and lymphatic involution (shrinkage), and 3) bleeding ulcers of the digestive tract. The same stress syndrome was found to result from such diverse stressors as illness, traumatic injury, heavy exercise, and emotional upset.

Furthermore, this triad of symptoms—which Selye called the *general adaptation syndrome* (GAS) (65)—seems to go through three stages: 1) the alarm reaction, 2) the stage of resistance, and 3) the stage of exhaustion. Thus the alarm reaction (AR) elicits the typical triad of symptoms, but if the stressor is of long duration, the organism enters the stage of resistance (SR), during which the stress syndrome (or GAS) seems to disappear but the resistance of the organism to stress actually is greater. Finally after the acquired adaptation is lost, the stage of exhaustion (SE) is entered, the original stress syndrome reappears, and death eventually ensues from the exhaustion of "adaptational energy."

Selye defined stress as the "state manifested by a specific syndrome which consists of all the nonspecifically induced changes within a biologic system" or, more simply, as the "rate of wear and tear in the body." The reaction of the organism to stressors, regardless of type, therefore involves the same stress syndrome in which the pituitary gland is alerted by the hypothalamus. The pituitary secretes the adrenocorticotrophic hormone (ACTH), which stimulates the adrenal cortex to secrete its glucocorticoids (mainly cortisone and cortisol). The glucocorticoids produce the syndrome described above, in which the lymphatic tissues shrink (these glucocorticoids are anti-inflammatory) and ulceration occurs in the digestive tract.

At the same time, the alarm reaction can be brought about by the coordinating efforts of the nervous system. This system also seems to act by secreting hormones, but it acts more directly on the tissues, for example, at the nerve endings. The nerve endings of the sympathetic nervous system are of two types: *adrenergic,* so called because their stimulation releases the catecholamine noradrenaline, and *cholinergic,* whose stimulation releases acetylcholine.

Implications of the Selye Theory for Health and Physical Education

The cortex (outer rind) of the adrenal glands secretes many hormones, and each of the hormones may have several effects. However, our discussion will be confined to two classes of corticoids (hormones from the adrenal cortex): *pro-inflammatory corticoids* (PC) and *anti-inflammatory corticoids* (AC). In general, the PCs of Selye belong to the group of hormones referred to by physiologists as *mineralocorticoids* (MC) because they affect mineral metabolism, causing sodium retention and potassium excretion. The most important of this group are aldosterone and desoxycorticosterone. The anti-inflammatory corticoids belong to the group physiologists call *glucocorticoids* (GC) because they can increase blood-sugar levels. The most important of these are cortisone and cortisol.

In many diseases the processes of inflammation may be essential to wall off infectious agents that are invading the tissues and prevent them from spreading throughout the entire organism. On the other hand, it is Selye's contention that some diseases are simply an overreaction of the organism to a stressor that is not serious enough to merit a strong reaction of PC corticoids. In these cases, the disease is merely a manifestation of overactivity of the PC corticoids, and it can be relieved or ameliorated by AC corticoids, such as cortisone. Some of the diseases in which maladaptation of the adrenal cortex is thought to play a part are high blood pressure, various heart diseases, rheumatoid arthritis, and allergic reactions.

One of the most important implications of Selye's work lies in his hypothesis that every person inherits a certain amount of "adaptation energy" that cannot be appreciably changed. If we accept this hypothesis and Selye's hypothesis that heavy muscular work constitutes a strong stressor, we would be forced to conclude that heavy exercise (athletics) might well shorten life. For when adaptation energy runs out, the organism enters the stage of exhaustion and death ensues.

Fortunately, however, the story is not that simple. To begin with, the available evidence indicates that exercise produces a degree of protection against stress (the resistance stage of Selye?). We might then reason that even though the total "bank account" of adaptation energy might be depleted a little earlier through a life of heavy muscular exercise, the conditioning effect of the exercise might prevent an even earlier, sudden demise due to a very stressful situation.

deVries has produced evidence that even a short, moderate exercise bout reduces residual neuromuscular tension significantly (13). Thus it might be postulated that although adaptation energy is used up faster through a vigorous life that involves heavy exercise, the net effect might be advantageous in preventing nervous diseases and other diseases that are thought to be related to tension (such as high blood pressure).

Indeed, Selye's concept of "deviation" appears entirely compatible with deVries's viewpoint. Selye points out that humans seldom if ever die of old age. They die because of the weakness or uneven wear of one organ or system. For this reason, he emphasizes the importance of the stress quotient:

$$\frac{Local\ stress\ in\ any\ one\ part}{Total\ stress\ in\ the\ body}$$

He suggests that when stress is disproportionately great on one organ or system, "deviation"—changing the type of activity to better distribute the stress—may be beneficial. The ultimate example of deviation is the use of electroshock or insulin shock to bring about the necessary changes.

Selye's GAS theory seems to provide a rational basis for answering many of the perplexing questions that have puzzled medical science. It also poses many questions to be investigated by exercise physiologists.

Exercise and Stress

That exercise can improve the response to stress in rats has been demonstrated by Bartlett (2). It had previously been shown that

stress made laboratory animals thermolabile (more reactive to temperature change). The body temperature in rats exposed to a low temperature (5°C) was found to be significantly less if they had been conditioned by three to ten minutes of daily exercise for twelve days.

Even more important, Seyle (65) has shown that animals can be made less vulnerable to experimental heart attacks (brought on by sensitization—salt and hormone) and subsequent stress if they are conditioned by physical exercise. Furthermore, he feels that conditioning by the moderate stress of a reasonable program of physical exercise sets up a "cross-resistance to various forms of pathogenic stress. By exercising intelligently a man can train his heart to resist attacks that might otherwise kill him. It doesn't matter if he has been training with calisthenics and is later attacked not by physical but emotional stress. . . . Cross-resistance will help his heart stand off the attack in any case."

In an experiment on college women, Ulrich (77) found that the stress level in varsity basketball players was lower after a game than it was when they had been prepared for a game that did not materialize. It seems that the physiological effects of emotional stress can be "worked off" by vigorous physical activity.

Function of the Adrenal Cortex in Training and Conditioning

Exercise has been shown to cause significant drops in the eosinophil count (a measure of stress response) even when little emotional involvement occurs, as in an experimental gymnasium exercise program (80). It has also been shown that the emotional involvement alone can bring about this drop in eosinophil count (62). Thus the adrenal cortex increases its function in response to both the physical and the emotional components of exercise. It seems reasonable to assume that the effects are additive. Experience seems to bear out this conclusion in that a competitive athletic event seems to be more stressful if a large emotional component is present—such as a league championship game compared with a scrimmage.

There seems to be unanimity in the literature that the *onset* of a heavy work program (or training program) elevates corticoid secretion. However data for the effects of a *prolonged* training program has been neglected. There has been shown to be a highly significant hypertrophy of the adrenals in rats and hamsters that seems to require three weeks to occur (21,60). The secretion of corticoids paralleled the adrenal hypertrophy for approximately three weeks and then fell off toward pretraining levels, while the hypertrophy was maintained at the higher level. The hypertrophy of the adrenal was found to be almost entirely due to growth of the cortex. The medulla showed only a small increase in size. It is tempting to extrapolate this data to humans because it would explain many of the phenomena observed by trainers and coaches.

Prokop (60) has shown (with hamsters) that a training load of two-thirds maximum provides the best training stimulus for the adrenal gland. Prokop also pointed out that this two-thirds maximum load must not be increased by "extracurricular additive" stress, or overtraining will result.

Prokop provides a very interesting analogy between the three phases of Selye's GAS and the phases involved in the athlete's training regimen.

Phase of GAS	Phase of Training Regime
1. Alarm reaction	1. The phase of *adaptation* in which training is initiated and progresses toward peak performance (5–12 weeks)
2. Resistance	2. *Completed adaptation* or achievement of peak condition (additional 3–6 weeks)
3. Exhaustion	3. *Readaptation:* The loss of peak condition (starts 8–16 weeks after beginning of training)

Although no experimental evidence is provided for this concept, it corresponds to the facts observed by coaches and athletes during the training process.

If we classify athletes by their endocrine function in the training regime, there seem to be two types: the *sympathicotonics,* who achieve their peak rapidly but can hold it for only relatively short periods, and the *vagotonics,* who achieve their peak more slowly but can hold it longer.

Overtraining and the resulting "staleness" can also be best explained in terms of adrenal function and the GAS of Selye. If athletes enter the readaptation phase of Prokop (SE of Selye) and are encouraged to work harder to maintain their peak—fighting the natural endocrine cycle, as it were—they will show signs of adrenal exhaustion, such as hypertension, increased nervous tension, and a less effective metabolism that results in impaired performance. The fact that Prokop has been able to treat "staleness" by administering corticoids lends further support to his analogy between the GAS and the training regime.

Effect of Exercise on Endocrine Function

Hypothalamus-Pituitary-Adrenal Axis

The importance of the hypothalamus-pituitary-adrenal axis with respect to stress has been discussed. To recapitulate, stress (independent of the cause) stimulates the hypothalamus (nervous system) to secrete corticotropin-releasing factor (CRF). This in turn

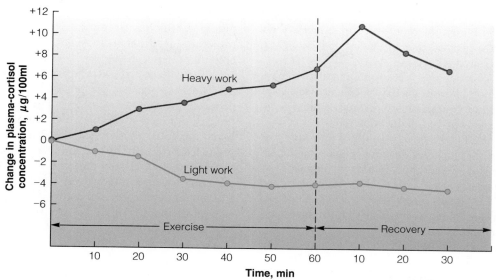

Figure 10.4 Time course of mean changes in ten male subjects of plasma-cortisol concentration during exercise at heavy work (60%–90% $\dot{V}O_2$ max) and light work (less than 50% $\dot{V}O_2$ max). (Redrawn from the data of Davies, C. T. M., and Few, J. D. *J. Appl. Physiol.* 35:887, 1973.)

stimulates the anterior pituitary to release adrenocorticotropin (ACTH), which causes the adrenal cortex to secrete glucocorticoids—most importantly, cortisol—into the circulation. With respect specifically to physical stress, ACTH has been shown to be elevated during physical activity (6, 16, 20, 26) and to mediate the exercise-induced increase in cortisol (68). Cortisol is also one of the factors that helps to maintain glucose homeostasis by stimulating hepatic gluconeogenesis and by mobilizing FFA from adipose tissue.

Of great interest is that cortisol level in the blood, which reflects the degree of stress under which the organism operates, increases significantly with high work loads, 60% to 90% $\dot{V}O_2$ max, but decreases very significantly with light work loads of less than 50% $\dot{V}O_2$ max. This is shown most clearly in the work of Davies and Few (11), which is illustrated in Figure 10.4. This finding helps to explain the work of deVries and Adams on the "tranquilizer" effect of exercise, in which exercise at

40% $\dot{V}O_2$ max was very effective in producing muscular relaxation, while exercise at 60% $\dot{V}O_2$ max produced an effect not significantly different from control (13). The results of studies relating plasma glucocorticoid (cortisol and corticosterone) level to exercise intensity have been quite consistent. During light to moderate work the plasma GC level was found to decrease or remain unchanged rather than rise. Only when the work level became heavy or exhaustive did the GC level rise significantly (75). Plasma levels of cortisol reflect the interaction between secretion into the blood and removal from circulation (73). During low intensity exercise, the rate of removal exceeds secretion while during high intensity exercise secretion is greater than removal (7, 19).

The importance of the psychological components of exercise (more importantly, athletic competition) has been shown by Raymond and colleagues (61) who found that for light, nonexhaustive exercise plasma-cortisol levels were elevated only in subjects with pre-exercise apprehension. In calm subjects their data supported that of Davies and Few (11), who found a decrease.

In moderately heavy to exhaustive exercise the plasma levels of GC increase in approximate proportion to exercise intensity (4, 16) and also to the duration (4).

ACTH is part of a family of pituitary peptides that includes the endogenous opioid peptide beta-endorphin (endo = endogenous; orphin = morphine). Beta-endorphin and ACTH result from the transcription and translation of a single gene that produces pro-opiomelanocortin (29).

Beta-endorphin consists of a 31 amino acid sequence from the total of 239 amino acids that make up pro-opiomelanocortin (29, 73). It has been suggested that the euphoric mood state experienced by some individuals during long term exercise called the "runner's high" is related to the action of circulating beta-endorphin (73). In addition, it has been hypothesized that during exercise, the endogenous opioids may produce an analgesic effect and increase the pain threshold (14, 76). These effects have not been demonstrated directly, however, and the validity of these hypotheses remains in question (14, 73, 76).

Most studies have shown that circulating beta-endorphin increases as a result of exercise (8, 17, 39, 69, 73). It appears that the response is intensity related with little or no change as a result of low to moderate work demands (17, 28, 39), but substantial increases during high intensity (greater than 70% $\dot{V}O_2$ max) exercise (18, 28, 39). It is presently unclear if there is a gender difference in the beta-endorphin response to exercise (8, 17, 27). Furthermore, the effect of endurance training on resting levels of beta-endorphin as well as the response to exercise is debatable (6, 18, 39, 47, 54, 58, 73).

In addition to the ACTH production of the pituitary, which is so important in the stress responses just discussed, the pituitary also secretes a protein called growth hormone (GH). In muscle tissue, GH acts to increase amino acid uptake, promote protein synthesis, and decrease glucose uptake (29). The growth-promoting effects of GH on skeletal muscle are likely mediated by somatomedins, which are produced primarily by the liver and released in response to GH stimulation (29, 73). GH secretion is also affected by exercise and training. Exercise of moderate intensity results in an increase in GH concentration (36, 44). During prolonged moderate work, GH levels fall toward resting values, but training causes these levels to be maintained (36). Interestingly, Stuart and coworkers (67) found no change in plasma somatomedin level following an exercise-induced increase in GH. The implications of these findings for child development are as yet unclear but suggest the need for further investigation.

Adrenal Medulla (Catecholamine Effects)

A second important pathway that mediates the stress response is through the catecholamines liberated under the influence of an acetylcholine discharge at autonomic nerve endings as well as in the adrenal medulla. The chromaffin cells of the adrenal medulla secrete mainly epinephrine (E), which provides readily available sources of energy by releasing glucose from glycogen depots and free fatty acids from the triglyceride stores of adipose tissue. Although some norepinephrine (NE) is produced in the adrenal medulla, the largest fraction is released from activation of adrenergic nerves. In any event, it is important to realize that while both the adrenal cortex and medulla are important in improving the level

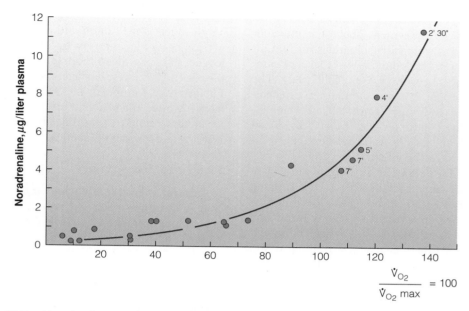

Figure 10.5   Norepinephrine levels in arterial blood plasma (ng/ml) in relation to the relative work load expressed as percent of individual maximal oxygen uptake. The number of minutes the subjects could stand the supramaximal work loads are indicated. (Redrawn from the data of Haggendal, Hartley, and Saltin. *Scand. J. Clin. and Lab Invest.* 26:338, 1970.)

of energy substrate to the muscles, the catecholamines E and NE are in themselves strong stressors when present in large dose (56). They elicit all the characteristic manifestations of the stress syndrome and in addition cause an immediate rise in heart rate and blood pressure and stimulate the sympathetic nervous system.

The effects of exercise on NE are well defined. There is only a very small rise up to 50% to 60% percent of $\dot{V}O_2$ max, with a large exponential rise with the heavier loads (24, 32, 40, 78). Thus, Howley (40) found a small rise in NE excretion at 49% $\dot{V}O_2$ max but a fivefold increase at the 82% level. Figure 10.5 illustrates the nature of the changes in plasma level of NE as related to exercise load (32). Again we see the importance of endocrine effects in allowing (if not to some extent causing)

the "tranquilizer" effect of exercise of low intensity, while heavy or exhausting exercise becomes an excitatory stressor (chap. 13). In contrast to NE responses, the E response is much smaller, with disagreement among investigators. However, Bannister and Griffiths (1) have provided strong evidence that the disagreement was probably due to methodology and that E increases parallel NE increases, though in smaller amounts. Recently, Hooker and colleagues (38) reported significant increases in E at 70% $\dot{V}O_2$ max during both leg and arm cranking ergometry. There was no difference in the E response for leg and arm exercise at the same relative percent (70%) of $\dot{V}O_2$ max. Thus, there appears to be an exponential rise in both E and NE with increasing work intensity (3, 22, 24, 73).

There *is* agreement about the effect of training upon the catecholamines, in that all investigators have found a lower level of catecholamine response (9, 35, 36, 37, 82). The importance of lowered circulating catecholamines in endurance work must be emphasized. The resulting lower heart rate, blood pressure, and rate pressure product (chaps. 14 and 15) have the effect of lowering the myocardial O_2 uptake at any given work load. These are important benefits to the training regimen in both health and disease. Interestingly, however, a recent review by Sothmann and coworkers (66) states "There is no evidence that fitness or exercise training is significantly associated with plasma epinephrine activity during short-term psychological stress."

Pancreatic Hormones

When exercise intensity exceeds approximately 50% of $\dot{V}O_2$ max, the insulin concentration in peripheral plasma decreases in direct proportion to the increases in work load (23, 35). On the other hand, plasma glucagon levels increase with exercise of different kinds but not until after one or more hours of duration (23, 31).

These changes are consistent with the needs of the organism in terms of the mobilization of stored energy substrate in response to exercise. The requirements for glucose in muscle during even moderate exercise tend to cause a decline in blood glucose. As blood glucose goes down, two things happen: the need for insulin declines, and the need for glucagon increases because of the need for release of glucose from the liver. Thus the observed decrease in insulin and the increase in glucagon are functional.

As a result of competitive swim training, plasma levels of glucagon were higher and insulin lower during a 1,000-yard swim after nine weeks of training (37, 82). This training effect on glucagon is maximum within three weeks of training. A recent review by Sutton and colleagues (73) provides a thorough discussion of the effects of exercise on pancreatic hormones. Furthermore, Lampman and Schteingart (52) have reviewed the effects of exercise training on factors related to insulin effectiveness in noninsulin dependent diabetics.

Thyroid Function

In general, plasma thyroxine levels do not change during exercise. At most, a small increase has been shown, which could be explained by the typical hemoconcentration resulting from exercise (74).

Parathyroid Hormone

Parathyroid hormone (PTH) is involved in calcium regulation. PTH increases blood calcium levels by: 1) mobilizing calcium from bone, 2) enhancing calcium reabsorbtion by the kidney, and 3) promoting intestinal calcium uptake (29). Recently, Ljunghall and coworkers (53) found that a seven day field exercise maneuver resulted in a mean increase of 25.4% in serum PTH. The authors further stated that "those who performed the largest amount of work also experienced the greatest stimulus for secretion of PTH." They found, however, no relationships between serum calcium levels and PTH concentrations.

Gonadal Hormones

Serum androgen levels in the adult male increase with exercise if the work intensity is strenuous (15, 25, 57). This effect, while shown in the adult male during treadmill exercise at 80% capacity, did not result in any significant increase in sperm production (57). Exercise-induced increases in testosterone are independent of changes in the pituitary luteinizing hormone (LH), which normally regulates testosterone secretion (12, 49, 50, 72, 73). Furthermore, ACTH, GH, catecholamines, and the endogenous opiates appear to have little effect on androgen levels in males during exercise (30, 70, 73). Apparently, testosterone concentrations measured during or following exercise reflect primarily a reduction in the metabolic clearance rate (71).

Serum testosterone increased significantly by 19% after a weight training session in college-age males, whereas no significant changes were seen in either college-age females or high school males (15). More recent studies have also reported increases in circulating testosterone with weightlifting (33, 34, 48). Kraemer (46) reviewed the endocrine responses to resistance training including the gonadal hormones.

The effect of exercise on ovarian hormones is relatively similar to its effect on gonadal hormones in the male. Exercise of sufficient intensity results in elevations in plasma estradiol, progesterone, and follicle-stimulating hormone but not in luteinizing hormone (43). The increases in estradiol and progesterone are related to the intensity of the exercise and appear to be independent of pituitary control. It is likely that the exercise-induced increase in circulating ovarian hormones is, in part, a function of decreased clearance from the blood due to a reduction in hepatic blood flow (45). In addition, the effects of exercise on ovarian hormones are influenced by the phase of the menstrual cycle (73). This confounding factor must be considered when interpreting the results of studies involving hormonal changes in females (5, 55).

Summary

1. There are essentially two systems for coordinating the physiological functions of the human organism: the nervous system provides the mechanism for quick homeostatic responses, and the endocrine system furnishes the longer-term control system.

2. Endocrine glands are ductless and secrete their hormone products (which may be steroids, proteins, or amines) directly into the bloodstream, which carries the hormones to their target organs or systems where they carry out their control functions.

3. The pancreatic hormones *insulin* and *glucagon* are important in increasing the mobilization of fuels necessary during prolonged physical work.

4. The *catecholamines, epinephrine* from the adrenal medulla and *norepinephrine* partly from the adrenal medulla but largely from the sympathetic adrenergic nerve endings, are likewise important in increasing availability of fuel to the active muscles. In addition, E and NE increase the tension and duration of the muscle twitch in FT muscle fibers, while ST muscle may respond with reduced tension and duration.

5. Animal experiments in the Soviet Union suggest that the increases in protein synthesis and lean body mass long associated with *testosterone* are the result of better transcription of ribosomal RNA in skeletal muscle, which brings about an increased synthesis of myofibrillar and sarcoplasmic protein.

6. The thyroid hormones, *thyroxine* and *triiodothyronine,* act to increase the rate of energy release from carbohydrates and also the rate of protein synthesis. Thus thyroid status is probably important in setting the thermoregulatory centers in exercise.

7. Selye's theory of stress postulates a specific syndrome of physiological effects of stress that are nonspecifically induced.

8. The *general adaptation syndrome* (GAS) of Selye proceeds through three stages: 1) the alarm reaction, 2) the stage of resistance, and 3) the stage of exhaustion.

9. Physical education and athletics can play an important part in lowering the stress quotient, defined as

$$\frac{Local\ stress\ in\ any\ one\ part}{Total\ stress\ in\ the\ body}$$

10. There is evidence that physical exercise can reduce stress under certain conditions. Selye's work also seems to indicate that exercise can condition the individual to better withstand stress of all kinds.

11. Many of the phenomena observed in training and conditioning athletes can be explained in terms of Selye's GAS.

12. Blood levels of cortisol, which reflect the stress level under which the organism operates, increase significantly with high exercise work loads (60% to 90% capacity) but decrease very significantly with light exercise work loads of less than 50% capacity.

13. Exercise of moderate intensity results in an increase in growth hormone concentration.

14. The catecholamines are in themselves strong stressors when present in large doses since they elicit all the characteristic manifestations of the stress syndrome. Thus, it is important to realize that there is only a very small rise during light exercise up to 60% capacity but a very large and rapid rise above that.

15. Physical training results in a lower level of catecholamine response to a given work-load level. This blunted response is an important benefit in both health and disease.

16. Physical training causes a rise in plasma glucagon and a fall in insulin level, both of which reflect better muscle energetics.

17. Weight training and strenuous endurance training increase the serum androgen levels in adult males but not in males of high school age or in females. In the female, heavy exercise results in elevations of plasma estradiol, progesterone, and follicle-stimulating hormone.

References

1. Bannister, E. W., and Griffiths, J. Blood levels of adrenergic amines during exercise. *J. Appl. Physiol.* 33:674–76, 1972.

2. Bartlett, R. G., Jr. Stress adaptation and inhibition of restraint-induced (emotional) hypothermia. *J. Appl. Physiol.* 8:661–63, 1956.

3. Bloom, S. R., Johnson, R. H., Park, D. M., Rennie, M. J., and Sulaiman, W. R. Differences in the metabolic and hormonal response to exercise between racing cyclists and untrained individuals. *J. Physiol.* (Lond.) 258:1–18, 1976.

4. Bonen, A. Effects of exercise on excretion rates of urinary free cortisol. *J. Appl. Physiol.* 40:155–58, 1976.

5. Bunt, J. C. Metabolic actions of estradiol: Significance for acute and chronic exercise responses. *Med. Sci. Sports Exerc.* 22:286–90, 1990.

6. Carr, D. B., Bullen, B. A., Skrinar, G. S., Arnold, M. A., Rosenblatt, M., Beitins, I. Z., Martin, J. B., and McArthur, J. W. Physical conditioning facilitates the exercise-induced secretion of beta-endorphin and beta-lipotropin in women. *N. Engl. J. Med.* 305:560–63, 1981.

7. Cashmore, G. C., Davies, C. T. M., and Few, J. D. Relationship between increases in plasma cortisol concentration and rate of cortisol secretion during exercise in man. *J. Endocrinol.* 72:109–10, 1977.

8. Colt, E. W. D., Wardlaw, S. L., and Frantz, A. G. The effect of running on plasma beta-endorphin. *Life Sci.* 28:1637–40, 1981.

9. Cousineau, D., Ferguson, R. J., de Champlain, J., Gauthier, P., Cote, P., and Bourassa, M. Catecholamines in coronary sinus during exercise in man before and after training. *J. Appl. Physiol.* 43:801–6, 1977.

10. Crass, M. F., Shipp, J. C., and Pieper, G. M. Effect of catecholamines on myocardial endogenous substrates and contractility. *Am. J. Physiol.* 228:618–27, 1975.

11. Davies, C. T. M., and Few, J. D. Effects of exercise on adrenocortical function. *J. Appl. Physiol.* 35:887–91, 1973.

12. Dessypris, A., Kuoppasalmi, K., and Adlercreutz, H. Plasma cortisol, testosterone, androstenedione and luteinizing hormone (LH) in a noncompetitive marathon run. *J. Steroid Biochem.* 7:33–37, 1976.

13. deVries, H. A., and Adams, G. M. Electromyographic comparison of single doses of exercise and meprobamate as to effects on muscular relaxation. *Am. J. Phys. Med.* 51:130–41, 1972.

14. Droste, C., Greenlee, M. W., Schreck, M., and Roskamm, H. Experimental pain thresholds and plasma beta-endorphin levels during exercise. *Med. Sci. Sports Exerc.* 23:334–42, 1991.

15. Fahey, T. D., Rolph, R., Moungmee, P., Nagel, J., and Mortara, S. Serum testosterone, body composition and strength of young adults. *Med. Sci. Sports* 8:31–34, 1976.

16. Farrell, P. A., Garthwaite, T. L., and Gustafson, A. B. Plasma adrenocorticotropin and cortisol responses to submaximal and exhaustive exercise. *J. Appl. Physiol.* 55:1441–44, 1983.

17. Farrell, P. A., Gates, W. K., Morgan, W. P., and Maksud, M. G. Increases in plasma beta-EP and beta-LPH immunoreactivity after treadmill running in humans. *J. Appl. Physiol.* 52:1245–49, 1982.

18. Farrell, P. A., Kjaer, M., Bach, F. W., and Galbo, H. Beta endorphin and adrenocorticotropin response to supramaximal treadmill exercise in trained and untrained males. *Acta Physiol. Scand.* 130:619–25, 1987.

19. Few, J. D. Effect of exercise on the secretion and metabolism of cortisol in man. *J. Endocrinol.* 62:341–53, 1974.

20. Fraioli, F., Moretti, C., Paolucci, D., Alicicco, E., Crescenzi, G., and Fortunio, G. Physical exercise stimulates marked concomitant release of beta-endorphin and ACTH in peripheral blood in man. *Experientia* 36:987–89, 1980.

21. Frenkl, R., and Csalay, L. On the endocrine adaptation to regular muscular activity. *J. Sports Med. Phys. Fitness* 10:151–56, 1970.

22. Galbo, H. Catecholamines and muscular exercise: Assessment of sympathoadrenal activity. *Biochemistry of Exercise IVB,* eds. J. R. Poortmans and G. Nisets. Baltimore: University Park Press, 1981.

23. Galbo, H. *Hormonal and Metabolic Adaptation to Exercise.* New York: Thieme-Stratton, 1983.

24. Galbo, H., Holst, J. J., and Christensen, N. J. Glucagon and plasma catecholamine responses to graded and prolonged exercise in man. *J. Appl. Physiol.* 38:70–76, 1975.

25. Galbo, H., Hummer, L., Petersen, I. B., Christensen, N. J., and Bie, N. Thyroid and testicular hormone responses to graded and prolonged exercise in man. *Eur. J. Appl. Physiol.* 36:101–6, 1977.

26. Gambert, S. R., Garthwaite, T. L., Pontzer, C. H., Cook, E. E., Tristani, F. E., Duthie, E. H., Martinson, D. R., Hagen, T. C., and McCarty, D. J. Running elevates plasma beta-endorphin immunoreactivity and ACTH in untrained human subjects. *Proc. Soc. Exp. Biol. Med.* 168:1–4, 1981.

27. Gambert, S. R., Hagen, T. C., Garthwaite, T. L., Duthie, E. H., and McCarty, D. J. Exercise and the endogenous opioids. *N. Engl. J. Med.* 305:1590–92, 1981.

28. Goldfarb, A. H., Hatfield, B. D., Armstrong, D., and Potts, J. Plasma beta-endorphin concentration: Response to intensity and duration of exercise. *Med. Sci. Sports Exerc.* 22:241–44, 1990.

29. Goodman, H. M. *Basic Medical Endocrinology.* New York: Raven Press, 1988.

30. Grossman, A., Bouloux, P., Price, P., Drury, P. L., Lam, K. S. L., Turner, T., Thomas, J., Besser, G. M., and Sutton, J. The role of opioid peptides in the hormonal responses to acute exercise in man. *Clin. Sci.* 67:483–91, 1984.

31. Gyntelberg, F., Rennie, M. J., Hickson, R. C., and Holloszy, J. O. Effect of training on the response of plasma glucagon to exercise. *J. Appl. Physiol.* 43:302–5, 1977.

32. Haggendal, J., Hartley, L. H., and Saltin, B. Arterial noradrenaline concentration during exercise in relation to the relative work levels. *Scand. J. Clin. Lab. Invest.* 26:337–42, 1970.

33. Hakkinen, K., Parkarinen, A., Alen, M., Kauhanen, H., and Komi, P. V. Daily hormonal and neuromuscular responses to intensive strength training in 1 week. *Int. J. Sports Med.* 9:422–28, 1988.

34. Hakkinen, K., Parkarinen, A., Alen, M., Kauhanen, H., and Komi, P. V. Neuromuscular and hormonal responses of elite athletes to two successive strength training sessions in one day. *Eur. J. Appl. Physiol.* 57:133–39, 1988.

35. Hartley, L. H. Growth hormone and catecholamine response to exercise in relation to physical training. *Med. Sci. Sports* 7:34–36, 1975.

36. Hartley, L. H., Mason, J. W., Hagan, R. P., Jones, L. G., Kotchen, T. A., Mougey, E. H., Wherry, F. E., Pennington, L. L., and Ricketts, P. T. Multiple hormonal responses to graded exercise in relation to physical training. *J. Appl. Physiol.* 33:602–6, 1972.

37. Hickson, R. C., Hagberg, J. M., Conlee, R. K., Jones, D. A., Ehsani, A. A., and Winder, W. W. Effect of training on hormonal responses to exercise in competitive swimmers. *Eur. J. Appl. Physiol.* 41:211–19, 1979.

38. Hooker, S. P., Wells, C. L., Manroe, M. M., Philip, S. A., and Martin, N. Differences in epinephrine and substrate responses between arm and leg exercise. *Med. Sci. Sports Exerc.* 22:779–84, 1990.

39. Howlett, T. A., Tomlin, S., Ngahfoong, L., Rees, L. H., Bullen, B. A., Skrinar, G. S., and McArthur, J. W. Release of beta-endorphin and met-enkephalin during exercise in normal women: Response to training. *Br. Med. J.* 288:1950–52, 1984.

40. Howley, E. T. The effect of different intensities of exercise on the excretion of epinephrine and norepinephrine. *Med. Sci. Sports* 8:219–22, 1976.

41. Issekutz, B. The role of hypoinsulinemia in exercise metabolism. *Diabetes* 29:629–35, 1980.

42. Jansson, E. Diet and muscle metabolism in man. *Acta Physiol. Scand. Suppl.* 487:1–24, 1980.

43. Jurkowski, J. E., Jones, N. L., Walker, W. C., Younglai, E. V., and Sutton, J. R. Ovarian hormonal responses to exercise. *J. Appl. Physiol.* 44:109–14, 1978.

44. Karagiorgos, A., Garcia, J. F., and Brooks, G. A. Growth hormone response to continuous and intermittent exercise. *Med. Sci. Sports* 11:302–7, 1979.

45. Keizer, H. A., Poortmans, J., and Bunniks, J. Influence of physical exercise on sex hormone metabolism. *Biochemistry of Exercise IV-B,* eds. J. Poortmans and G. Niset. Baltimore: University Park Press, 1981.

46. Kraemer, W. J. Endocrine responses to resistance exercise. *Med. Sci. Sports Exerc.* 20 (supplement):S152-S157, 1988.

47. Kraemer, W. J., Fleck, S. J., Callister, R., Shealy, M., Dudley, G. A., Maresh, C. M., Marchitelli, L., Cruthirds, C., Murray, T., and Falkel, J. E. Training responses of plasma beta-endorphin, adrenocorticotropin, and cortisol. *Med. Sci. Sports Exerc.* 21:146–53, 1989.

48. Kraemer, W., Gordon, S. E., Fleck, S. J., Marchitelli, L. J., Mello, R., Dziados, J. E., Friedl, K., Harman, E., Maresh, C., and Fry, A. C. Endogenous anabolic hormonal and growth factor responses to heavy resistance exercise in males and females. *Int. J. Sports Med.* 12:228–35, 1991.

49. Kuoppasalmi, K., Naveri, H., Harkonen, M., and Adlercreutz, H. Plasma cortisol, androstenedione, testosterone and luteinizing hormone in running exercise of different intensities. *Scand. J. Clin. Lab. Invest.* 40:403–9, 1980.

50. Kuoppasalmi, K., Naveri, H., Rehunen, S., Harkonen, M., and Adlercreutz, H. Effect of strenuous anaerobic running exercise on plasma growth hormone, cortisol, luteinizing hormone, testosterone, androsteredione, estrone, and estradiol. *J. Steroid Biochem.* 7:823–29, 1976.

51. Lamb, D. R. Androgens and exercise. *Med. Sci. Sports* 7:1–5, 1975.

52. Lampman, R. M., and Schteingart, D. E. Effects of exercise training on glucose control, lipid metabolism, and insulin sensitivity in hypertrigly-ceridemia and non-insulin dependent diabetes mellitus. *Med. Sci. Sports Exerc.* 23:703–12, 1991.

53. Ljunghall, S., Joborn, H., Roxin, L. E., Skarfors, E. T., Wide, L. E., and Lithell, H. O. Increase in serum parathyroid hormone levels after prolonged physical exercise. *Med. Sci. Sports Exerc.* 20:122–25, 1988.

54. Lobstein, D. D., and Ismail, A. H. Decreases in reating plasma beta-endorphin/-lipotropin after endurance training. *Med. Sci. Sports Exerc.* 21:161–66, 1989.

55. Loucks, A. B. Effects of exercise training on the menstrual cycle: Existence and mechanisms. *Med. Sci. Sports Exerc.* 22:275–80, 1990.

56. Mazzeo, R. S. Catecholamine responses to acute and chronic exercise. *Med. Sci. Sports Exerc.* 23:839–45, 1991.

57. McConnell, T. R., and Sinning, W. E. Exercise and temperature effects on human sperm production and testosterone levels. *Med. Sci. Sports Exer.* 16:51–55, 1984.

58. Mougin, C., Baulay, A., Henriet, M. T., Haton, D., Jacquier, M. C., Turnill, D., Berthelay, S., and Gaillard, R. C. Assessment of plasma opioid peptides, beta-endorphin and met-enkephalin at the end of an international Nordic ski race. *Eur. J. Appl. Physiol.* 56:281–86, 1987.

59. Nesher, R., Karl, I. E., and Kipnis, D. M. Epitrochlearis muscle. II. Metabolic effects of contraction and catecholamines. *Am. J. Physiol.* 239:E461–E467, 1980.

60. Prokop, L. Adrenals and sport. *J. Sports Med. Phys. Fitness* 3:115–21, 1963.

61. Raymond, L., Sode, J., and Tucci, J. Adrenocortical response to non-exhaustive muscular exercise. *Acta Endocrinol.* 70:73–80, 1972.

62. Renold, A. E., Quigley, T. B., Kenard, H. E., and Thorn, G. W. Reaction of the adrenal cortex to physical and emotional stress in college oarsmen. *New Eng. J. Med.* 244:754–57, 1951.

63. Rogozkin, V. Metabolic effects of anabolic steroid on skeletal muscle. *Med. Sci. Sports* 11:160–63, 1979.

64. Rogozkin, V., and Feldkoren, B. The effect of Retabolil and training on activity of RNA polymerase in skeletal muscles. *Med. Sci. Sports* 11:345–47, 1979.

65. Selye, H. *Stress in Health and Disease.* Boston: Butterworth, 1976.

66. Sothmann, M. S., Hart, B. A., and Horn, T. S. Plasma catecholamine response to acute psychological stress in humans: Relation to aerobic fitness and exercise training. *Med. Sci. Sports Exerc.* 23:860–67, 1991.

67. Stuart, M., Lazarus, L., and Sutton, J. Somatomedin: Changes following physiological and pharmacological stimuli to growth hormone secretion. *Proc. Endocrinol. Soc. Aust.* 15:21, 1972.

68. Sutton, J. R. Drugs used in metabolic disorders. *Med. Sci. Sports Exerc.* 13:266–71, 1981.

69. Sutton, J. R., Brown, G. M., Keane, P., Walker, W. H. C., Jones, N. L., Rosenbloom, D., and Besser, G. M. The role of endorphins in the hormonal and psychological responses to exercise. *Int. J. Sports Med.* 3:19, 1982.

70. Sutton, J. R., Coleman, M. J., and Casey, J. H. Adrenocorticol contribution to serum androgens during physical exercise. *Med. Sci. Sports* 6:72, 1974.

71. Sutton, J. R., Coleman, M. J., and Casey, J. H. Testosterone production rate during exercise. *Third International Symposium on Biochemistry of Exercise,* eds. F. Landry and W.A.R. Orban. Miami: Symposia Specialists, Inc., 1978.

72. Sutton, J. R., Coleman, M. J., Casey, J., and Lazarus, L. Androgen responses during physical exercise. *Br. Med. J.* 1:520–22, 1973.

73. Sutton, J. R., Farrell, P. A., and Harber, V. J. Hormonal adaptation to physical activity. *Exercise, Fitness, and Health,* eds. C. Bouchard, R. J. Shephard, T. Stephens, J. R. Sutton, and B. D. McPherson. Champaign: Human Kinetics Books, 1990.

74. Terjung, R. Endocrine response to exercise. *Exer. Sport Sci. Rev.* 7:153–80, 1979.

75. Tharp, G. D. The role of glucocorticoids in exercise. *Med. Sci. Sports* 7:6–11, 1975.

76. Thoren, P., Floras, J. S., Hoffman, P., and Seals, D. R. Endorphins and exercise: Physiological mechanisms and clinical implications. *Med. Sci. Sports Exerc.* 22:417–28, 1990.

77. Ulrich, A. C. Measurement of stress evidenced by college women in situations involving competition. Ph.D. diss., University of Southern California, 1956.

78. Von Euler, U.S. Sympatho-adrenal activity in physical exercise. *Med. Sci. Sports* 6:165–73, 1974.

79. Wahren, J., Felig, P., Ahlborg, G., and Jorfeldt, L. Glucose metabolism during leg exercise in man. *J. Clin. Invest.* 50:2715–25, 1971.

80. Wake, R. F., Graham, B. F., and McGrath, S. D. A study of the eosinophil response to exercise in man. *J. Aviation Med.* 24:127–30, 1953.

81. Waldeck, B. β-adrenoceptors in skeletal muscle. *Acta Pharmacol. et Toxicol.* 44 (suppl. 2):28–30, 1979.

82. Winder, W. W., Hickson, R. C., Hagberg, J. M., Ehsani, A. A., and McLane, J. A. Training-induced changes in hormonal and metabolic responses to submaximal exercise. *J. Appl. Physiol.* 46:766–71, 1979.

11

The Immune System and Exercise

The Immune System
  Leukocytes
Nonspecific Immune Mechanisms
  Phagocytosis
  Natural Killer Cells
  Complement Proteins
  Interferons
Specific Immune Mechanisms
  Antigens
  Humoral Immunity
  Cell-Mediated Immunity

The Effects of Exercise on Immune
    Function
  Exercise and Leukocytosis
  Exercise and Lymphocytosis
  Exercise and Antibodies
    (Immunoglobulins)
  Exercise and Complement Proteins
  Exercise and Interferons
Clinical Implications of Exercise and
    Immune Function
  Epidemiological Studies of Exercise
    and Upper Respiratory Infection
  Exercise during Infection

There is a popular belief that chronic exercise and improved physical fitness makes an individual "healthier." While much research has been conducted with regard to chronic illnesses such as coronary heart disease and obesity, relatively little is known about the effect of exercise on infectious diseases. Anecdotal evidence from athletes as well as nonathletes suggests that exercise enhances an individual's resistance to infection. However, coaches often express concerns about an increase in the number of infectious episodes in their athletes, particularly near the end of the competitive season. These conflicting testimonials indicate a need for systematic investigations to answer important questions regarding the interactions between exercise and immune function such as:

1. Does an acute bout of exercise affect immune function?

2. Does chronic exercise affect immune function?

3. Are the effects of exercise on immune function related to the metabolic characteristics (aerobic or anaerobic) of the activity?

4. What are the relationships between intensity, duration, and frequency of exercise and immune function?

5. What are the clinical implications of the interactions between exercise and immune function?

The Immune System

The term immune is derived from the Latin word *immunis,* meaning free. Therefore, the function of the immune system is to keep us free from invading organisms such as bacteria and viruses that may cause diseases. The immune system can be divided into two general classifications: nonspecific mechanisms and specific mechanisms. The estimated one trillion cells of the immune system (leukocytes) generally function within one of these two classifications but are, in some cases, involved in both nonspecific and specific immunity. Figure 11.1 describes the relationships among the cells of the immune system.

Leukocytes

Leukocytes (white blood cells) are formed from undifferentiated stem cells in bone marrow and can be classified as granular or agranular based on their staining characteristics. The population of granular leukocytes can be further classified into neutrophils, eosinophils, and basophils. Neutrophils are the most abundant of the granular leukocytes and make up approximately 50% to 75% of all blood leukocytes.

There are two major classifications of agranular leukocytes: lymphocytes and monocytes. Lymphocytes make up approximately 20% to 40% of blood leukocytes while monocytes constitute about 5%. Monocytes can be transformed into macrophages, and the population of lymphocytes includes T cells, B cells, and natural killer (NK) cells. There are four subclassifications of T cells (killer, helper, suppressor, and memory T cells) and two of B cells (plasma cells and memory B cells).

Nonspecific Immune Mechanisms

The nonspecific immune mechanisms are the first lines of defense against potentially pathogenic (disease causing) organisms. Nonspecific immunity involves two mechanisms: external and internal. The external mechanisms include structures such as the skin, digestive tract, respiratory tract, and urinary tract. Although these physical barriers are effective in protecting the body from most invading organisms, they are reinforced by

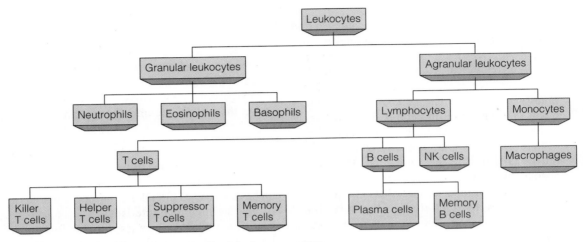

Figure 11.1   Relationships among cells of the immune system.

internal mechanisms designed to destroy those pathogens which penetrate the first (external) lines of defense. The internal mechanism associated with nonspecific immunity include the actions of phagocytic cells, NK cells, complement proteins, and interferons.

Phagocytosis

Two major groups of cells are involved in the nonspecific phagocytic process: neutrophils and mononuclear phagocytes such as monocytes, macrophages, and tissue-specific phagocytes in the liver, spleen, lymph nodes, lungs, and central nervous sytem. Phagocytosis is a process by which unwanted particles are engulfed and destroyed by digestive enzymes (fig. 11.2). An extension of the phagocytic cell membrane (called a pseudopod) "reaches" for the particle and surrounds it. Once the particle is engulfed, it binds to a cell organelle called the lysosome which contains digestive enzymes, and is destroyed.

Natural Killer Cells

NK cells are non-T and non-B lymphocytes that are thought to be involved with immune surveillance against cancer by destroying certain cells before they can produce tumors. However, the exact association between NK cell activity and the risk of developing cancer in humans, is unclear. In addition, the precise method by which NK cells lyse virally-infected and tumor cells is presently unknown.

Complement Proteins

The complement system consists of nine protein components (C1 through C9), which exist in an inactive state in blood and other bodily fluids. The complement system destroys cells that have been "marked" for elimination by antibodies (substances produced by plasma cells and discussed later in this chapter). Activation of the complement protein system occurs when antibodies bind with specific chemical substances on the membrane of the invading cells called antigens (also discussed later in this chapter). Following activation, the complement system proceeds through a series of events including binding to the cell membrane (a process called fixation) and destroying the cell. Destruction of the cell is accomplished by proteins C5 through C9, which puncture the cell membrane allowing water to enter and causing the cell to burst.

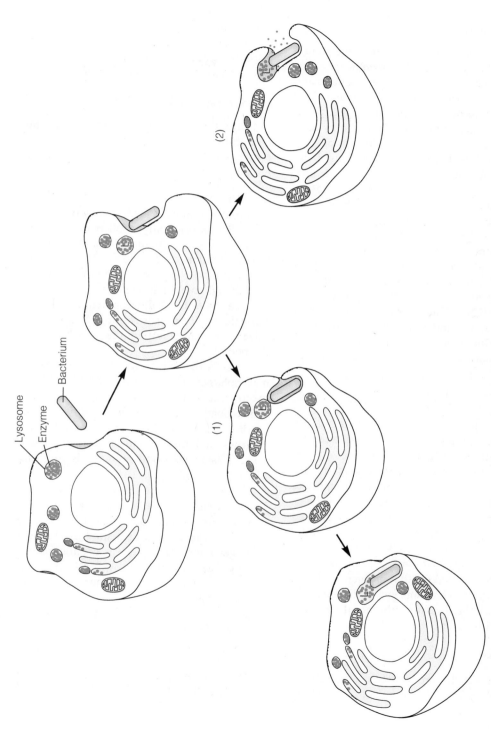

Figure 11.2 Phagocytosis by a neutrophil or macrophage. Phagocytic cell extends pseudopods around object to be engulfed (such as a bacterium). Dots represent lysosomal enzymes (L = lysosomes). If the pseudopods fuse to form a complete food vacuole (1), lysosomal enzymes are restricted to the organelle formed by the lysosome and food vacuole. If the lysosome fuses with the vacuole before fusion of the pseudopods is complete (2), lysosomal enzymes are released into the infected area of tissue. (From Stuart Ira Fox, *Human Physiology*. Copyright © 1984 Wm. C. Brown Communications, Inc., Dubuque, Iowa. All rights reserved. Reprinted by permission.)

Lysosome

Enzyme

Bacterium

Interferons

Interferons—polypeptides that "interfere" with the ability of viruses to replicate—are produced by cells infected with viruses and act on neighboring cells to prevent infection. The antiviral effects of interferons can be identified within hours following infection and may continue for several days (30). The association with virally infected cells has implicated interferons in immune surveillance against cancer. Many types of cells produce interferons including leukocytes, fibroblasts, and lymphocytes, which release alpha, beta, and gamma interferon, respectively. The mechanism of interferon action is both direct and indirect. The direct action involves the production of cellular enzymes that prevent viral protein synthesis and the destruction of viral messenger RNA. The indirect action involves stimulating NK and killer T cell activity as well as antibody production in plasma cells.

Specific Immune Mechanisms

While the nonspecific immune mechanisms are often successful in preventing disease, a second system called the specific immune mechanisms provides additional defenses against invading pathogens. The specific immune mechanisms involve the production of cells or a substance (called an antibody) to provide defense against a specific pathogen (called an antigen). Thus, if the body is exposed to a particular antigen, it will provide defenses specifically targeted for that antigen. The specific immune mechanisms can be divided into two general classifications: humoral and cell-mediated immunity.

Antigens

Antigen molecules are located on the cellular membrane of invading organisms and exhibit two unique characteristics: 1) they stimulate antibody production, and 2) they combine with a specific antibody. Most antigens are proteins but some are large polysaccharides.

Humoral Immunity

In Latin, the term *humor* means liquid. Thus, humoral immunity exists within the liquid components of the body such as blood and lymph.

B Cells

Humoral immunity is mediated by B cells. The letter B was originally applied to these cells because they were found in the Bursa of Fabricius of chickens. The name B cell is used in association with humoral immunity in humans even though mammals do not have a Bursa and the location of B cell development is unknown. Fully developed B cells reside in lymph nodes, spleen, and other lymphoid tissues throughout the body.

B cells respond to antigens presented by macrophages. The exact process by which the macrophages orient the antigen so that B cells will respond has not been fully identified. Once the B cell has been exposed to the antigen, it enlarges and divides into two subclassifications: plasma cells and memory B cells (fig. 11.3).

Plasma Cells and Antibodies.   Plasma cells secrete into circulation antibodies that are specific to the antigen presented by the macrophage. Each plasma cell is capable of producing approximately 2,000 antibody molecules per second for the four to seven day lifespan of the cell. Thus, a plasma cell can produce over 1 trillion antibody molecules in its short lifetime.

Antibodies (also known as immunoglobulins) are glycoproteins produced and secreted by plasma cells. The total number of antibody molecules within the human body is

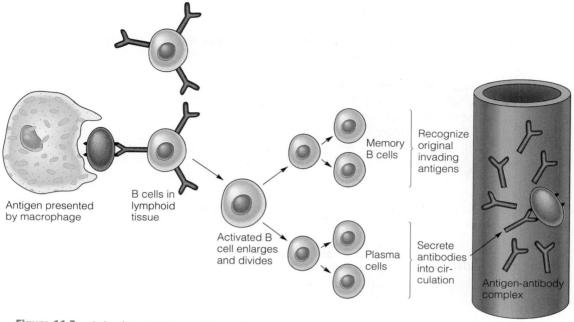

Figure 11.3   Role of B cells in humoral immunity. (Figures from *Principles of Anatomy and Physiology*, 4th ed., by Gerald Tortora and Nicholas Anagostakos. Copyright © 1984 by Biological Sciences Textbooks, Inc., and Elia-Sparta, Inc., A & P Textbooks. Reprinted by permission of HarperCollins Publishers.)

estimated at a staggering 100 million trillion. These antibodies are specific to millions of different antigens. There are five subclassifications of antibodies: immunoglobulin G (IgG), IgA, IgM, IgD, and IgE. The immunoglobulin subclasses are uniquely involved in the humoral defense mechanisms. For example, IgG and IgA are the most common antibodies found in serum and saliva, respectively, while IgM and IgD function as antigen receptors on the surface of lymphocytes prior to immunization. The IgE antibody subclass is involved in allergic reactions.

Antibodies are known to function in many ways although all of the mechanisms are not completely understood. It is important to recognize, however, that the antibody itself does not directly produce cell destruction but rather activates nonspecific immune mechanisms.

One of the primary mechanisms of antibody action involves the activation of the complement protein system. The antibody serves to identify the invading cell by binding with an antigen, which directs the complement system to destroy the invader.

In addition to activation of the complement system, antibodies have the ability to stimulate phagocytosis by binding with an antigen and macrophages through a process known as opsonization. As discussed earlier in this chapter, phagocytosis involves engulfing the invading organism and destroying it with lysosomal enzymes.

Antibodies are also involved in the destruction of cells through a process called antibody dependent cell-mediated cytotoxicity (ADCC). ADCC involves the binding of an antibody to an antigen on the cell surface, thus targeting the invader for destruction. The targeted cell is then lysed by certain lymphocytes, macrophages, neutrophils, and eosinophils. The mechanisms associated with the lysing of the targeted cells is not well understood but does not involve phagocytosis.

In addition to the more common mechanisms of antibody action discussed previously, specific antibodies work in diverse ways. For example, particular antibodies neutralize pathogenic chemicals called toxins, reduce the adherence of invading organisms to mucosal surfaces of the upper respiratory tract preventing colonization, and block antiphagocytic properties of some organisms.

Memory B Cells.   Memory cells are indistinguishable from the original B cells that enlarged and divided in response to an antigen. Memory cells are available to respond quickly and decisively to future exposure to the same antigen. In essence, memory cells remember a previous invader and act quickly to eliminate it.

Cell-Mediated Immunity

A class of lymphocytes called T cells provides defenses against specific antigens. Unlike B cells, however, this immunity does not involve the production and secretion of antibodies. When a macrophage presents an antigen to T cells located in lymphoid tissue that are programmed specifically for that antigen, the T cells become activated or sensitized. Sensitized T cells enlarge and divide into four subclassifications: killer T cells, helper T cells, suppressor T cells, and memory T cells (fig. 11.4). Each subclass has a unique function in cell-mediated immunity.

Killer T Cells
Unlike B cells, which secrete antibodies into circulation through the blood or lymph, killer T cells must be near or in contact with the cell targeted for destruction. Killer T cells provide both direct and indirect mechanisms for defense against invading organisms. The direct mechanisms include the production of cytotoxic polypeptides called lymphotoxins. Killer T cells migrate (from the lymphoid tissues in which they are stored) to the location of the invaders, attach to the targeted cells, and release lymphotoxins. Lymphotoxins are probably lysosomal enzymes that destroy the invading cell.

The indirect mechanisms of killer T cell action include the release of interferons as well as substances that enhance phagocytosis called macrophage chemotactic factor, macrophage activating factor, and macrophage migration inhibiting factor. As the names imply, these substances attract macrophages to the site of the invaders (chemotaxis), stimulate phagocytosis by macrophages (activation), and prevent macrophages from exiting the area (migration inhibiting).

Helper T Cells
Helper T cells have two main functions in cell-mediated immunity. Following activation by the macrophage-antigen complex, helper T cells stimulate the cytotoxic action of killer T cells and increase antibody production by plasma cells. Thus, there is an interaction between cell-mediated immunity and humoral immunity through the action of helper T cells.

Suppressor T Cells
Suppressor T cells regulate the action of killer T cells and the development of B cells into plasma cells. Thus, suppressor T cells modulate humoral immunity by inhibiting antibody production. The action of suppressor T cells helps keep the immune defense from exceeding the limits necessary for destruction of the invading organism.

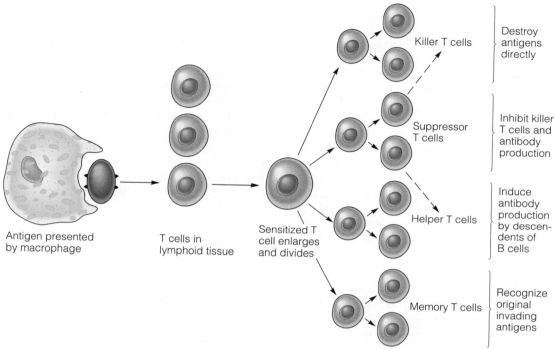

Killer T cells — Destroy antigens directly

Suppressor T cells — Inhibit killer T cells and antibody production

Helper T cells — Induce antibody production by descendents of B cells

Memory T cells — Recognize original invading antigens

Antigen presented by macrophage

T cells in lymphoid tissue

Sensitized T cell enlarges and divides

Figure 11.4   Role of T cells in cellular immunity. (Figures from *Principles of Anatomy and Physiology*, 4th ed., by Gerald Tortora and Nicholas Anagostakos. Copyright © 1984 by Biological Sciences Textbooks, Inc., and Elia-Sparta, Inc., A&P Textbooks. Reprinted by permission of HarperCollins Publishers.)

Memory T Cells

Memory T cells are capable of recognizing an antigen from a previous exposure. The ability to precisely identify potentially pathogenic invaders allows for a more rapid cell-mediated response. Usually the invading organism is destroyed before there are any outward symptoms of the disease.

The Effects of Exercise on Immune Function

Interest in the effect of exercise on immune function dates back at least to the 1920s when a series of studies were conducted to assess the impact of fatigue on susceptibility to infection (2, 24, 27). Even with this history of controlled investigations, we know relatively little about the impact of exercise on immune function in humans. It is likely, however, that advances in technology such as the electron microscope and sensitive assay techniques will lead to more conclusive research in this area.

Exercise and Leukocytosis

The majority of the presently available evidence indicates that exercise results in leukocytosis (1, 3, 4, 8, 10, 22, 28, 32), which is an increase in the number of circulating white blood cells (leukocytes). It appears, however, that the effect is transient, and the leukocyte number returns to normal within twenty-four hours following an acute bout of exercise (10,

19). Furthermore, the exercise-induced leukocytosis may be related to the intensity of exercise. Mackinnon and Tomasi (19) have stated that "maximal exercise in trained or untrained subjects and submaximal exercise in untrained subjects cause leukocytosis, whereas submaximal exercise in trained individuals does not."

The exercise-induced leukocytosis often exhibits a biphasic response (8, 19, 28). That is, there is an immediate increase in leukocyte number, followed by a period of normal values usually lasting approximately two hours and a second increase two to three hours following the exercise bout.

The mechanisms responsible for leukocytosis as a result of exercise have not been fully identified. It has been suggested that the immediate leukocyte response may be mediated by an increase in plasma levels of catecholamines, which are known to induce leukocytosis (19). The delayed mechanism underlying the response to exercise, however, is unknown. Furthermore, Mackinnon and Tomasi have suggested that exercise causes a release of leukocytes into circulation from storage areas of high blood flow such as the lungs. It is also likely that during exercise, leukocytes from the lymph vessels are redistributed into the blood stream. It does not appear, however, that changes in hemoconcentration or newly synthesized lymphoid cells account for the increase in circulating leukocytes as a result of exercise (19).

Exercise and Lymphocytosis

Most research studies have found that maximal and submaximal exercise results in a temporary increase (usually lasting less than forty-five minutes) in circulating lymphocytes, which ranges from approximately 35% to 180% (1, 12, 14, 19, 28, 31, 32). The disparity among investigations in the magnitude of the lymphocytosis is likely due to differences in the intensity and duration of exercise as well as the fitness level of the subjects. In addition, physical training affects the extent of the postexercise lymphocytosis (31). In general, there is less increase in the number of circulating lymphocytes as a result of a single bout of exercise following a training program than prior to it. That is, the lymphocyte response to physical activity is diminished as a result of exercise training. This is possibly due to a decrease in the catecholamine response (a potent stimulator of lymphocytosis) to exercise in a trained state compared to an untrained state (19).

Exercise affects the subclassifications of lymphocytes in a differential manner. Generally, total T cell numbers are less affected by exercise than B cells and NK cells which tend to increase substantially (14, 16, 19, 22, 32, 37). Within the total T cell population, however, exercise results in a redistribution in the number of circulating T suppressor cells and T helper cells such that there is an increase in the ratio of T suppressor to T helper cells (5, 7, 13, 16, 19).

Exercise and Antibodies (Immunoglobulins)

It is generally accepted that exercise has little or no effect on serum immunoglobulin levels (6, 9, 10, 17, 22, 26, 30). Cross-sectional studies have found that endurance athletes have levels within the normal range (9, 10). In addition, it is likely that the increases in serum immunoglobulin levels that have been reported following acute bouts of exercise can be explained by a change in plasma volume (23). Recently, Nehlsen-Cannarella and coworkers (23) reported a modest 20% increase in serum immunoglobulin levels following fifteen weeks of brisk walking in mildly obese females. This change, however, was not greater than that of the control group and thus the authors concluded that "exercise training has a minimal effect on serum immunoglobulin levels."

Secretory immunoglobulins are found in mucosal fluids such as saliva and provide a valuable line of defense against pathogens by preventing attachment and colonization. For example, the level of secretory immunoglobulin A is related to the occurrence of upper respiratory infection (18). Several recent studies have found that intense and prolonged bouts of acute exercise reduce salivary immunoglobulin A (sIgA) levels temporarily (one to twenty-four hours) and thus may increase susceptibility to upper respiration infection (17, 18, 29, 33, 34, 35). In addition, Tomasi and colleagues (35) reported that cross-country skiers involved in high volumes of exercise training have depressed resting levels of sIgA. Tharp and Barnes (34) reported a significant decrease in resting sIgA levels across a competitive season in collegiate swimmers. Interestingly, in a subsequent study, Tharp (33) found an increase in resting levels of sIgA in prepubescent and high school basketball players across a season. Perhaps the effect of exercise on sIgA is a function of the metabolic demands (aerobic versus anaerobic) of the sporting event. It should be noted, however, that in recent studies with nonathletes, moderate intensity (60% to 80% of maximal capacity) bouts of exercise for durations up to forty-five minutes had no effect on sIgA (20). This was also true for thirty minutes of running at 80% of maximal capacity at ambient temperatures between 6 and 35° C (15). In addition, ten weeks of moderate or high-intensity endurance training performed three times per week for twenty minutes per session had no effect on resting sIgA levels (21). Thus, the preponderance of the presently available evidence suggests that high-intensity, long duration bouts of exercise such as those performed by endurance athletes during practice

or competition result in a transient decrease in sIgA that lasts less than twenty-four hours. Repeated high-intensity endurance exercise sessions throughout a season may also result in depressed resting levels of sIgA. In general, however, acute bouts of submaximal exercise or moderate intensity endurance training have no effect on sIgA (15, 20, 21).

Few studies have examined the effect of exercise on secretory levels of immunoglobulins other than IgA. Mackinnon and coworkers (17) reported that a two hour maximal bicycle test resulted in reduced sIgA and sIgM but not sIgG levels. Additional research is needed to further examine if there is a differential response of the secretory immunoglobulin subclassifications to exercise.

Exercise and Complement Proteins

Few studies have examined the effect of exercise on complement proteins. Eberhardt (6) reported that twenty minutes of high-intensity cycle ergometry resulted in a small increase (14%) in certain complement proteins in untrained subjects, while Hanson and Flaherty (10) found no change in C3 or C4 following a 12.8 km run in trained subjects. Nieman and coworkers (26), however, found 15.3% and 11.3% increases in C3 and C4 in marathon runners following a maximal treadmill test. Interestingly, Nieman and coworkers also reported depressed resting levels of C3 and C4 in marathoners compared to age-matched sedentary controls, while Green and coworkers (9) found normal resting levels. Although much additional research is needed before conclusive evidence will be available, Simon (30) has stated that "it seems unlikely that exercise induces functionally important alterations in the complement system of athletes."

Exercise and Interferons

Viti and colleagues (36) found a small (3 IU pre-exercise versus 7 IU postexercise) but statistically significant increase in plasma interferon following sixty minutes of cycle ergometry at 70% of maximal oxygen consumption in untrained males. The increase was transient, however, and lasted less than two hours. Simon (30) has concluded "there is little evidence that exercise produces functionally important changes in circulating interferon levels."

Clinical Implications of Exercise and Immune Function

Few studies have examined the clinical implications of the effect of exercise on immune function. Mackinnon and Tomasi (19) have stated "Although many studies show that exercise alters several parameters central to immunity, it has not been shown conclusively that exercise influences resistance to disease." To fully address this issue would require long term, controlled investigations, which are expensive as well as difficult to conduct. There are, however, a limited number of studies that support the anecdotal evidence of a clinically important relationship between exercise and immune function.

Epidemiological Studies of Exercise and Upper Respiratory Infection

Recent epidemiological studies have examined the relationship between exercise and the incidence of upper respiratory infection (URI). Heath and coworkers (11) reported that subjects who ran more than 485 kilometers per year (an average of 9.3 kilometers per week) had a risk of developing URI (runny nose, sore throat, or cough on two consecutive days) that

was 2.0 to 3.5 times greater than those subjects who ran less than 485 kilometers per year. Nieman and colleagues (25) found that the risk of developing URI during the two month period prior to competing in a marathon race was 2.0 times greater in those competitors whose training distance was greater than 97 kilometers per week compared to those who ran less than 32 kilometers per week. In addition, the risk of developing URI during the week following the marathon was 5.9 times greater in participants than subjects who had trained for but chose not to run in the race. Interestingly, Mackinnon and coworkers (18) found that episodes of URI in squash and hockey players were preceded (within two days) by exercise-induced decreases in sIgA of 22% to 27%. Those athletes who did not develop URI exhibited markedly less change ($\pm 10\%$) in sIgA following exercise. The authors concluded that there is a temporal relationship between exercise-induced decreases in sIgA and subsequent appearance of URI and stated that "large changes in mucosal IgA occurring during exercise may be related to an increased incidence of URI in elite athletes." These findings have implications for both coaches and athletes who are concerned with "overtraining." Excessive training and highly demanding competitive events are likely to increase the risk of developing URI and adversely affect the health and performance of athletes. It is also possible that the additive effect of multiple stressors such as excessive training, caloric restriction, dehydration, and the psychological stress of competition may exacerbate the problem. This may be especially problematic for athletes such as wrestlers, gymnasts, boxers, and body builders.

Exercise during Infection

Coaches are often unsure about training and competition while an athlete is exhibiting signs of infection. While there is presently no definitive information in this area, Simon (30) has suggested that "It is probably not necessary for athletes with minor upper respiratory infections to restrict exercise, including competition and exposure to cold ambient temperatures. However, it does seem prudent to avoid vigorous exertion in the presence of fever, myalgia, and other constitutional symptoms suggestive of systemic infection." Simon further states that "Mild upper respiratory infections generally do not require interruption of exercise schedules. In fact, some individuals report relief of symptoms, probably because of the increased mucus flow associated with exercise." These suggestions provide useful guidelines for considering the appropriateness of training and/or competition during infection.

Summary

1. The function of the immune system is to keep us free from potentially pathogenic (disease causing) organisms such as bacteria and viruses.

2. The immune system can be divided into two general classifications: nonspecific and specific mechanisms.

3. Leukocytes (white blood cells) are formed in the bone marrow and can be classified as granular (neutrophils, eosinophils, and basophils) or agranular (lymphocytes and monocytes).

4. Monocytes can be transformed into macrophages, and lymphocytes include three primary subclassifications (T cells, B cells, and natural killer (NK) cells).

5. The nonspecific immune mechanisms are the first lines of defense and involve internal and external mechanisms.

6. The external nonspecific mechanisms include structures that serve as barriers to invading organisms such as the skin, digestive tract, respiratory tract, and urinary tract.

7. The internal nonspecific mechanisms include the actions of phagocytic cells, NK cells, complement proteins, and interferons.

8. Phagocytosis is a process by which unwanted particles are engulfed and destroyed by the digestive enzymes of the lysosome.

9. The specific immune mechanisms involve the production of cells or an antibody to provide defense against a specific pathogen (called an antigen).

10. The specific immune mechanisms can be divided into two general classifications: humoral and cell-mediated immunity.

11. Humoral immunity exists within the liquid components of the body such as blood and lymph and is mediated by B cells.

12. B cells that have been exposed to an antigen enlarge and divide into two subclassifications: plasma cells and memory cells.

13. Plasma cells release antibodies (also known as immunoglobulins) into circulation that activate nonspecific immune mechanisms to destroy specific invaders.

14. Memory cells remember previous invaders and act quickly to eliminate them.

15. Cell-mediated immunity involves the action of the four subclassifications of T lymphocytes: killer, helper, suppressor, and memory T cells.

16. Generally, exercise results in leukocytosis (increased number of leukocytes) and lymphocytosis (increased number of lymphocytes) but has little effect on serum immunoglobulin levels.

17. Acute and chronic high intensity exercise for a long duration has been shown to decrease salivary levels of immunoglobulin A and therefore may increase an individuals susceptibility to upper respiratory infection (URI).

18. Moderate intensity exercise has no effect on sIgA.

19. Mild URI generally does not require interruption of exercise schedules, but vigorous exercise should be avoided in the presence of fever, myalgia, and other constitutional symptoms of systemic infection.

References

1. Ahlborg, B., and Ahlborg, G. Exercise leukocytosis with and without beta-andrenergic blockade. *Acta. Med. Scand.* 187:241–46, 1970.

2. Bailey, G. H. The effect of fatigue upon the susceptibility of rabbits to intratracheal injections of type I pneumococcus. *Am. J. Hygiene* 5:175–95, 1925.

3. Berk, L. S., Nieman, D., Tan, S. A., Nehlsen-Cannarella, S., Kramer, J., Eby, W. C., and Owens, M. Lymphocyte subset changes during acute maximal exercise. *Med. Sci. Sports Exerc.* 18:706, 1986.

4. Busse, W. W., Anderson, O. L., Hanson, P. G., and Fots, J. D. The effect of exercise on the granulocyte response to isoproterenol in the trained athlete and unconditioned individual. *J. Allergy Clin. Immunol.* 65:358–64, 1980.

5. Calabrese, L. H. Exercise, immunity, cancer, and infection. *Exercise, Fitness, and Health,* eds. C. Bouchard, R. J. Shephard, T. Stephens, J. R. Sutton, and B. D. McPherson. Champaign: Human Kinetic Books, 1990.

6. Eberhardt, A. Influence of motor activity on serum serologic mechanisms of nonspecific immunity of the organism. II. Effect of strenuous physical effort. *Acta. Physiol. Pol.* 22:185–94, 1971.

7. Edwards, A. J., Bacon, T. H., Elms, C. A., Verardi, R., Felder, M., and Knight, S. C. Changes in the population of lymphoid cells in human peripheral blood following physical exercise. *Clin. Exp. Immunol.* 58:420–27, 1984.

8. Eskola, J., Ruuskanen, O., Soppi, E., Viljaner, M. K., Jarvinen, M., Toivoren, H., and Kouvalainen, K. Effect of stress on lymphocyte transformation and antibody formation. *Clin. Exp. Immunol.* 32:339–45, 1978.

9. Green, R. L., Kaplan, S. S., Rabin, B. S., Stanitski, C. L., and Zdziarski, U. Immune function in marathon runners. *Ann. Allergy* 47:73–75, 1981.

10. Hanson, P. G., and Flaherty, D. K. Immunological responses to training in conditioned runners. *Clin. Sci.* 60:225–28, 1981.

11. Heath, G. W., Ford, E. S., Craven, T. E., Macera, C. A., Jackson, K. L., and Pate, R. R. Exercise and the incidence of upper respiratory tract infections. *Med. Sci. Sports Exerc.* 23:152–57, 1991.

12. Hedfors, E., Biberfeld, P., and Wahren, J. Mobilizaton of the blood of human non-T and K lymphocytes during physical exercise. *J. Clin. Lab. Immunol.* 1:159–62, 1978.

13. Hedfors, E., Holm, G., Ivansen, M., and Wahren, J. Physiological variation of blood lymphocyte reactivity: T-cell subsets, immunoglobulin production, and mixed lymphocyte reactivity. *Clin. Immunol. Immunopath.* 27:9–14, 1983.

14. Hedfors, E., Holm G., and Ohnell, B. Variations of blood lymphocytes during work studied by cell surface markers, DNA synthesis and cytotoxicity. *Clin. Exp. Immunol.* 24:328–35, 1976.

15. Housh, T. J., Johnson, G. O., Housh, D. J., Evans, S. A., and Tharp, G. D. The effect of exercise at various temperatures on salivary levels of immunoglobulin A. *Int. J. Sports Med.* 12:498–500, 1991.

16. Landmann, R. M. A., Muller, F. B., Perini, C. H., Wesp, M., Erne, P., and Buhler, F. R. Changes of immunoregulatory cell induced by psychological and physical stress: Relationship to plasma catecholamines. *Clin. Exp. Immunol.* 58:127–35, 1984.

17. Mackinnon, L. T., Chick, T. W., van As, A., and Tomasi, T. B. The effect of exercise on secretory and natural immunity. *Adv. Exp. Med. Biol.* 216:869–76, 1987.

18. Mackinnon, L. T., Ginn, E., and Seymour, G. Temporal relationship between exercise-induced decreases in salivary IgA concentration and subsequent appearance of upper respiratory illness in elite athletes. *Med. Sci. Sports Exerc.* 23 (Suppl.):S45, 1991.

19. Mackinnon, L. T., and Tomasi, T. B. Immunology of exercise. *Sports Medicine, Fitness, Training, Injuries,* ed. O. Appenzeller. Baltimore: Urban and Schwarzenberg, 1988.

20. McDowell, S. L., Chaloa, K., Housh, T. J., Tharp, G. D., and Johnson, G. O. The effect of exercise intensity and duration on salivary immunoglobulin A. *Eur. J. Appl. Physiol.* 63:108–11, 1991.

21. McDowell, S. L., Hughes, R. A., Hughes, R. J., Housh, T. J., and Johnson, G. O. The effect of exercise training on salivary immunoglobulin A and cortisol responses to maximal exercise. *Int. J. Sports Med.* 13:577–580, 1992.

22. Moorthy, A. V., and Zimmerman, S. W. Human leukocyte response to an endurance race. *Eur. J. Appl. Physiol.* 38:271–76, 1978.

23. Nehlsen-Cannarella, S. L., Nieman, D. C., Balk-Lamberton, A. J., Markoff, P. A., Chritton, D. B., Gusewitch, G., and Lee, J. W. The effect of moderate exercise training on immune response. *Med. Sci. Sports Exerc.* 23:64–70, 1991.

24. Nicholls, E. E., and Spaeth, R. A. The relation between fatigue and the susceptibility of guinea pigs to infections of type I pneumococcus. *Am. J. Hygiene* 2:527–35, 1922.

25. Nieman, D. C., Johanssen, L. M., Lee, J. W., and Arabatzis, K. Infectious episodes in runners before and after the Los Angeles Marathon. *J. Sports Med. Phys. Fitness* 30:316–28, 1990.

26. Nieman, D. C., Tan, S. A., Lee, J. W., and Berk, L. S. Complement and immunoglobulin levels in athletes and sedentary controls. *Int. J. Sports Med.* 10:124–28, 1989.

27. Oppenheimer, E. H., and Spaeth, R. A. The relation between fatigue and the susceptibility of rats towards a toxin and an infection. *Am. J. Hygiene* 2:51–66, 1922.

28. Robertson, A. J., Ramesar, K. C. R. B., Potts, R. C., Gibbs, J. H., Browning, M. C. K., Brown, R. A., Hayes, P. C., and Beck, J. S. The effect of strenuous physical exercise on circulating blood lymphocytes and serum cortisol levels. *J. Clin. Lab. Immunol.* 5:53–57, 1981.

29. Schouten, W. J., Verschuur, R., and Kemper, H. C. G. Habitual physical activity, strenuous exercise, and salivary immunoglobulin A levels in young adults: The Amsterdam growth and health study. *Int. J. Sports Med.* 9:289–93, 1988.

30. Simon, H. B. Exercise and infection. *Phys. Sportsmed.* 15:135–41, 1987.

31. Soppi, E., Varjo, P., Eskola, J., and Laitinen, L. A. Effect of strenuous physical stress on circulating lymphocyte number and function before and after training. *J. Clin. Lab. Immunol.* 8:43–46, 1982.

32. Steel, C. M., and Evans, J. Physiological variation in circulating B cell: T cell ratio in man. *Nature* 247:387–89, 1974.

33. Tharp, G. D. Basketball exercise and secretory immunoglobulin-A. *Med. Sci. Sports Exerc.* 22:S125, 1990.

34. Tharp, G. D., and Barnes, M. W. Reduction of saliva immunoglobulin levels by swim training. *Eur. J. Appl. Physiol.* 60:61–64, 1990.

35. Tomasi, T. B., Trudeau, F. B., Czerwinski, D., and Erredge, S. Immune parameters in athletes before and after strenuous exercise. *J. Clin. Immunol.* 2:173–78, 1982.

36. Viti, A., Muscettola, M., Paulesu, L., Cocci, V., and Almi, A. Effect of exercise on plasma interferon levels. *J. Appl. Physiol.* 59:426–28, 1985.

37. Yu, D. T. Y., Clements, P. J., and Pearson, C. M. Effects of corticosteroids on exercise-induced lymphocytosis. *Clin. Exp. Immunol.* 28:326–31, 1977.

12

Exercise Metabolism

Definition of Terms
  Work
  Power
  Energy
  Efficiency
Methods for Standardizing and
    Measuring Exercise Loads
  Bench-Stepping
  Treadmill
  Cycle Ergometer
Methods for Measuring Energy
    Consumption
  Direct Calorimetry
  Indirect Calorimetry
  Gas Analysis
Oxygen Deficit and Recovery Oxygen

New Concepts Concerning Recovery
    Oxygen
Training Effect on Anaerobic Metabolism
    and Recovery Oxygen
Intermittent Work (Interval Training)
Maximal O_2 Consumption as a Measure
    of Physical Fitness
  Increasing Work Load
  O_2 Pulse
Respiratory Quotient
The Anaerobic Threshold Controversy
Theoretical Problems with the Anaerobic
    Threshold Concept
Negative Work

The essence and the uniqueness of the study of physiology of exercise lie in its concern with physiological mechanisms in operation not during rest but while the organism is stressed by physical activity. This physical activity may be work, physical education activity, athletics, or informal play. By observing the stress of vigorous physical activity, the exercise physiologist gains insight into physiology that is withheld when the organism is at rest. Questions about how well various organ systems can function under stress can be answered only in terms of the functional capacity an individual has with respect to his cardiovascular system, respiratory system, heat dissipation system, and so on. An individual may show no cardiac abnormality in a physician's diagnostic examination, but this does not tell us anything about that person's cardiac capacity for running a good time in the 440 or the mile. Functional tests are needed here, and these are in the domain of the exercise physiologist. To make these functional tests meaningful to other professions the exercise physiologist uses a vocabulary of terms that is taken from physics as well as physiology.

There is a movement among exercise scientists to use the Système International (SI) units for expressing data (table 12.1). While utilizing SI units would facilitate communication between scientists of various nations, most physical education students and coaches in the United States are more familiar with imperial and/or metric units. Therefore, for best communication with the intended readership, the imperial and metric systems have been retained in this text.

Definition of Terms

Work

Work is defined by the physicist as the product of force times the distance through which that force acts: $W = F \times D$. For example, a person who lifts a weight of 100 pounds to a height of 3 feet has done work of 100 pounds $\times$ 3 feet, or 300 ft-lb of work. In the metric system (which is commonly used internationally in exercise physiology, as in other sciences), an individual who weighs 100 kg and climbs up to stand on the 3-meter diving board performs 100 kg $\times$ 3 meters, or 300 kg-m of work. Note that no mention has been made of the time it takes to do the work. This is not a relevant factor in the concept of work. The same amount of work is performed regardless of how long it takes.

Unfortunately, the physicist's definition leaves something to be desired when the muscular activity is isometric, as in the case where one merely holds 100 pounds motionless. Here, since the distance is zero, the work must also be zero. However, there are other methods for evaluating the effort involved.

Power

If two individuals can each lift 100 pounds a distance of 3 feet but one does it twice as fast as the other, we have introduced the concept of power, which is work per unit of time (P = W/t). The person who does it twice as fast is twice as powerful. Power can be defined in terms of horsepower, just as in rating an automobile engine.

1 hp = 33,000 ft-lb/min = 550 ft-lb/sec

Power is distinct from *strength*. Power is composed of strength and speed. Thus an athlete's power in an event (such as the shot put)

Table 12.1   Système International (SI) Units.

Physical Quantity	Unit	Symbol
1. Acceleration	meters per second per second	$m \cdot sec^{-2}$
2. Amount of substance	mole	mol
3. Distance	meter	m
4. Force	newton	N
5. Mass	kilogram	kg
6. Power	watt	W
7. Time	second	sec
8. Torque	newton-meter	N-m
9. Velocity	meters per second	$m \cdot sec^{-1}$
10. Volume	liter	L
11. Work	joule	J

can be increased either by improving the strength of the muscles involved—as by heavy resistance training—or by improving the speed with which the movement is made.

To illustrate the calculation of horsepower, let us consider an individual performing the Harvard Step Test. In this test of physical fitness, one lifts one's body weight (150 pounds, let us say) onto a 20-inch-high bench 30 times per minute. Thus the work done per minute is as follows:

$$W = 150 \text{ lb} \times 1\tfrac{2}{3} \text{ ft } (20 \text{ in}) \times 30$$
$$= 7,500 \text{ ft-lb}$$

In terms of power, the subject has worked at the level of:

$$\frac{7,500 \text{ ft-lb/min}}{33,000 \text{ ft-lb/min}} = 0.227 \text{ hp}$$

A very powerful person can produce as much as three or four horsepower but only for very short periods of time (five to ten seconds).

Two other methods for expressing the magnitude of an exercise load are commonly used. Since many of the bicycle ergometers now in use are electrical devices, we often refer to the exercise load in *watts*.

For example:

$$1 \text{ W} = 6.12 \text{ kgm/min or approx. 6 kgm/min}$$
$$50 \text{ W} = \text{approximately } 300 \text{ kgm/min}$$
$$746 \text{ W} = 1 \text{ hp}$$

From a more physiological viewpoint the exercise load is often expressed in terms of METs, which is simply a number expressing the ratio of the exercise metabolic load to resting metabolic rate. Resting metabolic rate is approximately 3.5 ml of O_2 consumption per minute/per kilogram body weight. Thus the METs required for a given exercise load are calculated as follows:

$$\text{METs} = \frac{O_2 \text{ required for exercise}}{O_2 \text{ required for rest}}$$
$$= \frac{\dot{V}O_2 \text{ at exercise in ml/kg} \cdot min^{-1}}{3.5 \text{ ml/kg} \cdot min^{-1}}$$

Expressing the intensity of an exercise load in foot-pounds per minute, kilogram-meters per minute, or in watts results in a measure of power output. METs, on the other hand, are a measure of energy consumption.

Energy

Energy is defined as the capacity for doing work and can be expressed in the same units. Energy can be stored, in which case it is *potential energy*. The energy involved in the production of work is *kinetic energy*. Because humans are ultimately dependent on food for their energy, it is obvious that energy can be transformed from one form to another. This is done in accord with the *law of conservation of energy,* which states that in the conversion of energy from one form to another, energy is neither created nor destroyed. The energy in food is chemical energy, and it is converted into mechanical and heat energy by the muscles in bringing about movement and doing work.

The energy of food, which produces work, and the work itself can also be described in terms of calories (or kilocalories). One kilocalorie represents the heat required to raise the temperature of 1 kg of water $1°$ C. To convert heat units to mechanical units:

$$1 \text{ kcal} = 3,087 \text{ ft-lb} = 427 \text{ kgm}$$

Thus a one-ounce chocolate bar that contains 150 kilocalories can theoretically produce energy for some 463,000 ft-lb of work, or enough to keep a 150-pound person doing the Harvard Step Test for more than one hour at 100% efficiency. (However, the actual efficiency of such an exercise is not over 25%.)

Efficiency

Efficiency is usually defined as the percentage of energy input that appears as useful work. Thus if a person requires 4,000 kcal input of energy to perform a muscular activity that represents 1,000 kcal work output, efficiency is 25%.

Most of the experimentation in this area indicates that muscular performance under favorable circumstances achieves a mechanical efficiency of 20% to 25%. However, recent evidence suggests that efficiency may be much higher in running (chap. 23, "Efficiency of Muscle Activity"). It must be realized that the other energy, which does not appear as work, is not lost; it appears as heat, is dissipated, and tends to raise the body temperature during exercise.

Methods for Standardizing and Measuring Exercise Loads

To make meaningful measurements of the physiological processes during exercise, the exercise work load must be set up in such fashion as to be measurable and repeatable, and it should require little skill. Much of our athletic activity does not lend itself well to these requirements. Measuring the energy or work output of a football player, for instance, would be most difficult because bursts of activity are interspersed with variable periods of relative inactivity, such as huddles. Furthermore, the work done varies from moment to moment.

Three methods for establishing a standard measurable work load are in common use. Each has its advantages and disadvantages.

Bench-Stepping

Subjects lift their weight to a known height (the height of the bench). The rate can be easily set with a metronome. This activity requires minimum skill and lends itself well to large groups, but it is subject to several sources of inaccuracy. First, subjects, particularly when they are tired, tend not to straighten their bodies at the hip and knee joints and consequently have not lifted their center of gravity to the full height of the bench. Second, they are doing positive work (stepping up) and negative work (stepping down). Negative work requires considerably less energy expenditure than positive work but is difficult to assess.

Treadmill

A treadmill consists of a motor-driven conveyor belt that is large and strong enough for subjects to walk and run on. This device is usually constructed so that the speed of the belt and the incline are adjustable. The treadmill is advantageous since it requires a skill with which everyone is familiar (walking or running). Furthermore, it seems to bring about a slightly better involvement of large muscle masses than any other device since the arms and shoulders can and do enter into the activity.

It has two major disadvantages. First, the subject's movements make instrumentation somewhat difficult. Second, and more important, the units of work must be stated in arbitrary fashion—as running at 7 mph on a 10% incline—because much of the work is done in a horizontal direction, and this does not allow evaluation in the standard units of foot-pounds, kilogram-meters, or watts.

Cycle Ergometer

This instrument is a stationary bicycle whose front or back wheel is driven by subjects pedaling (figs. 12.1a, 12.1b, and 12.1c). The resistance against which subjects pedal is provided by a frictional band or by electromagnetic braking. The work load can be quickly and easily adjusted by changing the tension (and hence the frictional load) of the brake band or the electromagnetic load across the generator. Work is calculated easily from a scale reading, which provides the frictional resistance (force), and from a counter that records the number of times the wheel has turned and thus allows calculation of distance: $D = 2\pi r \times N$. The wheel's circumference, $2\pi r$, is the distance traveled by any point on the wheel in one revolution. N is the number of revolutions during the work period. Then, since $W = FD$, the total work done may be expressed as $W = F (2\pi r \times N)$.

This piece of equipment has several advantages. First, it is relatively inexpensive. Second, the subject's upper body is relatively motionless, facilitating instrumentation for electrocardiograph leads and so on. Third, and most important, the exercise load is expressed in standard units of work, foot-pounds, kilogram-meters, or watts. Thus work comparisons can be made more easily with the cycle ergometer than with the treadmill.

An international team of work physiologists compared the maximal O_2 consumption measured by the three ergometric methods in the same twenty-four healthy young subjects. They found that the terminal pulse rates and arterial lactate levels two minutes after exercise are very similar for step, bicycle, and treadmill exercise (3). However, the maximal O_2 uptake in the treadmill test was 7% greater than that in the bicycle test, while the step test values were between the treadmill and bicycle ergometer values. It has been suggested that these differences may be due to a lower blood flow in the lower limb during cycling (40). It has also been found that cardiac output and stroke volume are approximately 5% higher on the treadmill than on the ergometer (24). A comparison of stair climbing and cycling has shown that at similar work rates ventilatory volume is some 20% lower during stair climbing (similar to bench stepping), a difference that results in a fall in arterial O_2 saturation (43).

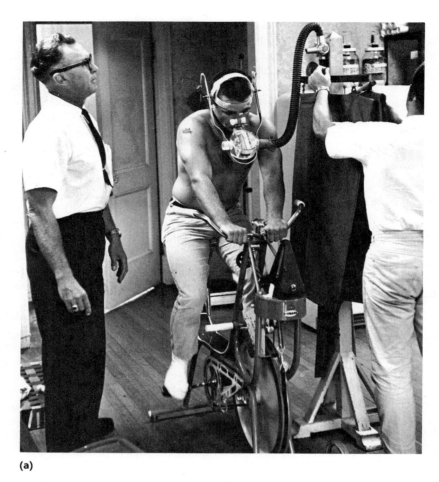

(a)

Figure 12.1   Figures 12.1a, 12.1b, and 12.1c describe a chronology of gas collection procedure. Figure 12.1a shows gas collection by the "classic" Douglas bag method using a simple frictional bicycle ergometer. Figure 12.1b shows deVries's laboratory using semiautomated electronic methods for gas collection and an electronically controlled and programmed bicycle ergometer. Figure 12.1c shows the use of a modern metabolic cart and an electronically braked bicycle ergometer.

These differences in physiological response suggest that in evaluating athletes' maximal aerobic power it is important to select a work situation that allows movement as similar as possible to the subjects' specific sports activity.

The consensus of an international group of experts reporting to the World Health Organization (WHO) was that the "order of preference of exercise tests is considered to be as follows: upright bicycle ergometer, step test, and treadmill" (54).

It must be recognized that in setting work loads on the bicycle ergometer equal work loads can have very different physiological effect if pedal frequency is allowed to vary (7, 26). Highest values of maximum O_2 consumption are obtained using between 60 and 70 rpm (25).

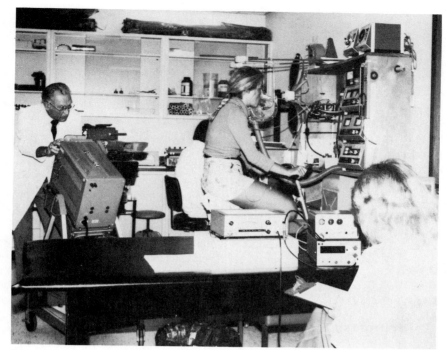

(b)

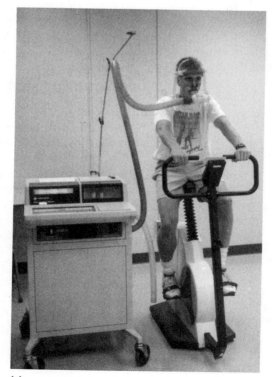

(c)

Figure 12.1   *Continued.*

It is also important to consider the effects of learning and habituation on the performance, particularly when measurements such as heart rate at submaximal work loads are of concern. Most subjects experience anxiety in a new test situation, and this of course affects observed heart rate. There is also a learning effect that produces small increases in efficiency. These effects must be controlled or balanced out in any test-retest experiment, whether the exercise is on a cycle ergometer, treadmill, or stepping bench.

Methods for Measuring Energy Consumption

Direct Calorimetry

Because the human organism is essentially a heat engine, the direct approach to measurements of energy consumption is to measure the heat produced by an individual's metabolic processes. This has been done in specially constructed chambers, where all metabolic heat is accumulated by the air and walls of the chamber and changes in their temperature are used to calculate the energy output. This method is called *direct calorimetry*. However, the equipment is expensive and difficult to use and consequently is seldom used in exercise physiology.

Indirect Calorimetry

Because the body's metabolic processes utilize oxygen and produce carbon dioxide (either during activity or immediately after), the energy output is directly related to the quantity of these respiratory gasses. The gasses can be collected from the expired air and measured. This is a much simpler process than

direct calorimetry and is therefore commonly used in exercise physiology. There are two methods for accomplishing indirect calorimetry: the *closed-circuit* and the *open-circuit* methods.

In the closed-circuit method illustrated in figure 12.2, the subject inspires from a face mask that is connected to an oxygen chamber charged from an O_2 cylinder. Expired air is conducted back to the oxygen chamber by way of a soda lime cannister, where the CO_2 produced is absorbed. Thus only the O_2 that remains after the respiratory exchange is returned to the oxygen chamber, and the changes in the volume of the O_2 that remains in the chamber are recorded from breath to breath. Each peak in the kymogram in figure 12.2 represents one respiration. By measuring the downward slope of the bottom points of the record per unit time, the value of O_2 consumed can be calculated.

This method has the advantage of simplicity, but its accuracy is not much better than plus or minus 10% of the true value. Furthermore, no value for the CO_2 produced is obtained, and consequently the respiratory quotient (to be discussed below) cannot be calculated.

In the classic open-circuit method, the subject inspires directly from the atmospheric air and expires into a rubberized canvas bag called a *Douglas bag* (fig. 12.3). After an exercise period during which gas collection is accurately timed, samples of the expired gas are taken from the bag for analysis, and the volume of expired gasses is measured by a gas meter similar to that used for metering the gas used in a home (fig. 12.3). The concentrations of O_2 and CO_2 in the atmosphere are very constant—20.93% and 0.03%, respectively. On the assumption that the remaining gasses (79.04%) lumped together as N_2 do not enter

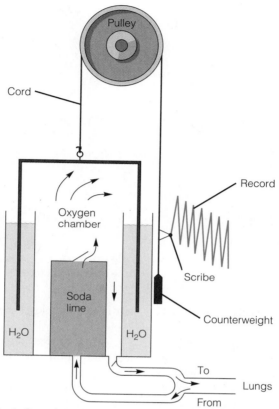

Figure 12.2   Apparatus for indirect determination of heat production by measuring oxygen consumption. The subject breathes into and from the oxygen chamber through the tubes at the bottom. The slope of the curve recorded by the movements of the upper cylinder is a measure of the rate at which oxygen is used by the subject. Arrows indicate direction of oxygen movement as the subject breathes. (From Carlson, A. J., and Johnson, R. E. *The Machinery of the Body.* © 1953 University of Chicago Press. Courtesy of The University of Chicago Press, Chicago.)

into physiological reactions, the volume of inspired air can be calculated from the volume of expired air as follows:

$$\frac{\text{Volume inspired}}{\text{Volume expired}} = \frac{\substack{\text{Percent of } N_2 \\ \text{in expired air}}}{79.04}$$

or

$$\text{Volume inspired} = \frac{\substack{\text{Percent of } N_2 \text{ in expired} \\ \text{air} \times \text{Volume expired}}}{79.04}$$

This calculation is necessary because the volume of CO_2 produced is not usually equal to the volume of O_2 consumed, and consequently the total volume of expired air also differs from the total inspired.

To calculate the O_2 consumed, one need only subtract the volume of O_2 remaining in the expired air (percent of O_2 expired times volume expired) from the volume of O_2 in the inspired air (20.93 times volume inspired). The same sort of calculation will also provide the

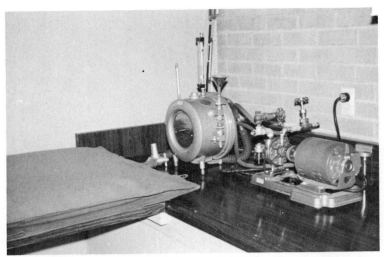

Figure 12.3   Measuring the volume of expired respiratory gasses from the Douglas bag with a wet-test gas meter. Gasses are drawn through the meter at a constant rate by an electrical vacuum pump.

volume of CO_2 produced during the exercise. This method is obviously somewhat more involved than the closed-circuit method, but the gain in precision is commensurate. In the open-circuit method, the error may be less than $\pm 1.0\%$, compared with $\pm 10\%$ for the closed-circuit. Furthermore, data are obtained for the percent of CO_2, which enables computation of the respiratory quotient (RQ).

Gas Analysis

The percentage of O_2 remaining and CO_2 produced in the expired air are analyzed either by biochemical or electronic methods. The classic biochemical method—the *Haldane apparatus* and *procedure*—uses the absorption of CO_2 by potassium hydroxide from a sample of known size. The change in volume of the sample by absorption of CO_2 is observed. The proportion this change represents in the total volume of the sample represents the proportion or percent of CO_2 in the sample. The O_2 is then absorbed out by a strong reducing solution and the same reasoning is applied. All of the gasses

left in the sample at this point are considered N_2.

A more recent development of the chemical (absorptiometric) method is the *Scholander apparatus* (fig. 12.4). It uses the same principle described above but is a considerably faster procedure. (Both methods are capable of a precision of better than $\pm 0.02\%$ in the range of respiratory gasses.)

Still more recently, electronic methods have been developed for measuring respiratory gasses, and they have advantages in both speed and simplicity of operation. Indeed, on-line computer analysis and breath-by-breath graphic display of exercise function tests are now available (fig. 12.1c). The electronic methods compare favorably with the precision of the Haldane and Scholander apparatus.

Oxygen Deficit and Recovery Oxygen

In the normal, resting individual, the supply of O_2 to the tissues is sufficient for the complete breakdown of glycogen to CO_2 and H_2O,

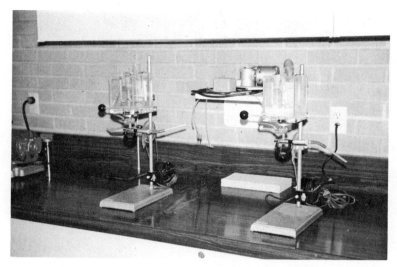

Figure 12.4   Micro Scholander gas analyzers used for estimating the percentage of O_2 and CO_2 in the expired gas volume.

with no accumulation of lactic acid. This situation also applies when the rate of work is such that the metabolic demands can be met aerobically.

In any exercise bout there is a transition period between rest and exercise, involving a short period during which the circulatory and respiratory adjustments lag behind.

The amount by which the O_2 supply fails to meet need by virtue of this lag in the organism's adjustment to the rise in metabolic rate is called the *oxygen (O_2) deficit.* Function of the organism under O_2 deficit conditions is made possible by several energy sources not dependent on O_2 transport. Most important are 1) the splitting of ATP and CP; 2) anaerobic breakdown of glycogen (glycolysis) to lactic acid; and 3) use of O_2 bound to muscle myoglobin and blood O_2 stores as shown in figure 12.5.

When exercise creates a metabolic need for greater O_2 than can be supplied by the cardiorespiratory processes, part of the energy of muscular activity is supplied by the anaerobic

mechanism described in chapter 3. Lactic acid accumulates as the end product of metabolism. Whenever the supply of O_2 is insufficient to meet demands, an individual is said to contract an *oxygen debt* (a term coined by A. V. Hill, a pioneer in exercise physiology).

However, the term *oxygen debt* is no longer acceptable to some investigators because of mounting evidence that the excess O_2 during recovery is not related to "paying off" an O_2 debt in terms of simply metabolizing lactate built up during the exercise, as had been postulated by earlier investigators. The student should be familiar with the term *oxygen debt* because of its widespread use over some five decades in scientific literature. However, in view of the recent evidence to be discussed below, we shall use instead the term *recovery oxygen,* defined loosely as the excess oxygen consumption during recovery due to a combination of phenomena that are not yet completely understood (9, 18, 20, 21, 22).

In light exercise, where a steady level of O_2 consumption is attained as shown in figure

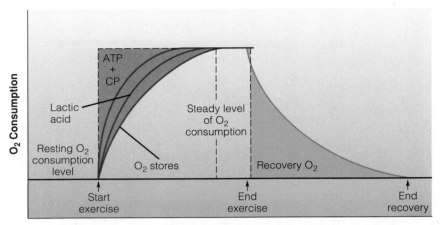

Figure 12.5   Diagram of the relationship of O_2 consumption and time before, during, and after submaximal exercise. The crosshatched area represents O_2 deficit, which depends on at least three factors: (1) breakdown of high energy phosphates ATP + CP; (2) glycolysis to form lactic acid; and (3) use of O_2 stores such as oxymyohemoglobin and O_2 of the venous blood. The stippled area represents the recovery oxygen used during recovery. All values of O_2 consumption are measured above the resting value as a baseline.

12.5, the recovery oxygen may be due entirely to the O_2 deficit at the beginning of exercise. At the end of exercise then, there must be a recovery period during which the O_2 deficit is repaid. This is why the heart and the ventilation rates remain elevated after exercise ceases.

When an exercise represents a true overload in which a steady state cannot be achieved, the duration of the effort (or the level of performance) is limited by the athlete's ability to sustain anaerobic metabolism. In maximum work load situations where energy supply is predominately from anaerobic sources, duration is limited to one to two minutes and recovery may take forty-five minutes or even longer.

To illustrate, let us consider a typical experiment on the cycle ergometer (outlined in table 12.2).

It is clear that this individual had a metabolic demand for 4 liters of O_2 per minute, 3 liters of which were provided by aerobic mechanisms and 1 liter by anaerobic mechanisms. This necessitated a recovery oxygen of more O_2 per minute than the resting state would have demanded until the equilibrium was reestablished. The length of time for monitoring recovery O_2 consumption is determined by observations of heart rate and minute-by-minute O_2 consumption. When these values have returned to their preexercise values, recovery is complete.

New Concepts Concerning Recovery Oxygen

The older literature had established that, under overload conditions (work loads greater than aerobic capacity), for every liter of O_2 debt the lactic acid level increased by 7 gm. However, the classic work of Margaria, Edwards, and Dill (39) had shown that for the first 2.5 liters of O_2 debt no increase in lactate could be demonstrated. On this basis, O_2 debt was thought

Table 12.2

Time	Activity	Total Liters of O_2 Consumed	Liters of O_2 Consumed per Minute
8:00–8:05	Resting (seated on cycle ergometer)	1.50	.30
8:05–8:10	Riding (at 1,500 kgm/min)	16.50	3.30
8:10–8:40	Recovery (seated on cycle ergometer)	14.00	.47

Calculations (in liters)

1. Total gross O_2 cost $=O_2$ during ride $+ \ O_2$ recovery
   $= 16.50$ liters $+ \ 14.00$ liters $= 30.50$ liters
2. Total net O_2 cost $= O_2$ during ride $+ \ O_2$ recovery $- \ O_2$ for equivalent period of rest (35 min)
   $= 16.50$ liters $+ \ 14.00$ liters $- \ (35 \times 0.30) = 20.0$ liters

3. Net O_2 cost per min of ride $= \dfrac{20.00 \text{ liters}}{5 \text{ min}} = 4.00$ liters/min

4. Net O_2 intake during ride $= O_2$ during $- \ O_2$ for equivalent rest period
   $= 16.50 - (5 \times 0.30) = 15.00$ liters

5. Net O_2 intake during ride, per min $= \dfrac{15.00 \text{ liters}}{5 \text{ min}} = 3.00$ liters/min

6. "O_2 debt" incurred per min $=$ net O_2 cost per min of ride $-$ net O_2 intake during ride, per min
   $= 4.00$ liters $- \ 3.00$ liters $= 1.00$ liters/min

7. Total "O_2 debt" incurred $= 5 \times 1.00$ liters $= 5.00$ liters

From Carpenter, T. M., *Tables, Factors, and Formulas for Computing Respiratory Exchange and Biological Transformations of Energy,* 4th ed., 1948. Reprinted by permission of Carnegie Institute of Washington.

to have two components: *lactacid,* which was represented by proportional increases in blood lactate, and *alactacid,* for which no lactate increase was found. Furthermore, Margaria and colleagues also demonstrated a great difference in the repayment of these two components of the O_2 debt. The alactacid debt was repaid approximately thirty times faster than the lactacid debt. Thus the fast component (alactacid) was ascribed to replacement of O_2 and energy stores, and the slow or lactacid component was thought to be used to remove lactate from the blood.

While the two components of O_2 debt with respect to rate of repayment are well verified,

the *lactacid-alactacid* explanation of the physiology involved has proved to be an oversimplification. It is now clear that many processes besides the elimination of lactate may be involved in the delayed return of O_2 uptake to the resting value after cessation of exercise (recovery oxygen):

1. During exercise, O_2 stores of the body are greatly reduced, and part of the recovery O_2 is used to

   a. restore muscle myoglobin to resting values

   b. restore venous oxyhemoglobin levels

   c. replenish O_2 dissolved in tissue fluids

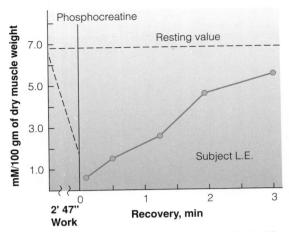

Figure 12.6   Phosphocreatine concentration (mM per 100 gm dry muscle) before and after a maximal work load. (From Hermansen, L. *Medicine and Science in Sports* 1:32, 1969.)

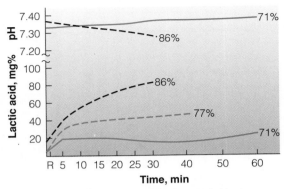

Figure 12.7   Mean lactic acid values and pH values over duration of runs at 82%–89% $\dot{V}O_2$ max, 74%–79% $\dot{V}O_2$ max, and 67%–74% $\dot{V}O_2$ max. (From Nagle, F. *Medicine and Science in Sports* 2:185, 1970.)

2. The rise in body temperature resulting from vigorous exercise creates a demand for more O_2.

3. Neither heart rate nor cardiac output returns immediately to resting values, and thus excess O_2 is required for cardiac metabolism.

4. What is true for heart rate and cardiac output is also true for pulmonary function.

5. The output of catecholamines is probably still above resting values, and this augments O_2 consumption.

6. The high energy phosphate breakdown (fig. 12.6) must be reversed at a considerable cost of O_2 consumption (36).

The fast component (formerly alactacid debt) may be largely accounted for by the energy required to reverse the changes in CP and ATP (item 6) (18). The available evidence suggests that the most important factors operative in the slow component (formerly lactacid debt) are probably the higher than normal core and muscle temperature together with oxidation of lactate (18, 20, 21). Lactate metabolism (in classic concepts thought to account entirely for the slow component) probably accounts for no more than 30% of the total recovery oxygen (22). Consequently the terms *lactacid debt* and *alactacid debt* are no longer appropriate.

To further complicate the relationship of lactate level to O_2 debt as measured by excess recovery O_2, Rowell and coworkers (44) have shown that even during moderate exercise as much as 50% of the lactate production may be removed by hepatic splanchnic tissues. It has also been shown that the nonexercising muscles may be consuming lactate even as the exercising muscles are producing it (2). Obviously, this precludes any neat 7 gm lactate per liter O_2 debt relationship as had been suggested by earlier workers. Thus a lactate buildup in the blood is unlikely at any but the heaviest work loads, as shown in figure 12.7. Of course, no proportionality between blood lactate and level of anaerobic metabolism could be expected.

Training Effect on Anaerobic Metabolism and Recovery Oxygen

In football, baseball, basketball, and probably most athletic activities that find favor in our country, one important determinant of success is *anaerobic power,* the ability to get moving quickly for short distances. Relatively few sports events in the United States require a sustained effort longer than thirty to sixty seconds. Consequently the vast majority of events depend on anaerobic power, which has been given very little attention by researchers in physiology of exercise.

Fortunately, a simple and practical method for measuring this important parameter was developed by Margaria, Aghemo, and Rovelli (38). The test consists of measuring the vertical component of the maximal speed with which an individual can run up an ordinary staircase. More recently, cycle ergometer tests of anaerobic power have been developed by Katch and coworkers (32) and Bar-Or (8).

There is evidence to show that endurance training enables a person to adjust to the energy requirements of a constant load of submaximal work more rapidly, resulting in a smaller O_2 deficit (20). Considerable evidence also supports the notion that endurance training reduces the recovery O_2 required for the same work load or permits sustaining higher blood lactate levels after maximal effort (23).

Intermittent Work (Interval Training)

At this point it is of interest to examine the work of the Astrands, Christensen, and their coworkers (5, 6, 10), since it seems to have large implications for the planning of training

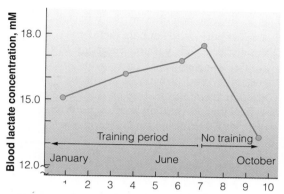

Figure 12.8   Blood lactate concentration (peak value) after maximal exercise (100 meters swimming) during the training period and after twenty-four months with no training. (From Hermansen, L. *Medicine and Science in Sports* 1:37, 1969.)

regimens. In one experiment, for example, a well-trained subject was able to work for thirty minutes at a very high work load (4.4 liters of O_2 per minute) by alternating five seconds of work with five seconds of rest. This appeared to be something like a steady state in that very little lactic acid accumulated. Even for a highly trained athlete, a work load of that size done continuously would result in a high level of blood lactate (fig. 12.8).

In another experiment a subject alternately ran ten seconds and rested five seconds, for a total of thirty minutes and 6.67 km. His O_2 intake for the thirty-minute period averaged 5.0 liters/min (his maximum capacity was 5.6 liters/min). His actual O_2 uptake for the twenty minutes of running was 101 liters, and his uptake during the accumulated rest periods was 49 liters. Subtracting a resting O_2 consumption of 4.0 liters for the ten minutes of rest from the total 49 liters leaves a tremendous recovery O_2 requirement of 45 liters, which had been eliminated in some fashion during the five-second rest periods. The largest O_2 requirement ordinarily reported after continuous work varies from 15 to 20 liters of O_2. These experimenters suggest that O_2 is stored as oxymyohemoglobin in the muscles during the rest periods to support metabolism during the work periods without resorting to the anaerobic mechanisms. This is an interesting possibility and provides a scientific basis for interval training of athletes. Indeed, there is now evidence that intermittent exercise can train both aerobic and anaerobic capacity (33).

Maximal O_2 Consumption as a Measure of Physical Fitness

The maximal O_2 consumption ($\dot{V}O_2$ max) for any individual is a good criterion of how well various physiological functions can adapt to the increased metabolic needs of work or exercise. At least the following functions are involved and contribute to the magnitude of an athlete's ability to maintain a steady state:

1. Lung ventilation
2. Pulmonary diffusion
3. O_2 and CO_2 transport by the blood
4. Cardiac function
5. Vascular adaptation (vasodilatation of active tissues and vasoconstriction of inactive tissues)
6. Physical condition of the involved muscles

Increasing Work Load

The method for measuring maximal O_2 consumption (aerobic power) involves working subjects at ever-increasing work loads, during each of which steady state level O_2 consumption is measured (usually by open-circuit spirometry). When an increase in work load fails to elicit a significant increase in O_2 consumption, the highest value attained represents the maximum O_2 consumption, as shown in figure 12.9.

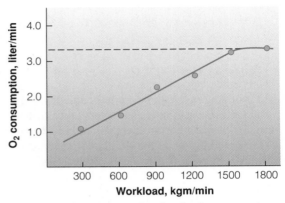

Figure 12.9   Diagram showing the O_2 consumption work load relationship when the subject was tested at repeated five-minute workouts with rest intervals. The maximum O_2 consumption is indicated by the dashed line at 3.30 liters/min.

Any of the ergometric methods discussed earlier can be used. The test can be administered either on a continuous or discontinuous protocol. In the discontinuous method, subjects are worked at each load until a steady O_2 level is attained (at least five minutes), with rest periods between work loads sufficient to allow recovery. Unfortunately, this method usually involves at least two or three visits to the laboratory and requires a great deal of technician and lab time in addition. Fortunately, the results obtained by the continuous method, where the load is increased every minute or every two minutes, are closely comparable to those obtained in the discontinuous method (2). This procedure can be completed in one half-hour visit to the laboratory. The error of the measurement of aerobic power has been reported to be about 2.5% (49).

Saltin and Astrand (45) tested ninety-five male and thirty-eight female members of the Swedish national teams and found the mean maximal O_2 uptake for the best fifteen males to be 5.75 liters/min and for the best ten females 3.6 liters/min. The highest values found were 6.17 liters/min and 4.07 liters/min for the male and female, respectively. The highest values were achieved by the cross-country ski team.

A clever experiment was designed by Klissouras (34) to determine to what extent aerobic power is determined genetically. He tested fifteen monozygous and ten dizygous twins and found that in these young boys aged seven through thirteen the variability in aerobic power was determined 93% by genetic factors. In a subsequent experiment (35) in which comparisons were made of a trained and an untrained monozygous twin, the trained twin was found to be superior in aerobic capacity by 37%. But the absolute value after training was still only in the average category, leading to the conclusion that while training can bring about substantial improvement, the ceiling is set by genetic factors. However, Klissouras did not control all of the statistical variables, and more recent work attributed to Bouchard suggests that genetic makeup explains only about 50% of the variability in $\dot{V}O_2$ max (17).

O₂ Pulse

The measurement of maximal O_2 consumption requires a willingness on the part of the subject to work to exhaustion, plus a sufficiently conditioned musculature to fully load the O_2 transport systems. In sedentary middle-aged or older adults neither of these conditions is apt to be satisfied. Furthermore, exhaustive physical tests are not completely without hazard for sedentary older populations where unrecognized heart disease may complicate matters. Under such conditions, considerable information can be derived from measuring O_2 pulse at a standardized submaximal level that can be attained by all members of the group to be tested. O_2 pulse is derived by simply dividing O_2 consumption by the heart rate at the time of measurement, thus giving the dimension of O_2 transport per heartbeat.

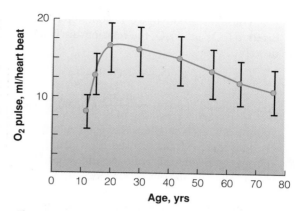

Figure 12.10   Maximum O_2 pulse as a function of age. Mean ± S.E.M. (Drawn from the data of Hollmann, W. *Internationales Seminar für Ergometrie*, 1965, p. 186. Inst. für Leistungsgrenzen, Berlin.)

It has been shown that at any given work rate the subject with the greatest maximum work capacity (aerobic power) has the highest O_2 pulse. Conversely the lowest work capacity is associated with the lowest O_2 pulse (52). O_2 pulse under exercise conditions is, of course, largely determined by stroke volume and arteriovenous O_2 difference (42). Norms for this measurement are shown in figure 12.10.

Respiratory Quotient

The relationship of CO_2 produced to O_2 consumed—RQ, the *respiratory quotient*—is an important physiological concept because it provides information that tells which foodstuff is being used for energy supply, if the subject is resting or in a steady state of moderate exercise. The RQ is sometimes termed the respiratory exchange ratio or R value (chap. 14).

$$RQ = \frac{\text{Volume } CO_2 \text{ produced}}{\text{Volume } O_2 \text{ consumed}}$$

Thus, if carbohydrate is completely oxidized to CO_2 and H_2O, the relationship can be described as:

$$C_6H_{12}O_6 + 6O_2 \rightarrow 6CO_2 + 6H_2O$$

And it follows that $RQ = \dfrac{6CO_2}{6O_2} = 1.00$, if one volume of CO_2 is produced for each volume of O_2 consumed. If fat is used as a source of energy, however, the ratio is somewhat different. The fats and oils of our foods are largely mixtures of palmitin, stearin, and olein. These substances are of similar chemical compositions, and their oxidation can be simplified as follows.

$$2C_{51}H_{98}O_6 + 145O_2 \rightarrow 102CO_2 + 98H_2O$$
$$RQ = \frac{102}{145} = 0.70$$

Since the exact structure of the extremely large protein molecules has not yet been completely elucidated, the RQ for protein metabolism is estimated from known amino acid structures as approximately 0.80. However, protein plays a small part in energy metabolism, and because its participation can be closely estimated from urine analysis, it is not important for the present discussion.

Consequently, if a subject is in a steady state, a reasonably valid deduction of the foodstuff being oxidized can be made on the basis of the observed value of the RQ. For example, if analysis of the respired gasses yielded an RQ of 1.00, the subject could be considered to be utilizing only carbohydrate for energy. A value between 0.70 and 1.00 would indicate a mixture of fat and carbohydrate being burned. The exact amounts of each of the latter are shown in table 12.3.

Table 12.3 The Caloric Equivalents of Oxygen and Carbon Dioxide for Nonprotein Respiratory Quotients

Nonprotein respiratory quotient	Kcal/liter	
	Oxygen	Carbon dioxide
0.70	4.686	6.694
0.72	4.702	6.531
0.74	4.727	6.388
0.76	4.752	6.253
0.78	4.776	6.123
0.80	4.801	6.001
0.82	4.825	5.884
0.84	4.850	5.774
0.86	4.875	5.669
0.88	4.900	5.568
0.90	4.928	5.471
0.92	4.948	5.378
0.94	4.973	5.290
0.96	4.997	5.205
0.98	5.022	5.124
1.00	5.047	5.047

From T. M. Carpenter. *Tables, Factors, and Formulas for Computing Respiratory Exchange and Biological Transformation of Energy,* 4th ed., 1948. Reprinted by permission of Carnegie Institute of Washington.

The Anaerobic Threshold Controversy

As was pointed out earlier in this chapter, maximal O_2 consumption ($\dot{V}O_2$ max) has long been recognized as an important determinant of performance in events requiring endurance. It has been shown, however, that an even more important determinant with respect to distance running is the fraction of $\dot{V}O_2$ max that can be utilized over the distance without incurring a large buildup in blood lactate.

Costill (11) has shown that highly trained distance runners are capable of utilizing more than 90% of their $\dot{V}O_2$ max for twenty-five to thirty minutes with only a moderate accumulation of blood lactate. Later work from the same laboratory showed a correlation of -0.91 between performance in a ten-mile race and $\dot{V}O_2$ max, while the correlation with percentage of $\dot{V}O_2$ max utilized at a given speed was even greater, $-.94$ (12). Similar data have been presented for a 1½-mile run (41). More recent data from other laboratories support these findings (13, 14, 48).

It has also been pointed out by Londeree and Ames (37) that since $\dot{V}O_2$ max is largely determined by hereditary factors, one should not use it as a measure of training status. For a given $\dot{V}O_2$ max it is impossible to know whether the subject has a lot of inherited ability and is out of shape, or has little ability and is in good shape. Their work showed that training status is best reflected in the percentage of $\dot{V}O_2$ max and maximal heart rate that can be maintained without greatly exceeding resting blood lactate values. However, these findings do not preclude the fact that *changes* in $\dot{V}O_2$ max can serve as excellent indices of *change* in condition.

For all of the aforementioned reasons, the concept of an anaerobic threshold (AT) has become important in exercise physiology. The anaerobic threshold is defined as the level of work, or O_2 consumption, just below that at which metabolic acidosis and associated changes in gas exchange occur (53). That is, when the exercise load is ever increasing, at some point the O_2 demand exceeds the O_2 supply, and at this point (AT) the energy release from anaerobic metabolism increases, with a subsequent increase in lactate formation. Wasserman and his colleagues have developed noninvasive methods for estimating AT, using the point of a nonlinear increase in ventilation, CO_2 production, and a sudden increase in RQ and other gas exchange parameters (53). Figure 12.11 shows the application of these concepts by Davis and others (15) using instrumentation typically available in well-equipped exercise physiology labs. The AT can be estimated from gas exchange without drawing blood for lactate concentration analysis.

Use of the AT concept offers many potential advantages for evaluating work capacity in healthy athletes, as well as for clinical evaluation of cardiovascular-respiratory disease in the general public.

Theoretical Problems with the Anaerobic Threshold Concept

The "anaerobic threshold" has become the center of considerable controversy. As conceptualized by Wasserman and his colleagues (51), anaerobic threshold is the O_2 consumption level above which aerobic energy production must be supplemented by anaerobic metabolism and which results in a significant increase in lactate.

First there is the problem that blood lactate, the criterion against which respiratory and other noninvasive methods have been evaluated, is itself not well defined. As has been pointed out earlier, lactate is not only produced by the active muscle but may be consumed simultaneously by both the active muscle and other inactive muscle as well as by the liver and kidney. Thus the blood lactate concentration represents a balance between lactate entry into and exit from the plasma. Besides this problem, it has been shown that there is at best a poor relationship between lactate in the plasma and its concentration in muscle—which is really the matter of interest (19, 50). Another factor to be considered in interpreting blood lactate concentration is the time delay for lactate transfer from the site of production in the muscle tissue to the site of blood sampling, which may be a matter of several minutes (31). In light of these considerations, it is not surprising that several investigators have found little correlation between the excess $\dot{V}O_2$ (above steady state) or ventilatory parameters and blood lactate concentration (21, 22, 27, 28, 29, 46, 47).

Davis and colleagues (14) have shown that changes in anaerobic threshold as the result of endurance training in men are much larger than the concurrent changes in $\dot{V}O_2$ max, thus making it a more sensitive measure of training effects. Until recently it was accepted that the reduced lactate accumulation in trained persons results from a greater oxidative capacity and lesser lactate production in skeletal muscle. However, this explanation has seemed inadequate because trained and untrained subjects have similar O_2 consumption at any given work load. Because of this, animal studies were undertaken in which radioactive isotopic carbon tracers were used to follow the course of the carbon skeleton of the lactate molecule. Thus, turnover rate and production versus consumption could be evaluated. The results suggest that endurance training affects not the production of lactate but its clearance from the blood (16).

The most serious criticisms of the classical concept of anaerobic threshold are twofold: 1) Since lactate in the plasma is the result of an equilibrium struck between production and clearance from the blood, it cannot be considered a true measure of the magnitude of *anaerobic* metabolism per se. 2) Carefully collected data by two different groups of investigators (18, 55) has shown that the relationship of lactate to time with incremental work loads is represented by a smooth curvilinear rise rather than a breaking point or *threshold* as shown in figure 12.11. Thus there is a semantic problem with the term *anaerobic threshold*. For these reasons, the term *lactate threshold* seems more appropriate and is rapidly replacing the older term (30). The finding of a "threshold," while problematical, is probably dependent on the methods used.

While the physiological basis for the lactate threshold is still debated, most investigators agree that it represents an increased use of the glycolytic metabolic pathway. In spite of the theoretical objections to a literal application of the anaerobic threshold concept, a remarkable consistency of plasma lactate concentration can be demonstrated in a person performing a given exercise (15).

In an incremental test of relatively short duration, the relationship between changes in ventilation and changes in plasma lactate concentration is usually close enough to allow the lactate threshold to be estimated from ventilation measurements (fig. 12.11) as long as care is taken to not let the effects of diet, previous heavy exercise, and acid-base abnormalities affect the findings. For a review of these methods and the theoretical arguments pro and con, the reader is referred to Jones and Ehrsam (30) and Wasserman (51).

Negative Work

So far, our main concern has been with exercise loads involving predominantly concentric contraction in which the muscle shortens to do work. This can be called *positive work*.

But effort also involves the muscular activity of resisting lengthening, as in eccentric contraction, and the physicist's definition of

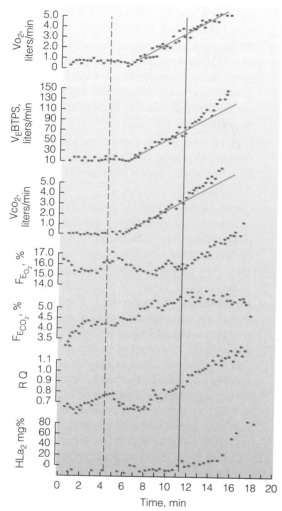

Figure 12.11 Measurements of respiratory gas exchange and venous blood lactate during an incremental leg cycling test. Solid vertical line denotes anaerobic threshold. Dashed vertical line indicates onset of incremental work. Exercise duration was sixteen minutes. Lactate levels during four minutes of recovery are also shown. (From Davis, J. A. et al., "Anaerobic Threshold and Maximal Anaerobic Power for Three Modes of Exercise" in *Journal of Applied Physiology* 41:544. © 1976 American Physiological Society. Reprinted by permission.)

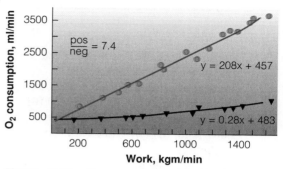

Figure 12.12 The oxygen consumption in milliliters per minute of a man bicycling "uphill" and "downhill" on a motor-driven treadmill plotted against the rate of work in kilograms per minute. (From Asmussen, E., in *Ergonomics Society Symposium on Fatigue*, 1953. Courtesy of H. K. Lewis, London.)

work can no longer be applied. It has become common to refer to the work done by eccentric contraction as *negative work,* and to compute it as if it were positive: $W = F \times D$. However, the work calculated in this fashion cannot be used interchangeably with the work of positive work; the energy involved per unit work is quite different.

This was ingeniously demonstrated by Abbott, Bigland, and Ritchie (1) who coupled two bicycle riders in opposition, one of whom pedaled concentrically while the other pedaled eccentrically. Although the forces developed exactly balanced each other, the O_2 consumption of the subject doing positive work was 3.7 times higher. Asmussen (4) confirmed this and plotted negative and positive work loads versus O_2 consumption (fig. 12.12). Although negative work was linearly related to O_2 consumption, the ratio of the slope lines was 7.4 for their rate of pedaling. For varying rates of pedaling, the ratio of O_2 consumption for positive/negative work varied from three to nine, the ratio increasing with the speed of pedaling. Thus it would seem that positive work is from three to nine times more costly in terms of energy expenditure than negative work.

Summary

1. Here are some of the terms needed for discussing exercise metabolism intelligently: (a) *work:* $W = F \times D$; (b) *power* (in hp): 1 hp = 33,000 ft-lb/min; (c) *energy* (in kcal): 1 kcal = 3,087 ft-lb; (d) *efficiency* (in ratio or percentage):

$$\text{Efficiency} = \frac{\text{Energy input}}{\text{Work output}}$$

2. Three methods are commonly used for setting up standard work loads: *bench-stepping, treadmill,* and *bicycle ergometer.*

3. The two methods for measuring energy expenditures are *direct* and *indirect calorimetry.* The latter uses either the *closed-circuit* or the *open-circuit* method.

4. Muscular work can be performed *aerobically,* if the energy source is completely oxidized to CO_2 and H_2O, or *anaerobically,* if the biochemical breakdown of glycogen ends at the lactic acid stage.

5. When exercise begins, there is a lag in the response of the O_2 transport systems. The amount by which the O_2 supply lacks being adequate until the O_2 transport catches up with the demand is called O_2 *deficit.*

6. Recovery oxygen is defined as the amount of O_2 taken up in excess of the resting value during the recovery period. This constitutes the repayment of the O_2 deficit plus any anaerobic metabolism that may have occurred.

7. Anaerobic capacity is an important determinant of success in many American athletic contests. Improvement in this parameter can be brought about by appropriate training directed to short, sprint-type activity.

8. When equal loads of continuous and intermittent work are compared, much lower stress seems to result from intermittent work. Storage of O_2 as oxymyohemoglobin has been postulated to explain this phenomenon.

9. If physical fitness is defined as physical working capacity, the best single measure of this factor is maximal O_2 consumption.

10. Under resting and steady-state exercise conditions, the *respiratory quotient* (RQ) accurately reflects the foodstuff being utilized.

11. Though a useful concept for predicting endurance performance, the *anaerobic threshold,* now termed the *lactate threshold,* rests on insecure bases, both conceptually and theoretically. It does not indicate the onset of "anaerobiosis," and a "threshold" exists only under certain prescribed exercise protocols. Under appropriate testing conditions, the lactate threshold appears to be useful in predicting performance in endurance events and in assessing exercise capacity in patients with cardiovascular-respiratory disease.

12. Work in which muscular contraction is eccentric is called *negative work.* Depending on the rate, negative work can be performed from three to nine times more economically than *positive work.*

References

1. Abbott, B. C., Bigland, B., and Ritchie, J. M. Physiological cost of negative work. *J. Physiol.* 117:380–90, 1952.

2. Ahlborg, G., Hagenfeldt, L., and Wahren, J. Substrate utilization by the inactive leg during one-leg or arm exercise. *J. Appl. Physiol.* 39:718–23, 1975.

3. Anderson, K. L., Shephard, R. J., Denolin, H., Varnauskas, E., and Masironi, R. *Fundamentals of exercise testing.* Geneva: World Health Organization, 1971.

4. Asmussen, E. Experiments on positive and negative work. *Ergonomics Society Symposium on Fatigue,* eds. W. F. Floyd and A. T. Welford. London: Lewis and Co., 1953.

5. Astrand, I., Astrand, P-O., Christensen, E. H., and Hedman, R. Intermittent muscular work. *Acta Physiol. Scand.* 48:448–53, 1960a.

6. ———. Myohemoglobin as an oxygen-store in man. *Acta Physiol. Scand.* 48:454–60, 1960b.

7. Bannister, E. W., and Jackson, R. C. The effect of speed and load changes on oxygen intake for equivalent power outputs during bicycle ergometry. *Int. Z. Angew. Physiol.* 24:284–90, 1968.

8. Bar-Or, O. The wingate anaerobic test: An update on methodology, reliability and validity. *Sports Med.* 4:381–94, 1987.

9. Brooks, G. A., and Gaesser, G. A. End points of lactate and glucose metabolism after exhausting exercise. *J. Appl. Physiol.* 49:1057–69, 1980.

10. Christensen, E. H., Hedman, R., and Saltin, B. Intermittent and continuous running. *Acta Physiol. Scand.* 50:269–86, 1960.

11. Costill, D. L. Metabolic responses during distance running. *J. Appl. Physiol.* 28:251–55, 1970.

12. Costill, D. L., Thomason, H., and Roberts, E. Fractional utilization of the aerobic capacity during distance running. *Med. Sci. Sports* 5:248–52, 1973.

13. Coyle, E. F., Martin, W. H., Ehsani, A. A., Hagberg, J. M., Bloomfield, S. A., Sinacors, D. R., and Holloszy, J. O. Blood lactate threshold in some well-trained ischemic heart disease patients. *J. Appl. Physiol.* 54:18–23, 1983.

14. Davis, J. A., Frank, M. H., Whipp, B. J., and Wasserman, K. H. Anaerobic threshold alterations caused by endurance training in middle aged men. *J. Appl. Physiol.* 46:1039–46, 1979.

15. Davis, J. A. Vodak, P., Wilmore, J. H., Vodak, J., and Kurtz, P. Anaerobic threshold and maximal aerobic power for three modes of exercise. *J. Appl. Physiol.* 41:544–50, 1976.

16. Donovan, C. M., and Brooks, G. A. Endurance training affects lactate clearance, not lactate production. *Am. J. Physiol.* January 24, E83–E92, 1983.

17. Dunn, K. Twin studies and sports: Estimating the future? *Physician and Sportsmed.* 9:131–36, 1981.

18. Gaesser, G. A., and Brooks, G. A. Metabolic bases of excess post exercise oxygen consumption: a review. *Med. Sci. Sports Exer.* 16:29–43, 1984.

19. Green, H. J., Hughson, R. L., Orr, G. W., and Ranney, D. A. Anaerobic threshold, blood lactate and muscle metabolites in progressive exercise. *J. Appl. Physiol.* 54:1032–38, 1983.

20. Hagberg, J. M., Hickson, R. C., Ehsani, A. A., and Holloszy, J. O. Faster adjustment to and recovery from submaximal exercise in the trained state. *J. Appl. Physiol.* 48:218–24, 1980.

21. Hagberg, J. M., Mullin, J. P., and Nagle, F. J. Oxygen consumption during constant load exercise. *J. Appl. Physiol.* 45:381–84, 1978.

22. Hagberg, J. M., Mullin, J. P., and Nagle, F. J. Effect of work intensity and duration on recovery O_2. *J. Appl. Physiol.* 48:540–44, 1980.

23. Hermansen, L. Anaerobic energy release. *Med. Sci. Sports* 1:32–38, 1969.

24. Hermansen, L., Ekblom, B., and Saltin, B. Cardiac output during submaximal and maximal treadmill and bicycle exercise. *J. Appl. Physiol.* 29:82–86, 1970.

25. Hermansen, L., and Saltin, B. Oxygen uptake during maximal treadmill and bicycle exercise. *J. Appl. Physiol.* 26:31–37, 1969.

26. Hess, P., and Seusing, J. Der Einfluss der Tretfrequenz und des Pedaldruckes auf die Sauerstoff aufnahme die Untersuchungen am Ergometer. *Int. Z. Angew. Physiol.* 19:468–75, 1963.

27. Hogan, M. C., Cox, R. H., and Welch, H. G. Lactate accumulation during incremental exercise with varied inspired oxygen fractions. *J. Appl. Physiol.* 55:1134–40, 1983.

28. Hughes, E. F., Turner, S. C., and Brooks, G. A. Effects of glycogen depletion and pedaling speed on "anaerobic threshold." *J. Appl. Physiol.* 52:1598–1607, 1982.

29. Hughson, R. L., and Green, H. J. Blood acid-base and lactate relationships studied by ramp work tests. *Med. Sci. Sports Exer.* 14:297–302, 1982.

30. Jones, N. L., and Ehrsam, R. E. The anaerobic threshold. *Exer. Sports Sci. Rev.* 10:49–83, 1982.

31. Karlsson, J., and Jacobs, I. Onset of blood lactate accumulation during muscular exercise as a threshold concept. *Int. J. Sports Med.* 3:190–201, 1982.

32. Katch, V., Weltman, A., Martin, R., and Gray, L. Optimal test characteristics for maximal anaerobic work on the bicycle ergometer. *Res. Q.* 48:319–27, 1977.

33. Keul, J., and Doll, E. Intermittent exercise: metabolites, pO_2 and acid-base equilibrium in the blood. *J. Appl. Physiol.* 34:220–25, 1973.

34. Klissouras, V. Heritability of adaptive variation. *J. Appl. Physiol.* 31:338–44, 1971.

35. ———. Genetic limit of functional adaptability. *Int. Z. Angew. Physiol.* 30:85–94, 1972.

36. Knuttgen, H. G., and Saltin, B. Muscle metabolites and oxygen uptake in short term submaximal exercise in man. *J. Appl. Physiol.* 32:690–94, 1972.

37. Londeree, B. R., and Ames, S. A. Maximal steady state versus state of conditioning. *Eur. J. Appl. Physiol.* 34:269–78, 1975.

38. Margaria, R., Aghemo, P., and Rovelli, E. Measurement of muscular power (anaerobic) in man. *J. Appl. Physiol.* 21:1662–64, 1966.

39. Margaria, R., Edwards, H. T., and Dill, D. B. The possible mechanisms of contracting and paying the O_2 debt and the role of lactic acid in muscular contraction. *Am. J. Physiol.* 106:689–715, 1933.

40. Matsui, H., Kitamura, K., and Miyamura, M. Oxygen uptake and bloodflow of the lower limb in maximal treadmill and bicycle exercise. *Eur. J. Physiol. Occup. Physiol.* 40:57–62, 1978.

41. Mayhew, J. L., and Andrew, J. Assessment of running performance in college males from aerobic capacity percentage utilization coefficients. *J. Sports Med. Phys. Fitness* 15:342–46, 1975.

42. Musshoff, K., Reindell, H., Stein, H., and Konig, K. Die Sauerstoff aufnahme pro Herzschlag (O_2 puls) als Funktion des Schlagvolumens der Arterio-venosen Differenz Des Minuten volumens und Herzvolumens. *Z. Kreislaufforschung* 48:255–77, 1959.

43. Oldenburg, F. A., McCormack, D. W., Morse, J. L. C., and Jones, N. L. Comparison of exercise responses in stair climbing and cycling. *J. Appl. Physiol.* 46:510–16, 1979.

44. Rowell, L. B., Kraning, K. K., Evans, T. O., Kennedy, J. W., Blackmon, J. R., and Kusumi, F. Splanchnic removal of lactate and pyruvate during prolonged exercise in man. *J. Appl. Physiol.* 21:1773–83, 1966.

45. Saltin, B., and Astrand, P-O. Maximal oxygen uptake in athletes. *J. Appl. Physiol.* 23:353–58, 1967.

46. Scheen, A., Juchmes, J., and Cession-Fossion, A. Critical analysis of the "anaerobic threshold" during exercise at constant work loads. *Eur. J. Appl. Physiol. Occup. Physiol.* 46:367–77, 1981.

47. Simon, J., Young, J. L., Gutin, B., Blood, D. K., and Case, R. B. Lactate accumulation relative to the anaerobic and respiratory compensation thresholds. *J. Appl. Physiol.* 54:13–17, 1983.

48. Tanaka, K., Matsuura, Y., Matsuzaka, A., Hirakoba, K., Kumagai, S., Sun, S. O., and Asano, K. A longitudinal assessment of anaerobic threshold and distance running performance. *Med. Sci. Sports Exer.* 16:278–82, 1984.

49. Taylor, H. L., Buskirk, E., and Henschel, A. Maximal oxygen intake as an objective measure of cardiorespiratory performance. *J. Appl. Physiol.* 8:73–80, 1955.

50. Tesch, P. A., Daniels, W. L., and Sharp, D. S. Lactate accumulation in muscle and blood during submaximal exercise. *Acta Physiol. Scand.* 114:441–46, 1982.

51. Wasserman, K. The anaerobic threshold measurement to evaluate exercise performance. *Am. Rev. Resp. Dis.* 129 (suppl.): S35–S40, 1984.

52. Wasserman, K., Van Kessel, A. L., and Burton, G. G. Interaction of physiological mechanisms during exercise. *J. Appl. Physiol.* 22:71–85, 1967.

53. Wasserman, K., Whipp, B. J., Koyal, S., and Beaver, W. L. Anaerobic threshold and respiratory gas exchange during exercise. *J. Appl. Physiol.* 35:236–43, 1973.

54. World Health Organization. Exercise tests in relation to cardiovascular function. WHO Technical Report series no. 388. Geneva, Switzerland, 1968.

55. Yeh, M. P., Gardner, R. M., Adams, T. D., Yanowitz, F. G., and Crapo, R. O. "Anaerobic threshold": Problems of determination and validation. *J. Appl. Physiol.* 55:1178–86, 1983.

PART **2**

Physiology Applied to
Health and Fitness

Health Benefits: Prophylactic and Therapeutic Effects of Exercise

Physical Activity, Physical Fitness, and
    All-Cause Mortality

The Cardiovascular System and Exercise
    Physical Activity and Coronary
      Heart Disease
    Exercise and Coronary Circulation
    Exercise and the Peripheral
      Circulation
    Exercise Effect on Blood Pressure
    Changes in the Blood Accompanying
      Stress and Exercise

Lipid Metabolism and Exercise
    Cholesterol
    Triglycerides

Pulmonary Function Effects

Oxygen Transport Effects

Effects on Bones, Joints, and Connective
    Tissue

Effects of Exercise on Cancer

The "Tranquilizer Effect"
    State of Neuromuscular System
      Related to Anxiety and Tension
    Exercise and Relaxation

Effect of Exercise on Psychiatric State

The nature of the illnesses that beset our American population has in recent years undergone a transition from a predominance of infectious diseases to the present predominance of degenerative diseases. This change represents the contributions of the medical profession, both in research and clinical practice, toward the virtual control and the imminent eradication of a large portion of the formerly dreaded infectious scourges.

The increase of such degenerative diseases as cardiovascular incidents (heart attacks and strokes), hypertension, neuroses, and malignancies offers a challenge not only to medicine but to physical education as well. It seems that as improvements in medical science allow us to escape decimation by such infectious diseases as tuberculosis, diphtheria, and poliomyelitis, we live longer only to fall prey to the degenerative diseases at a slightly older age. Whether this involvement with the degenerative problems follows from our living longer or is the result of our simultaneous change in life-style cannot yet be answered.

Along with our newly acquired control over the infectious diseases, we have made at least three other changes that seem likely to affect adversely our physical and mental well-being:

1. We have learned to produce and eat more food than we need.

2. We have learned to control our environment with very little expenditure of physical energy.

3. We have so constituted our society that most of us are subjected to unusual stresses for which our biological responses are inadequate or, indeed, deleterious.

Our grandparents labored hard and long physically in agriculture or industry. We now use automobiles to go to the corner drugstore. Adults have power lawn mowers, automatic washers, and dishwashers, and children get motor scooters at the earliest possible age. On weekends we stage athletic spectacles in which our population gets its exercise vicariously by watching its hired athletes perform. The result of this sedentary life-style appears to be the growth of degenerative diseases and an increasing involvement with neuroses and psychoses for which our grandparents just did not have time.

No one advocates a return to the long, tedious drudgery of manual work, but we cannot deny that we need to learn how to adjust in better fashion to our newly found leisure time. The U.S. Preventive Services Task Force has recommended that physicians council their patients to perform regular physical activity (32). The *fun* of exercise, sport, and physically vigorous recreation must replace the *tedium* of hard work that kept our grandparents physically fit. Herein is the challenge to the medical and physical education professions.

Physical Activity, Physical Fitness, and All-Cause Mortality

The influence of life-style on the health and illnesses of a lifetime has been suggested in the past, but hard, scientific evidence has only recently become available. In a survey of 6,928 adults of Alameda County, California (5, 6), individual health practices were related to health and also to mortality statistics. The health practices surveyed included 1) smoking, 2) weight in relation to desirable standards, 3) use of alcohol, 4) hours of sleep, 5) breakfast eating, 6) regularity of meals, and 7) physical activity. It was found that the average life expectancy of men age forty-five who reported six or seven "good" practices was more than eleven years greater than that of men reporting fewer than four. For women, the difference in life expectancy was seven years.

It was also found that the good health practices were reliably associated with positive health and that the relationship of the different health practices was cumulative: those who followed all of the good practices, even though older, were in better health than those who failed to follow them. This association was found to be independent of age, gender, and economic status.

Recent epidemiological evidence also suggests that individuals who are physically active and/or physically fit tend to live longer than their sedentary, unfit peers (7, 60). Data from the Harvard Alumni study by Paffenbarger and colleagues (60) indicated that men who engaged in physical activity (recreational activities, sports play, stair climbing, walking, and so on), which resulted in the expenditure of greater than 2,000 kcal per week from thirty-five to eighty years of age, had a life expectancy that was 1.5 years greater than men who had been less active (less than 2,000 kcal per week). The added years of life appear to be related to the age at which the physical activity program begins. That is, the later in life one begins to participate in physical activity, the fewer years that are added to the life expectancy. Interestingly however, beginning a 2,000 kcal per week physical activity program at sixty years of age adds approximately one year to the average male life expectancy. These findings clearly indicate that it is never too late to gain the benefits of regular exercise.

Blair and coworkers (7) examined the relationship between physical fitness (measured by a maximal treadmill test) and all-cause mortality during an eight year period in 10,224 males (mean age 41.7 years) and 3,120 females (41.0 years). For both genders, the age-adjusted death rates decreased as physical fitness increased. The death rates (males and females) for the lowest fit 20% of samples were approximately two to five times greater than the moderate to highly fit subjects. The authors concluded that "Higher levels of physical fitness appear to delay all-cause mortality

primarily due to lowered rates of cardiovascular disease and cancer."

The Cardiovascular System and Exercise

Physical Activity and Coronary Heart Disease

Since World War II, several large-scale statistical surveys have been conducted to evaluate the relationships between activity level and coronary heart disease (CHD).

Probably the most widely known study was conducted by Morris and associates (53) on bus drivers and conductors of the London Transport Authority. They found, among 31,000 drivers and conductors, that the drivers suffered significantly more coronary heart disease than the conductors. Since the drivers might be considered sedentary, while the conductors (of double-decker busses) did considerable walking and stair-climbing, it would seem that men in active jobs suffer less CHD. However, we cannot deduce from this that the exercise involved was the causative factor, because it is possible that coronary-prone people selected the driver jobs.

Taylor and his colleagues at the Laboratory of Physiological Hygiene at the University of Minnesota conducted a similar study on American railway employees (84). They found that in 191,609 man-years of risk and 1,978 reported deaths, the age-adjusted deaths for arteriosclerotic heart disease were 5.7, 3.9, and 2.8 for clerks, switchmen, and section men, respectively. Since the clerks' jobs were sedentary, the switchmen's moderately active, and the section men's very active, this data supports that of the Morris group.

In a Framingham, Massachusetts, study a team of investigators from the U.S. Public Health Service classified men by habitual level of physical activity (42). In the ten years following the physical activity assessments, 207 men developed some manifestation of a coronary attack, and those who had been classified as most sedentary in each age group had an incidence almost twice that of the group which was at least moderately active. These findings were corroborated by Leon and coworkers (48) in the Multiple Risk Factor Intervention Trial (MRFIT) who found that during seven years of follow-up "men at high risk for CHD who self-selected moderate amounts of predominately light and moderate non-work physical activity had lower rates of CHD mortality, sudden death, and overall mortality than more sedentary men." The results of the MRFIT study indicated that leisure time physical activity was inversely related to CHD and overall mortality in middle-age men.

Brunner (10) studied 5,279 men and 5,229 women in Israeli kibbutzim. The kibbutzim are run as communes and consequently allow comparison of physical activity effects uncontaminated by the effects of income, diet, and other factors, since all members regardless of the nature of their work have the same income and eat in the same communal dining room. He found the incidence of the anginal syndrome, myocardial infarction, and fatalities due to CHD was 2.5 to 4 times higher in sedentary than in physically active workers. Cooper and associates (16), after studying some 3,000 men at the Aerobics Center in Dallas, concluded that physical fitness is related to lower coronary risk factors.

Until recently it was not possible to attribute the protective effects of exercise directly to the physical activity itself since it could have acted by lessening other risk factors such as smoking, hypertension, obesity, glucose intolerance, and so on. However, the work of Paffenbarger and his coworkers at Stanford provides strong evidence that physical activity is in fact a primary factor (8, 58, 59). They studied a group of 3,975 San Francisco longshoremen over a period of twenty-two years and found that after statistical adjustments were made for age, race, blood pressure, smoking, body mass, glucose intol-

erance, and EKG status, the men with a heavy work activity still had a fatal heart attack rate only one-half that of the men with a low work activity.

In a study on 16,936 Harvard alumni, Paffenbarger and associates (61) also provided evidence regarding the question, How much physical activity is required to significantly lessen the risk of heart attack? They found that as the history of physical activity increased from 500 kcal per week to 2,000 to 3,000 kcal, heart attacks (both fatal and nonfatal) decreased steadily to a plateau value (2,000 to 3,000 kcal per week) at which point the low-activity men were at 64% greater risk than classmates with higher activity levels. On this basis, the optimal effect could be obtained by approximately 30 to 60 minutes of jogging or equivalent exercise five times per week. It should be recognized, however, that the figure of 2,000 kcal per week included normal daily activities such as walking and stair climbing. In this regard, LaPorte and associates (46) have stated "It is likely that only 5 to 8 miles of running a week in addition to the normal activities of daily living would bring the total to 2,000."

It is important for physical educators and allied health professionals to know that CHD has its origin during childhood. As discussed earlier in this chapter, degenerative diseases such as CHD normally are manifested (heart attacks) late in life but develop gradually for many years. Thus, although children and adolescents are usually asymptomatic, atherosclerosis may be progressing.

Children often exhibit the beginnings of atherosclerotic development (fatty streaks) by three years of age (37, 70). These fatty streaks are thought to develop into fiberous plaques and eventually calcify (70). Fiberous plaques that decrease lumen size are clearly evident by early adulthood (27).

The implications for physical educators are clear. Rowland (70) has stated "The signal to health caretakers of children is a strong one: Getting youngsters started early in habits of regular exercise can provide a lifelong means of helping to prevent chronic cardiovascular disease in adulthood."

Up to this point all the evidence cited might be considered circumstantial. However, there is now excellent experimental evidence supporting the epidemiological data. In a study on rats in which myocardial infarction (heart attack) was brought about by injection of isoproterenol, no rat in the group of thirty-three who were trained at 65% of maximum died, while 24% of the unexercised control group of sixty-three died from the experimental heart attack (19).

An even more convincing study was reported recently by Kramsch and associates (45) who fed an atherogenic diet to monkeys for twenty-four months. One group of nine was conditioned by treadmill running (equivalent to jogging for the human) for eighteen months prior to the twenty-four months of high lipid diet. Another group of nine remained sedentary. Postmortem examination revealed that although the exercised group also developed atherosclerotic plaque formation in the coronary arteries, it was considerably less than in the sedentary group. Even more importantly, the exercised monkeys showed an increase in coronary vessel diameter and a decrease in lesion size, which acted together to reduce the substantial coronary artery narrowing induced in the sedentary group to "clinically inapparent" levels in the exercised group.

Exercise and Coronary Circulation

Eckstein (26) operated on 117 dogs to produce various degrees of narrowing of the circumflex coronary artery. This simulated the narrowing brought about in coronary disease by deposition of cholesterol in the intima of the coronary arteries. When the dogs with constricted arteries were exercised, coronary blood flow capacity increased significantly by virtue of increased collateral circulation.

Raab (62, 63) provided considerable data on the importance of the autonomic control of the heart. The rate and metabolism of the heart are established as the result of a balance between the parasympathetic system (vagus nerve) and the sympathetic system (accelerator nerve). This balance is established in the midbrain and is mediated through release of neurohormonal (chemical) transmitters. The sympathogenic effects are brought about by the catecholamines, epinephrine and norepinephrine, while the vagal effects are brought about through acetylcholine.

In general, athletic training brings about vagal preponderance, as indicated by the slower heart rate in the athlete both at rest and under any given work load. A state of nervous excitement (emotional upset) causes a sympathogenic preponderance. The sympathogenic catecholamines were shown (63) to have undesirable effects on the myocardium, such as an excessive increase in O_2 consumption. Raab and others demonstrated that the combination of coronary constriction (as in atherosclerosis) and a sympathogenic supply of catecholamines brings about the typical ECG changes of coronary disease. He felt that this neurohormonal imbalance (sympathetic preponderance) is caused jointly by "1) hypothalamic-stimulating emotional socioeconomic pressures, and 2) a deficiency of vagal and sympathoinhibitory counterregulation resulting from lack of physical exercise."

In an experiment by Heusner and coworkers (35), it was shown that similar myocardial damage can be produced by 1) epinephrine injection, 2) anoxia, 3) severe emotional stress, and 4) *severe* exercise. Most interestingly they also showed that appropriate physical conditioning can protect against the stressor effect of extreme anxiety or emotional stress.

Results from two different laboratories agree in showing increased coronary tree size to result from physical conditioning in rats (83, 85). Stevenson and associates extended their investigation to include the question of the effect of intensity and frequency on the increase in coronary vessel size. They found that moderate exercise (twice weekly) had a more beneficial effect than extremely severe exercise (four hours per day, four days per week) (83).

More recent work on rats has confirmed that endurance training results in the growth of capillary blood vessels in the myocardium but only if the training is heavy enough to bring about cardiac hypertrophy (49).

Exercise and the Peripheral Circulation

The effect of exercise training on the capillary bed of skeletal muscles is not quite so clear. While older work had suggested an increase in the capillary density of exercising skeletal muscles in experimental animals, this has not been confirmed by more modern methods such as electron microscopy (34, 49). In a study comparing well-trained and untrained humans, no difference in capillary density was found either, but the muscle fibers were larger in the well-trained subjects, and consequently the number of capillaries per fiber was increased (34).

Clarke (14) reports on work done at the Longevity Research Institute in Santa Barbara, California, on patients with severe peripheral vascular disease. Walking exercise over a six-month period resulted in a dramatic improvement of 300% in treadmill walking distance, which strongly suggests an improvement in peripheral circulation for these patients for whom other therapies have not been encouraging. A combination of walking and vigorous dietary control was even more effective.

Exercise Effect on Blood Pressure

In a recent review of the literature, Seals and Hagberg (73) found that of twelve investigations dealing with the effect of exercise on blood pressure, eight reported modest reductions in systolic and/or diastolic blood pressure at rest. The average reduction in blood pressure for these studies was 9 mm Hg for systolic and 7 mm Hg diastolic. Epidemiological evidence suggests that reductions of this magnitude could have clinical implications for the hypertensive individual by lowering the risk of stroke and cardiovascular disease.

The variability in findings cited above may be explained in part by the work of Tipton and associates with rats (87), in which they explored the importance of exercise intensity on blood pressure response to training. They found no difference between trained and untrained rats when training intensity was greater than 75% of capacity but found consistently lower resting blood pressure after training at 40% to 60% of capacity.

Changes in the Blood Accompanying Stress and Exercise

Thus far we have discussed the effects of stress and exercise on the blood vessels and muscle tissue of the heart. However, another factor is thought to be of considerable importance in the etiology of heart disease: the *physicochemical properties* of the blood that courses through these coronary vessels. It is obvious that changes in the blood that lead to quicker coagulation or clotting time might also be more likely to result in thrombus formation, the plugging of a coronary artery in a heart attack.

The work of Schneider and Zangari (72) demonstrated the effects of stress on the blood. Anxiety, tension, fear, anger, and hostility were associated with shorter clotting times, increased viscosity, and blood pressure. It was suggested that this pattern was appropriate as a protective reaction when the organism was under attack because excessive blood loss would be prevented by the shortened clotting time and O_2 transport would be enhanced by the increased viscosity. If this pattern occurred chronically, however—as seemed to be the case in their hypertensive subjects—it could prove detrimental by favoring intravascular thrombosis and by increasing the work of the heart (because of the increased viscosity of the blood). Their work has since been corroborated by Friedman (28) and others.

Since moderate exercise has been shown to have significant tranquilizer effects, it is reasonable to believe that these undesirable effects of stress might be relieved to some extent by appropriate exercise.

Another important effect of exercise training is the reduction of serum uric acid (SUA) (17). Reports from the Tecumseh Project involving over 1,200 men showed that physically active men had significantly lower SUA levels than sedentary men (50). SUA is important because of its causal relationship to gout and its suggested relationship to coronary artery disease.

Increases of *total blood volume* (TBV) that had been reported earlier were considered equivocal because of methodological questions, but evidence has been presented to confirm the fact that endurance training can increase the blood volume by as much as 6% (56). The increased TBV was found to be due to increased plasma volume; red cell volume did not change significantly. These facts are important to cardiac function because of the implications for improved venous return without increased flow resistance.

Lipid Metabolism and Exercise

The lipids include the *typical fats*, which are esters of fatty acids and glycerol (triglycerides), and *sterols* such as cholesterol (as well as other categories). Our interest in these members of the lipid family stems from the fact that both are found in the deposits that narrow the lumen of arteries in atherosclerosis. The physician's concern with the blood cholesterol level as a predisposing factor to heart disease

is well known. It is based on statistical evidence that indicates a strong relationship (though possibly not causal) between cholesterol level and heart disease. For these reasons, the effect of exercise on blood triglyceride and cholesterol is of interest.

Cholesterol

Cholesterol is transported in the blood in combination with special proteins to form lipoprotein. Three different lipoproteins are responsible for this transport, and they are differentiated by their densities: 1) alpha lipoprotein, also called high density lipoprotein (HDL) because it has the greatest density; 2) beta lipoprotein, also called low density lipoprotein (LDL) because of its lower density; and 3) pre-beta lipoprotein, also called very low density lipoprotein (VLDL) because it is the least dense. It is now known that only about 17% of the cholesterol in fasting plasma is carried by the HDL, whereas the remainder is carried by the LDL and VLDL. Furthermore, there is agreement among several epidemiologic studies that ischemic heart disease is associated with high levels of LDL and VLDL, whereas high levels of HDL appear to protect against coronary artery disease and seem to be related to longevity. There seems to be little doubt that LDL and VLDL are the transport mechanisms by which cholesterol is transported from the periphery into the smooth muscle cells of the arteries where it collects, plugging the arteries and causing the disease we call atherosclerosis. On the other hand, the HDL works against this atherosclerotic process, either by 1) resisting the movement of LDL cholesterol into the arterial wall, or 2) promoting the efflux of cholesterol from the tissues to the liver where it is broken down and excreted. The mechanism of the HDL protective effect is not yet completely clear, and it is possible that both mechanisms are operative. In any event the HDLs are the "good guys" and the LDL and VLDLs are the "bad guys." This is important to us because there is now considerable evidence that exercise is one of the important means by which HDL can be increased (2, 33, 64, 68, 69, 89).

Triglycerides

Holloszy and colleagues (36) have shown that six months of physical conditioning by calisthenics and distance running reduced serum triglycerides by 40%. However, this effect appeared to last only about two days. Thus it may be inferred from their work that serum triglycerides can be maintained at a significantly lower level by exercise, but the exercise must be done at least every other day. More recent work has supported their data and has also shown that exercise is effective in correcting certain abnormalities of fat metabolism (55).

Pulmonary Function Effects

Until recently, the only beneficial effects of physical conditioning on pulmonary function seemed to be improvements in static lung volumes, in capacities such as functional residual capacity, residual volume, vital capacity, and the ratio of residual volume to total lung capacity (4), and in lung diffusion (38).

Although the muscles involved in breathing are skeletal muscles, no one had thought to investigate the trainability of these muscles until relatively recently. Leith and Bradley (47) have shown that in normals the respiratory muscles respond to strength and endurance training just as we might expect— that is, by increases in these measures of approximately 55% and 14%, respectively. More recent work has supported these findings (67). Subsequently, it has been shown that cystic fibrosis patients improve their respiratory muscle endurance by even greater percentages and that the training can be accomplished equally well by specific breathing exercise or by upper body endurance exercise (43).

A considerable volume of literature has developed concerning the effects of exercise on

chronic obstructive lung disease. To sum up the evidence, there is no reason to believe that exercise can restore destroyed alveolar tissue. However, the improvements in respiratory muscle strength and endurance bring about a much improved exercise or work tolerance and for some individuals considerable symptomatic relief.

Oxygen Transport Effects

The benefits to the systems that determine the capacity for oxygen transport have been supported by experiments too numerous to cite. In general, improvements in maximal O_2 consumption from appropriate physical conditioning have been shown to occur in all ages and both genders. Improvements reported have ranged from approximately 5% to 30%. Differences in training effect would be expected according to the fitness level at the start of an experiment and the intensity-duration-frequency characteristics of the training regimen.

Effects on Bones, Joints, and Connective Tissue

It is well known that disuse of the skeletal system results in its atrophy, with the eventual development of osteoporosis. Loading of the bones of the skeletal framework is necessary for normal bone metabolism, which consists of both anabolic and catabolic processes such as those occurring in other living tissues. In bone, both mineral and organic metabolic processes are involved, and studies using animals have provided evidence that the stress of exercise exerts a conservatory influence on both the mineral and the collagenous (organic) components of bone (3, 44).

Osteoporosis results in an estimated 1.2 million fractures per year at a total cost of approximately 6.1 billion dollars (12, 66). The majority of these fractures occur in older adults, particularly postmenopausal women. Most research (57, 75, 77, 78, 79, 80, 81, 91) indicates that weight bearing exercises such as walking, jogging, and aerobic dance have a favorable effect on bone density in males and females. This appears to be the case for vertebra as well as the bones of the limbs (18, 78, 91).

Work from several independent investigations has shown the importance of physical conditioning on connective tissues such as ligaments. It was shown in rats that the strength of ligaments of the knee joint improves with physical activity (1, 93). Tipton and coworkers have performed a series of experiments in which the same ligament strength results were shown in large animals (dogs). In addition they demonstrated that the collagen content and fiber bundle size were significantly greater in trained dogs (86). Interestingly, they also showed the beneficial exercise effects on ligament strength after surgical repair. This, of course, has important implications for the postsurgical treatment of knee injuries in athletes. In another investigation Tipton and colleagues questioned whether these effects were hormonal, since connective tissues are known to be responsive to hormonal effects. They found that the mechanical stresses of training can act independently of the hormonal effect, which was verified. An excellent review of this work is available (88).

In deVries's laboratory, Chapman (13) showed that the resistance to movement in a joint can be significantly reduced both in the old and in the young by appropriate exercise.

Effects of Exercise on Cancer

As long ago as 1921, it was reported from a study of 86,838 men in Minnesota (76) that the death rate from cancer was roughly inversely proportional to the amount of muscular effort required on the job.

Rigan (65) has summarized research reports for the years 1920 until 1963 that relate to the effects of exercise on cancer. The reported evidence showed an inverse relationship between physical activity and the cancer death rate in men. In various animal experiments over these forty years, the following observations were reported.

1. Caloric restriction inhibited the growth rate of malignancies.

2. In mice, two hours of daily exercise reduced the incidence of mammary gland carcinoma.

3. Three studies indicated a retarded tumor growth rate in exercised mice.

4. Tumor growth rate was reported to be inhibited in rats when they were injected with saline solution that had bathed excised rat muscle fatigued by exercise.

More recent evidence has been supplied by Colacino and Balke (15) who found only half the number of tumors in exercising mice compared with controls when both groups had been subjected to carcinogenic agents. Since there were no differences in food intake or weight, their study supports the older work with respect to the effect of exercise on tumor growth.

A growing body of evidence suggests that physical activity influences the risk of developing some forms of cancer in humans. Recent studies (30, 31, 90) have reported an inverse relationship between physical activity and colon cancer. It is possible that the favorable effect of exercise on colon cancer is related to increased peristalsis of the digestive tract and reduced transit time (11). Frisch and colleagues (29) found that women who had competed in athletics in college exhibited lower incidences of cancers of the uterus, ovaries, cervix, vagina, and breasts than nonathletes. These findings are particularly interesting because they describe a relationship between physical activity and cancers which, usually, are not diagnosed for twenty years or more

(11). Although far from conclusive, these results suggest that activity patterns during adolescence and early adulthood influence the risk of developing cancer later in life. In addition, Paffenbarger and associates (60) reported an increased incidence of all cancers in a group of very sedentary Harvard alumni, and Blair and associates (7) found that the mortality rates from cancer decreased as the level of physical fitness increased for both males and females. Thus, epidemiological evidence suggests that physical activity and physical fitness are associated with a reduced risk of cancer.

It must be emphasized that none of these studies provides evidence of a direct cause-and-effect relationship between exercise and prevention of cancer. Exercise is *not* being advanced as a panacea for cancer prevention. However, if a life of hygienic exercise can make a contribution—no matter how small in a statistical sense—to the prevention of this dread disease, this information (even though causal relationships are not scientifically valid) may be extremely important.

The "Tranquilizer Effect"

The importance of being able to achieve neuromuscular relaxation is shown by the many references to this topic in popular literature. More than $300 million are spent yearly in the United States on tranquilizers to quiet jangled nerves. Many books and articles have been written on the subject, and physical educators often voice the opinion that a good workout can relieve nervous tension. Until recently, however, little scientifically acceptable evidence had been submitted that relates exercise to relief of residual neuromuscular tension.

State of Neuromuscular System Related to Anxiety and Tension

Overwhelming evidence supports the concept of a neuromuscular manifestation of various psychologically induced *anxiety* and *tension* states. The classic work, and much of the evidence, was provided by Edmund Jacobson (39, 40, 41), who was the first to recognize this relationship and to apply it to the need for making objective measurements of previously unmeasurable symptoms. Thus, by making electronic measurements of the activity of the skeletal muscles (electromyography or EMG), it was possible to gain an objective insight into subjects' emotional states and nervousness. Later investigators have supported the work of Jacobson, and, on the basis of the work of Sainsbury and Gibson (71) and Nidever (54), it would appear that sampling even one or two representative muscles in the resting state can provide good evidence on the state of the entire organism at any given moment. Indeed, work in deVries's laboratory has shown a correlation of $r = 0.58$ between resting oxygen consumption (total body) and the EMG activity in one muscle group, the right elbow flexors (23). Significant relationships have been shown to exist between these EMG measurements on selected skeletal muscles and such clinical states as headache, backache, mental activity, and emotional states.

Exercise and Relaxation

The earliest objective work relative to exercise and relaxation was done by Jacobson (39), who compared the ability of college athletes with normal control subjects. He found that the athletes could relax more quickly and completely than the untrained controls. However, controls who were trained in the art of relaxation were superior to the athletes (as a group). Obviously, this experiment does not tell us whether an athletic program contributes to relaxation ability or whether more relaxed persons take up athletics.

In deVries's laboratory, twenty-nine young, healthy subjects were studied for EMG changes after five minutes of bench-stepping as standard exercise. Neuromuscular tension was decreased significantly in the experimental situation, dropping 58% in electrical activity one hour after exercise. No significant change was seen in the same subjects on the control day. A chronic effect of conditioning was also shown (20). More recent work in deVries's laboratory was directed toward comparison of the exercise effect with that of a recognized tranquilizer drug, *meprobamate* (22). To make the experiment more sensitive, older people with complaints of nervous tension acted as subjects. EMG measurements were made before and after (immediately, thirty minutes, and sixty minutes after) each of the five following treatment conditions:

1. Meprobamate 400 mg (normal dosage)
2. Placebo, 400 mg lactose
3. Fifteen minutes of walking-type exercises at a heart rate of 100
4. Fifteen minutes of the same exercise at a heart rate of 120
5. Resting control

Conditions 1 and 2 were administered double-blind. It was found that exercise at a heart rate of 100 lowered electrical activity in the musculature by 20%, 23%, and 20% at the first, second, and third posttests, respectively. These changes were highly significant ($p < .01$). Neither meprobamate nor placebo treatments were significantly different from controls. Exercise at the higher heart rate was only slightly less effective, but the data were more variable and approached, but did not achieve, significance.

Similar results have been found by Morgan and Horstman (52), who showed a reduction in anxiety in normals as well as in clinically anxious individuals, and by Sime (74), who found brief, mild exercise to have a potent effect in reducing the physiological response to an acute stressor.

Work from deVries's laboratory has confirmed the EMG findings. Hoffmann reflexes were used to show a lower activation level in the anterior horn of the spinal cord as the result of 15 to 20 minutes of bicycle exercise at 40% $\dot{V}O_2$ max (24, 25). A review of this literature is available (21).

In recent years, investigators using the methods of psychology have also evaluated the tranquilizer effect of exercise, with results that are essentially consistent with the physiological findings discussed above. Morgan and Goldston have provided an excellent review of this literature (51).

The data suggest that exercise should not be overlooked when a tranquilizer effect is desired, since exercise has no undesirable side effects, whereas tranquilizer drugs used in sufficient repeated dosage to bring about the same effect also impair motor coordination, reaction time, and so on, resulting in subsequent hazards while driving an automobile and performing any other activity requiring normal reactions.

Effect of Exercise on Psychiatric State

There is growing interest in the effects of exercise and fitness level on mood and psychiatric state. Morgan and Horstman (52) were among the first to show the important effect of exercise therapy in bringing about significant reductions in depression. Brown and others (9) at the University of Virginia also show significant improvements in various depressive disorders from ten weeks of jogging.

A study by Young and Ismael (92) has shown an interesting relationship between fitness and emotional stability in middle-age men, and Stamford and associates (82) found both physiological and psychiatric improvement in institutionalized elderly mental patients as a result of daily exercise.

The wisdom of the ages that suggested that vigorous exercise makes you feel good is now supported by laboratory evidence. The importance of this issue is such that the National Institute for Mental Health (NIMH) convened a meeting of scientists from around the country to discuss the role of exercise in the development and maintenance of mental health. The results of this meeting furnish an excellent review of this subject (51).

Summary

Although much evidence has been furnished that supports the value of exercise as a prophylactic and therapeutic measure, exercise is not a panacea. In none of the areas we have discussed in this chapter is the evidence final and conclusive, but we can confidently say that the evidence indicates that a vigorous life maintains optimum levels of health and well-being. All physical educators should be dedicated to this principle, both in their personal and in their professional lives. In no other way can the youth of this nation be led into the full life that only vigorous activity can bring.

References

1. Adams, A. Effect of exercise on ligament strength. *Res. Q.* 37:163–67, 1966.

2. Altekruse, E. B., and Wilmore, J. H. Changes in blood chemistries following a controlled exercise program. *J. Occup. Med.* 15:110–13, 1973.

3. Anderson, J. J. B., Milin, L., and Crackel, W. C. Effect of exercise on mineral and organic bone turnover in swine. *J. Appl. Physiol.* 30:810–13, 1971.

4. Bachman, J. C., and Horvath, S. M. Pulmonary function changes which accompany athletic conditioning programs. *Res. Q.* 39:235–39, 1968.

5. Belloc, N. B. Relationship of health practices and mortality. *Prev. Med.* 2:67–81, 1973.

6. Belloc, N. B., and Breslow, L. Relationship of physical health status and health practices. *Prev. Med.* 1:409–21, 1972.

7. Blair, S. N., Kohl, H. W., Paffenbarger, R. S., Clark, D. G., Cooper, K. H., and Gibbons, L. W. Physical fitness and all-cause mortality. A prospective study of healthy men and women. J.A.M.A. 262:2395–2401, 1989.

8. Brand, R. J., Paffenbarger, R. S., Shultz, R. I., and Kampert, J. B. Work activity and fatal heart attack studied by multiple logistic risk analysis. *Am. J. Epidemiol.* 110:52–62, 1979.

9. Brown, R. S., Ramirez, D. E., and Taub, J. M. The prescription of exercise for depression. Paper read at ACSM meeting, May 24, 1978, Washington, D.C.

10. Brunner, D. The influence of physical activity on incidence and prognosis of ischemic heart disease. *Prevention of Ischemic Heart Disease,* ed. W. Raab, pp. 236–43. Springfield, IL.: Charles C. Thomas, 1966.

11. Calabrese, L. H. Exercise, immunity, cancer, and infection. *Exercise, Fitness, and Health,* ed. C. Bouchard, R. J. Shephard, T. Stephens, J. R. Sutton, B. D. McPherson, pp. 567–79. Champaign, IL.: Human Kinetics Books, 1990.

12. Carlucci, D., Goldfine, H., Ward, A., Taylor, P., and Rippe, J. M. Exercise: Not just for the healthy. *Phys. Sportsmed.* 19:46–54, 1991.

13. Chapman, E. A., deVries, H. A., and Swezey, R. Joint stiffness: Effects of exercise on young and old men. *J. Geront.* 27: 218–21, 1972.

14. Clarke, H. H. Diet and exercise related to vascular disease. *Phys. Fitness Res. Digest* 6:11–17, 1976.

15. Colacino, D., and Balke, B. Tumor reduction in endurance trained mice. Paper read at ACSM meeting, May 1972, Philadelphia.

16. Cooper, K. H., Pollock, M. L., Martin, R. P., White, S. R., Linnerud, A. C., and Jackson, A. Physical fitness levels versus selected coronary risk factors. *J.A.M.A.* 236:166–69, 1976.

17. Cronau, L. H., Rasch, P. J., Hamby, J. W., and Burns, H. J. Effects of strenuous physical training on serum uric acid levels. *J. Sports Med.* 12:23–25, 1972.

18. Dalsky, G. P., Stocke, K. S., Ehsani, A. A., Slatopolsky, E., Lee, W. C., and Birge, S. J. Weight-bearing exercise training and lumbar bone mineral content in postmenopausal women. *Ann. Intern. Med.* 108:824–28, 1988.

19. Darrah, M. I., and Engen, R. L. Beneficial effects of exercise on l-isoproterenol induced myocardial infarction in male rats. *Med. Sci. Sports Exer.* 14:76–80, 1982.

20. deVries, H. A. Immediate and long-term effects of exercise upon resting muscle action potential level. *J. Sports Med. Phys. Fitness* 8:1–11, 1968.

21. ———. Tranquilizer effect of exercise: A critical review. *Physician and Sportsmed.* Nov. 1981 (pp. 46–55).

22. deVries, H. A., and Adams, G. M. Electromyographic comparison of single doses of exercise and meprobamate as to effects on muscular relaxation. *Am. J. Phys. Med.* 51:130–41, 1972.

23. deVries, H. A., Burke, R. K., Hopper, R. T., and Sloan, J. H. Relationship of resting EMG level to total body metabolism with reference to the origin of "tissue noise." *Am. J. Phys. Med.* 55:139–47, 1976.

24. deVries, H. A., Simard, C., Wiswell, R. A., Heckathorne, E., and Carabetta, V. Fusimotor system involvement in the tranquilizer effect of exercise. *Am. J. Phys. Med.* 61:111–22, 1982.

25. deVries, H. A., Wiswell, R. A., Bulbulian, R., and Moritani, T. Tranquilizer effect of exercise: Acute effects of moderate aerobic exercise on spinal reflex activation level. *Am. J. Phys. Med.* 60:57–66, 1981.

26. Eckstein, R. W. Effect of exercise on coronary artery narrowing and coronary collateral circulation. *Circ. Res.* 5:230–35, 1957.

27. Enos, W. F., Beyer, J. C., and Holmes, R. H. Pathogenesis of coronary disease in American soldiers killed in Korea. J.A.M.A. 158:912–14, 1955.

28. Friedman, M. *Pathogenesis of Coronary Artery Disease.* New York: McGraw-Hill Book Co., 1969.

29. Frisch, R. E., Wyshak, G., Albright, N. L., Albright, T. E., Schiff, I., Jones, K. P., Witschi, J., Shiang, E., Koff, E., and Marguglio, M. Lower prevalence of breast cancer and cancers of the reproductive system among former college athletes compared to nonathletes. *Br. J. Cancer* 52:885–91, 1985.

30. Garabrunt, D. H., Peters, J. M., Mack, T. M., and Bernstein, L. Job activity and colon cancer risk. *Am. J. Epidemiol.* 119:1005–14, 1984.

31. Gerhardsson, M., Norell, S. E., Kiviranta, H., Pedersen, N. L., and Ahlbom, A. Sedentary jobs and colon cancer. *Am. J. Epidemiol.* 123:775–80, 1986.

32. Harris, S. S., Caspersen, C. J., DeFriese, G. H., and Estes, E. H. Physical activity counseling for healthy adults as a primary preventive intervention in the clinical setting. Report for the U.S.

Preventive Services Task Force. J.A.M.A. 261:3590–98, 1989.

33. Hartung, G. H., Foreyt, J. P., Mitchell, R. E., Vlasek, I., and Gotto, A. M. Relation of diet to high-density-lipoprotein cholesterol in middle-aged marathon runners, joggers and inactive men. *New Eng. J. Med.* 302:357–61, 1980.

34. Hermansen, L., and Wachtlova, M. Capillary density of skeletal muscle on well-trained and untrained men. *J. Appl. Physiol.* 30:860–63, 1971.

35. Heusner, W. W., Van Huss, W. D., Carrow, R. E., Wells, R. L., Anderson, D. J., and Ruhling, R. O. Exercise, anxiety, and myocardial damage. Paper read at ACSM meeting, May 1, 1972, Philadelphia.

36. Holloszy, J. O., Skinner, J. S., Toro, G., and Cureton, T. K. Effects of a 6-month program of endurance exercise on the serum lipids of middle-aged men. *Am. J. Cardiol.* 14:748–55, 1964.

37. Holman, R. L., McGill, H. C., Strong, J. P., and Geer, J. C. The natural history of atherosclerosis: The early aortic lesions as seen in New Orleans in the middle of the 20th century. *Am. J. Pathol.* 34:209–35, 1958.

38. Holmgren, A. On the variation of DL_{CO} with increasing oxygen uptake during exercise in healthy trained young men and women. *Acta Physiol. Scand.* 65:207–20, 1965.

39. Jacobson, E. The course of relaxation of muscles of athletes. *Am. J. Psychol.* 48:98–108, 1936.

40. ———. *Progressive Relaxation.* Chicago: University of Chicago Press, 1938.

41. ———. The cultivation of physiological relaxation. *Ann. Intern. Med.* 19:965–72, 1943.

42. Kannel, W. B., Sorlie, P., and McNamara, P. The relation of physical activity to risk of coronary heart disease: the Framingham study. *Coronary Heart Disease and Physical Fitness,* eds. O. A. Larson and R. O. Malmborg, p. 256. Baltimore: University Park Press, 1971.

43. Keens, T. G., Krastins, I. R. B., Wannamaker, E. M., Levison, H., Crozier, D. N., and Bryan, A. C. Ventilatory muscle endurance training in normal subjects and patients with cystic fibrosis. *Am. Rev. Respir. Dis.* 116:853–60, 1977.

44. Kiiskinen, A., and Heikkinen, E. Physical training and connective tissues in young mice: Biochemistry of long bones. *J. Appl. Physiol.* 44:50–54, 1978.

45. Kramsch, D. M., Aspen, A. J., Abramowitz, B. M., Kreimendahl, T., and Hood, W. B. Reduction of coronary atherosclerosis by moderate conditioning exercise in monkeys on an atherogenic diet. *New Eng. J. Med.* 305:1483–89, 1981.

46. LaPorte, R. E., Dearwater, S., Cauley, J. A., Slemenda, C., and Cook, T. Physical activity or cardiovascular fitness: Which is more important for health? *Phys. Sportsmed.* 13:145–50, 1985.

47. Leith, D. E., and Bradley, M. Ventilatory muscle strength and endurance training. *J. Appl. Physiol.* 41:508–16, 1976.

48. Leon, A. S., Connett, J., Jacobs, D. R., and Rauramaa, R. Leisure-time physical activity levels and risk of coronary heart disease and death. J.A.M.A. 258:2388–95, 1987.

49. Ljungqvist, A., and Unge, G. Capillary proliferative activity in myocardium and skeletal muscle of exercised rats. *J. Appl. Physiol.* 43:306–7, 1977.

50. Montoye, H. J., Mikkelsen, W. M., Metzner, H. L., and Keller, J. B. Physical activity, fatness, and serum uric acid. *J. Sports Med. Phys. Fitness* 16:253–60, 1976.

51. Morgan, W. P., and Goldston, S. E. Exercise and mental health. Washington, D.C.: Hemisphere Publishing Corporation, 1987.

52. Morgan, W. P., and Horstman, D. H. Anxiety reduction following acute physical activity. Abstracted in *Med. Sci. Sports* 8:62, 1976.

53. Morris, J. N., Heady, J. A., Raffle, P. A. B., Roberts, C. G., and Parks, J. W. Coronary heart disease and physical activity of work. *Lancet* 2:1053–1111, 1953.

54. Nidever, J. E. A factor analytic study of general muscular tension. Ph.D. diss., University of California at Los Angeles, 1959.

55. Oscai, L. B., Patterson, J. A., Bogard, D. C., Beck, R. J., and Rothermel, B. L. Normalization of serum triglycerides and lipoprotein electrophoretic patterns by exercise. *Am. J. Cardiol.* 30:775–80, 1972.

56. Oscai, L. B., Williams, B. T., and Hertig, B. A. Effect of exercise on blood volume. *J. Appl. Physiol.* 24:622–24, 1968.

57. Oyster, N., Morton, M., and Linnell, S. Physical activity and osteoporosis in post-menopausal women. *Med. Sci. Sports Exer.* 16:44–50, 1984.

58. Paffenbarger, R. S., and Hale, W. E. Work activity and coronary heart mortality. *New Eng. J. Med.* 292:545–50, 1975.

59. Paffenbarger, R. S., Hale, W. E., Brand, R. J., and Hyde, R. T. Work-energy level, personal characteristics, and fatal heart attack: a birth-cohort effect. *Am. J. Epidemiol.* 105:200–213, 1977.

60. Paffenbarger, R. S., Hyde, R. T., Wing, A. L., and Hsieh, C. C. Physical activity, all-cause mortality, and longevity of college alumni. *N. Engl. J. Med.* 314:605–613, 1986.

61. Paffenbarger, R. S., Wing, A. L., and Hyde, R. T. Physical activity as an index of heart attack risk in college alumni. *Am. J. Epidemiol.* 108:161–75, 1978.

62. Raab, W. Metabolic protection and reconditioning of the heart muscle through habitual physical exercise. *Ann. Intern. Med.* 53:87–105, 1960.

63. Raab, W., van Lith, P., Lepeschkin, E., and Herrlick, H. C. Catecholamine-induced myocardial hypoxia in the presence of impaired coronary dilatability independent of external cardiac work. *Am. J. Cardiol.* 9:455, 1962.

64. Ratliff, R., Elliott, K., and Rubenstein, C. Plasma lipid and lipoprotein changes with chronic training. *Med. Sci. Sports* 10:55, 1978.

65. Rigan, D. Exercise and cancer, a review. *J. Am. Osteopathic Assoc.* 62:596–99, 1963.

66. Riggs, B. L., and Melton, L. J. Involutional osteoporosis. *N. Engl. J. Med.* 314:1676–84, 1986.

67. Robinson, E. P., and Kjeldgaard, J. M. Improvement in ventilatory muscle function with running. *J. Appl. Physiol.* 52:1400–6, 1982.

68. Rotkis, T. C., Cote, R., and Coyle, E. Relationship between high-density lipoprotein cholesterol and weekly running mileage. *J. Cardiac Rehab.* 2 (March):109–12, 1982.

69. Roundy, E. S., Fisher, G. A., and Anderson, S. Effect of exercise on serum lipids and lipoproteins. *Med. Sci. Sports* 10:55, 1978.

70. Rowland, T. W. *Exercise and Children's Health.* Champaign: Human Kinetics Books, 1990.

71. Sainsbury, P., and Gibson, J. G. Symptoms of anxiety and the accompanying physiological changes in the muscular system. *J. Neurol. Neurosurg. Psychiatry* 17:216–24, 1954.

72. Schneider, R. A., and Zangari, V. M. Variations in clotting time, relative viscosity and other physicochemical properties of the blood accompanying physical and emotional stress in the normotensive and hypertensive subject. *Psychosom. Med.* 13:289–303, 1951.

73. Seals, D. R., and Hagberg, J. M. The effect of exercise training on human hypertension: A review. *Med. Sci. Sports Exer.* 16:207–15, 1984.

74. Sime, W. E. A comparison of exercise and meditation in reducing physiological response to stress. *Med. Sci. Sports* 9:55, 1977.

75. Sinaki, M. Exercise and osteoporosis. *Arch. Phys. Med. Rehabil.* 70:220–29, 1989.

76. Sivertsen, I., and Dahlstrom, A. W. Relation of muscular activity to carcinoma; preliminary report. *J. Cancer Res.* 6:365–78, 1921.

77. Smith, E. L. Exercise for prevention of osteoporosis; a review. *Physician and Sportsmed.* 10 (March):72–82, 1982.

78. Smith, E. L., Gilligan, C., McAdam, M., Ensign, C. P., and Smith, P. E. Deterring bone loss by exercise intervention in premenopausal and postmenopausal women. *Calcif. Tissue Int.* 44:312–21, 1989.

79. Smith, E. L., and Raab, D. M. Osteoporosis and physical activity. *Acta Med. Scand.* 711 (Suppl):149–56, 1986.

80. Smith, E. L., and Reddan, W. Physical activity—a modality for bone accretion in the aged. *Am. J. Roentgen. Radium Ther. Nucl. Med.* 126:1297, 1977.

81. Smith, E. L., Reddan, W., and Smith, P. E. Physical activity and calcium modalities for bone mineral increase in aged women. *Med. Sci. Sports Exer.* 13:60–64, 1981.

82. Stamford, B. A., Hambacher, W., and Fallica, A. Effects of daily physical exercise on the psychiatric state of institutionalized geriatric mental patients. *Res. Q.* 45:34–41, 1974.

83. Stevenson, J. A., Feleki, V., Rechnitzer, P., and Beaton, J. R. Effect of exercise on coronary tree size in the rat. *Circ. Res.* 15:265–69, 1964.

84. Taylor, H. L., Klepetar, E., Keys, A., Parlin, W., Blackburn, H., and Puchner, T. Death rates among physically active and sedentary employees of the railway industry. *Am. J. Public Health* 52:1697–1707, 1962.

85. Tepperman, J., and Pearlman, D. Effects of exercise and anemia on coronary arteries of small animals as revealed by the corrosion-cast technique. *Circ. Res.* 9:576–84, 1961.

86. Tipton, C. M., James, S. L., Mergner, W., and Tcheng, T. K. Influence of exercise on strength of medial collateral knee ligaments of dogs. *Am. J. Physiol.* 218:894–901, 1970.

87. Tipton, C. M., Matthes, R. D., Marcus, K. D., Rowlett, K. A., and Leininger, J. R. Influence of exercise intensity, age, and medication on resting systolic blood pressure of SHR populations. *J. Appl. Physiol.* 55:1305–10, 1983.

88. Tipton, C. M., Matthes, R. D., Maynard, J. A., and Carey, R. A. The influence of physical activity on ligaments and tendons. *Med. Sci. Sports* 7:165–75, 1975.

89. Tran, Z. V., Weltman, A., Glass, G. V., and Mood, D. P. The effects of exercise on blood lipids and lipoproteins: a meta-analysis of studies. *Med. Sci. Sports Exer.* 15:393–402, 1983.

90. Vena, J. E., Graham, S., Zielezny, M., Brasure, J., Swanson, M. K. Occupational exercise and risk of cancer. *Am. J. Clin. Nutr.* 45:318–27, 1987.

91. Williams, J. A., Wagner, J., Wasnich, R., and Heilbrun, L. The effect of long-distance running upon the appendicular bone mineral content. *Med. Sci. Sports Exer.* 16:223–27, 1984.

92. Young, R. J., and Ismael, A. H. Relationship between anthropometric, physiological, biochemical and personality variables before and after a four-month conditioning program for middle-aged men. *J. Sports Med. Phys. Fitness* 16:267–76, 1976.

93. Zuckerman, J., and Stull, G. A. Effects of exercise on knee ligament separation force in rats. *J. Appl. Physiol.* 26:716–19, 1969.

14

Physical Fitness Testing

Measurement of Physical Working
    Capacity (PWC) by Maximum O_2
    Consumption
    Medical Examination—Informed
      Consent
    Personnel
    Emergency Equipment
    Exercise Protocol
    Environmental Considerations
    Time of Day, Diet, and Other
      Variables
    Parameters to Be Measured
    Criteria for Ending the Test
    Extrapolation of Submaximal $\dot{V}O_2$
      Data to Estimate $\dot{V}O_2$ Max
Estimation of PWC from Heart Rate at
    Submaximal Loads
    PWC-170 Test
    Astrand-Ryhming Nomogram
    Harvard Step Test
    Canadian Home Fitness Test
    Cooper Twelve-Minute Run-Walk
      Test
    Twelve-Minute Swimming Test
    Treadmill Walking Test

    Rockport Walking Test
    Estimation of $\dot{V}O_2$ Peak without
      Exercise Testing
Measurement of Anaerobic Capabilities
    Margaria Step-Running Anaerobic
      Power Test
    Wingate Anaerobic Test
New Concepts in Measuring Physical
    Fitness
    The Critical Power Test
    Physical Working Capacity at the
      Fatigue Threshold (PWC_{FT}) from
      Supramaximal Power Outputs
    PWC_{FT} from Submaximal Power
      Outputs
Motor Fitness Tests
    Army/Air Force Physical Fitness
      Test
    AAHPER Youth Fitness Test Battery
The New AAHPERD Health-Related
    Physical Fitness Test
Physical Fitness Evaluation as a Function
    of Age Groups

Hardly a day goes by without a newspaper reference to physical fitness or the lack of it. We hear frequently from the medical profession that obesity is our most common disease, that we suffer from a softness brought about by our highly mechanized lives, and that our complex civilization is producing ever-increasing levels of nervous and mental disease. On the other hand, sportswriters have a field day after our Olympic successes, enthusiastically rebutting allegations of *our* lack of physical fitness because our *athletes* demonstrated superb fitness.

Herein lies one of the greatest fallacies of American physical education. We do indeed develop outstanding athletes to represent us in international competition, but they are in no way typical of the population. It is unfortunate that the spectator sports—football, basketball, and baseball—occupy such a prominent place in physical education, for there is little opportunity to pursue them in adult life. In fact, this emphasis is probably also responsible for the neglect of our less physically talented children; our culture encourages them to be spectators rather than participants.

Despite all the interest shown in physical fitness, by nonprofessionals and professionals alike, we are not yet prepared to offer a universally acceptable definition of the term, much less an operational definition. It must be realized that not all definitions can be couched in terms of absolutes; sometimes a definition must be arbitrary and arrived at by consensus. Thus a nautical mile is based on an absolute measure, one minute of latitude, but the statute mile, which we use much more frequently, is an arbitrary 5,280 feet. It is necessary that we define physical fitness arbitrarily so that we may proceed with an operational definition and with the most important work of all: improving physical fitness at all levels in our population.

The best possible definition of physical fitness encompasses the work that has been performed and accepted by the two professions most interested in this area: physical education and medicine. Thus physical educators have developed many fine tests, which include such items as running, jumping, throwing, pull-ups, and push-ups. These test batteries, which are categorized as tests of *motor fitness,* attempt to measure the following *elements* of physical fitness: strength, speed, agility, endurance, power, coordination, balance, flexibility, and body control.

The concept of *physical working capacity* (PWC), a measure of aerobic power, has gained wide acceptance as a measure of fitness among physiologists, pediatricians, cardiologists, and other members of the medical profession. PWC may be defined as the maximum level of metabolism (power) of which an individual is capable. PWC is measured by objective and accurate means (maximal O_2 consumption), and simpler but valid methods are available for predicting PWC from the submaximal heart rate tests described below.

Much could be gained by wider use of the PWC concept in the physical education profession. First, a unification of thought between the physical education and medical professions would greatly benefit both. Second, PWC testing would provide a motivating factor for students in physical activity classes who are not skillful enough to compete successfully in athletics with their peer groups. The need for health-related physical fitness testing is now recognized—a new AAHPERD test reflects this need. Furthermore, we are coming to appreciate the fact that testing should primarily concern the needs of the individual and the progress made in physical education class rather than position in relation to the norms.

That the PWC concept is not widely used in physical education is probably due to three factors:

1. The inability of physical educators to perform these analyses.

2. Lack of facilities.
3. Classes that are too large to permit sufficient attention to individual testing.

We suggest that some of the tests described in this chapter, such as the Astrand-Ryhming nomogram, which requires only one inexpensive piece of equipment, the cycle ergometer, ought to be at least part of every corrective physical education program. It is also to be hoped that eventually an enlightened public will demand smaller size physical education classes, at which time PWC testing should become an integral part of the general program.

An individual's PWC ultimately depends on his or her capacity to supply oxygen to the working muscles. This, in turn, means that PWC probably evaluates, directly or indirectly, at least the following elements of physical fitness: 1) cardiovascular function, 2) respiratory function, 3) muscular efficiency, 4) strength, 5) muscular endurance, and 6) obesity. Obesity becomes a factor because the final score in maximal O_2 consumption is usually expressed in milliliters of O_2 per kilogram of body weight.

It is readily seen that PWC and motor fitness testing are needed in a well-rounded physical education curriculum. The relative importance of the elements tested by the two major components varies with the age group under consideration, and this factor will be considered later in this chapter.

Measurement of Physical Working Capacity (PWC) by Maximum O_2 Consumption

Work by human muscular effort can be produced by aerobic and anaerobic metabolic processes, as discussed earlier. However, anaerobic processes, when fully loaded, can function only for approximately forty seconds. For this reason it is really *aerobic power* that we measure when we measure PWC, and it is sometimes referred to in these terms.

The measurement of maximal O_2 consumption ($\dot{V}O_2$ max) requires going not only to the exercise load that elicits $\dot{V}O_2$ max but at least one step beyond to assure that a true maximal value has been reached (fig. 12.9). Although this causes little concern in tests on healthy college age or younger subjects, this discussion will deal with adult fitness testing as well and consequently safety measures are emphasized. Where feasible it is sensible to employ the same precautions for the school age subjects, since there are occasionally undiagnosed cases of heart disease among them.

Medical Examination— Informed Consent

Persons over thirty-five years of age and anybody of any age who 1) has any question about his or her health status, 2) develops symptoms during testing, or 3) has not had a medical examination in two years, must be cleared for testing by a personal physician (3). The medical referral form recommended by the American College of Sports Medicine (ACSM) is shown in table 14.1.

For all subjects undergoing maximal exercise testing, the procedures listed in table 14.2 must be carefully explained. Above all, participants must know exactly what is expected of them and must be allowed to ask questions about the procedures. After all questions are answered to their satisfaction, participants must sign an informed consent form such as the one recommended by ACSM and shown in table 14.2.

Personnel

For testing healthy school age subjects and adults under thirty-five with no known primary coronary heart disease (CHD) risk

Table 14.1   Medical Referral Form for Participation in Graded Exercise Test and Exercise Program

Patient's name _____ Date _____

                        Last   First   Initial

Address _____ Age _____ Phone _____

I consider the above individual as:

             _____ Normal
             _____ Cardiac patient
             _____ Prone to coronary heart disease
             _____ Other (Explain) _____

Diagnostic Data Etiologic	*Present Physical Activity*	*ECG*	*Rhythm*
1. No heart disease	1. Very active	1. Normal	1. Sinus
2. Rheumatic heart disease	2. Normal	2. Dig. effect only	2. Atrial fib.
3. Congenital heart disease	3. Limited	3. Abnormal	3. Other
4. Hypertension	4. Very limited	4. Infarct	
5. Ischemic heart disease			
6. Other			

Specific cardiac diagnosis _____

_____

Additional abnormalities you are aware of _____

_____

Date of last complete physical examination _____

Present medication _____

Please fill in the information below if it is available:

1. Urine, sp.gr. _____ Alb. _____ Glucose _____ Micro. _____

2. Complete blood count: Hbg. _____ Hct. _____ WBC _____ Diff. _____

3. ECG, 12 lead (enclose copy) _____

4. Blood pressure, syst. _____ diast. _____

5. Glucose _____ mg%

6. 2-hr post-Dexicola _____ mg%

7. Cholesterol _____ mg% Lipoprotein electrophoresis _____
   Triglyceride _____ mg%

8. Graded exercise test results (If available, enclose.)

Impression of above information _____

_____

    The above listed person is capable of participating in an exercise program as well as periodic laboratory evaluations, under the guidance and supervision of a

( ) Physician
( ) Exercise leader (_____) Check appropriate supervision (_____).

Signed: _____ M.D.

Type or Print
Name of Physician _____

Table 14.2	Informed Consent for Graded Exercise Test*

1. *Explanation of the Graded Exercise Test*
    You will perform a graded exercise test on a bicycle ergometer and/or a motor-driven treadmill. The work levels will begin at a level you can easily accomplish and will be advanced in stages, depending on your work capacity. We may stop the test at any time because of signs of fatigue, or you may stop when you wish to because of personal feelings of fatigue or discomfort. We do not wish you to exercise at a level which is abnormally uncomfortable for you.

2. *Risks and Discomforts*
    There exists the possibility of certain changes occurring during the test. They include abnormal blood pressure, fainting, disorders of heartbeat, and very rare instances of heart attack. Every effort will be made to minimize them by the preliminary examination and by observations during testing. Emergency equipment and trained personnel are available to deal with unusual situations which may arise.

3. *Benefits to be Expected*
    The results obtained from the exercise test may assist in the diagnosis of your illness or in evaluating what types of activities you might carry out with no or low hazards.

4. *Inquiries*
    Any questions about the procedures used in the graded exercise test or in the estimation of functional capacity are welcome. If you have any doubts or questions, please ask us for further explanations.

5. *Freedom of Consent*
    Permission for you to perform this graded exercise test is voluntary. You are free to deny consent if you so desire.
    I have read this form and I understand the test procedures that I will perform and I consent to participate in this test.

_____
Signature of Patient

_____   _____
Date   Witness

*Where test is for a purpose other than prescription, e.g., experimental interest, this should be indicated on the Informed Consent Form.

From "Guidelines for Graded Exercise Testing and Exercise Prescription," by American College of Sports Medicine. © 1975 Lea & Febiger. Reprinted by permission.

factors* or symptoms, testing may be conducted by a trained exercise technician without the presence of a physician. The exercise technicians must have had training in cardiopulmonary resuscitation (CPR) and mouth-to-mouth breathing techniques.

A physician's presence is required when testing a participant of any age who has shown symptoms of CHD, either suspected or documented. A physician should be available at

*Primary CHD risk factors are hypertension, hyperlipidemia, and cigarette smoking. Secondary risk factors are family history, obesity, physical inactivity, diabetes mellitus, and asymptomatic hyperglycemia. The participant's status in the last two risk factors need not be determined in young (less than thirty-five) asymptomatic participants with no risk factors. In participants thirty-five and over and in participants with risk factors or symptoms, blood lipids and blood glucose levels should be measured (2).

least in the general testing area if the subject is over thirty-five or if the subject exhibits major risk factors or has documented CHD (asymptomatic).

Emergency Equipment

Minimal emergency equipment should include 1) a defibrillator, 2) an oxygenator with intermittent positive pressure capability, 3) oral and endotrachial airways, and 4) a bag-valve-mask respirator. When a physician is required or available for testing, many medical instruments and pharmaceuticals would also be provided at the physician's discretion and preferably set up as an emergency cart that would be available at all times.

Exercise Protocol

As discussed in chapter 12, at least three exercise modalities can serve for testing $\dot{V}O_2$ max. The cycle ergometer is probably the most popular because of its advantages of objectively and accurately measured power output and relative lack of movement of the upper body, which greatly lessens the problems of instrumentation, producing a "cleaner" electrocardiogram, fewer leaks around the mouthpiece, and other advantages. The treadmill is almost as popular because it allows the use of the familiar movements of running and walking. It also involves a slightly larger muscle mass, and consequently $\dot{V}O_2$ max is usually found to be 5%–8% higher on the treadmill. The third technique, bench-stepping, is the least desirable choice because of the great amount of body movement and its relatively small potential range of power outputs.

With any of the three exercise modalities, the protocol may be as follows:

1. *Intermittent incremental loading.*
   Exercise loads are usually started at a low level, and each load is applied for three to six minutes to allow an approximate steady state to develop. Rest intervals are allowed between exercise loads to prevent undue fatigue. Exercise loads are raised in some systematic fashion until two consecutive loads result in either a downturn in $\dot{V}O_2$, a leveling to a plateau, or at least an insignificant increase (less than 150 ml O_2 is commonly used as a criterion). This protocol often requires participants to make two visits to the laboratory to complete the test.

2. *Continuous step-incremental loading.*
   This procedure is typified on the cycle ergometer by the Luft protocol in which the power output required for the first three minutes is 50 watts. Each minute thereafter the load is increased by 12.5 watts (approximately 75 kgm/min) until the subject is unable to continue. This much simpler procedure results in values for $\dot{V}O_2$ max that are still within 5% of values obtained by the more cumbersome method described above and can be completed in most cases in twenty to twenty-two minutes (33). This protocol can also be modified to use step increments in loading such as 10 W/min, 20 W/2 min, 25 W/2 min, or 30 W/3 min without substantial differences in result (12). On the treadmill the Balke protocol is commonly used, in which the subject walks at 3.3 mph for the first two minutes on the horizontal treadmill. Every minute thereafter the incline is increased by 1% until either the heart rate reaches 180 bpm or until exhaustion. Balke considered a heart rate of 180 as the aerobic crest load, with work beyond this largely accomplished via anaerobic metabolism. However, results are more comparable with other protocols if continued until exhaustion.

3. *Continuously incremented loading (ramp loading)*. Figure 14.1 shows the difference in these exercise protocols with respect to the way in which exercise intensity is increased with time The continuously incremented or ramp-loading protocol, although not widely used yet, is becoming more popular as interest in such phenomena as lactate threshold and other points in the time history of the workout become more important. Breath-by-breath analyses of the gas parameters also greatly enhance the values to be derived from ramp loading. This method obviously has the advantage of providing an infinitely gentle progression of work load (no sudden increments to disturb the subject's equilibrium), but it also requires an electronic ergometer that must be modified in most cases to provide a ramp program.

Environmental Considerations

Environmental conditions such as ambient temperature, relative humidity, and air movement have a considerable effect on how the available cardiac output is divided between the active muscles and the cutaneous vessels for cooling. Thus, for example, lengthy heat exposure may lead to reduction of the central blood volume, concomitant loss of cardiac output, and spuriously low values of $\dot{V}O_2$ max. To make either intraindividual or interindividual comparisons of PWC, environmental conditions should be controlled. The World Health Organization recommends that the testing environment be maintained in the range 18°–22° C (64°–72° F), with the relative humidity below 60%, and in still air. The upper limit can be increased by about 2° C if the effective temperature is reduced by the use of a large fan (3). Normally, exercise tests are not conducted in a cold environment, and testing should be discouraged if the room temperature is below 10° C (50° F).

Time of Day, Diet, and Other Variables

Since many of the physiological functions entering into the determination of $\dot{V}O_2$ max are affected by time of day (circadian rhythm), this factor should be recorded and maintained constant in test-retest evaluations.

Ingestion of food results in a rise in both heart rate and ventilation for an hour or more, while a complete fast may result in low blood sugar during testing. Therefore a compromise is necessary, and the subject is instructed to eat only a light meal at least an hour before testing.

Unusually strenuous exertion should be avoided on the day prior to testing, and on the day of testing no other strenuous activity should precede the test. A rest period in the laboratory of at least one hour prior to testing is highly desirable. Anxiety concerning the test procedure can be a significant problem in submaximal tests, which depend on heart rate, but there is little if any effect on $\dot{V}O_2$ max. Indeed, recent work suggests it may not be a consideration even in submaximal tests (43).

Parameters to Be Measured

Since this text is directed to physical education students, the parameters to be measured

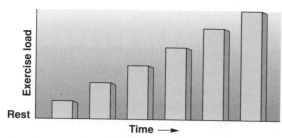

A. Intermittent incremental loading

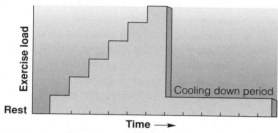

B. Continuous step increment loading

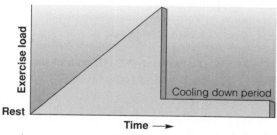

C. Continuously incremented loading (Ramp loading)

Figure 14.1   Three commonly used protocols for $\dot{V}O_2$ max testing.

will be limited to noninvasive (bloodless) techniques. In spite of this limitation, a great deal of important information can be extracted with respect to cardiovascular and respiratory function. Ideally, the following primary parameters, from which many secondary parameters can be derived, should be recorded at each exercise load:

A. Primary Data
1. F_{O2_E}—% O_2 in expired gas for calculation of $\dot{V}O_2$
2. F_{CO2_E}—% CO_2 in expired gas for calculation of $\dot{V}O_2$
3. V_E—minute ventilation
4. HR—preferably from cardiotachometer, but can be taken later from recorded ECG
5. BP—systolic is obtained clearly; diastolic may be difficult
6. ECG—lead CM_5 if only one lead can be taken

B. Derived Data (calculated from primary data)
1. $R = \dot{V}_{CO_2}/\dot{V}_{O_2}$
2. O_2 pulse = $\dot{V}_{O_2}$ per heart beat
3. Double product = HR $\times$ BPsyst/100
4. Ventilation equivalent for O_2 = $\dot{V}_E/\dot{V}_{O_2}$
5. Ventilatory anaerobic threshold (chap. 12)

The significance of the primary data is probably obvious. Of the derived data, the respiratory exchange ratio (R) is of greatest interest in helping define the point when anaerobic metabolism becomes prominent. As such, it is also useful as one criterion that $\dot{V}O_2$ max has indeed been achieved. Various authorities use different criteria, but in the absence of an $R > 1.05$, it would be unlikely that a true $\dot{V}O_2$ max had been achieved. Before the onset of the lactate threshold, R is of course a reflection of the energy substrate utilized.

O_2 pulse provides some insight into the behavior of stroke volume and arteriovenous O_2 difference (chap. 12).

The double product of heart rate and systolic blood pressure (HR $\times$ BPsyst/100) has been found to be well correlated with myocardial O_2 consumption and therefore reflects the work of the heart at each level. This will be important in our subsequent discussion of cardiac rehabilitation (chap. 16).

The ventilation equivalent for O_2 tells us how many liters of lung ventilation are required for one liter of O_2 uptake by the tissues. Thus this is an important reflection of the efficiency of O_2 transport mechanisms.

Lactate threshold, or its noninvasive analogue, ventilatory threshold, appears to be a very important determinant of the level of endurance performance that can be sustained in distance running events. Recent evidence suggests that it has important implications independent of the $\dot{V}O_2$ max (chap. 12).

Criteria for Ending the Test

According to ACSM recommendations (2), when an exercise test is being conducted by a nonphysician, it should be stopped for the following reasons. If a physician is conducting the test, he or she may decide to use other criteria.

1. Symptoms of significant exertional intolerance
   a. dizziness or near-syncope
   b. angina
   c. unusual or intolerable fatigue
   d. intolerable claudication or pain
2. Signs of intolerance
   a. staggering or unsteadiness
   b. mental confusion
   c. facial expression signifying disorders (strained or blank faces)
   d. cyanosis or pallor (facial or elsewhere)
   e. rapid, distressful breathing

   f. nausea or vomiting
   g. a definite fall in systolic blood pressure with increasing work load
3. Electrocardiographic changes
   a. S-T segment displacement of 0.2 mV below the base line
   b. supraventricular or ventricular dysrhythmias or ectopic ventricular activity occurring before the end of a T-wave (R-on-T phenomenon). *It is recommended that a test be terminated in the presence of three or more successive ectopic ventricular complexes or with a significant increase in their occurrence—about ten per minute—depending on clinical judgment.*
   c. major left intraventricular conduction disturbances
4. Inappropriate blood pressure responses, such as a decrease in systolic blood pressure with an increase in work load

Extrapolation of Submaximal $\dot{V}O_2$ Data to Estimate $\dot{V}O_2$ Max

If heart rate and metabolic rate ($\dot{V}O_2$) are both measured at steady state, the relationship is approximately linear, as shown in figure 14.2. Thus, if two or more paired $\dot{V}O_2$-HR values are plotted, as in figure 14.2, the resulting straight line can be extrapolated to the predicted maximum heart rate (220 − age), and the $\dot{V}O_2$ max can then be read off the graph.

Estimation of PWC from Heart Rate at Submaximal Loads

It has long been known that heart rate rises linearly with increasing work loads (within limits). Furthermore, the rate of rise in heart rate for the same increments of work has been

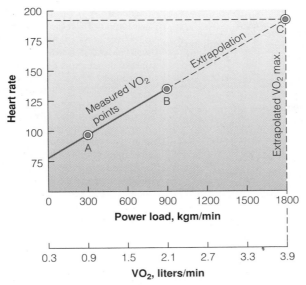

Figure 14.2   Extrapolation of submaximal $\dot{V}O_2$ data to estimate $\dot{V}O_2$ max. Linear extrapolation of the two measured $\dot{V}O_2$—HR points (A and B) to point C, the intersection with the estimated maximum heart rate line, provides an estimate of $\dot{V}O_2$ max = 3.9 liters/min.

used in several different methods for evaluating PWC. Figure 14.3 illustrates this principle for two middle-age men, one in good athletic condition, the other untrained.

PWC-170 Test

The PWC-170 test consists of two consecutive six-minute bicycle ergometer rides in which the work loads are selected to produce heart rates of approximately 140 and 170 per minute. The working capacity is calculated by plotting (on graph paper) the heart rate against the work load at the end of each trial. A straight line is drawn through the two points to intersect the line of 170 bpm. The estimated power output that corresponds to a heart rate of 170 is then recorded as the individual's PWC-170. The heart rate of 170 is used rather arbitrarily as a point beyond which little increase in aerobic metabolism is expected. Use of this principle for the unconditioned subject in figure 14.3 would thus give an estimated PWC-170 of 975 kgm/min.

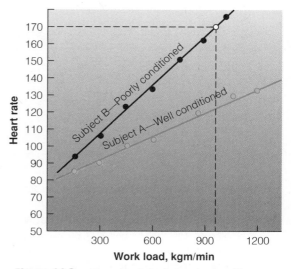

Figure 14.3   The rate of rise in heart rate with increasing exercise load as a function of physical condition.

This PWC-170 test has been found to correlate rather well with the measured maximal O_2 consumption of college men in deVries's laboratory: $r = 0.88$. The standard error of

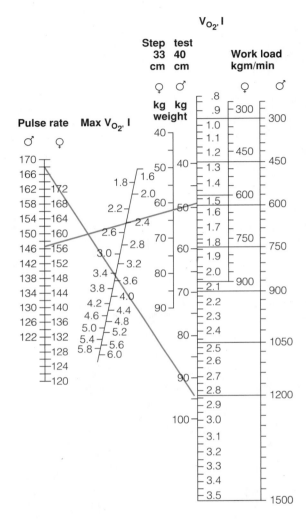

V_{O_2}, l

Figure 14.4 The adjusted nomogram for calculation of aerobic work capacity from submaximal pulse rate and O_2 uptake values (cycling, running or walking, and step test). In tests without direct O_2 uptake measurement, it can be estimated by reading horizontally from the body weight scale (step test) or work load scale (cycle test) to the O_2 uptake scale. The point on the O_2 uptake scale (V_{O_2}, 1) shall be connected with the corresponding point on the pulse rate scale, and the predicted maximal O_2 uptake should be read on the middle scale. A female subject (61 kg) reaches a heart rate of 156 at step test; predicted maximal V_{O_2} = 2.41. A male subject reaches a heart rate of 166 at cycling test on a work load of 1,200 kg-m/min; predicted maximal V_{O_2} = 3.61 (exemplified by dotted lines). (From Astrand, I., in *Acta Physiologica Scandinavica* 49 [suppl. 169]. © 1960 Scandinavian Physiologica Society. Reprinted by permission.)

of healthy male subjects averaged 128 after six minutes of work. The corresponding heart rate for female subjects was 138. When their subjects worked with a heavier load, thus demanding oxygen consumption of 70% of their aerobic capacity, the average heart rate was 154 for males and 164 for females. The standard deviation was eight or nine beats per minute.

Astrand and Ryhming used these data to develop a nomogram (fig. 14.4) for predicting maximal O_2 consumption from heart rate for one six-minute submaximal work load. They found that the accuracy of prediction varied with the level of the work load selected. On the bicycle ergometer at 900 kgm/min, the standard error of prediction for men was ± 10.4%, and at 1,200 kgm/min it was ± 6.7%. deVries and Klafs (18) found a correlation of 0.74 between predicted maximal O_2 consumption by the Astrand-Ryhming method and maximal O_2 consumption as measured in deVries's laboratory. These data yielded an error of prediction of ± 9.3%, which agrees with their figures. Tables 14.3 and 14.4 provide the nomogram data for young men and young women in more easily used form.

prediction of maximal O_2 consumption from the PWC-170 test was found to be ± 9.4%, which seems to be an entirely acceptable value for this type of test (18). The test eliminates all of the laboratory technique of maximal O_2 consumption tests but is not practical for use with large groups.

Astrand-Ryhming Nomogram

Astrand and Ryhming (5) found, when working at a load that required 50% of maximal O_2 consumption, that the heart rate for a group

Table 14.3 Calculation of Maximal Oxygen Uptake from Pulse Rate and Exercise Load on a Cycle Ergometer (Men)

Working Pulse	Maximal Oxygen Uptake Liters/min					Working Pulse	Maximal Oxygen Uptake Liters/min				
	300 kgm/min	600 kgm/min	900 kgm/min	1200 kgm/min	1500 kgm/min		300 kgm/min	600 kgm/min	900 kgm/min	1200 kgm/min	1500 kgm/min
120	2.2	3.5	4.8			148		2.4	3.2	4.3	5.4
121	2.2	3.4	4.7			149		2.3	3.2	4.3	5.4
122	2.2	3.4	4.6			150		2.3	3.2	4.2	5.3
123	2.1	3.4	4.6			151		2.3	3.1	4.2	5.2
124	2.1	3.3	4.5	6.0		152		2.3	3.1	4.1	5.2
125	2.0	3.2	4.4	5.9		153		2.2	3.0	4.1	5.1
126	2.0	3.2	4.4	5.8		154		2.2	3.0	4.0	5.1
127	2.0	3.1	4.3	5.7		155		2.2	3.0	4.0	5.0
128	2.0	3.1	4.2	5.6		156		2.2	2.9	4.0	5.0
129	1.9	3.0	4.2	5.6		157		2.1	2.9	3.9	4.9
130	1.9	3.0	4.1	5.5		158		2.1	2.9	3.9	4.9
131	1.9	2.9	4.0	5.4		159		2.1	2.8	3.8	4.8
132	1.8	2.9	4.0	5.3		160		2.1	2.8	3.8	4.8
133	1.8	2.8	3.9	5.3		161		2.0	2.8	3.7	4.7
134	1.8	2.8	3.9	5.2		162		2.0	2.8	3.7	4.6
135	1.7	2.8	3.8	5.1		163		2.0	2.8	3.7	4.6
136	1.7	2.7	3.8	5.0		164		2.0	2.7	3.6	4.5
137	1.7	2.7	3.7	5.0		165		2.0	2.7	3.6	4.5
138	1.6	2.7	3.7	4.9		166		1.9	2.7	3.6	4.5
139	1.6	2.6	3.6	4.8		167		1.9	2.6	3.5	4.4
140	1.6	2.6	3.6	4.8	6.0	168		1.9	2.6	3.5	4.4
141		2.6	3.5	4.7	5.9	169		1.9	2.6	3.5	4.3
142		2.5	3.5	4.6	5.8	170		1.8	2.6	3.4	4.3
143		2.5	3.4	4.6	5.7						
144		2.5	3.4	4.5	5.7						
145		2.4	3.4	4.5	5.6						
146		2.4	3.3	4.4	5.6						
147		2.4	3.3	4.4	5.5						

Modified from I. Astrand's *Acta Physiologica Scandinavica* 49 (suppl. 169), 1960 by P-O. Astrand in *Work Test with the Bicycle Ergometer.* Varberg, Sweden: Monark, 1965.

Table 14.4 Calculation of Maximal Oxygen Uptake from Pulse Rate and Exercise Load on a Cycle Ergometer (Women)

Working Pulse	Maximal Oxygen Uptake Liters/min					Working Pulse	Maximal Oxygen Uptake Liters/min				
	300 kgm/min	450 kgm/min	600 kgm/min	750 kgm/min	900 kgm/min		300 kgm/min	450 kgm/min	600 kgm/min	750 kgm/min	900 kgm/min
120	2.6	3.4	4.1	4.8		148	1.6	2.1	2.6	3.1	3.6
121	2.5	3.3	4.0	4.8		149		2.1	2.6	3.0	3.5
122	2.5	3.2	3.9	4.7		150		2.0	2.5	3.0	3.5
123	2.4	3.1	3.9	4.6		151		2.0	2.5	3.0	3.4
124	2.4	3.1	3.8	4.5		152		2.0	2.5	2.9	3.4
125	2.3	3.0	3.7	4.4		153		2.0	2.4	2.9	3.3
126	2.3	3.0	3.6	4.3		154		2.0	2.4	2.8	3.3
127	2.2	2.9	3.5	4.2		155		1.9	2.4	2.8	3.2
128	2.2	2.8	3.5	4.2	4.8	156		1.9	2.3	2.8	3.2
129	2.2	2.8	3.4	4.1	4.8	157		1.9	2.3	2.7	3.2
130	2.1	2.7	3.4	4.0	4.7	158		1.8	2.3	2.7	3.1
131	2.1	2.7	3.4	4.0	4.6	159		1.8	2.2	2.7	3.1
132	2.0	2.7	3.3	3.9	4.5	160		1.8	2.2	2.6	3.0
133	2.0	2.6	3.2	3.8	4.4	161		1.8	2.2	2.6	3.0
134	2.0	2.6	3.2	3.8	4.4	162		1.8	2.2	2.6	3.0
135	2.0	2.6	3.1	3.7	4.3	163		1.7	2.2	2.6	2.9
136	1.9	2.5	3.1	3.6	4.2	164		1.7	2.1	2.5	2.9
137	1.9	2.5	3.0	3.6	4.2	165		1.7	2.1	2.5	2.9
138	1.8	2.4	3.0	3.5	4.1	166		1.7	2.1	2.5	2.8
139	1.8	2.4	2.9	3.5	4.0	167		1.6	2.1	2.4	2.8
140	1.8	2.4	2.8	3.4	4.0	168		1.6	2.0	2.4	2.8
141	1.8	2.3	2.8	3.4	3.9	169		1.6	2.0	2.4	2.8
142	1.7	2.3	2.8	3.3	3.9	170		1.6	2.0	2.4	2.7
143	1.7	2.2	2.7	3.3	3.8						
144	1.7	2.2	2.7	3.2	3.8						
145	1.6	2.2	2.7	3.2	3.7						
146	1.6	2.2	2.6	3.2	3.7						
147	1.6	2.1	2.6	3.1	3.6						

Modified from I. Astrand's *Acta Physiologica Scandinavica* 49 (suppl. 169), 1960 by P-O. Astrand in *Work Test with the Bicycle Ergometer*. Varberg, Sweden: Monark, 1965.

Table 14.5	Norms for Maximal O_2 Consumption (Aerobic Working Capacity)				
Women					
Age	Low	Fair	Average	Good	High
20–29	1.69	1.70–1.99	2.00–2.49	2.50–2.79	2.80+
	28	29–34	35–43	44–48	49+
30–39	1.59	1.60–1.89	1.90–2.39	2.40–2.69	2.70+
	27	28–33	34–41	42–47	48+
40–49	1.49	1.50–1.79	1.80–2.29	2.30–2.59	2.60+
	25	26–31	32–40	41–45	46+
50–65	1.29	1.30–1.59	1.60–2.09	2.10–2.39	2.40+
	21	22–28	29–36	37–41	42+
Men					
Age	Low	Fair	Average	Good	High
20–29	2.79	2.80–3.09	3.10–3.69	3.70–3.99	4.00+
	38	39–43	44–51	52–56	57+
30–39	2.49	2.50–2.79	2.80–3.39	3.40–3.69	3.70+
	34	35–39	40–47	48–51	52+
40–49	2.19	2.20–2.49	2.50–3.09	3.10–3.39	3.40+
	30	31–35	36–43	44–47	48+
50–59	1.89	1.90–2.19	2.20–2.79	2.80–3.09	3.10+
	25	26–31	32–39	40–43	44+
60–69	1.59	1.60–1.89	1.90–2.49	2.50–2.79	2.80+
	21	22–26	27–35	36–39	40+

Lower figure = milliliters of O_2 per kilogram body weight per minute (ml/kg·min^{-1}).
From I. Astrand, *Acta Physiologica Scandinavica* 49 (suppl. 169), 1960. Reprinted by permission.

The Astrand-Ryhming nomogram has proved a very usable method for small groups and requires about ten minutes per subject. Norms, which are given in table 14.5, have been provided (4). The test can be performed with no equipment other than a stopwatch (for taking heart rate), since the nomogram includes step-test data as well as data for cycle ergometer use.

This widely used test has been much criticized because of its error in predicting $\dot{V}O_2$ max (recognized by Astrand as well as by critics). However, the simplicity with which it can be administered makes it a very valuable field test. Furthermore, while the error in predicting $\dot{V}O_2$ max at any given point in time is recognized, its error in following training effect in the same subject over a period of time is no greater than that in the actual measurement of $\dot{V}O_2$ max (49).

Ambient temperatures, which impose a heat stress on individuals being tested, will obviously invalidate the procedure. For subjects

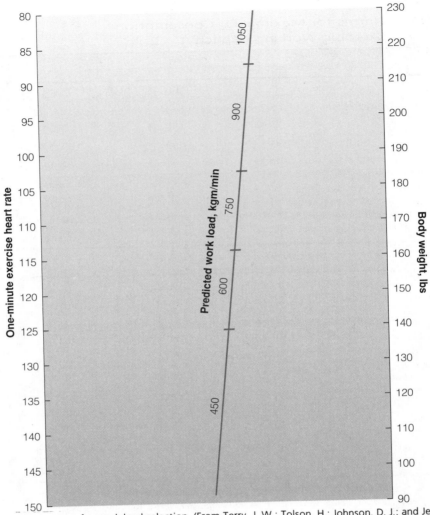

Figure 14.5   Nomogram for work load selection. (From Terry, J. W.; Tolson, H.; Johnson, D. J.; and Jessup, G. T., in *Journal of Sports Medicine and Physical Fitness* 12:361–66. © 1977 Federation Internationale de Medicine Sportive. Reprinted by permission.)

over twenty-five years of age, an age correction factor must be applied (47).

One question that arises in the use of this test is, "What is a suitable test exercise load for any given subject?" The errors of prediction are least when a working heart rate of 160–165 is achieved. To help the selection of an appropriate exercise load, a nomogram has been developed by Terry and others (46) and is provided in figure 14.5. The subject is tested for one minute at 600 kgm/min. The heart rate achieved and the body weight are then used to calculate the appropriate exercise load for the test.

Zuti and Corbin (50) have used the Astrand test on over 3,000 freshman men and women at Kansas State University, and their

| Table 14.6 | Physical Fitness Norms for Females and Males |

Female

Percentiles	Height		Weight		$\dot{V}O_2max$		% Fat
	cm	in	kg	lb	l/min	ml/kg·min^{-1}	
100	188.0	74.0	92.3	203.0	3.80	65.0	11.0
90	173.2	68.2	69.1	152.0	2.90	49.5	18.3
80	170.2	67.0	65.0	143.0	2.60	45.0	19.8
70	167.9	66.1	62.0	136.5	2.41	41.8	20.9
60	166.4	65.5	59.7	131.3	2.35	40.3	22.0
50	164.6	64.8	58.0	127.5	2.16	37.2	23.2
40	162.6	64.0	56.2	123.7	2.05	35.0	24.1
30	160.8	63.3	54.2	119.3	1.93	32.9	25.3
20	158.8	62.5	52.1	114.7	1.70	30.5	26.8
10	156.0	61.4	49.5	109.0	1.60	27.7	29.3
0	132.0	52.0	37.7	83.0	1.10	18.0	40.0

Male

100	200.7	79.0	110.9	244.0	4.80	65.0	3.0
90	186.4	73.4	84.5	186.0	3.60	51.5	6.5
80	183.1	72.1	79.5	175.0	3.33	46.7	7.7
70	181.4	71.4	76.9	169.2	3.13	43.6	8.6
60	179.3	70.6	74.1	163.0	2.95	41.0	9.6
50	177.5	69.9	71.7	157.7	2.79	38.8	10.8
40	176.0	69.3	69.5	153.0	2.65	36.7	12.0
30	174.2	68.6	67.7	149.0	2.45	34.4	13.5
20	172.0	67.7	65.0	143.0	2.33	32.3	15.3
10	168.4	66.3	61.4	135.0	2.13	29.3	19.0
0	147.3	58.0	51.4	113.0	1.50	21.0	35.0

From W.B. Zuti and C.B. Corbin. "Physical Norms for College Freshmen," in *College Quarterly* 48:499. © 1977 American Alliance for Health, Physical Education, and Recreation. Reprinted by permission.

data provide norms that better reflect the fitness of American student populations than Astrand's norms do (table 14.6). Comparison of the Zuti-Corbin norms with those of Astrand in table 14.5 suggests that Scandinavian students are somewhat more fit, at least for cycle ergometer exercise.

Harvard Step Test

The two tests we have described use heart rate *during* exercise as a criterion of PWC. Exercise on a cycle ergometer is best suited for this approach since the subject's upper body is relatively stationary. To eliminate the need for a cycle ergometer, tests have been devised that use bench-stepping as exercise and measure heart rate *after* exercise (during recovery). The principle is that the better the PWC of the individual, the greater the proportion of the cardiac cost that is paid during exercise, the smaller the recovery cardiac cost, and the lower the rate during recovery.

The Harvard step test was devised for use with large groups. It is simple and easily administered. However, its error in predicting maximal oxygen consumption in deVries's laboratory was ±12.5%. The test requires only a stepping bench or benches (twenty inches high and eighteen inches deep) adequate for the number of subjects (who are to step simultaneously), a stopwatch for each observer, and a metronome.

Subjects are lined up in front of the stepping bench (thirty inches of width are allowed for each), and there is one observer for each subject. The person in charge counts cadence to a metronome set at 120 counts per minute: "up—two—three—four," and so on. On *up,* subjects place one foot on the bench; on *two,* they bring the other foot up and *straighten their back and legs;* on *three,* they step down with the foot that was placed on the bench first; and on *four,* they return to the starting position. Thus subjects complete one step every two seconds, or thirty steps per minute. Subjects lead off with the same foot each time, although one or two changes may be made in the course of the five-minute stepping period.

If subjects fall behind the cadence because of exhaustion, they are stopped twenty seconds after falling behind the pace. When they stop (either at completion of five minutes or due to exhaustion), they sit down quietly, and observers restart their stopwatches, having recorded the duration of the stepping. Observers then take the pulse rate at the carotid artery in the neck from sixty to ninety seconds after exercise. On the basis of the duration and the recovery pulse rate, the score (in arbitrary units) is taken from table 14.7. Interpretation of the score is as follows: below 50, poor; 50 to 80, average; above 80, good.

Canadian Home Fitness Test

Subjects are required to climb and descend the bottom two steps of a domestic staircase at a pace set by a long-playing record. Fitness is classified on the test duration (three, six, or nine minutes of a progressive rhythm) and the immediate post-exercise pulse count. During initial validation of the test, an attempt was made to recruit a randomly selected sample of the Saskatoon population. Over 2,800 names were taken from the telephone directory, but unfortunately only about a third of those contacted agreed to participate. It was thus necessary to supplement the sample from such sources as the local police and fire departments. Particular difficulty was encountered in recruiting older subjects, and this may have biased the results toward an overestimation of average levels of fitness in the elderly.

The principle involved in this test is that if one chooses a load that represents a fixed percentage of capacity for the average sedentary person of given gender and age, then the exercise response in terms of duration of work and/or the resultant heart rate reflects that person's physical fitness level. Validation data and norms have been provided (6).

Cooper Twelve-Minute Run-Walk Test

Cooper (14) developed a twelve-minute modification of the original Balke fifteen-minute run-walk field test, which he validated on 115 young air force men (mean age, twenty-two). He found that his test results on the distance covered in twelve minutes correlated 0.897

| Table 14.7 | Scoring for the Harvard Step Test |

Duration of Effort (Minutes)	Total Heart Beats 1 to 1½ Minutes in Recovery											
	40–44	45–49	50–54	55–59	60–64	65–69	70–74	75–79	80–84	85–89	90–94	95–99
	Score (Arbitrary Units)											
0–½	6	6	5	5	4	4	4	4	3	3	3	3
½–1	19	17	16	14	13	12	11	11	10	9	9	8
1–1½	32	29	26	24	22	20	19	18	17	16	15	14
1½–2	45	41	38	34	31	29	27	25	23	22	21	20
2–2½	58	52	47	43	40	36	34	32	30	28	27	25
2½–3	71	64	58	53	48	45	42	39	37	34	33	31
3–3½	84	75	68	62	57	53	49	46	43	41	39	37
3½–4	97	87	79	72	66	61	57	53	50	47	45	42
4–4½	110	98	89	82	75	70	65	61	57	54	51	48
4½–5	123	110	100	91	84	77	72	68	63	60	57	54
5	129	116	105	96	88	82	76	71	67	63	60	56

From C.F. Consolazio et al. *Physiological Measurements of Metabolic Function in Man.* Copyright © 1963. McGraw-Hill Book Company. Used by permission.

with measured maximal O_2 consumption. To achieve good results with this test, motivation must be high. As Cooper pointed out, "this study indicates that in young, well-motivated subjects, field testing can provide a good assessment of maximum O_2 consumption; but the accuracy of the estimate is related directly to the motivation of the subjects."

Doolittle and Bigbee (21) used the test on 153 ninth grade boys and found the validity to be equally good for them ($r = 0.90$), and the test-retest data correlated $r = 0.94$. They also found the twelve-minute run-walk to be a more valid test for this age group than a 600-yard run-walk test ($r = 0.62$).

Maksud and Coutts (34) found the test equally reproducible with boys eleven to fourteen, but the validity correlation with maximum O_2 consumption was lower ($r = 0.65$).

Shaver measured both $\dot{V}O_2$ max and performance at various distances in running for thirty untrained college men. The results show

clearly that distances over one-half mile are required to produce significant correlations with $\dot{V}O_2$ max, while distances below that are better related to anaerobic work capacity (table 14.8) (45).

Buono and coworkers (11) compared the validity and reliability of a one mile run, step test, and submaximal cycle ergometer test for predicting $\dot{V}O_2$ max in ninety children and adolescents age ten to eighteen years. The results indicated that the one mile run was the most valid (validity compared to $\dot{V}O_2$ max from a treadmill test, $r = -0.73$ for the one mile run versus $r = -0.48$ and 0.49 for the step test and cycle test, respectively) and reliable (test-retest, $r = 0.95$ for the one mile run versus $r = 0.82$ and 0.77 for the step test and cycle test, respectively). These findings suggest the maximal run-walk tests are preferred over submaximal step tests or cycle ergometer tests for estimating $\dot{V}O_2$ max in children and adolescents.

Table 14.8	Correlations between Various Running Performances and $\dot{V}O_2$ Max	
Running Distance	**$\dot{V}O_2$ Max (r)**	**Anaerobic Power (r)**
100 yards	−.08	−.85
220 yards	−.25	−.82
440 yards	−.29	−.79
880 yards	−.35	−.32
1 mile	−.43	−.28
2 miles	−.76	−.15
3 miles	−.82	−.05

Compiled from the data of L.G. Shaver, *Journal of Sports Medicine and Physical Fitness* 15:147–50, 1975.

Since the net metabolic cost of running when referred to body weight and distance covered is essentially a constant, independent of speed, Margaria, Aghemo, and Limas (35) have provided a nomogram from which one can estimate $\dot{V}O_2$ max from best run time over distances long enough to allow reaching steady state (fig. 14.6). For example, it can be seen from the nomogram that a subject who can run 6 km in approximately 21 minutes would have to have an aerobic capacity ($\dot{V}O_2$ max) of 60 ml/kg·min^{-1}. This nomogram can be quite useful because it applies not only to male and female athletes but to the whole population, including the elderly and children, since the energy cost of running when referred to distance covered and to the body weight is essentially the same for all reasonably fit people. It cannot, however, be applied to those who are not fit enough to run continuously for at least 2 to 3 km, because the oxygen costs of walking and running are not the same.

Twelve-Minute Swimming Test

The twelve-minute swimming test involves swimming as far as possible in twelve minutes.

Table 14.9 provides normative fitness categories for various age groups and both genders based on the distance swum during the test (15).

Jackson and coworkers (29) reported that the twelve-minute swim test was a valid measure of swimming endurance. However, Conley and coworkers (13) examined the validity of the twelve-minute swim test and found a low correlation ($r = 0.40$) with $\dot{V}O_2$ max determined during tethered swimming. The authors concluded that "the twelve-minute swim has relatively low validity as a field test of peak aerobic power and that should not be considered an equally valid alternative to the twelve-minute run in young male recreational swimmers." Interestingly, the twelve-minute run was more highly correlated ($r = 0.74$ to 0.88) than the twelve-minute swim ($r = 0.38$ to 0.40) with $\dot{V}O_2$ max determined from both tethered swimming and treadmill running. These findings were likely a result of variability in swimming economy, since some of the subjects were more skilled swimmers than others.

Treadmill Walking Test

Ebbeling and others (22) developed an equation for estimating $\dot{V}O_2$ max from a single-stage submaximal treadmill walking test. The

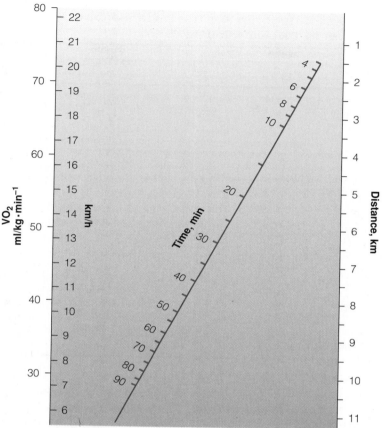

Figure 14.6   Nomogram to relate the maximal aerobic power of the subject $\dot{V}O_2$ max with the minimal time necessary in minutes when running at maximal speed to cover the distance in kilometers. On the $\dot{V}O_2$ max line the corresponding maintenance speed of running due to aerobic energy is also indicated. (From Margaria, R.; Aghemo, P.; and Limas, F. P., in *Journal of Applied Physiology* 38:351–52. © 1975 American Physiological Society. Reprinted by permission.)

equation uses treadmill speed, heart rate, treadmill speed times age, heart rate times age, and gender to predict $\dot{V}O_2$ max. The test protocol involves walking for four minutes at a constant pace of 2.0, 3.0, 4.0, or 4.5 mph and 5% grade. A brisk walking pace that elicits a heart rate between 50% and 70% of age predicted maximum (220-age) is selected during a four minute warm-up at 0% grade and used for the test.

$\dot{V}O_2$ max (ml/kg·min^{-1})
= 15.1 + 21.8 (treadmill speed) − 0.327 (heart rate) − 0.263 (treadmill speed × age) + 0.00504 (heart rate × age) + 5.98 (female = 0; males = 1)

The predicted $\dot{V}O_2$ max from the equation correlated highly (R = 0.96; SEE = 4.85 ml/kg·min^{-1}) with measured $\dot{V}O_2$ max from a graded treadmill test to exhaustion. The authors (22) concluded "the equation to estimate $\dot{V}O_2$ max (ml/kg·min^{-1}) from a single

Table 14.9	Fitness Categories for the Distance (Yards) Swum in Twelve Minutes					
Fitness Category	**Age (Years)**					
	13–19	**20–29**	**30–39**	**40–49**	**50–59**	**60+**
I. Very poor (men)	<500*	<400	<350	<300	<250	<250
(women)	<400	<300	<250	<200	<150	<150
II. Poor (men)	500–599	400–499	350–449	300–399	250–349	250–299
(women)	400–499	300–399	250–349	200–299	150–249	150–199
III. Fair (men)	600–699	500–599	450–549	400–499	350–449	300–399
(women)	500–599	400–499	350–449	300–399	250–349	200–299
IV. Good (men)	700–799	600–699	550–649	500–599	450–549	400–499
(women)	600–699	500–599	450–549	400–499	350–449	300–399
V. Excellent (men)	>800	>700	>650	>600	>550	>500
(women)	>700	>600	>550	>500	>450	>400

*<Means "less than"; >means "more than."
The Swimming test requires you to swim as far as you can in twelve minutes, using whatever stroke you prefer and resting as necessary, but trying for a maximum effort. The easiest way to take the test is in a pool with known dimensions, and it helps to have another person record the laps and time. Be sure to use a watch with a sweep second hand.
From *The Aerobics Way*, by Kenneth H. Cooper. Copyright © 1977 by Kenneth H. Cooper. Used by permission of Bantam Books, a division of Bantam Doubleday Dell Publishing Group, Inc.

stage at 5% grade during a submaximal treadmill test provides a valid and time-efficient method for assessing aerobic power in individuals who are at low risk, free from heart disease, and not taking medications known to affect heart rate."

Rockport Walking Test

Kline and others (31) developed and validated the Rockport Walking Test. The equation below was derived to predict $\dot{V}O_2$ max in adults between 30 and 69 years of age from the results of a timed one mile walk completed as fast as possible.

$\dot{V}O_2$ max (ml/kg·min⁻¹)
= 132.853 − 0.0769 (weight) − 0.3877 (age) − 3.2649 (one mile walk time) − 0.1565 (heart rate for the final 0.25 mile of the one mile walk) + 6.3150 (female = 0; male = 1)

Validation of the test was accomplished using a sample of 174 subjects (82 males and 92 females) and cross-validation was performed on 169 subjects (83 males and 86 females) who had completed treadmill tests to exhaustion for the determination of $\dot{V}O_2$ max. The validation and cross-validation analyses resulted in identical correlations of $r = 0.88$ and standard error of estimates of 5.0 and 4.4 ml/kg·min⁻¹, respectively.

The authors recommended the test for use based on the following:

1. The equation was developed and validated on relatively large samples.

2. The validation and cross-validation groups were homogeneous for all independent variables.

3. The generalized equation appears to be valid across a wide age range.

4. There were no differences between observed and estimated $\dot{V}O_2$ max or standard deviations in the cross-validation groups.

5. Accuracy of estimation represented by the standard error of estimate (SEE) was comparable to most of the other submaximal protocols reviewed.

6. As a field test, this protocol has the advantage of being simple, easy, and needing only a measured, flat one-mile surface, a stop watch, and the ability to measure pulse accurately.

7. The test requires only fast walking, which makes it useful in testing older or sedentary subjects.

Estimation of $\dot{V}O_2$ Peak without Exercise Testing

Jackson and colleagues (28) developed equations for estimating functional aerobic capacity ($\dot{V}O_2$ peak) without the necessity of performing an exercise test. Two equations were developed to predict $\dot{V}O_2$ peak using a physical activity rating scale (PA-R), age and gender with either percent body fat (% fat) or body mass index (BMI). $\dot{V}O_2$ peak was defined as the highest full-minute $\dot{V}O_2$ value during the final minute of a graded treadmill test continued to voluntary exhaustion with a respiratory quotient > 1.0.

Generalized (nongender specific) equation using % fat ($R = 0.812$; SEE $= 5.35$ ml/kg·min^{-1}):

$\dot{V}O_2$ peak (ml/kg·min^{-1}) $= 50.513 + 1.589$ (PA-R) $- 0.289$ (age) $- 0.552$ (% fat) $9 + 5.863$ (female $= 0$; male $= 1$)

Generalized equation using BMI ($R = 0.783$; SEE $= 5.70$ ml/kg·min^{-1}):

$\dot{V}O_2$ peak (ml/kg·min^{-1}) $= 56.363$ (PA-R) $- 0.381$ (age) $- 0.754$ (BMI) $+ 10.987$ (female $= 0$; male $= 1$)

Based on the results of cross-validation analyses, the authors concluded "The accuracy of the N-Ex (nonexercise) models exceeds the accuracy obtained with popular submaximal prediction models and is only slightly less accurate than the Rockport Walk Test." Generally the equations were found to be accurate for all subjects except the highly fit ($\dot{V}O_2$ peak ≥ 55 ml/kg·min^{-1}) and, therefore, should be considered acceptable alternatives to standard submaximal tests for estimating the aerobic endurance capacity of low to moderately fit males and females.

Measurement of Anaerobic Capabilities

Many sports involve short duration, high-intensity work. Track and field activities such as sprinting, high jumping, and long jumping as well as team sports such as basketball, football, and volleyball use energy produced primarily through anaerobic processes. Because direct measurement of anaerobic energy production is difficult, functional tests are often used as indirect indicators of anaerobic capabilities. Described below are two of the most widely accepted tests for estimating anaerobic capabilities: the Margaria Step-Running Anaerobic Power Test and the Wingate Anaerobic Test.

Margaria Step-Running Anaerobic Power Test

Margaria and coworkers (36) developed a test of maximal anaerobic power that involved measuring the time for subjects to run up stairs. The subject runs at top speed on a flat surface for approximately 2 meters prior to the stairs. The steps (each approximately 17.5 cm in height) are climbed two at a time as fast as possible. Photo-electric cells are used to determine the time between the fourth and sixth

Table 14.10	Mean Maximal Anaerobic Power for Various Groups		
Sample	**Reference**	**Gender**	**Mean Maximal Anaerobic Power (hp)**
1. Untrained college men	(45)	males	1.39
2. College women	(44)	females	0.98
3. Runners and walkers	(48)	males	1.30
4. Basketball players	(48)	males	1.58
5. Hockey players	(48)	males	1.52
6. Soccer players	(48)	males	1.65

jump (70 cm vertical distance). The subject's maximal anaerobic power is calculated as (30):

Maximal anaerobic power (horsepower)
= ((body weight (kg) × vertical distance (meters))/time (seconds))/76.07

Margaria and coworkers found that there was less than ± 2% variability for several repeated tests over a period of five weeks and Shaver (45) reported a test-retest reliability coefficient of $r = 0.94$ for the Margaria step-running anaerobic power test. In addition, maximal anaerobic power has been shown to correlate significantly with 100 ($r = -0.85$), 220 ($r = -0.83$), and 440 ($r = -0.79$) yard sprints (45) as well as to discriminate among athletic groups (48) and between athletes and untrained nonathletes (36). Thus, the Margaria step-running test is a reliable, valid, and sensitive method for estimating maximal anaerobic power. Table 14.10 provides mean data for untrained college-age men and women, runners and walkers, basketball players, hockey players, and soccer players.

Wingate Anaerobic Test

One of the most commonly used tests of anaerobic capabilities is the Wingate Anaerobic Test, which has been shown to be reliable, valid, and sensitive to changes in anaerobic fitness (8, 9). The name was derived from the Wingate Institute in Israel where the test was developed (9).

The Wingate Anaerobic Test involves leg pedaling or arm cranking at maximal speed for thirty seconds with the resistance determined based on the body weight of the subject (8). Originally, it was recommended that the resistance be calculated as 0.075 kp per kg of body weight for leg pedaling and 0.050 kp per kg of body weight for arm cranking (8). Recently, it has been recommended that the resistance for leg pedaling be calculated as 0.100 kp per kg of body weight (9). The question of the optimal resistance for subjects who vary in age, size, and athletic specialty, however, is still unresolved (9).

The number of pedal revolutions is monitored continuously throughout the test. At the beginning of the test, the subject pedals as fast as possible against an unloaded flywheel for approximately two to three seconds while the appropriate resistance is set.

The results of the Wingate Anaerobic Test can be used to derive three parameters: mean power, peak power, and fatigue index (8).

Mean power (formerly called anaerobic capacity (8)) is the total work performed during the thirty second workout expressed as a power output in watts ((total work in thirty seconds × 2)/6.12). Mean power reflects the ability of the limb muscles to sustain extremely high power outputs (9).

Peak power (formerly called maximal anaerobic power (8)) is the highest five second work output during the thirty second test expressed in watts ((highest work output in any five second period $\times$ 12)/6.12). Peak power reflects the ability of the limb muscles to produce high mechanical power in a short time (9).

Fatigue index is the percentage drop off in work output between the highest and lowest five second periods (9). For example, if the peak power (highest five second work output) was 300 watts, and the lowest five second work output (likely during the last five seconds of the thirty-second test) was 165 watts, then the fatigue index would be 45% ((((300–165)/300) x 100) = 45%). Bar-Or (9) has stated "Most research has focused on peak power and mean power. Much less is known on the relevance of the fatigue indices to anaerobic fitness."

Tables 14.11, 14.12, and 14.13 provide normative data (leg cranking ergometry) for mean power, peak power, and fatigue index derived from samples of 112 males and 74 females between eighteen and twenty-eight years of age (37). Mean power and peak power are expressed in watts, watts per kilogram of body weight ($W \cdot kgBW^{-1}$), and watts per kilogram of lean body mass ($W \cdot kgLBM^{-1}$).

New Concepts in Measuring Physical Fitness

At this point it would be helpful to consider that our most commonly accepted approach to the measurement of PWC, that is, the measurement of maximal O_2 consumption itself, has some serious problems. Although this measure, $\dot{V}O_2$ max, has come to be the criterion against which all other PWC test procedures are evaluated, it can be criticized on at least four grounds: 1) the subject must be taken to a state of exhaustion, 2) the results of the test vary considerably with test method and protocol, 3) the results are couched in chemical terms when the physical educator or coach is working with the physical parameters of work and power, and 4) the test requires an expensive laboratory and considerable testing time.

Furthermore, for purposes of health counseling, exercise prescription, and in athletics where endurance is a factor, we are really more interested in the level of performance that can be maintained without fatigue, rather than the aerobic power ($\dot{V}O_2$ max) available at the point of exhaustion. It has been suggested that the anaerobic threshold (now called lactate or ventilatory threshold—chap. 12) provides such a measurement, but this is still being debated on both conceptual and empirical bases. For these reasons deVries and his coworkers have developed a simple test requiring nothing more than a cycle ergometer and a stop watch, which provides estimates of both the lactate threshold and the aerobic power ($\dot{V}O_2$ max) from two or three short workouts of one to four minutes duration each (7,19,38).

The Critical Power Test

Two or more workouts to the onset of fatigue are performed at different power loads (27). When the total work (for example, watts $\times$ minutes on a cycle ergometer for each of two or more loads) is plotted against time before fatigue (fig. 14.7), a straight line is generated ($W_{max} = a + bT_{max}$). It is postulated on the basis of the available evidence (12, 19) that the intercept (a) represents the subject's energy reserve, and the slope (b) represents the ability of the subject's cardiovascular-respiratory systems to replenish the muscles' energy. If a line with slope (b) is drawn through the origin so that the energy reserve factor drops out of the equation, then all work rates below the line can be accomplished without fatigue and loads above the line will surpass the threshold of fatigue or critical power. Therefore the test provides the critical power

Table 14.11   Percentile Norms and Descriptive Statistics for Mean Power for the Wingate Anaerobic Test Males (N = 60) and Females (N = 69)

Percentile Rank	Watts		$W \cdot kgBW^{-1}$		$W \cdot kgLBM^{-1}$	
	Male	Female	Male	Female	Male	Female
95	676.6	483.0	8.63	7.52	9.30	9.43
90	661.8	469.9	8.24	7.31	9.03	9.01
85	630.5	437.0	8.09	7.08	8.88	8.88
80	617.9	419.4	8.01	6.95	8.80	8.76
75	604.3	413.5	7.96	6.93	8.70	8.68
70	600.0	409.7	7.91	6.77	8.63	8.52
65	591.7	402.2	7.70	6.65	8.50	8.32
60	576.8	391.4	7.59	6.59	8.44	8.18
55	574.5	386.0	7.46	6.51	8.24	8.13
50	564.6	381.1	7.44	6.39	8.21	7.93
45	552.8	376.9	7.26	6.20	8.14	7.86
40	547.6	366.9	7.14	6.15	8.04	7.70
35	534.6	360.5	7.08	6.13	7.95	7.57
30	529.7	353.2	7.00	6.03	7.80	7.46
25	520.6	346.8	6.79	5.94	7.64	7.32
20	496.1	336.5	6.59	5.71	7.46	7.11
15	484.6	320.3	6.39	5.56	7.28	7.03
10	470.9	306.1	5.98	5.25	6.83	6.83
5	453.2	286.5	5.56	5.07	6.49	6.70
M	562.7	380.8	7.28	6.35	8.11	7.96
SD	66.5	56.4	.88	.73	.82	.88
Minimum	441.3	235.4	4.63	4.53	5.72	5.12
Maximum	711.0	528.6	9.07	8.11	9.66	9.66

This table is reprinted with permission from *Research Quarterly for Exercise and Sport*, vol. 60, no. 2 (June 1989). *The Research Quarterly for Exercise and Sport* is a publication of the American Alliance for Health, Physical Education, Recreation and Dance, 1900 Association Drive, Reston, VA 22091.

Table 14.12   Percentile Norms and Descriptive Statistics
for Peak Power of the Wingate Anaerobic Test
Males (N = 62) and Females (N = 68)

Percentile Rank	Watts		$W \cdot kgBW^{-1}$		$W \cdot kgLBM^{-1}$	
	Male	Female	Male	Female	Male	Female
95	866.9	602.1	11.08	9.32	12.26	11.87
90	821.8	560.0	10.89	9.02	11.96	11.47
85	807.1	529.6	10.59	8.92	11.67	11.28
80	776.7	526.6	10.39	8.83	11.47	10.79
75	767.9	517.8	10.39	8.63	11.38	10.69
70	757.1	505.0	10.20	8.53	11.28	10.39
65	744.3	493.3	10.00	8.34	11.08	10.30
60	720.8	479.5	9.80	8.14	10.79	10.10
55	706.1	463.9	9.51	7.85	10.30	9.90
50	689.4	449.1	9.22	7.65	10.20	9.61
45	677.6	447.2	9.02	7.16	10.10	9.41
40	670.8	432.5	8.92	6.96	10.00	8.92
35	661.9	417.8	8.63	6.96	9.90	8.83
30	656.1	399.1	8.53	6.86	9.51	8.73
25	646.3	396.2	8.34	6.77	9.32	8.43
20	617.8	375.6	8.24	6.57	9.12	8.34
15	594.3	361.9	7.45	6.37	8.53	8.04
10	569.8	353.0	7.06	5.98	8.04	7.75
5	530.5	329.5	6.57	5.69	7.45	6.86
M	699.5	454.5	9.18	7.61	10.18	9.54
SD	94.7	81.3	1.43	1.24	1.46	1.51
Minimum	500.1	239.3	5.31	4.58	6.55	5.20
Maximum	926.7	622.7	11.90	10.64	12.96	12.90

This table is reprinted with permission from *Research Quarterly for Exercise and Sport*, vol. 60, no. 2 (June 1989). *The Research Quarterly for Exercise and Sport* is a publication of the American Alliance for Health, Physical Education, Recreation and Dance, 1900 Association Drive, Reston, VA 22091.

Table 14.13	Percentile Norms and Descriptive Statistics for Fatigue Index	

| Percentile Rank | Fatigue Index[a] | |
	Male	Female
95	55.01	48.05
90	51.69	47.33
85	47.40	44.25
80	46.67	43.57
75	44.98	42.19
70	43.51	40.33
65	41.93	39.04
60	39.92	38.21
55	39.48	36.69
50	38.39	35.15
45	36.77	34.36
40	35.04	33.70
35	34.07	30.70
30	31.09	28.74
25	30.23	28.11
20	29.55	26.45
15	26.86	25.00
10	23.18	25.00
5	20.77	19.65
M	37.67	35.05
SD	9.89	8.32
Minimum	14.71	17.86
Maximum	57.51	48.94

Note. N = Males 52, Females 50
[a]Fatigue index as a percent change calculated as peak power minus minimum power, divided by peak power, and multiplied by 100.
This table is reprinted with permission from *Research Quarterly for Exercise and Sport*, vol. 60, no. 2 (June 1989). *The Research Quarterly for Exercise and Sport* is a publication of the American Alliance for Health, Physical Education, Recreation and Dance, 1900 Association Drive, Reston, VA 22091.

(b) below which any power output can be accomplished without the occurrence of fatigue, which is defined as a slowing of pedal rpm from the 70 required to below 60 rpm.

It has been shown (19, 38) that the critical power so measured correlates well with the anaerobic threshold as calculated by the method of Davis and associates ($r = 0.93$) (fig. 12.11). That it relates well to the onset of fatigue measured objectively by EMG fatigue curves has been demonstrated by the finding of $r = 0.87$ (19). Recent studies, however, have reported that the critical power test overestimated the power output that can be maintained for one hour by approximately 17% (26) and that the critical power was 28% greater than the power output corresponding to OBLA (onset of blood lactate accumulation = 4.0 mMol blood lactate level) (23).

Further work with respect to the critical power concept is needed to better define the potential uses for exercise prescription and to develop training regimens for athletes as well as to corroborate the data from the authors' laboratories. The simplicity of the procedure and the need for relatively inexpensive equipment make it a very attractive test for physical education and athletics.

Physical Working Capacity at the Fatigue Threshold (PWC$_{FT}$) from Supramaximal Power Outputs

In 1982, deVries and others (19) proposed an electromyographic (EMG) technique for identifying the power output associated with the onset of muscular fatigue called the physical working capacity at the fatigue threshold (PWC$_{FT}$) test. The test was based on the concept that during a fatiguing workbout on a cycle ergometer there is a linear rise in the integrated electromyogram (IEMG) from the vastus lateralis that reflects an increase in the number of muscle fibers recruited and the frequency of impulses to those fibers. Theoretically, any power output below the fatigue

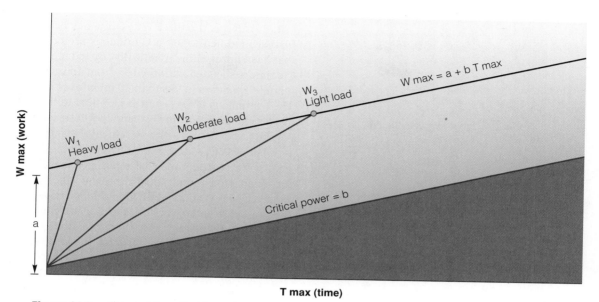

Figure 14.7   The graphic method for estimating the critical power. Points W_1, W_2, and W_3 represent the time to fatigue (pedal rpm drops from 70 to below 60) for three different workouts (power loadings). The y intercept (a) represents the subject's energy reservoir, while the slope of the line (b) represents the energy replacement rate. Theoretically any work rate below the critical power (shaded area) can be performed indefinitely. (From deVries, H. A.; Moritani, T.; Nagata, A.; and Magnussen, K. *Ergonomics* 25:783–91, 1982.)

threshold (PWC_{FT}) can be maintained for an extended period of time without an increase in the electrical activity (IEMG) of the thigh muscles.

The original PWC_{FT} test used three or four supramaximal workouts at power outputs that ranged from 150 to 400 watts. During each exhaustive ride, the electrical activity (IEMG) from the vastus lateralis was monitored. As shown in figure 14.8, the IEMG values (microvolts) were plotted as a function of time, and linear relationships that ranged from $r^2 = 0.66$ to 0.99 were found. The power output for each workout was then plotted as a function of the slope coefficients for each IEMG versus time relationship (fig. 14.8). Theoretically, the y-intercept of the power output versus slope coefficient plot represents the maximal power output (PWC_{FT}) that can be maintained with no increase in the electrical activity of the vastus lateralis (slope = 0). The PWC_{FT} determined in this manner was

found to be highly correlated with anaerobic threshold ($r = 0.903$) and critical power ($r = 0.869$) (19).

PWC_{FT} from Submaximal Power Outputs

The original PWC_{FT} test used supramaximal power outputs and therefore was most appropriate for young healthy subjects. To extend the usefulness of the PWC_{FT} test to low fit and elderly subjects, deVries and coworkers (20) modified the PWC_{FT} technique to use submaximal power outputs. The modified procedure involved a series of discontinuous two minute workouts beginning at approximately 70 watts (fig. 14.9). Subsequent workouts were performed at 70 watt increments separated by a sufficient rest interval to allow the subject's heart rate to return to within 10 beats per minute of the pre-exercise level. During each workout, the electrical activity from the

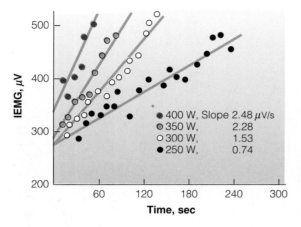

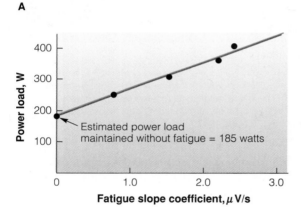

A

B

Figure 14.8   Diagram of the method used to determine PWC$_{FT}$ from supramaximal power outputs. (From deVries, H. A. et al. *Ergonomics* 25:783–91, 1982. Reprinted by permission.)

vastus lateralis was monitored and the IEMG values for six ten-second integrals (expressed in microvolts) were plotted over time to determine the rate of rise (fig. 14.9). The PWC$_{FT}$ was defined as the highest power output that resulted in a nonsignificant increase in IEMG over time. The PWC$_{FT}$ derived from submaximal power outputs has been shown to be valid, reliable (20), and sensitive to fitness changes as a result of training (16). In addition, it has been used to examine the physiological mechanisms underlying neuromuscular fatigue

(24, 25). Recently, the PWC$_{FT}$ test has been further modified to use a continuous protocol that has improved the practicality by reducing the time associated with the test from approximately 1.5 hours to less than 30 minutes (17). The continuous PWC$_{FT}$ test is identical to the discontinuous procedure except there are no rest intervals between the incremental stages.

The PWC$_{FT}$ determined from submaximal power outputs may be especially useful for monitoring the physical fitness of elderly subjects. Many elderly individuals do not have the muscular endurance to fully tax the cardiorespiratory system and therefore do not provide valid data during tests for the determination of maximal oxygen uptake. Furthermore, the appropriateness of $\dot{V}O_2$ max as a criterion for functional physical fitness in older adults is questionable since most elderly individuals rarely perform maximal activity. It is likely that a more appropriate criterion is the level of submaximal work that can be maintained for an extended period of time as measured by the PWC$_{FT}$ test.

Motor Fitness Tests

Many excellent tests of motor fitness have been devised. The elements of motor fitness are so many, however, and some are so difficult to define, that each motor performance test battery must be considered a compromise between the ideal of measuring all identifiable elements and the practical need to choose a number of representative elements that will allow the measuring to be done in reasonable amounts of time. Obviously, testing programs that intrude unnecessarily on instructional time cannot be tolerated.

For this reason, only examples of some of the best compromises will be offered here. For illustrative purposes, an example of the approach used by the armed forces during World War II and one example of test batteries for school age children will be offered.

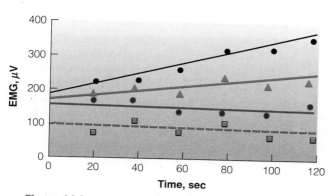
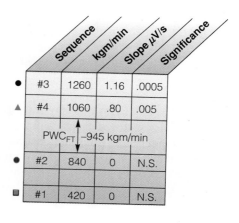

	Sequence	kgm/min	Slope μV/s	Significance
●	#3	1260	1.16	.0005
▲	#4	1060	.80	.005
	PWC$_{FT}$ –945 kgm/min			
●	#2	840	0	N.S.
▫	#1	420	0	N.S.

Figure 14.9   Diagram of the method used to determine PWC$_{FT}$ from submaximal power outputs. (From deVries, H. A. et al. *Ergonomics* 30:1195–1204, 1987. Reprinted by permission.)

Army/Air Force Physical Fitness Test

The items for the Army/Air Force physical fitness test were selected to evaluate the motor fitness elements of muscle strength and endurance, cardiorespiratory endurance, speed, coordination, and power. The test items selected were sit-ups, pull-ups, and a 300-yard shuttle run (five lengths of 60 yards each). It was deVries's experience during World War II that several hundred men could be tested per hour by four experienced physical training instructors. This test is one of the best for handling very large groups of adults.

AAHPER Youth Fitness Test Battery

After the much publicized results of the Kraus-Weber test (32) and other research findings pointed out the need for a national concern about fitness, a committee of members of the national research council of the American Association for Health, Physical Education, and Recreation was set up under the direction of Paul A. Hunsicker. As a result of this group's work on the Youth Fitness Project, the Youth Fitness Test was developed, designed for boys

and girls from the fifth through the twelfth grade. National norms are available for these age groups and also for college men and women and young adults from eighteen to thirty (1). This test battery consists of the following items (all for grades five through twelve).

1. Pull-up for boys; modified pull-up for girls
2. Sit-up for boys and girls
3. Shuttle run for boys and girls
4. Standing broad jump for boys and girls
5. Fifty-yard dash for boys and girls
6. Softball throw for distance for boys and girls
7. 600-yard run and walk for boys and girls

Additional tests in aquatics are recommended where facilities permit.

Interestingly, Olree and associates (40) showed that three items correlated 0.925 with the results of the entire test. Thus much time can be saved by using only pull-ups, sit-ups, and the fifty-yard run, with a loss in accuracy of less than 15%.

The New AAHPERD Health-Related Physical Fitness Test

The philosophy regarding physical fitness for our youth is undergoing profound change. It has been pointed out that motor fitness as exemplified by the AAHPER Youth Fitness Test Battery described above is important in evaluating the qualities needed in athletics, but "health related physical fitness" is for everyone (10, 41, 42). Consequently the new Health Related Physical Fitness Test consists of the following test items: 1) the nine-minute run for distance or the one mile run for time, 2) the sum of the triceps and subscapular skinfolds, 3) the number of bent-knee sit-ups accomplished in one minute, and 4) the sit-and-reach test.

It is obvious that these test elements evaluate the factors of cardiorespiratory endurance, body composition, abdominal wall strength, and endurance and flexibility, all of which are important to the maintenance of good health.

Physical Fitness Evaluation as a Function of Age Groups

It is obvious that the various criteria of physical fitness do not have equal importance for all age groups, and several criteria that seem likely to be very important for middle-age and elderly groups have not yet been mentioned. Because very little experimental work has been done to identify the most important elements of physical fitness for the older age groups, much of what follows is based on the authors' survey of medical and physical education opinion.

There seems little doubt that the motor fitness elements discussed above are important in elementary and secondary school age children. PWC is at least as important for secondary school age groups as it is for elementary groups and possibly somewhat less important for those at the elementary level since elementary school age children participate in vigorous physical activity by nature. It would, however, be difficult to justify many of the elements of motor fitness as necessary or essential for middle-age and elderly populations. For example, it is unlikely that a businessperson needs high levels of speed, strength, or agility.

For the older age brackets a much better case can be made for the importance of 1) normal body weight, 2) cardiovascular fitness, 3) respiratory fitness, 4) neuromuscular relaxation, and 5) flexibility. The value of the first four elements is probably self-evident. The last, flexibility, becomes more important as aging proceeds because connective tissues tend to lose their elasticity with age, and this in turn seems to be related to many of the aches and pains of old age. Considerable evidence exists that maintaining range of motion exerts a beneficial effect in this regard. Table 14.14 lists the factors of greatest importance in physical fitness by age groups.

Summary

1. Physical fitness can be conceptualized in two ways: (a) the *motor fitness* concept in which the elements of performance are measured, and (b) the *physical working capacity* (PWC) concept in which the capacity for O_2 transport is evaluated.

2. The following elements constitute motor fitness: strength, speed, agility, endurance, power, coordination, balance, flexibility, and body control.

3. PWC is determined by the following physiological components: cardiovascular function, respiratory function, muscular efficiency, strength,

| Table 14.14 | Suggested Values of the Components of Physical Fitness by Age Groups (in Order of Importance) | | | |

Prepuberty	Adolescence	Young Adult	Older Adult
Motor fitness	Motor fitness	PWC	PWC
PWC	PWC	Body composition	Body composition
	Body composition	Relaxation	Flexibility
		Flexibility	Relaxation

muscular endurance, and maintenance of proper body weight.

4. A screening medical examination is necessary prior to testing $\dot{V}O_2$ max for (a) anyone over thirty-five, (b) anyone who has questions about personal health status or who develops symptoms during testing, or (c) anyone who has not had a medical exam in two years.

5. All subjects for $\dot{V}O_2$ max testing must have the testing procedures carefully explained to them, and after all questions are answered they must sign an informed consent form.

6. Physical education personnel, trained as exercise technicians, may conduct maximal tests on healthy school age subjects and adults under thirty-five who have no known primary CHD risk factors.

7. $\dot{V}O_2$ max testing can be accomplished on a cycle ergometer, a treadmill, or a step bench. Using any of these three exercise modalities, the protocol may be: (a) intermittent incremental loading, (b) continuous step-incremental loading, or (c) continuously incremented loading (ramp loading).

8. Environmental conditions, such as time of day, diet, and prior activity, must all be carefully controlled if either intraindividual or interindividual comparisons are to be made.

9. The primary physiological parameters to be measured and recorded are (a) percent of O_2 in expired gas; (b) percent of CO_2 in expired gas; (c) minute ventilation; (d) heart rate; (e) blood pressure; and (f) electrical activity of the heart as shown on the electrocardiogram.

10. From the primary physiological parameters one can calculate (a) respiratory exchange ratio (R); (b) oxygen pulse; (c) heart rate-blood pressure product; (d) ventilation equivalent for O_2; and (e) the anaerobic threshold (AT).

11. PWC is best evaluated by *measuring* maximum O_2 consumption. PWC can also be *estimated* from submaximal tests if errors of measurement ranging from 10% to 15% are acceptable as a trade-off for the savings of time and effort by both subject and investigator.

12. The relative importance of the elements of physical fitness changes with increasing age. Motor fitness, which is important to children, is no longer of great importance to adults. For middle-age and older adults, maintaining high levels of PWC, appropriate body weight, good flexibility, and a relaxed musculature are much more important, since these factors contribute to good health.

References

1. American Association for Health, Physical Education and Recreation. *Youth Fitness Test Manual.* Washington, D.C.: The Association, 1958.

2. American College of Sports Medicine. *Guidelines for Graded Exercise Testing and Exercise Prescription.* Philadelphia: Lea & Febiger, 1975.

3. Andersen, K. L., Shephard, R. J., Denolin, H., Varnauskas, E., and Masironi, R. *Fundamentals of exercise testing.* Geneva: World Health Organization, 1971.

4. Astrand, I. Aerobic work capacity in men and women with special reference to age. *Acta Physiol. Scand.* 49 (suppl. 169), 1960.

5. Astrand, P. O., and Ryhming, I. A nomogram for calculation of aerobic capacity (physical fitness) from pulse rate during submaximal work. *J. Appl. Physiol.* 7:218–21, 1954.

6. Bailey, D. A., Shephard, R. J., and Mirwald, R. L. Validation of a self-administered home test of cardio-respiratory fitness. *Can. J. Appl. Sports Sci.* 1:67–78, 1976.

7. Barnes, L. Measuring anaerobic threshold simplified. *Physician and Sportsmed.* 8 (July):15–16, 1980.

8. Bar-Or, O. A new anaerobic test-characteristics and applications. Presented at the 21st World Congress in Sports Medicine, Brasilia, 1978.

9. Bar-Or, O. The Wingate Anaerobic Test: An update on methodology, reliability and validity. *Sportsmed.* 4:381–94, 1987.

10. Blair, S. N., Falls, H. B., and Pate, R. R. A new physical fitness test. *Physician and Sportsmed.* 11 (April):87–95, 1983.

11. Buono, J. M., Roby, J. J., Micale, F. G., Sallis, J. F., and Shepard, W. E. Validity and reliability of predicting maximum oxygen uptake via field tests in children and adolescents. *Ped. Exer. Sci.* 3:250–55, 1991.

12. Cherchi, A. A. A synthetic triangular exercise test. *Ergometry in Cardiology,* eds. H. Denolin, K. Konig, R. Messin, and S. Degre, pp. 65–86. Mannheim, Germany: Boehringer Mannheim, 1968.

13. Conley, D. S., Cureton, K. J., Dengel, D. R., and Weyand, P. G. Validation of the 12-minute swim as a field test of peak aerobic power in young men. *Med. Sci. Sports Exerc.* 23:766–73, 1991.

14. Cooper, K. H. A means of assessing maximal O_2 intake. *J.A.M.A.* 203:201–4, 1968.

15. Cooper, K. H. *The Aerobics Way.* Toronto: Bantam Books, 1977.

16. deVries, H. A., Brodowicz, G. R., Robertson, L. D., Svoboda, M. D., Schendel, J. S., Tichy, A. M., and Tichy, M. W. Estimating physical working capacity and training changes in the elderly at the fatigue threshold (PWC_{FT}). *Ergonomics* 32:967–77, 1989.

17. deVries, H. A., Housh, T. J., Johnson, G. O., Evans, S. A., Tharp, G. D., Housh, D. J., and Hughes, R. J. Factors affecting the measurement of physical working capacity at the fatigue threshold. *Ergonomics* 33:25–33, 1990.

18. deVries, H. A., and Klafs, C. E. Prediction of maximal O_2 intake from submaximal tests. *J. Sports Med. Phys. Fitness* 5:207–14, 1965.

19. deVries, H. A., Moritani, T., Nagata, A., and Magnussen, K. The relationship between critical power and neuromuscular fatigue as estimated from electromyographic data. *Ergonomics* 25:783–91, 1982.

20. deVries, H. A., Tichy, M. W., Housh, T. J., Smyth, K. D., Tichy, A. M., and Housh, D. J. A method for estimating physical working capacity at the fatigue threshold (PWC$_{FT}$). *Ergonomics* 30:1195–1204, 1987.

21. Doolittle, T. L., and Bigbee, R. The twelve-minute run-walk: a test of cardiorespiratory fitness of adolescent boys. *Res. Q.* 39:491–95, 1968.

22. Ebbeling, C. B., Ward, A., Puleo, E. M., Widrick, J., and Rippe, J. M. Development of a single-stage submaximal treadmill walking test. *Med. Sci. Sports Exerc.* 23:966–73, 1991.

23. Housh, T. J., deVries, H. A., Housh, D. J., Tichy, M. W., Smyth, K. D., and Tichy, A. M. The relationship between critical power and the onset of blood lactate accumulation. *J. Sports Med.* 31:31–36, 1991.

24. Housh, T. J., deVries, H. A., Johnson, G. O., Evans, S. A., and McDowell, S. L. The effect of ammonium chloride and sodium bicarbonate ingestion on the physical working capacity at the fatigue threshold. *Eur. J. Appl. Physiol.* 62:189–92, 1991.

25. Housh, T. J., deVries, H. A., Johnson, G. O., Evans, S. A., Tharp, G. D., Housh, D. J., and Hughes, R. J. The effect of glycogen depletion and supercompensation on the physical working capacity at the fatigue threshold (PWC$_{FT}$). *Eur. J. Appl. Physiol.* 60:391–94, 1990.

26. Housh, D. J., Housh, T. J., and Bauge, S. M. The accuracy of the critical power test for predicting time to exhaustion during cycle ergometry. *Ergonomics* 32:997–1004, 1989.

27. Housh, D. J., Housh, T. J., and Bauge, S. M. A methodological consideration for the determination of critical power and anaerobic work capacity. *Res. Quart. Exerc. Sport* 61:406–9, 1990.

28. Jackson, A. S., Blair, S. N., Mahar, M. T., Weir, L. T., Ross, R. M., and Stuteville, J. E. Prediction of functional aerobic capacity without exercise testing. *Med. Sci. Sports Exerc.* 22:863–70, 1990.

29. Jackson, A., Jackson, A. S., and Frankiewicz, R. G. The construct and concurrent validity of a 12-minute crawl stroke swim as a field test of swimming endurance. *Res. Quart.* 50:641–48, 1979.

30. Johnson, B. L., and Nelson, J. K. The measurement of power. *Practical Measurements for Evaluation in Physical Education,* 4th ed., Chap. 12. Edina, MN: Burgess Publishing, 1986.

31. Kline, G. M., Porcari, J. P., Hintermeister, R., Freedson, P. S., Ward, L.A., McCarron, R. F., Ross, J., and Rippe, J. M. Estimation of $\dot{V}O_2$ max from a one-mile track walk, gender, age, and body weight. *Med. Sci. Sports Exerc.* 19:253–59, 1987.

32. Kraus, H., and Hirschland, R. P. Minimum muscular fitness in schoolchildren. *Res. Q.* 25:178–88, 1954.

33. Luft, U. C., Cardus, D., Lim, T. P. K., Howarth, J. L., and Anderson, E. C. Physical performance in relation to body size and composition. *Ann. N.Y. Acad. Sci.* 110:795–808, 1963.

34. Maksud, M. G., and Coutts, K. D. Application of the Cooper twelve-minute run-walk test to young males. *Res. Q.* 42:54–59, 1971.

35. Margaria, R., Aghemo, P., and Limas, F. P. A simple relation between performance in running and maximal aerobic power. *J. Appl. Physiol.* 38:351–52, 1975.

36. Margaria, R., Aghemo, P., and Rovelli, E. Measurement of muscular power (anaerobic) in man. *J. Appl. Physiol.* 21:1661–64, 1966.

37. Maud, P. J., and Schultz, B. B. Norms for the Wingate Anaerobic Test with comparison to another similar test. *Res. Quart. Exerc. Sport* 60:144–51, 1989.

38. Moritani, T., Nagata, A., deVries, H. A., and Muro, M. Critical power as a measure of physical work capacity and anaerobic threshold. *Ergonomics* 24:339–50, 1981.

39. Moritani, T., Tanaka, H., Yoshida, T., Ishii, C., Yoshida, T., and Shindo, M. Relationship between myoelectric signals and blood lactate during incremental forearm exercise. *Am. J. Phys. Med.* 63:122–32, 1984.

40. Olree, H., Stevens, C., Nelson, T., Agnerik, G., and Clark, R. T. Evaluation of the AAHPER youth fitness test. *J. Sports Med. Phys. Fitness* 5:67–71, 1965.

41. Pate, R. R. A new definition of youth fitness test. *Physician and Sportsmed.* 11 (April):77–83, 1983.

42. Plowman, S. Health related physical fitness. *J.O.P.E.R.* Jan. 1981, p. 26.

43. Purvis, J. W., and Morgan, J. P. Influence of repeated maximal testing on anxiety and work capacity in college women. *Res. Q.* 49:512–19, 1978.

44. Sawka, M. N., Tahamont, M. V., Fitzgerald, P. I., Miles, and Knowlton, R. G. Alactic capacity and power. *Eur. J. Appl. Physiol.* 45:109–16, 1980.

45. Shaver, L. G. Maximal aerobic power and anaerobic work capacity prediction from various running performances of untrained college men. *J. Sports Med. Phys. Fitness* 15:147–50, 1975.

46. Terry, J. W., Tolson, H., Johnson, D. J., and Jessup, G. T. A workload selection procedure for the Astrand-Ryhming test. *J. Sports Med. Phys. Fitness* 17:361–66, 1977.

47. Von Dobeln, W., Astrand, I., and Bergstrom, A. An analysis of age and other factors related to maximal oxygen uptake. *J. Appl. Physiol.* 22:934–38, 1967.

48. Withers, R. T., Roberts, R. G. D., and Davies, G. J. The maximum aerobic power, anaerobic power and body composition of South Australian male representatives in athletics, basketball, field hockey and soccer. *J. Sports Med.* 17:391–400, 1977.

49. Wright, G. R., Sidney, K., and Shephard, R. J. Variance of direct and indirect measurements of aerobic power. *J. Sports Med. Phys. Fitness* 18:33–42, 1978.

50. Zuti, W. B., and Corbin, C. B. Physical fitness norms for college freshmen. *Res. Q.* 48:499–503, 1977.

15

Physical Conditioning for Health and Fitness (Prescription of Exercise)

Principles Involved in Scientific Prescription of Exercise

Need for Medical Evaluation and Exercise Testing Prior to Participation in Endurance Exercise
- *Apparently Healthy Individuals*
- *Individuals at Higher Risk*
- *Individuals with Disease*
- *Contraindications to Exercise Testing*
- *Physiological Pretest and Monitoring of Progress*

Training Curves

Interval Training versus Continuous Exercise

Recommendations of the American College of Sports Medicine (ACSM) for Developing Cardiorespiratory Fitness in Healthy Adults

Mode of Exercise (ACSM Recommendation: Aerobic in Nature)

Intensity of Exercise
- *Dose or Response*
- *Target Oxygen Consumption Rate Range (ACSM Recommendation: 50% to 85% $\dot{V}O_2$ max)*
- *Target Heart Rate Range (ACSM Recommendation: 60% to 90% of Maximum HR or 50% to 85% of HRR)*
- *Target Rating of Perceived Exertion Range (ACSM Recommendation: 12 to 15, "Somewhat Hard" to "Hard")*
- *Target Range for Metabolic Equivalents (METs) (ACSM Recommendation: 60% to 70% of Maximal METs)*

Duration of Exercise (ACSM Recommendation: Twenty to Sixty Minutes of Continuous Aerobic Exercise)

Frequency of Exercise (ACSM Recommendation: Three to Five Days Per Week)

Exercise Prescription
- *Daily Workout Plan*
- *Elements of the Ex Rx*

Effect of Gender and Age on Training Adaptations

Specificity of Training

Potential Physiological Changes Resulting from Training

Training as a Stressor

In this chapter we will deal with how to use exercise to improve health and fitness. In the light of the evidence cited in chapter 13 and that to come in chapter 16, it seems entirely likely that the physical education profession will be called upon to expand its interests beyond that of teaching skills and games to children and adolescents to that of service to the community at large. As advisors in the use of exercise to improve health and fitness, we can serve not only schoolchildren but also young, middle-age, and elderly adults, and females as well as males.

In a letter from the President's Council on Physical Fitness and Sports (PCPFS) to physical fitness leaders in the United States (10), the following health and fitness problems were pointed out:

1. Fifty million of the 110 million adults in the United States never engage in physical activity for exercise.

2. Old, poor, and less-educated Americans frequently do not understand the contributions that exercise can make to health, performance, and the quality of life.

3. Millions of Americans are willing victims of "get-fit-quick" schemes that promise fitness in a few minutes a day (thirty minutes a week) without sweat or strain.

4. The nation has a debit of well over 100,000 tons of fat.

5. The American Medical Association estimates that one-third of all American children are overweight.

6. The performances of the youth on the National Physical Fitness Tests have not improved since 1965, and in the opinion of the Council the fitness levels at that time were very low!

More recent information (43, 44) from the National Children and Youth Fitness Study (NCYFS) further emphasizes the lack of improvement in the health related physical fitness of American children between the early 1960s and mid 1980s. In fact, Ross and Gilbert (43) stated "The NCYFS shows that American young people have become fatter since the 1960s."

This information from the PCPFS and NCYFS shows the great need for greater motivational efforts and better instruction on the part of the physical education profession in helping people apply the basics of exercise physiology to the improvement of health and fitness.

While we do not yet understand all there is to know about the prescription of exercise, we do have considerable information based on laboratory studies that can help us, as the professionals in this field, guide the layperson to better use of exercise as a replacement for the physical work that has disappeared in our modern life-style. That at least some of the lay public recognizes the need for activity is borne out by the tremendous growth in popularity of jogging and such sports as tennis and racquetball.

Unfortunately, it is still common for a physician to prescribe to a patient, "You must get some exercise." This, of course, is roughly analogous to prescribing, "You must get some drugs," without specifying which pharmaceutical and how much and how often to take it. Just as the medicine prescribed for a headache is quite different from that for diabetes, the exercise prescribed for developing maximal strength and muscle bulk is quite different from that needed for optimal cardiorespiratory endurance. Thus there is exercise, and there is exercise, just as there is medicine, and medicine. With exercise, there are also the questions, How much is enough? How much is too much? How much is optimal? How often? For how long?

Principles Involved in Scientific Prescription of Exercise

The following aspects of a proposed exercise program must be considered and where possible defined on the basis of scientifically derived data.

1. *Objective of the exercise program.*
   There is good evidence that we can bring about very desirable adaptations in human functional capacities and health related parameters such as (a) muscular strength, (b) muscular endurance, (c) cardiorespiratory endurance, (d) muscular efficiency, (e) speed of movement, and (f) flexibility. However, each of these goals requires a different and specific exercise program.

2. *Mode of exercise.* For strength gain one would prescribe progressive resistance exercise (PRE), whereas for enhancement of cardiorespiratory function one would prescribe one of many endurance-type exercise programs such as jogging.

3. *Intensity of exercise.* Here we are concerned with the dose-response relationship, or the level of exercise work load (power output) to the amount of adaptation brought about in the human organism.

4. *Duration of exercise.* How long must the exercise be continued to bring about the desired result? Is more always better, or is there a practical limit or desirable amount that optimizes the gain for time spent?

5. *Frequency of exercise.* How many times a week should one work out for best training effect?

6. *Intensity threshold for training effect.* Is there some minimal value of exercise training intensity below which no training adaptations occur?

7. *Rate of training adaptation as a function of pretraining fitness level.* Do all individuals progress at the same rate in a conditioning program, or is progress dictated by the level of fitness at entry into the program?

Our discussion in this chapter will be limited to the development of cardiorespiratory fitness since the other elements of human performance are treated in great detail in part 3 of this text, which is devoted to the training and conditioning of athletes. Furthermore we can consider cardiorespiratory fitness of three-fold importance to health and fitness because the type of exercise program (endurance exercise) used for its development also contributes significantly to weight control and to relief from neuromuscular tension (relaxation). Thus we achieve three important health benefits for the price of one workout. This is not to deny the importance of muscular strength, muscular endurance, or flexibility in the overall health and fitness picture. It is merely to stress the overriding importance of cardiorespiratory fitness to our lifelong good health.

Need for Medical Evaluation and Exercise Testing Prior to Participation in Endurance Exercise

The American College of Sports Medicine (ACSM) has provided guidelines for exercise testing and prescription (1). A careful examination of an individual's current health as well as health and exercise history should precede exercise testing and the initiation of an exercise program. This examination serves to:

1. Assure the safety of exercise testing and subsequent exercise program.

2. Decide on the appropriate type of exercise test.

3. Identify those in need of more comprehensive medical evaluation.

4. Prescribe the appropriate type of exercise program following the exercise testing.

According to the ACSM (1), exercise testing is generally performed to:

1. Aid in the diagnosis of coronary heart disease in asymptomatic or symptomatic individuals.

2. Assess the safety of exercise prior to starting an exercise program.

3. Assess the cardiopulmonary functional capacity of apparently healthy or diseased individuals.

4. Follow the progress of known coronary or pulmonary disease.

5. Assess the efficiency of various medical and surgical procedures including the effect of medications.

Exercise testing is normally performed on individuals who fall into three major groups: apparently healthy individuals, individuals at higher risk, and individuals with disease.

Apparently Healthy Individuals

This group includes those who are apparently healthy and have no major coronary risk factors such as hypertension, hyperlipidemia, smoking, abnormal resting ECG, family history of heart disease, or diabetes mellitus. Apparently healthy individuals under forty-five years of age can begin a progressive exercise program without exercise testing. The ACSM recommends that individuals who are equal to or greater than forty-five years of age have a maximal exercise test prior to beginning an exercise program. Maximal testing is also recommended for apparently healthy forty-five-year-olds who exercise regularly.

Individuals at Higher Risk

Individuals at higher risk include those who have symptoms suggestive of possible coronary disease and/or at least one major coronary risk factor. Exercise testing prior to the initiation of an exercise program is not necessary for asymptomatic individuals at higher risk who are less than thirty-five years of age. For symptomatic individuals or those greater than or equal to thirty-five years of age, maximal exercise testing is recommended.

Individuals with Disease

Individuals with disease include those with known cardiac, pulmonary, or metabolic disease. At any age, individuals in this category should have a maximal exercise test prior to beginning an exercise program.

Contraindications to Exercise Testing

Individuals who are at substantial risk from exercise testing should not be exposed to the potential dangers. Tables 15.1 and 15.2 list the contraindications and relative contraindications to exercise testing. These factors should be considered prior to exercise testing.

Physiological Pretest and Monitoring of Progress

The type of screening test used at entry into a conditioning program will vary in level of sophistication and test parameters required with the type of population to be involved in the program. For healthy school age groups with which there is virtually no concern for CHD risk factors and in which large numbers must be tested in a short time, the step tests described in chapter 14 will serve. On the other hand, in adult conditioning programs, time must be taken to provide better physiological data, including $\dot{V}O_2$ max and as many of the derived parameters as the sophistication of the laboratory allows. This is necessary not only

Table 15.1	Contraindications to Exercise Testing

1. A recent significant change in the resting ECG suggesting infarction or other acute cardiac event
2. Recent complicated myocardial infarction
3. Unstable angina
4. Uncontrolled venticular dysrhythmia
5. Uncontrolled atrial dysrhythmia that compromises cardiac function
6. Third-degree A-V block
7. Acute congestive heart failure
8. Severe aotic stenosis
9. Suspected or known dissecting aneurysm
10. Active or suspected myocarditis or pericarditis
11. Thrombophlebitis or intracardiac thrombi
12. Recent systemic or pulmonary embolus
13. Acute infection
14. Significant emotional distress (psychosis)

Table 15.2	Relative Contraindications to Exercise Testing

1. Resting diastolic blood pressure over 120 mm Hg or resting systolic blood pressure over 200 mm Hg
2. Moderate valvular heart disease
3. Known electrolyte abnormalities (hypokalenia, hypomagnesemia)
4. Fixed-rate pacemaker (rarely used)
5. Frequent or complex ventricular ectopy
6. Ventricular aneurysm
7. Cardiomyopathy including hypertrophic cardiomyopathy
8. Uncontrolled metabolic disease (e.g., diabetes, thyrotoxicosis, myxedema)
9. Chronic infectious disease (e.g., mononucleosis, hepatitis, AIDS)
10. Neuromuscular, musculoskeletal, or rheumatoid disorders that are exacerbated by exercise
11. Advanced or complicated pregnancy

From American College of Sports Medicine: *Guidelines for Exercise Testing and Prescription*, 4th ed. Philadelphia: Lea and Febiger, 1991. Reproduced with permission.

for safety reasons but also to enhance the level of motivation of the participants. For the participants in physical fitness programs, nothing is more gratifying than the feedback from repeated testing that shows them the rewards for their efforts in terms of objectively derived health-related measurements. The discussion of the test results with the participants both individually and in groups offers excellent opportunities for educating lay people about the physiology of exercise with special emphasis on the health benefits derived from well-conceived scientific exercise programs.

Training Curves

The points in time and the frequency of re-testing can be defined from study of figures 15.1 and 15.2. Figure 15.1 shows the training curve for a young male previously decondi-tioned by bed rest (46). The data fit an ex-ponential curve very well ($r^2 = .997$). This type of curve has practical meaning for us be-cause the mathematical nature of an exponen-tial is such that the rate of change (training effect) is inversely proportional to the level of achievement at any given point in the training program. In other words the progress is most rapid when the fitness is poorest (at the begin-ning of training from a deconditioned state). Progress grows slower and slower as the fitness level is improved by conditioning.

Figure 15.2 shows the training curve for five older men who were monitored over forty-two weeks (14). This group shows a curve of the same exponential type ($r^2 = .969$), but in-terestingly the rate of improvement is much slower. The half-time ($t_{1/2}$), or time to achieve one-half the potential improvement, is 1.3 weeks for the young and 12 weeks for the old men. More recent work by Hickson and as-sociates on young men is in close agreement (24). Whether this is a true age difference or simply a result of even greater deconditioning in the old men after a lifetime of sedentary living is not known. In any event, it is obvious from the two figures that the first retest should be at about six weeks to show the dramatic early improvement. After that, retesting at six-month intervals for healthy normals is prob-ably sufficient.

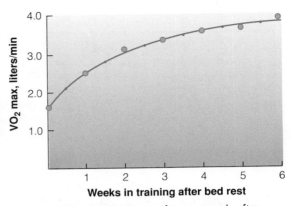

Figure 15.1   Training curve for young male after bed rest. Subject made 31% improvement over pre-bed-rest control value. (Drawn from the data of Saltin, B. et al., in *Circulation* [suppl. VII], vols. 37–38, November 1968. Reprinted by permission of the American Heart Association, Inc.)

Interval Training versus Continuous Exercise

In recent years considerable enthusiasm has developed about using interval training for training athletes. Much of the interest gener-ated probably resulted from the very inter-esting study of intermittent work done by Scandinavian investigators and discussed in chapter 12. Their work showed that subjects could handle very heavy exercise loads with surprisingly low accumulations of O_2 debt and lactic acid when work and rest intervals were interspersed.

However, Saltin (45), who is one of the Scandinavian authorities in this area of inves-tigation, reviewed the evidence and came to the conclusion that interval training does not appear to have an advantage over continuous training in enhancing endurance capacity.

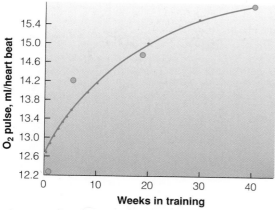

Figure 15.2 Training curve for old men ($N = 5$) who made 29% improvement in O_2 transport ($P <$ .05). (Reprinted by permission of *The Journal of Gerontology*. Volume 25, Number 4, October 1970.)

Roskamm (42), a German pioneer in this area, performed a carefully controlled experiment comparing the training effect of continuous and interval training. He found very small differences when testing the training response at maximal exercise. When heart rate at moderate exercise loads was used as the criterion for testing, continuous exercise produced far better results.

Perhaps even more important for our interests in adult fitness, Pollock (35, 38) has found that the dropout rate in a high intensity interval training program for adults was double that of a continuous jogging program.

It should be pointed out that interval training for athletes may have an advantage over continuous training, in that the faster pace of interval training may come closer to game conditions and therefore involve using the same muscles, fiber types, and muscle recruitment patterns used in the competitive situation.

Until more scientific evidence is available, we must conclude that although interval training may have some small advantages (as yet unproven) over continuous training for the competitive athlete, continuous exercise at lower intensity levels is both safer and better received for purposes of health and fitness in both young and older adults.

Recommendations of the American College of Sports Medicine (ACSM) for Developing Cardiorespiratory Fitness in Healthy Adults

There are four main factors that must be considered when prescribing an endurance training program: mode, intensity, duration, and frequency of exercise. Table 15.3 includes the ACSM (1, 2) recommendations with respect to these factors for developing cardiorespiratory fitness in healthy adults.

Mode of Exercise (ACSM Recommendation: Aerobic in Nature)

The modes of exercise commonly used to improve cardiorespiratory fitness are jogging, walking, swimming, cycling, cross-country skiing, rope skipping, stair climbing, skating, and various endurance game activities (2). Many other activities of an endurance nature can be used. Recent evidence shows that singles tennis (19) and vigorous rowing (6) can also provide an aerobic training effect. Even dancing, when developed as an aerobic endurance exercise through control of rhythm and cadence can elicit a $\dot{V}O_2$ as high as 40 ml/kg·min^{-1} (20). Among the modalities commonly used—jogging, walking, swimming, and cycling—there is probably little difference in training effect if equal levels of total work are used (38, 41). The inclusion of walking may

Table 15.3	ACSM Recommendations for Developing Cardiorespiratory Fitness in Healthy Adults

Mode of Exercise
1. Utilizes large muscle groups
2. Can be maintained continuously
3. Must be rhythmical
4. Must be aerobic in nature

Intensity of Exercise
1. 60%–90% of maximum heart rate (HR)
2. 50%–85% of heart rate reserve (HRR)
3. 50%–85% of maximal oxygen uptake ($\dot{V}O_2$ max)
4. Rating of perceived exertion of approximately 12–15 (somewhat hard to hard)
5. Approximately 60%–70% of maximal METs

Duration of Exercise
1. 20–60 minutes of continuous aerobic exercise
2. Low-intensity exercise should be continued for a longer duration (i.e., 45–60 minutes)
3. High intensity exercise can be continued for a shorter duration (i.e., 20–30 minutes)
4. Generally, low to moderate intensity with longer duration is recommended for most individuals

Frequency of Exercise.
1. 3–5 days per week

be surprising, but Pollock and associates (40) found large and very significant improvement in $\dot{V}O_2$ max in healthy, middle-age, sedentary men from walking. It would, of course, be an insufficient challenge for a young person of average fitness. This will be discussed in the next section.

When choosing a mode of exercise, one important consideration, particularly for older adults, is getting the most exercise for the least heart strain (work of the heart). deVries and Adams (17) provided data (fig. 15.3) that show clearly the differing effects of walking, cycling, and a crawling type of exercise on the relationship of heart strain to total body work in older men (mean age sixty-nine). At all levels of total body work, crawling required more work of the heart than cycling, and the work of the heart rose with increasing total

work more rapidly in both crawling and cycling than in walking. Obviously, when working with sedentary, middle-age, and older people, it is desirable to minimize the ratio of cardiac effort to total body effort for maximum conditioning at minimum risk. The most important determinant of the work of the heart is the amount of rise in blood pressure caused by the exercise. This is least when large muscles are used rhythmically in dynamic contractions (16). It is greatest when small muscles are used at high fractions of their capacity or when muscles are held in static contraction. Thus the crawling exercise is worst because it involves heavy use of the small muscles in the shoulder girdle and upper limbs, and it also involves static contractions of the trunk muscles to maintain the crawling posture. Cycling also caused greater blood pressure effects than walking because, as deVries and Adams

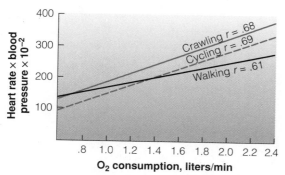

Figure 15.3 The relationship of cardiac effort to total body effort for the three different types of exercise (crawling, cycling, and walking). Each regression line represents the data on twelve subjects at five levels of O_2 consumption. (From deVries, H. A., and Adams, G. M., in *Journal of Sports Medicine and Physical Fitness* 17:41, 1977. Federation Internationale de Medicine Sportive. Reprinted by permission.)

showed by EMG techniques (16), there is considerable static contraction in the upper limb muscles. Research with young men supports these findings: they showed greater blood pressure responses to the bicycle ergometer than to the treadmill at equal, heavy exercise loads (3).

Intensity of Exercise

Dose or Response

The intensity of exercise can be determined on the basis of dose or response. For example, we can define the intensity of the exercise in the case of jogging by spelling out the distance to be accomplished and the rate of running (time for each mile). This is prescription by dose. On the other hand we can also spell out the intensity of the exercise in terms of physiological responses such as $\dot{V}O_2$, HR, RPE, or METs. The use of a physiological parameter is the safer and more effective method because the physiological strain or challenge of any given workout defined as distance and rate can vary

greatly with such factors as weather, changing physical fitness, or incipient illness.

Target Oxygen Consumption Rate Range (ACSM Recommendation: 50% to 85% $\dot{V}O_2$ max)

Oxygen consumption rate ($\dot{V}O_2$) is the physiological parameter most commonly used to measure the cardiorespiratory response to exercise. Therefore, it is logical that $\dot{V}O_2$ is an important parameter upon which to base criteria for the improvement of cardiorespiratory endurance. Unfortunately, $\dot{V}O_2$ is not widely understood by most of the exercising public and therefore is not as practical to use for exercise prescription as other criteria such as heart rate. Furthermore, to prescribe the intensity of exercise based on $\dot{V}O_2$ requires knowledge of the individuals $\dot{V}O_2$ max as well as the oxygen cost of various activities. These factors limit the practical application of $\dot{V}O_2$ as a means of assigning an appropriate training intensity.

Target Heart Rate Range (ACSM Recommendation: 60% to 90% of Maximum HR or 50% to 85% of HRR)

In using heart rate to determine intensity of exercise we are faced with two choices. We can express heart rate (HR) as a percent of maximum HR or as a percent of heart rate reserve (HRR). Later in the chapter there are examples of the calculation of the target heart rate range using the HRR method. Because we start with a resting HR, which is a large fraction of the maximum HR, there is not a very good proportionality between percent maximum HR and the exercise $\dot{V}O_2$ (13). Figure 15.4 demonstrates the difference in expressing the exercise target HR in percent HRR. It can be seen that percent HRR relates quite accurately to the actual $\dot{V}O_2$. That is to say, 50% HRR is about the same as 50% of max $\dot{V}O_2$. But it would require about 68% of max HR in a young subject to produce an actual $\dot{V}O_2$ of 50%, and in the elderly the percent max HR would be about 75 to produce the 50% $\dot{V}O_2$ max.

Since the classic study of Karvonen and colleagues (28) in 1957, we have been aware that some threshold or certain minimal level of exercise intensity must be reached before measurable training effects are achieved. Karvonen showed that to achieve a training effect required 60% of HRR. However, his findings were based on the study of only six young male subjects, and no consideration could be given to the possible effects of age, gender, and physical fitness differences. In general, later work has supported the threshold concept, and the 60% HRR seems to be well supported with respect to young subjects of average fitness (5, 9, 48, 50). However, deVries (15) found considerable difference with respect to age and fitness. The threshold value for men in their sixties and seventies is only 40% HRR, and there is a well-defined effect of level of fitness at the beginning of the training program. On the basis of the available evidence, figure 15.5 seems to provide the best conceptualization of the dose-response relationship. The important points to be noted are 1) there is a point in the HRR below which no training effect is achieved (intensity threshold); 2) the intensity threshold grows higher with higher levels of fitness; 3) once the threshold is reached, the response is relatively proportional to the dose but with somewhat less response per unit dose as fitness improves; and 4) the percentage improvement potential grows smaller with increasing fitness at the beginning of training, as would be expected from the nature of the training curves shown in figures 15.1 and 15.2.

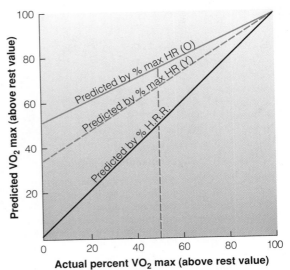

Figure 15.4   Illustration of the errors in using percent maximum heart rate for exercise prescription compared with the use of percent heart rate range. Y = college ages, O = 80-year-old.

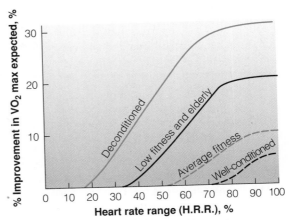

Figure 15.5   Family of curves showing exercise intensity threshold, dose-response relationship, and probable maximum results as related to pretraining $\dot{V}O_2$ max. (Conceptualization based on data of deVries, H. A., *Geriatrics* 26:94–101, 1971, and Saltin, B. et al., *AHA Monograph #23*, 1968.)

Target Rating of Perceived Exertion Range (ACSM Recommendation: 12 to 15, ''Somewhat Hard'' to ''Hard'')

The use of rating of perceived exertion (RPE) to monitor the intensity of exercise is gaining acceptance (7). The advantages include the simplicity and the lack of necessity for measuring a physiological parameter. On the negative side, to accurately use RPE requires that the true relationship between HR and RPE for the individual be known. Furthermore, the individual must be familiar with the Borg Scale (fig. 15.6), and precise identification of intensity cannot be critical since RPE is a subjective estimation. RPE is often used in conjunction with HR (1, 2) until the individual develops a clear understanding of the relationship between HR and RPE. As the exercise program progresses, the individual can usually rely less on HR and more on RPE (1). Furthermore, a recent study by Williams and colleagues (52) reported that "RPE is readily learned by older children and adolescents and is a potentially useful frame of reference when self-regulating effort intensity during vigorous exercise."

Target Range for Metabolic Equivalents (METs) (ACSM Recommendation: 60% to 70% of Maximal METs)

METs are multiples of the resting oxygen consumption rate ($\dot{V}O_2$). A value of 3.5 ml/kg·min^{-1} is considered the average resting $\dot{V}O_2$ value and is defined as 1 MET. Intensity of exercise can be described as a multiple of the resting $\dot{V}O_2$ such as 1 MET, 2 METs, and so on. Once the individual's maximal functional capacity (maximal METs) has been determined from a pretraining exercise test, the appropriate intensity in METs can be calculated. Table 15.4 provides the average MET value for various activities.

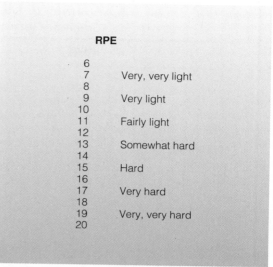

RPE	
6	
7	Very, very light
8	
9	Very light
10	
11	Fairly light
12	
13	Somewhat hard
14	
15	Hard
16	
17	Very hard
18	
19	Very, very hard
20	

Figure 15.6   The rating of perceived exertion scale. (G. V. Borg, "Physiophysical Bases of Perceived Exertion," *Medicine and Science in Sports and Exercise,* vol. 14, pp. 377–381, 1982 © by the American College of Sports Medicine.) Reprinted by permission.

Duration of Exercise (ACSM Recommendation: Twenty to Sixty Minutes of Continuous Aerobic Exercise)

The dose-response data presently available do not yet allow a precise graphic presentation of the relationship between exercise duration and fitness improvement, but figure 15.7 shows a conceptualization based on a review of the literature, with heavy emphasis on the work of Hartung and associates (23) and of Pollock (35), both of whose data points are shown. In general, it appears that a minimum duration of approximately fifteen minutes is required at an optimal intensity before significant training changes are brought about (23). Best results probably require thirty to sixty minutes at optimal intensity (40).

Table 15.4   Leisure Activities in METs: Sports, Exercise Classes, Games, Dancing

	Mean	Range
Archery	3.9	3–4
Backpacking	—	5–11
Badminton	5.8	4–9+
Basketball		
Gameplay	8.3	7–12+
Non-game	—	3–9
Billiards	2.5	—
Bowling	—	2–4
Boxing		
In-ring	13.3	—
Sparring	8.3	—
Canoeing, Rowing and Kayaking	—	3–8
Conditioning Exercise	—	3–8+
Climbing Hills	7.2	5–10+
Cricket	5.2	4.6–7.4
Croquet	3.5	—
Cycling		
Pleasure or to work	—	3–8+
10 mph	7.0	—
Dancing (Social, Square, Tap)	—	3.7–7.4
Dancing (Aerobic)	—	6–9
Fencing	—	6–10+
Field Hockey	8.0	—
Fishing		
from bank	3.7	2–4
wading in stream	—	5–6
Football (Touch)	7.9	6–10
Golf		
Power cart	—	2–3
Walking (carrying bag or pulling cart)	5.1	4–7
Handball	—	8–12+
Hiking (Cross-country)	—	3–7
Horseback Riding		
Galloping	8.2	—
Trotting	6.6	—
Walking	2.4	—
Horseshoe Pitching	—	2–3

	Mean	Range
Hunting (Bow or Gun)		
Small game (walking, carrying light load)	—	3–7
Big game (dragging carcass, walking)	—	3–14
Judo	13.5	—
Mountain Climbing	—	5–10+
Music Playing	—	2–3
Paddleball, Racquetball	9	8–12
Rope Jumping	11	—
60–80 skips/min	9	—
120–140 skips/min	—	11–12
Running		
12 min per mile	8.7	—
11 min per mile	9.4	—
10 min per mile	10.2	—
9 min per mile	11.2	—
8 min per mile	12.5	—
7 min per mile	14.1	—
6 min per mile	16.3	—
Sailing	—	2–5
Scubadiving	—	5–10
Shuffleboard	—	2–3
Skating, Ice and Roller	—	5–8
Skiing, Snow		
Downhill	—	5–8
Cross-country	—	6–12+
Skiing, Water	—	5–7
Sledding, Tobogganing	—	4–8
Snowshoeing	9.9	7–14
Squash	—	8–12+
Soccer	—	5–12+
Stair climbing	—	4–8
Swimming	—	4–8+
Table Tennis	4.1	3–5
Tennis	6.5	4–9+
Volleyball	—	3–6

From American College of Sports Medicine: Guidelines for Exercise Testing and Prescription, 4th ed. Philadelphia: Lea and Febiger, 1991. Reproduced with permission.

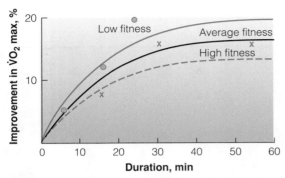

Figure 15.7 Relationship of percent improvement in VO₂ max to duration of exercise. (Curves based on data of Hartung, G. H. et al., *Journal of Human Ergology* 6:61, 1977 (o), and Pollock, M. L., *Physician and Sports Medicine* 6:6 June 1978 (x). Hartung data at intensity of 65% HRR, Pollock data at intensity of 85%–90% HRR.)

It must be emphasized, however, that with previously sedentary or deconditioned subjects, one may not achieve even the fifteen-minute duration in continuous exercise. Progressive development to even that low level of duration may be required.

There is also some reason to believe that there is an interaction between intensity and duration. Pollock (40) has shown that for middle-age men (forty to fifty-seven) walking for forty minutes per day, four days a week produced a training effect equal to that gained from jogging thirty minutes a day, three days a week, where the weekly energy cost of the two programs was equal. Similar results have been demonstrated with older men (14).

In a well-controlled study, Pollock and associates (38) provided some interesting data showing that the injury rate was more than double in subjects who trained for forty-five minutes as compared with those who trained for thirty minutes (54% and 24%, respectively). The injuries were largely shin splints and knee problems. As indicated in chapter 26, shin splints can be controlled and virtually eliminated by use of static stretching. In any event the data suggest that to hold injury rates to a minimum the duration should be limited

to thirty minutes or less for beginning joggers. As aerobic capacity and general fitness improve, duration can be increased. On the other hand, after a training effect (increased V̇O₂ max) has been gained, it appears that the improvement can be maintained with as little as one-third the duration used in the original training period if intensity and frequency (six days/week) are maintained (26). If training is discontinued, a significant reduction in cardiorespiratory fitness occurs in as little as two weeks (2).

Although this chapter is directed to cardiorespiratory fitness, note that the endurance exercise prescribed here is also one of the best means of weight control (to be discussed in chap. 17), and of course, all other things being equal, the caloric expenditure is directly proportional to the duration.

It has been observed that in a typical physical education class lasting fifty minutes, children were active for only five to ten minutes, and of that short period, HR was above 150 for only one to two minutes (22). Similar findings with respect to elementary school children suggest that they do not voluntarily engage in sufficient aerobic activity during recess to be likely to improve their fitness level (27). Clearly, competent and dedicated leadership is required at all levels if we are to improve the fitness of our youth.

Frequency of Exercise (ACSM Recommendation: Three to Five Days Per Week)

Figure 15.8 shows the dose-response curve for exercise frequency using data from several sources (5, 21, 37, 39). In general, the available data suggest little if any improvement from one workout per week. Improvement accelerates rapidly when workouts are increased to three or five per week, with smaller payoffs for increases to six or seven per week.

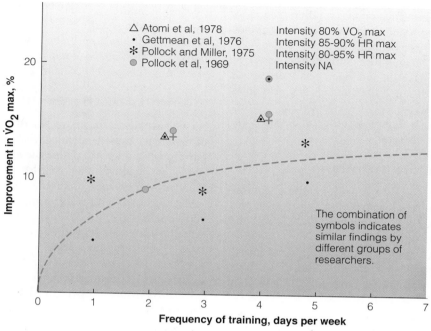

Figure 15.8   Relationship of percent improvement in $\dot{V}O_2$ max to frequency of workout. (Curves based on data from references shown above.)

It seems almost certain that seven heavy workouts per week would be counterproductive, since there would be no opportunity for the muscle glycogen overshoot phenomenon to occur (chap. 3).

It appears that the optimal payoff for time spent occurs with three to five workouts per week (2). What effect does the spacing of the workouts have? Moffatt and associates (33) have shown that there is no difference in training effect in young males when the training is conducted on Monday, Tuesday, and Wednesday as compared with Monday, Wednesday, and Friday. It has also been shown that a conditioning effect once accomplished can be maintained with as little as two workouts per week if intensity and duration are maintained (24).

Again, for the novice jogger, injury rate is three times greater for five workouts per week than it is for three workouts per week (39). But there are significant advantages in longer and more frequent workouts for weight reduction. Thus on the basis of available evidence it would seem prudent to prescribe no more than three workouts of thirty minutes duration per week of jogging until good fitness has been realized, at which time dosage could be increased, if desired, for weight reduction purposes to five workouts of forty-five to sixty minutes each. As the workouts become longer and more frequent, intensity would need to be reduced commensurately to prevent overtraining (staleness).

Exercise Prescription

From the preceding discussion it is obvious that, to the greatest extent possible, exercise prescription (Ex Rx) should be given on an individual basis. Even though the Ex Rx is individual, large numbers of normals can be separated into four or five smaller groups by fitness category and can then exercise together as a homogeneous unit.

The following discussion will be based on the use of jog-walk and jogging as the exercise modality, although the methods and principles applied will be equally effective if cycling, swimming, walking, or other endurance exercises are chosen.

Daily Workout Plan

Every workout must include three components: 1) the warm-up period, 2) the main part of the workout, the endurance activity, and 3) the cool-down.

Warming up is so important to the health and safety of participants that a separate chapter (chap. 27) is devoted to this topic in part 3 of this text. Suffice to say, both the cardiovascular-respiratory and the neuromuscular systems must be brought to a state of readiness for vigorous activity by very gradual increases in intensity until myocardial blood flow and deep muscle temperatures are suitable for the challenge of the endurance workout. However, endurance activity such as jogging can be one of the safest and most effective warm-ups in itself if simply started at a rate that is slow and easy for the participant. Calisthenics so often used as a warm-up can be more effective at the end of the jogging workout as a means of improving muscle tone and flexibility. This is especially true when static stretching routines are used for preventing muscle problems such as shin splints and soreness in the calf muscles.

In the case of jogging workouts, the cooldown period is typically a period of brisk walking until HR returns to about 120 for young and 110 and 100 for middle-age and older adults, respectively. Thus the daily workout plan would start with five to ten minutes of slow jogging leading into the jogging workout designed to achieve target HR, followed by ten to fifteen minutes of appropriate calisthenics designed to improve muscle

strength, endurance, and flexibility of the shoulder girdle and the chest as well as the abdominal wall and upper and lower back. Finally, the workout is completed with static stretching (chaps. 25, 26, and 27).

Elements of the Ex Rx

As we have discussed above, the four elements of the Ex Rx must be defined. For purposes of our discussion, we will define the *exercise modality* as jogging. The ACSM has recommended a *frequency* of three to five times a week (fig. 15.8) and a *duration* of twenty to sixty minutes (fig. 15.7). However, previously sedentary individuals will require from six to ten weeks of gradual increases to achieve this duration. The remainder of our discussion will be directed to the most important factor of *intensity* for which we will need the following definitions:

$$RHR = \text{resting HR}$$
$$EHR = \text{exercise HR}$$
$$MHR = \text{maximum HR (from table 15.6)}$$
$$HRR = \text{HR reserve} = MHR - RHR$$
$$\%HRR = \frac{EHR - RHR}{MHR - RHR} \times 100$$

Using these definitions, we now need to define three HR values for the participant:

Min HR—the intensity threshold value of HR, below which improvement is unlikely.

Target HR—the HR to which the participant should work to assure optimal training progress with minimum hazard.

Do-not-exceed HR—the HR above which intensity may be too high for optimal results and that may be counterproductive for some.

Since significant negative correlations between training response and initial fitness level have been found (15), it is necessary to adjust the Ex Rx to the fitness level of the participant as shown in table 15.5.

Let us now calculate the intensity for a twenty-one-year-old participant who is to start

Table 15.5	Exercise Prescription by Fitness Level		
	Low Fitness	**Average Fitness**	**High Fitness**
Minimum HR	40% HRR	60% HRR	70% HRR
Target HR	60% HRR	75% HRR	80% HRR
Do-not-exceed HR	75% HRR	85% HRR	90% HRR

Table 15.6   Age-Fitness Adjusted Predicted MHR for Three Levels of Fitness Based on Balke Treadmill Stress Testing

Age	Predicted MHR, bpm			Age	Predicted MHR, bpm		
	Below Average	**Average**	**Above Average**		**Below Average**	**Average**	**Above Average**
20	201	201	196	45	174	183	183
21	199	200	196	46	173	182	183
22	198	199	195	47	172	181	182
23	197	198	195	48	171	181	182
24	196	198	194	49	170	180	181
25	195	197	194	50	168	179	180
26	194	196	193	51	167	179	180
27	193	196	193	52	166	178	179
28	192	195	192	53	165	177	179
29	191	193	192	54	164	176	178
30	190	193	191	55	163	176	178
31	189	193	191	56	162	175	177
32	188	192	190	57	161	174	177
33	187	191	189	58	160	174	176
34	186	191	189	59	159	173	176
35	184	190	188	60	158	172	175
36	183	189	188	61	157	172	175
37	182	189	187	62	156	171	174
38	181	188	187	63	155	170	174
39	180	187	186	64	154	169	173
40	179	186	186	65	152	169	173
41	178	186	185	66	151	168	172
42	177	185	185	67	150	167	171
43	176	184	184	68	149	167	171
44	175	184	184	69	148	166	170
				70	147	165	170

From Cooper, K.H., Purdy, J.G., White, S.R., Pollock, M.L., and Linnerud, A.C. "Age-Fitness Adjusted Maximum Heart Rates," in *Medicine and Sport* 10: "The Role of Exercise in Internal Medicine," D. Brunner and E. Jokl, eds. Basel: Karger, 1977, 78–88.

in a conditioning program having been tested and found to have a $\dot{V}O_2$ max in the average category for his age. First check table 15.6 and find that the maximum HR would be predicted at 200 (11). The resting HR in this example is 70.

$$HRR = MHR - RHR = 200 - 70 = 130$$

For training purposes

$$Min\ HR = 60\%\ HRR + Resting\ HR$$
$$= 78 + 70 = 148$$
$$Target\ HR = 75\%\ HRR + RHR$$
$$= 97.5 + 70 \cong 168$$
$$Do\text{-}not\text{-}exceed\ HR = 85\%\ HRR + RHR$$
$$= 110.5 + 70 \cong 181$$

Note that these values are quite different for an individual of low fitness at age sixty with a resting HR of 70. At age sixty, MHR from table 15.6 is 158.

$$Target\ HR = .60\ (158 - 70) + 70 = 123$$

For an individual, age twenty-one, already of better than average fitness with a resting HR of 70,

$$Target\ HR = .80\ (196 - 70) + 70 = 171$$

Heart rate can be taken most accurately by monitoring the apical heartbeat on the lower left side of the chest wall by stethoscope. A common method for estimating exercise heart rate is to count the number of heartbeats for six seconds and add a zero. That is, if 12 heartbeats are counted in six seconds, the heart rate in beats per minute is 120. Although this procedure is accurate enough for most situations, it should be recognized that there is some error because it is not possible to count a fraction of a heartbeat. In addition, counting heartbeats for a ten-second period has been shown to be a valid method when used within ten to fifteen seconds of cessation of exercise, providing HR within 2% of the true value taken during the exercise by radio telemetry (36).

It had been thought that palpation of the pulse rate at the carotid artery did not provide valid heart rate estimates because pressure on the carotid sinus can induce a reflex slowing of heart rate. Errors of 11 and 15 bpm had been reported at rest and during recovery (51). However, three more recent investigations have shown that there is no significant error from such palpation if carefully performed (12, 34, 47). Proper instruction in technique is necessary, with particular emphasis on the following points: 1) palpate lightly; 2) palpate at a point one-third way between the thyroid cartilage and the angle of the mandible; and 3) obviously, only one side should be palpated (34).

Recently, highly accurate cardiomonitors have been marketed for use in determining exercise heart rate (30). These devices are becoming less costly and provide a practical method for determining the intensity of exercise.

It should be noted that using the aforementioned HR methods have the following very significant advantages over the prescription of a jogging rate and distance:

1. In hot, humid weather, working to a target HR automatically protects participants from overdoing, because the stress of the heat load will be reflected in the observed exercise HR. To avoid exceeding the THR, the individual will need to slow down, thus maintaining training stress as a constant rather than rate and distance.

2. Physiological changes due to incipient illness will similarly be corrected for.

3. As fitness improves there is no need to change the Ex Rx because, again, the exercise HR, which grows less for any given exercise bout, forces the individual to increase rate to maintain the target HR.

Effect of Gender and Age on Training Adaptations

Until recently, virtually all of the research dealing with the training parameters of intensity, duration, and frequency had been conducted on males. Recently, however, studies have been conducted to better elucidate the training adaptations of females. While the data are still sparse, there appears to be no great gender difference in training responses with respect to intensity threshold (29), duration (55), or the magnitude of response (4, 6, 49). Thus the principles just discussed appear to apply equally well to both genders (8).

With respect to age, work from deVries's laboratory has shown that the trainability of older men (14) and women (4) is just as good as that of the young if looked at on a relative basis. Although the elderly start at a much lower fitness level, the percentage by which fitness can be improved is not significantly different in the old than it is in the young (14), nor is there apparently any great difference in trainability between the genders in old age (4).

Specificity of Training

As was discussed in chapter 3, training results in adaptations that are specific to exercise type, intensity, and duration. Indeed, even the use of energy substrate was seen to be specific to these factors. A good review of the subcellular bases for the specificity of training is available (32). It is not surprising that when the training effect of jogging is measured ($\dot{V}O_2$ max) on the treadmill, it may be almost threefold greater than that measured during a maximal swim test (31). However, there are also central circulatory adaptations to training such that training in one modality such as jogging can result in highly significant and relatively similar reductions in heart rate during other modes of *submaximal* exercise. For example, it has been shown that ten weeks of training at jogging resulted in approximately equal reductions in submaximal HR at such dissimilar activities as treadmill walking, leg cycling, arm cycling, and load carrying (48).

It can be concluded that the training effects for high level performance are highly specific but that the health benefits with respect to reduced heart stress at submaximal work are quite general.

Potential Physiological Changes Resulting from Training

It has been found in many well-controlled experiments that very significant physiological changes are brought about by conditioning previously sedentary subjects. One of the better experiments (18) showed, for example, that sixteen weeks of training (cross-country running and interval training) three times a week produced the following benefits:

1. Fifty-two percent increase of total work output at exhaustion

2. Decrease in heart rate at a submaximal task from 170 to 144 bpm

3. Increase of 16.2% in maximal O_2 uptake

4. Maximal cardiac output increase of almost 2 liters/min

5. Stroke volume increase of 13.4%

6. Significant arteriovenous oxygen difference increase

7. Lower blood lactate levels at a given submaximal load

8. Significant improvements in mechanical efficiency at the higher submaximal work loads

Training as a Stressor

As with all other good things in life, exercise and training can be carried to extremes, and the resulting stress may be detrimental instead of beneficial. The time course of normal training challenges shows an adaptive response. In the case of the endocrine system, the sympathoadrenal response to the training workout may show a gradual lowering in the level of blood catecholamines. It has been shown, for example, that the adaptation to a standard exercise challenge of thirty to fifty minutes per day for six days per week can result in plasma epinephrine dropping to one-third and norepinephrine to one-half their pretraining values. This must be considered a beneficial response in that the organism appears to be under less stress after the training period of seven weeks (54).

On the other hand, if the exercise is overdone the opposite may be the case. Williams and Ward (53) performed hematological studies before and after a relay marathon race in which each team member ran approximately one mile all out every hour for twenty-four hours. They found significant increases in white blood cell counts and percentage of polymorphonuclear leucocytes, and significant decreases in lymphocytes and eosinophils after the twenty-four hourly runs. These changes are typical of the response to high levels of stress. In addition they found highly significant increases in bilirubin, which suggest red blood cell damage, and certain muscle enzymes, which suggest muscle tissue damage.

Thus we may conclude that while exercise or training in appropriate amounts can result in better responses to a stressful environment, excessive exercise of too heavy intensity and duration may result in very high levels of stress with possibilities for tissue damage.

Summary

1. There is a need for physical education professionals to help the lay public learn how to use exercise for health and fitness purposes.

2. To use exercise for improving fitness requires consideration of objectives, mode of exercise, intensity, duration, frequency, intensity threshold for training effect, and rate of training adaptation as a function of pretraining fitness level.

3. The need for medical evaluation prior to participation in endurance exercise depends on age, symptomatology, and risk factors. Medical screening examinations should be required for all persons over thirty-five and also for those younger if they are symptomatic or at high risk for cardiovascular disease.

4. The type of physiological screening and monitoring performed must vary in sophistication with the type of population to be evaluated.

5. The change in cardiovascular fitness ($\dot{V}O_2$ max) during the course of a training program appears to be well described as an exponential relationship. This means that at any point the rate of gain varies inversely with the fitness status at that time.

6. Interval training may have some small advantage over continuous training (as yet unproven) for the competitive athlete. However, continuous exercise at lower intensity levels is equally effective, safer, and better received for purposes of health and fitness in both young and older adults.

7. Among the exercise modalities commonly used (jogging, walking, swimming, and cycling), there is probably little difference in training effect if equal levels of total work are used.

8. When working with previously sedentary, middle-age, and older people, it is desirable to minimize the ratio of cardiac effort to total body effort to produce maximum conditioning at minimum risk. This is done by using exercise modalities that use large muscles rhythmically in dynamic contractions.

9. Using dose-response relationships when prescribing exercise requires consideration of the factors of *intensity, duration,* and *frequency.*

10. The intensity threshold below which no cardiorespiratory training effect is likely is about 60% of aerobic power for the young individual of average fitness. The threshold is lower for the unfit and elderly and higher for those at better levels of fitness.

11. A minimal exercise *duration* of about fifteen to twenty minutes at optimal intensity is required before significant training changes are realized. Best results probably require thirty to sixty minutes at optimal intensity.

12. There is likely to be little or no improvement from one workout per week. The rate of gain grows rapidly by increasing the frequency to four or five per week, with smaller payoff for time spent beyond that.

13. The daily workout plan must include three components: (a) warm-up, (b) the body of the workout (endurance activity in the case of cardiorespiratory conditioning), and (c) the cool-down period.

14. Procedures based on the monitoring of heart rate are described for the prescription of exercise in terms of minimum HR, target HR, and do-not-exceed HR.

15. Exercise can be prescribed either on the basis of dose (rate and distance of run, for example) or on the basis of physiological response (heart rate). The latter is preferable because the use of heart rate, for example, automatically adjusts the work load dosage for such variables as weather, personal well-being, and changes in fitness.

16. There appear to be no great differences between the genders in training responses with respect to intensity threshold, duration, or magnitude of response.

17. The trainability of older men and women is equally as good as that of the young if looked at on a relative basis.

18. The training effects for high level performance are highly specific, but the health benefits with respect to reduced heart rate at submaximal work are quite general.

19. Physiological benefits derived from a conditioning program that improves cardiorespiratory fitness include at least the following: (a) large increases in physical working capacity, (b) significant gains in aerobic power, (c) increased capacity for cardiac output, and (d) more efficient achievement of submaximal work loads at lower heart rates.

20. While exercise in appropriate amounts can result in better responses to a stressful environment, excessive exercise of too heavy intensity and duration may result in very high levels of stress and possible tissue damage.

References

1. American College of Sports Medicine. *Guidelines for Exercise Testing and Prescription,* 3d ed. Philadelphia: Lea and Febiger, 1986.

2. ACSM Position Statement. The recommended quantity and quality of exercise for developing and maintaining cardiorespiratory and muscular fitness in healthy adults. *Med. Sci. Sports Exerc.* 22:265–74, 1990.

3. Adams, G. E., Bonner, E. A., Ribisl, P. M., and Miller, H. S. Blood pressure during heavy work on the treadmill and bicycle ergometer. *Med. Sci. Sports* 10:50, 1978.

4. Adams, G. M., and deVries, H. A. Physiological effects of an exercise training regimen upon women aged 52–79. *J. Gerontol.* 28:50–55, 1973.

5. Atomi, Y., Ito, K., Iwasaki, H., and Miyashita, M. Effects of intensity and frequency of training on aerobic work capacity of young females. *J. Sports Med. Phys. Fitness* 18:3–9, 1978.

6. Bassett, D. R., Smith, P. A., and Getchell, L. H. Energy cost of simulated rowing using a wind-resistance device. *Physician and Sportsmed.* 12 (August):113–18, 1984.

7. Borg, G. A. V. Psychophysical bases of perceived exertion. *Med. Sci. Sports Exerc.* 14:377–81, 1982.

8. Burke, E. J. Physiological effects of similar training programs in males and females. *Res. Q.* 48:510–17, 1977.

9. Burke, E. J., and Franks, B. D. Changes in $\dot{V}O_2$ max resulting from bicycle training at different intensities holding total mechanical work constant. *Res. Q.* 46:31–37, 1975.

10. Conrad, C. C. Progress report of the President's Council on Physical Fitness and Sports. December 31, 1975.

11. Cooper, K. H., Purdy, J. G., White, S. R., Pollock, M. L., and Linnerud, A. C. Age-fitness adjusted maximal heart rates. *Med. Sci. Sports* 6:1–11, 1976.

12. Couldry, W., Corbin, C. B., and Wilcox, A. Carotid versus radial pulse counts. *Physician and Sportsmed.* 10 (December):67–72, 1982.

13. Davis, J. A., and Convertino, V. A. A comparison of heart rate methods for predicting endurance training intensity. *Med. Sci. Sports* 7:295–98, 1975.

14. deVries, H. A. Physiological effects of an exercise training regimen upon men aged 52–88. *J. Geront.* 25:325–36, 1970.

15. ———. Exercise intensity threshold for improvement of cardiovascular-respiratory function in older men. *Geriatrics* 26:94–101, 1971.

16. deVries, H. A., and Adams, G. M. Total muscle mass activation versus relative loading of individual muscles as determinants of exercise response in older men. *Med. Sci. Sports* 4:146–54, 1972.

17. ———. Effect of the type of exercise upon the work of the heart in older men. *J. Sports Med. Phys. Fitness* 17:41–48, 1977.

18. Ekblom, B., Astrand, P. O., Saltin, B., Stenberg, J., and Wallstrom, B. Effect of training on circulatory response to exercise. *J. Appl. Physiol.* 24:518–28, 1968.

19. Friedman, D. B., Ramo, B. W., Gray, G. J. Tennis and cardiovascular fitness in middle-aged men. *Physician and Sportsmed.* 12 (July):87–92, 1984.

20. Foster, C. Physiological requirements of aerobic dancing. *Res. Q.* 46:120–22, 1975.

21. Gettman, L. R., Pollock, M. L., Durstine, J. L., Ward, A., Ayres, J., and Linnerud, A. C. Physiological responses of men to 1, 3, and 5 day per week training programs. *Res. Q.* 47:638–46, 1976.

22. Goode, R. C., Virgin, A., Romet, T. T., Crawford, P., Duffin, J., Pallandi, T., and Woch, Z. Effects of a short period of physical activity in adolescent boys and girls. *Can. J. Appl. Sports Sci.* 1:241–50, 1976.

23. Hartung, G. H., Smolensky, M. H., Harrist, R. B., Rangel, R., and Skrovan, C. Effects of varied durations of training on improvement in cardiorespiratory endurance. *J. Human Ergol.* 6:61–68, 1977.

24. Hickson, R. C., Hagberg, J. M., Ehsani, A. A., and Holloszy, J. O. Time course of the adaptive responses of aerobic power and heart rate to training. *Med. Sci. Sports Exer.* 13:17–20, 1981.

25. Hickson, R. C., Kanakis, C., Davis, J. R., Moore, A. M., and Rich, S. Reduced training duration effects on aerobic power, endurance and cardiac growth. *J. Appl. Physiol.* 53:225–29, 1982.

26. Hickson, R. C., and Rosenkoetter, M. A. Reduced training frequencies and maintenance of increased aerobic power. *Med. Sci. Sports Exer.* 13:13–16, 1981.

27. Hovell, M. F., Bursick, J. H., Sharkey, R., and McClure, J. An evaluation of elementary students voluntary physical activity during recess. *Res. Q.* 49:460–74, 1978.

28. Karovonen, M. J., Kentala, E., and Mustala, O. The effects of training on heart rate. *Ann. Med. Exper. Fenn.* 35:307–15, 1957.

29. Kearney, J. T., Stull, G. A., Ewing, J. L., and Strein, J. W. Cardiorespiratory responses of sedentary college women as a function of training intensity. *J. Appl. Physiol.* 41:822–25, 1976.

30. Leger, L., and Thivierge, M. Heart rate monitors: Validity, stability, and functionality. *Physician and Sportsmed.* 16:143–51, 1988.

31. McArdle, W. D., Magel, J. R., Delio, D. J., Toner, M., and Chase, J. M. Specificity of run training on $\dot{V}O_2$ max and heart rate changes during running and swimming. *Med. Sci. Sports* 10:16–20, 1978.

32. McCafferty, W. B., and Horvath, S. M. Specificity of exercise and specificity of training: a subcellular review. *Res. Q.* 48:358–71, 1977.

33. Moffatt, R. J., Stamford, B. A., and Neill, R. D. Placement of tri-weekly training sessions: Importance regarding enhancement of aerobic capacity. *Res. Q.* 48:583–91, 1977.

34. Oldridge, N. B., Haskell, W. L., and Single, P. Carotid palpation coronary heart disease and exercise rehabilitation. *Med. Sci. Sports Exer.* 13:6–8, 1981.

35. Pollock, M. L. How much exercise is enough? *Physician and Sportsmed.* 6 (June):50–64, 1978.

36. Pollock, M. L., Broida, J., and Kendrick, Z. Validity of the palpation technique of heart rate determination and its estimation of training heart rate. *Res. Q.* 43:77–81, 1972.

37. Pollock, M. L., Cureton, T. K., and Greninger, L. Effects of frequency of training on working capacity, cardiovascular function, and body composition of adult men. *Med. Sci. Sports* 1:70–74, 1969.

38. Pollock, M. L., Gettman, L. R., Milesis, C. A., Bah, M. D., Durstine, L., and Johnson, R. G. Effects of frequency and duration of training on attrition and incidence of injury. *Med. Sci. Sports* 9:31–36, 1977.

39. Pollock, M. L., and Miller, H. S. Frequency of training as a determinant for improvement in cardiovascular function and body composition of middle-aged men. *Arch. Phys. Med. Rehabil.* 56:141–45, 1975.

40. Pollock, M. L., Miller, H. S., Janeway, R., Linnerud, A. C., Robertson, B., and Valentino, R. Effects of walking on body composition and cardiovascular function of middle aged men. *J. Appl. Physiol.* 30:126–30, 1971.

41. Roberts, J. A., and Morgan, W. P. Effect of type and frequency of participation in physical activity upon physical working capacity. *Am. Corr. J.* 25:99–104, 1971.

42. Roskamm, H. Optimum patterns of exercise for healthy adults. *Can. Med. Assoc. J.* 96:895, 1967.

43. Ross, J. G., and Gilbert, G. G. The national children and youth fitness study: A summary of findings. *JOPERD* 56:45–50, 1985.

44. Ross, J. G., and Pate, R. R. The national children and youth fitness study II: A summary of findings. *JOPERD* 58:51–56, 1987.

45. Saltin, B. Intermittent exercise: Its physiology and practical application. John R. Emens Lecture, Ball State University, Muncie, Ind., February 20, 1975.

46. Saltin, B., Blomquist, G., Mitchell, J. H., Johnson, R. L., Wildenthal, K.; and Chapman, C. B. Response to exercise after bed rest and after training. American Heart Association,

Monograph 23. New York: The Association, 1968.

47. Sedlock, D. A., Knowlton, R. G., Fitzgerald, P. I., Tahamont, M. V., and Schneider, D. A. Accuracy of subject-palpated carotid pulse after exercise. *Physician and Sportsmed.* 11 (April):106–16, 1983.

48. Shephard, R. J. The development of cardiorespiratory fitness. *Med. Services J. Canada,* 21:533–44, 1965.

49. Van Handel, P. J., Costill, D. L., and Getchell, L. H. Central circulatory adaptations to physical training. *Res. Q.* 47:815–23, 1976.

50. Wenger, H. A., and MacNab, R. B. J. Endurance training: The effects of intensity, total work, duration and initial fitness. *J. Sports Med. Phys. Fitness* 15:199–211, 1975.

51. White, J. R. EKG changes using carotid artery for heart rate monitoring. *Med. Sci. Sports* 9:88–94, 1977.

52. Williams, J. G., Eston, R. G., and Stretch C. Use of the rating of perceived exertion to control exercise intensity in children. *Ped. Exerc. Sci.* 3:21–27, 1991.

53. Williams, M. H., and Ward, A. J. Hematological changes elicited by prolonged intermittent aerobic exercise. *Res. Q.* 48:606–16, 1977.

54. Winder, W. W., Hagberg, J. M., Hickson, R. C., Ehsani, A. A., and McLane, J. A. Time course of sympathoadrenal adaptation to endurance exercise training in man. *J. Appl. Physiol.* 45:370–74, 1978.

55. Yeager, S. A., and Brynteson, P. Effects of varying training periods on the development of cardiovascular efficiency of college women. *Res. Q.* 41:589–92, 1970.

16

Exercise Physiology in the Prevention and Rehabilitation of Cardiovascular Disease

Anatomy and Physiology of the Coronary
   Arteries

Nature of Coronary Heart Disease
   (CHD)
   Angina Pectoris
   Myocardial Infarction
   Sudden Death
   Congestive Heart Failure

Theories Regarding Causation of CHD

The Risk Factor Concept in CHD

Physiological Bases for Use of Exercise in
   CHD Prevention

Exercise Physiology in Cardiac
   Rehabilitation

Principles of Exercise Testing in Cardiac
   Rehabilitation
   Parameters to Be Measured
   Safety and Litigation Experience

Exercise Prescription for Cardiac
   Rehabilitation
   Phase I Exercise Programs
   Phase II Exercise Programs
   Phase III Exercise Programs

Weight Training for Cardiac
   Rehabilitation

Program Development

To those of us who have been involved with exercise physiology for the last several decades, it seems like only yesterday that we were defending participation in competitive athletics and heavy physical training against the charges that such activity would result in dire consequences such as "athlete's heart." We are now likely to be more concerned with moderating the claims for exercise as a panacea for all ills by some of our lay enthusiasts in the pseudoscientific health areas. The truth, of course, lies at neither extreme but somewhere in between.

This change in attitude toward the effects of exercise on the cardiovascular system, and on the heart in particular, probably came about largely as a result of cardiologists being inspired by the work of Eckstein (17). He simulated the effect of coronary disease in dogs by surgically restricting blood flow in the coronary arteries. His experiments showed that while this arterial narrowing by itself failed to initiate collateral vessel growth to take over as a result of the partially occluded vessels, the addition of exercise did in fact promote an effective collateral circulation. Although this work was published in 1957, we do not yet have any clear evidence of this physiological adaptation in humans. Much evidence has been presented pro and con, and the issue is still in question. However, there are other physiological bases upon which one can construct a case for the use of exercise in preventing coronary heart disease (CHD) and rehabilitating CHD patients. We have already presented in chapter 13 much of the epidemiological evidence for the importance of exercise in preventing CHD. In this chapter we will consider the contribution that exercise physiology can make to the prevention of CHD and to the rehabilitation of CHD patients. This discussion will involve the theoretical bases as well as the how-to concepts in the realization that the future will probably bring demands for ever greater numbers of physical educators who can work with

cardiologists and other physicians in the scientific application of exercise to the needs of CHD patients and, even more important, in the preventive aspects of this serious health problem. The beginnings of CHD are present in the form of fatty streaks by three years of age (33). Furthermore, it has been reported (19) that 77.3% of the autopsies on Korean battle casualties showed gross evidence of coronary arteriosclerosis in spite of the fact that mean age was only twenty-two. It has also been pointed out that the most common mode of death in persons with either symptomatic or presymptomatic CHD is sudden death, which accounts for over half of all coronary fatalities under age sixty-five. Furthermore, of these fatalities, over 65% have shown no prior symptoms, and death occurs totally unexpectedly outside the hospital before cardiac resuscitation teams can reach the victims (27). These facts underscore the need for preventive measures on a population basis since the physician may never have the opportunity to work his art in 65% of the cases.

Health and physical education professionals can help improve the life-style of our American people at all ages, particularly through teaching the appropriate use of physical conditioning, the optimization of body weight and nutrition, and relaxation skills.

Although the evidence for the benefits to be derived from exercise in CHD remains somewhat controversial, we would do well to consider the rules under which we accept or reject scientific evidence, as pointed out so well by Dr. Sam Fox, the former director of the National Heart Disease and Stroke Control Program (24). Levels of acceptance of evidence beyond proven versus unproven do exist: 1) proven beyond reasonable doubt; 2) of probable benefit, but not above question; 3) a prudent action, on the basis of a good chance of benefit and acceptably low hazard; and 4) promising but more good data needed. In 1969, Dr. Fox concluded that the evidence is such that it is prudent to include increased habitual physical activity in a program to prevent or manage nonacute CHD. If anything, the evidence appears to have strengthened in the years since Dr. Fox's conservative estimate.

In any event, it is important to realize from the outset that there is little evidence to suggest a *curative* effect from physical conditioning alone after the CHD process has become established. It is clear, however, that exercise can serve to relieve or alleviate some of the symptoms. Furthermore, a recent study (49) has reported some degree of regression of atherosclerosis with life-style changes including a low-fat vegetarian diet, smoking cessation, stress management, and moderate exercise. It should also be recognized that this chapter does not propose to train physical educators in cardiology. But we hope to instill interest and sufficient knowledge to allow physical educators to communicate and interact successfully with the physicians who must always bear the ultimate responsibility for the welfare of their patients.

Anatomy and Physiology of the Coronary Arteries

Figure 16.1 shows the larger coronary arteries of the anterior wall of the heart. These arteries arise directly from the aorta as the right and left coronary arteries, which with their subdivisions supply the blood necessary to support myocardial metabolism and thus the muscular work of the heart.

With respect to CHD, the blood supply to the left ventricle is most important since this chamber is responsible for the total systemic circulation. Therefore any major interruption of blood flow in the left coronary artery must have serious functional consequences.

As has been noted in the earlier chapters, the skeletal muscles can function for short

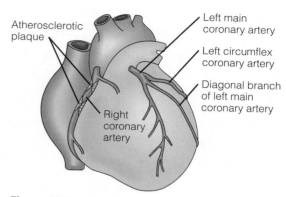

Figure 16.1   Illustration of the larger coronary arteries showing the partial occlusion of the right coronary artery by atherosclerotic plaque formation.

periods of time in the absence of O_2, that is, anaerobically. The myocardium, however, is capable of very little anaerobic metabolism. In addition, the heart already extracts the largest part of the O_2 supply available to it while at rest, in contradistinction to the skeletal muscles whose extraction at rest is very low. Thus virtually the only reserve in function for the heart muscle depends on increasing the O_2 supply through increasing coronary blood flow when the body's demands for O_2 are increased as in exercise. In the normal heart, any increase in myocardial O_2 demand ($M\dot{V}O_2$) is precisely balanced by increases in coronary blood flow, which is affected by mechanical, neural, humoral, and metabolic factors that together reduce coronary vascular resistance and increase coronary blood flow as a consequence.

Because of its almost complete dependence on a pay-as-you-go O_2 supply, the heart muscle is vulnerable to any imbalance between supply and demand. Thus any tendency toward hypoxia, whether because of too much demand or too little supply, is associated with rapid deterioration of function such as losses in contractility and cardiac output, which thus compromise the heart's ability to meet either the pressure or volume requirements of the general circulation. These losses in function are accompanied by abnormal electrophysiology, which the physician sees as an abnormal electrocardiogram. If the cellular hypoxia is sufficiently severe, irreversible structural and functional damage can occur (heart attack) within minutes.

Nature of Coronary Heart Disease (CHD)

When the coronary arteries become rigid and narrow through atherosclerosis (the process of deposition of lipids in the intima of the arteries), or if the arteries in the inner layers of the heart muscle are being compressed from inside the left ventricle by high pressure, they can no longer adequately compensate for increased amounts of O_2 consumed by the myocardium. A critical ischemia (decreased blood supply) will result, leading to various functional and ultimately structural disturbances discussed below.

Angina Pectoris

Angina pectoris is a severe constricting pain in the chest, often radiating from the precordium (the anterior wall of the chest overlying the heart and great vessels) to the left shoulder and down the left arm. It is due to ischemia of the heart muscle, usually, but not always, caused by coronary disease. This condition is typically transient and reversible in terms of symptoms and associated functional alteration.

The medical diagnostic technique of angiography provides X-ray–type evidence of the closing down of the coronary arteries by the lipid deposits of the atherosclerotic process. Such evidence has shown that clinically manifest myocardial ischemia is usually the result of occlusion of more than 70% of the lumen of one or more arteries (5). A majority of patients with diagnosed CHD such as angina pectoris have major stenoses (narrowing) in

two or three of the major coronary arteries. In less than 30% only one vessel is involved.

The process of atherosclerosis is long term, as the data from autopsies of battle casualties from the Korean War have shown (19). It is obvious that we must become concerned with life-style modifications throughout childhood, adolescence, and adulthood if we are to have optimal chances for success in the prevention of CHD.

Myocardial Infarction

When the myocardial ischemia is of sufficient severity and duration to cause cell death (necrosis), the individual is said to have suffered a myocardial infarction (MI), which the layperson refers to as a heart attack. The area of necrosis has, of course, suffered irreversible damage. The necrotic part of the heart muscle is replaced by noncontractile, fibrous tissue during the healing process. If this area of scar tissue is small, appropriate rehabilitative procedures can improve the contractile function of the remaining muscle tissue so that normal function can be regained. Indeed, one case has been reported in which a well-motivated man not only reversed his loss of function post-MI but succeeded in achieving a work capacity some 44% greater than his pre-MI level (47). This must, of course, be considered an unusual case in which the myocardial damage could not have been extensive, combined with great motivation on the part of the patient. This improvement was maintained over the following fourteen-year period. This case seems to define the outside limits for rehabilitation of CHD patients.

Sudden Death

As was pointed out earlier in this chapter, sudden death accounts for the majority of deaths from CHD. This catastrophic event seems to be the result of ischemic changes that affect the rhythm of the heart, causing such potentially lethal effects as ventricular tachycardia and fibrillation. That such cases of sudden death are, in fact, caused by severe CHD has been shown by postmortem studies in which 75% of the cases were found to have had multivessel involvement (53).

Congestive Heart Failure

Congestive heart failure is a clinical condition resulting from failure of the heart to maintain adequate circulation of the blood. It can happen in the later stages of CHD when tissue loss has resulted in mechanical or pumping inadequacies that lead to venous congestion and edema in the tissues affected by the venous congestion.

Theories Regarding Causation of CHD

Thus far we have exemplified the CHD processes as occurring because of the accumulation of lipid deposits in the walls of the coronary arteries, the process we call atherosclerosis, which was discussed in chapter 13. We pointed out that the level of total serum cholesterol is probably not the most important factor in CHD risk, but rather that the levels of the subfractions of total cholesterol including low density lipoprotein (LDL), very low density lipoprotein (VLDL), and high density lipoprotein (HDL) are crucial in the deposition of lipid plaque on the interior of the coronary vessels. Furthermore, the total cholesterol-HDL ratio is a valuable predictor of CHD (10) and can be favorably modified by exercise training (44, 46). While this atherogenic process probably accounts for much if not most of the prevalent CHD, it must be recognized that there is a considerable fraction of infarction cases in which the coronary arteries are found to be only moderately or even quite insignificantly involved at autopsy.

Wilhelm Raab, a pioneer in preventive cardiology, spent much of his professional lifetime calling our attention to the importance of neurogenic and metabolic factors in the etiology of CHD (*ischemic heart disease* in his terms, since he objected to the term *coronary heart disease* for reasons that will become clear in this discussion). Figure 16.2 illustrates his conception of the pathophysiology involved in CHD. While he recognized the importance of atherosclerosis as the most common predisposing factor in the origin of degenerative heart disease, he deplored the lack of attention directed to the heart muscle's own nerve and hormone regulated metabolic processes. Thus in figure 16.2 one sees the possibilities for interaction among 1) the vascular mechanical factor, 2) the neurogenic-metabolic factors, and 3) the hormonal metabolic factor (56). Note that in this conceptualization, the effect of the decreased O_2 supply brought about by the atherosclerotic process is *potentiated* by the increased O_2 demand due to the sympathetic adrenergic preponderance, thereby exacerbating the myocardial hypoxia. In addition, the increased secretion of cortisol due to emotional stress is synergistic with the myocardial hypoxia in bringing about the electrolyte imbalance that ultimately causes the clinical events seen as angina, myocardial infarction, or sudden death. Raab has presented abundant evidence for the reasonableness of each step, but the total theory remains to be fully tested. Evidence from animal studies has shown that 1) stimulation of certain brain areas can induce cardiac ischemic changes and arrythmias (45); 2) prolonged electrical stimulation of the stellate ganglia produces systolic hypertension and subendocardial hemorrhages in dogs (38); 3) certain types of acute cardiac necroses can be prevented by pretreatment with such stressors as physical exercise and cold baths.

In the human, it has been shown that the first day of imprisonment (serious stress) resulted in consistent findings of ECG changes suggestive of ischemia (41), and there seems to be a consistent relationship between an individual's emotional arousal, whatever its quality, and catecholamine output (42).

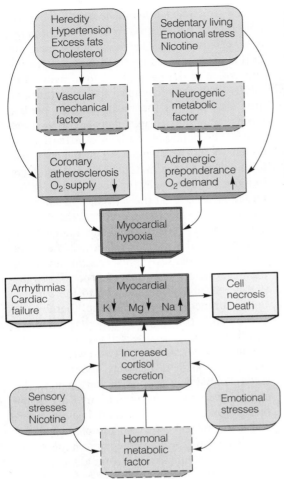

Figure 16.2   Structural formula of pluricausal degenerative, so-called coronary, heart disease. Coordination and integration of today's available clinical and experimental data reveals three interrelated main categories of potentially pathogenic interferences in the heart muscle's electrolyte-dependent functions and structure. Vascular, neurogenic, and hormonal factors appear to be jointly, and in various combinations and degrees, responsible for a typical pattern of electrolyte imbalance throughout the ventricular myocardium—namely: low potassium, magnesium, and K^+/Na^+ ratio; high sodium. Qualitatively uniform, but widely varying in degree, this pattern is characteristically present at autopsy in the following forms of cardiac pathology; subclinical and overt coronary insufficiency, ventricular hypertrophy, congestive heart failure, and myocardial infarction (including the noninfarcted tissue). (From *Annals of the New York Academy of Sciences* 147:666, 1969.)

Friedman and his collaborators at the Harold Brunn Institute in San Francisco have built a case for the importance of personality type A in the predisposition to the development of CHD. It is their position that the major cause of coronary artery and heart disease is a complex of emotional reactions that they designate Type A behavior pattern, which is observed in an "individual who is *aggressively* involved in a *chronic incessant* struggle to achieve more and more in less and less time, and if required to do so, against the opposing efforts of other things or other persons" (26).

Since the inception of this concept in the mid-fifties, they have done voluminous research that supports the importance of individual emotional patterns as strong contributing factors to the etiology of CHD. Friedman has summarized their findings as follows: "Extraordinarily efficient prevention could be achieved if *each of these four* measures was adopted: 1) *drastic* elimination of dietary cholesterol and animal fat, 2) avoidance of behavior pattern A, 3) lifetime participation in an *extensive* degree of physical activity, and 4) exclusion of cigarette smoking" (26).

There is basic agreement between Raab and Friedman in that both accept the importance of the atherosclerotic factor but feel that this is an incomplete picture of what should be considered a pluricausal disease entity, in that neural, hormonal, and metabolic factors (and their emotional antecedents) are important contributors to its cause.

The Risk Factor Concept in CHD

The Framingham study (28) and other epidemiological studies have shown that the likelihood of developing CHD can be predicted for *groups of persons* well in advance of the appearance of symptoms. Among the risk factors are male gender, age over thirty-five, cigarette smoking, elevated blood pressure, high level of serum cholesterol, glucose intolerance, and ECG abnormalities. These are not all-inclusive, as later discussion will show, but they are a set of proven merit widely used by physicians because they can be readily measured by an office nurse or technician without hazard or trauma to the patient (27).

In general, in the use of these risk factor tables, the more risk factors present, or the greater the degree of abnormality of any one factor, the greater the risk. As an example, a forty-year-old man who does not smoke cigarettes, does not have glucose intolerance or ECG abnormalities, but who has a systolic blood pressure of 165 and cholesterol of 285 mg/100 ml, has a probability of 4.9 in 100 of developing CHD within six years. On the other hand a man of the same age who smokes cigarettes, is glucose intolerant, with ECG abnormalities, blood pressure of 195, and cholesterol of 335 mg/100 ml has a probability of 37.1 in 100 of developing CHD in the next six years. These figures compare with the average Framingham male of this age with average values for the risk factors who has a probability of only 2.3 in 100. Even this value is probably much higher than it would be

were we all to live optimal life-styles. Indeed, the work of Paffenbarger and his coworkers suggests strongly that physical inactivity deserves consideration as a primary risk factor (50, 51, 52).

It will be noted in light of the previous discussion that emotional stress and personality factors were not included in the Framingham study. This was apparently because "investigation of a possible relation between 'emotional stress' and CHD has been severely hampered by methodological problems" (35). However, Kannel, a principal in the Framingham study, and his colleagues go on to say, "In spite of these basic difficulties, the concept of emotional stress as a potent force of morbidity and mortality in cardiovascular disease has gained increased prominence and acceptance" (35).

As a follow-up to the Framingham study, the Western Collaborative Group Study (WCGS) considered the same risk factors but also evaluated the effect of personality type A (9). This was a prospective, epidemiological study of 3,154 initially well men. Using the Framingham risk prediction equation, their data over an 8½-year follow-up for CHD correlated well with those taken at Framingham. In addition, they estimated that removal of the excess risk associated with type A behavior would correspond to a 31% reduction of CHD incidence in their WCGS study.

Physiological Bases for Use of Exercise in CHD Prevention

The question may well be asked: On what physiological bases, or through what physiological mechanisms, is physical conditioning likely to be beneficial in the prevention of CHD? Table 16.1 shows the factors that are thought to operate in the direction of such benefit. Recognizing the importance of maximizing the ratio of myocardial O_2 supply to O_2 demand, the table is broken down into those

| Table 16.1 | Physiological Mechanisms that May Have Potential Benefit in the Prevention (or Postponement of Symptomatology) of CHD |

Factors That May Increase Myocardial O_2 Supply	Factors That May Reduce Myocardial O_2 Demand
1. ↑ size of the coronary tree	1. ↓ HR × BP product
2. ↑ collateral circulation	2. ↑ ability to relax tension in skeletal muscles
3. ↑ arterial O_2 saturation	3. ↓ emotional responses
4. ↑ myocardial contractility	4. ↓ obesity
5. ↑ blood volume	5. ↓ resting O_2 consumption by skeletal muscles
6. ↓ blood viscosity	6. ↑ blood distribution
7. ↑ red blood cells	
8. ↑ ventricular pressure	
9. ↑ resting period of cardiac cycle	

Factors Thought to Act in Favor of CHD Risk
Factor Reduction

1. ↓ serum triglycerides
2. ↓ serum cholesterol (in the presence of weight loss)
3. ↑ high density lipoprotein fraction of serum cholesterol
4. ↓ blood coagulability
5. ↑ relaxation and resistance to emotional stress
6. ↓ blood pressure
7. ↑ glucose tolerance
8. ↓ ECG abnormalities

factors that could increase the former and those that may decrease the latter. It should be pointed out that the evidence supporting these various factors ranges from that which is well proven to that which is still largely controversial. For example, the decreased HR × BP product (work of the heart) at any given submaximal work load as a result of physical conditioning is well accepted, while such factors as increased arterial O_2 saturation and improved blood distribution are still controversial.

We must also consider the potential benefits to be derived from the postulated effects of exercise on the aforementioned CHD risk factors described. There seems little doubt that vigorous exercise regimens can have significant effect on some of the physiological mechanisms that are at least statistically related to CHD incidence.

Since the research literature in this area is voluminous, documentation for the above discussion would require hundreds of references. However, we are fortunate that reviews of this literature are available for the interested reader. For the general area of physical activity and cardiovascular health, the reader is referred to Fox, Naughton, and Gorman (23), Hartung (30), and Scheuer and Tipton (59) as well as a series of excellent reviews edited by Bouchard and others (8). For further insight into risk factor modification by chronic physical exercise see Bonanno (7). The control and modification of stress emotions through chronic exercise are well reviewed by Folkins and Amsterdam (22).

Exercise Physiology in Cardiac Rehabilitation

The term *cardiac rehabilitation* rather than the more limiting term *coronary rehabilitation* is used here because the principles and practices to be discussed are as appropriate for patients who have undergone heart surgery for correction of congenital defects or for coronary bypasses as they are for patients with coronary disease, whether they suffer angina pectoris or are postinfarction. Indeed, it is possible that the greatest good might come from including individuals without overt symptoms of CHD who are at high risk for its development.

Naughton (47) defines cardiac rehabilitation as "a form of longitudinal comprehensive care through which selected patients are restored to and maintained at their optimal medical, physiological, psychological, social, vocational, and recreational status." Since one of the more important sequelae of heart disease is usually impairment of physical working capacity (PWC), it is quite natural to see the developing interest of exercise physiologists in this domain. It has been estimated that 80% of the survivors of myocardial infarction should be able to return to work and normal levels of activity (63). However, we probably fall considerably short of this goal, and we hope that the assistance of skilled exercise management by trained physical educators will contribute to the ultimate rehabilitation of the greatest possible numbers.

We have discussed the physiological mechanisms that might be effective in the *prevention* of CHD. Let us now turn our attention to the potential for improvement in PWC and its attendant health benefits by bringing about improvement in general body function when the myocardium has already sustained some measure of insult and is compromised to greater or lesser extent in its functional capacity. We must consider two possible but not mutually exclusive routes to this end: 1) reversal of the losses in myocardial functional capacity, and 2) compensatory improvement in other tissues such as skeletal muscle and organ systems such as the pulmonary system.

In the light of reports that document the capability of CHD patients to run the full marathon (42.2 km) after appropriate training (16) and of the case alluded to earlier of the patient who was able to increase his $\dot{V}O_2$ max by 44% over its preinfarction value (47), it is tempting to believe that at least a partial reversal of myocardial functional losses has occurred. While many investigators have shown very significant improvement in PWC (13, 14, 20, 21, 48, 60), there is as yet no clear evidence for improvement of coronary collateral circulation in humans, although recent evidence suggests improved collateral circulation in dogs by daily exercise (39). Angiographic techniques have not as yet shown any improvement in vascularization; nor does there appear to be an improvement in myocardial O_2 supply (13, 20, 21, 60, 62). Ferguson and associates (20) have provided evidence that strongly suggests that the major effect of exercise training on angina pectoris patients is related to a reduction in O_2 demand (therefore lower coronary flow requirement). They found that symptom-limited exercise capacity improved by 43% with training in their patients. This appeared to be due to a decreased sympathetic drive to the heart and systemic arteries as reflected by lower HR and BP, and lower levels of catecholamines in arterial and coronary sinus blood for a given work load. It was postulated that peripheral adaptive changes in the trained skeletal muscles may be responsible for the decreased sympathetic drive. This is supported by earlier work that showed training to improve blood flow distribution in CHD patients.

Strong evidence to support the importance of physical activity as a prophylactic measure against CHD was provided by Kramsch and associates (40) who put monkeys on a severely atherogenic diet. They found that the monkeys that were exercised had an increase in coronary vessel caliber and a decrease in lesion size that together seemed to reduce, to clinically inapparent levels, the substantial coronary artery narrowing induced in sedentary monkeys by the diet.

Although we may not yet fully understand the physiological mechanisms, there is fairly good agreement about the benefits to be derived from improved functional capacity and reduction in clinical symptoms. To begin with, experience from many different locations around the world has shown that typically only 40% of the patients with MI who survive the acute attack recover sufficiently to resume their original work. On the other hand, it has been repeatedly reported that in groups of patients with MI where a rehabilitation program was applied, 80% or more were able to resume their original work or start a new job (54).

Even more important, Gottheiner (29), one of the pioneers in the use of vigorous exercise conditioning for CHD, showed that 1,103 trainees in his program in Israel had a mortality rate of only 3.6% compared with 12% in a similar series of physically inactive patients.

Data have now been reported from five other longitudinal studies with very similar results (31). However, Haskell (31) points out that there are serious questions as to the comparability of the active and nonactive groups in each study with respect to the severity of illness and the likelihood of reinfarction.

Virtually all investigators have agreed in finding that physical training does increase the exercise angina threshold of most patients who adhere to the program (11, 25, 32, 60). This is of great importance to patients because it may enable participation in everyday life activities that were formerly barred to them. Hellerstein (32), who was one of the American pioneers in this field, showed that ECG responses to exercise also improved in 79% of the rehabilitation patients at the Cleveland clinic who succeeded in improving their physical fitness. This, of course, is related to, and supports the findings of, the increased anginal threshold.

In a very interesting study by Adams, McHenry, and Bernauer (4), it was shown that most subjects trained after MI can achieve the performance levels of normal sedentary subjects, although some do not exhibit a classic training effect, probably because of residual myocardial dysfunction. Successful coronary artery bypass surgery, on the other hand, did not entirely normalize work performance, metabolic or hemodynamic function, but physical training after the bypass surgery resulted in further improvement.

Principles of Exercise Testing in Cardiac Rehabilitation

It should to be noted that the purposes of exercise testing in cardiac rehabilitation are somewhat different from those of exercise testing of normal, healthy individuals, which was discussed in chapter 14. The purposes here are twofold: 1) to *diagnose* ischemic heart disease and investigate physiologic mechanisms underlying cardiac symptoms (angina, arrhythmias, inordinate blood pressure rise, functional valve incompetence), and 2) to *measure functional capacity* for work, sport, or participation in a rehabilitation program or to estimate response to medical or surgical treatment (12).

Physicians often find it necessary to estimate the level of physical activity that is appropriate for a cardiac patient and to prescribe exercise on the basis of mode, intensity, duration, and frequency for those patients who may benefit from such a program. While this sort of exercise testing and prescription lies within the domain of the physician, many doctors have used the assistance of physical educators in the implementation of such programs, just as they were able to improve their effectiveness by employing medical technicians to provide other highly specialized services.

In this area, as with normals, exercise tests can be designed to use steps, treadmill, bicycle, or arm-cranking ergometers. But regardless of the instrumentation, the following principles (12) apply:

1. Continuous step-incremental loading should be used and load intensity should be measurable.

2. The test should start at an exercise load considerably below the estimated level of impairment.

3. Achievement of steady state at each exercise load level is desirable.

4. The minimal parameters to be monitored are blood pressure, heart rate, and the ECG. These must be monitored at rest, at each exercise load, and during recovery.

5. Informed consent should be obtained prior to testing.

6. Commonly used criteria for stopping a test include:

   a. Attainment of true maximum as described in chapter 14.

   b. Attainment of an end point based on emergence of signs or symptoms of a disease process.

   c. Attainment of a predetermined end point, such as 85% of age-related MHR, arbitrary HR as in PWC 150, or diagnostic ECG change.

The normal responses to exercise testing have been discussed in chapter 14. Recognizing abnormal responses is, of course, the primary responsibility of the physician who supervises the test, but the trained physical educator can function as the first line of defense and should have basic knowledge in this regard.

The American Heart Association lists the following responses to exercise testing as abnormal (12):

1. A decrease in, or failure to increase, systolic blood pressure in response to increasing load (indicative of inadequate pump function of the heart).

2. Bradycardia due to the onset of complete heart block or other abnormalities of sinus regulation may occur (generally, individuals with greater impairments of function respond with greater increases in HR to increasing load, even at very low loads).

3. Various ECG abnormalities that are diagnosed by the physician.

4. Symptoms such as chest discomfort or pain, severe dyspnea or faintness, or claudication (pain in exercising muscles due to ischemia).

5. Signs such as pallor, cyanosis, or cold sweat.

Whereas PWC tests on normals typically go to true maximal capacity as described in chapter 14, most clinical investigators use tests that terminate short of maximum. In fact, heart patients often reach a level of discomforting symptoms far below their physiologic maximum. Thus symptom-limited peak performance may and often does differ considerably from physiologic maximum.

While in exercise physiology we generally express exercise loads in terms of power output such as watts or kgm/min, in cardiac rehabilitation it is more common to use the O_2 cost associated with a specific task. The use of the

Table 16.2	Approximate Energy Expenditure in METs During Cycle Ergometry							
Body Weight	**Exercise Rate (kgm/min and Watts)**							
kg lbs	300 / 50	450 / 75	600 / 100	750 / 125	900 / 150	1050 / 175	1200 / 200	(kgm/min) (Watts)
50 110	5.1	6.9	8.6	10.3	12.0	13.7	15.4	
60 132	4.3	5.7	7.1	8.6	10.0	11.4	12.9	
70 154	3.7	4.9	6.1	7.3	8.6	9.8	11.0	
80 176	3.2	4.3	5.4	6.4	7.5	8.6	9.0	
90 198	2.9	3.8	4.8	5.7	6.7	7.6	8.6	
100 220	2.6	3.4	4.3	5.1	6.0	6.9	7.7	

NOTE: $\dot{V}O_2$ for zero load pedaling is approximately 550 ml/min for 70 to 80 kg subjects.
From *American College of Sports Medicine: Guidelines for Exercise Testing and Prescription*, 3d ed. Philadelphia: Lea and Febiger, 1986. Reproduced with permission.

MET as a measure has become popular because it allows better communication with the layperson. The resting $\dot{V}O_2$ is approximately 3.5 ml/kg·min^{-1} and is defined as one MET. Any level of physical activity can then be expressed as a multiple of the O_2 cost of rest, that is, 1 MET, 2 METs, 3 METs, and so on. Tables 16.2 and 16.3 show the energy costs in METs for cycle ergometry and walking, respectively.

According to the New York Heart Association functional class system (34) for evaluating performance of heart disease patients, a patient who becomes limited at 2.0 METs or less is class IV; 3 or 4 METs, class III; 5 or 6 METs, class II; and a patient who achieves 7.0 METs or more is considered class I. Thus class IV shows symptoms at rest, class III shows symptoms with less than ordinary activity, class II shows symptoms with ordinary activity, and class I is not symptom-limited, although clinical evidence such as an abnormal ECG is present.

Parameters to Be Measured

The single most important measurement recorded is, of course, the ECG. Recording and interpretation of the ECG lies in the domain of the physician (usually a cardiologist) who decides the lead system to be used and all pertinent methods and procedures. However, exercise program directors, leaders, and technicians should take every opportunity to learn the basics of ECG analysis. Many cardiologists have found it helpful to provide courses for paramedical personnel dealing with ECG interpretation.

The HR × BP product, sometimes called the double product or rate-pressure product, is a very important measurement because it shows a consistent relationship with angina under various kinds of work load, with anginal pain appearing time and again at the same value of double product (57). The reproducibility of this measurement is excellent (6), and it has now also been validated against measured myocardial O_2 consumption in humans with a correlation of $r = .90$ (37). Thus HR × BP is thought to provide a good estimate of the work of the heart, which is quite different from the total work of the whole body, as was discussed in chapter 15 (fig. 15.3). However, it has also been pointed out by Ellestad (18) that under certain conditions (some

Table 16.3	Approximate Energy Requirements in METs For Horizontal and Grade Walking					
% Grade	mi/hr	1.7	2.0	2.5	3.0	3.4	3.75
	m/min	45.6	53.7	67.0	80.5	91.2	100.5
0		2.3	2.5	2.9	3.3	3.6	3.9
2.5		2.9	3.2	3.8	4.3	4.8	5.2
5.0		3.5	3.9	4.6	5.4	5.9	6.5
7.5		4.1	4.6	5.5	6.4	7.1	7.8
10.0		4.6	5.3	6.3	7.4	8.3	9.1
12.5		5.2	6.0	7.2	8.5	9.5	10.4
15.0		5.8	6.6	8.1	9.5	10.6	11.7
17.5		6.4	7.3	8.9	10.5	11.8	12.9
20.0		7.0	8.0	9.8	11.6	13.0	14.2
22.5		7.6	8.7	10.6	12.6	14.2	15.5
25.0		8.2	9.4	11.5	13.6	15.3	16.8

From *American College of Sports Medicine: Guidelines for Exercise Testing and Prescription*, 3d ed. Philadelphia: Lea and Febiger, 1986. Reproduced with permission.

patients with hypertension and valvular disease) HR alone is a better estimate of the work of the heart than the double product.

It is becoming more common to make some estimate of $\dot{V}O_2$ max when assessing the responses of the postcoronary patient to an exercise rehabilitation program. Kavanagh and Shephard (36) performed tests to $\dot{V}O_2$ max on thirty-six postmyocardial infarction patients and concluded that in patients who have recovered sufficiently to enter an exercise rehabilitation program, predictions of $\dot{V}O_2$ max (as in chap. 14, Astrand test) have about the same accuracy ($\pm 10\%$) as in healthy subjects. They also concluded that direct measurements of $\dot{V}O_2$ max can often be pursued to an O_2 plateau without undue risk. Such a decision will, of course, rest with the physician responsible for each patient. Direct knowledge of the patient's aerobic power can be very helpful in formulating exercise prescription and in monitoring progress.

It should be pointed out that age-adjusted maximum heart rates as used in chapter 15, while valid for healthy subjects, do not hold for cardiac patients (47). Only about 15% of the cardiac population can achieve their age-adjusted MHR without other abnormalities intervening. The remaining 85% will be limited by some abnormality at an HR level 85% or less than age-predicted MHR (47). Some cardiac patients' HR response is lower than predicted at each work load (in the absence of training effect). Ellestad (18) uses the term chronotropic incompetence to describe such responses and has found this to have a bad prognostic implication.

Safety and Litigation Experience

The techniques, safety, and litigation experience of seventy-three medical centers have been surveyed and reported (58). The mortality rate was 16 deaths in 170,000 stress tests, or about 0.01%. The combined incidence of mortality and morbidity was about 0.04%. Successful litigation with an out-of-court settlement was reported in one instance.

For medically supervised cardiac rehabilitation exercise programs with appropriate emergency equipment and drugs available, the risk of a cardiovascular event is small. Recently, Van Camp and Peterson (61) reported one cardiac arrest per 111,996 patient-hours, one myocardial infarction per 293,000 patient-hours, and one fatality per 783,972 patient-hours of exercise.

Exercise Prescription for Cardiac Rehabilitation

In cardiac rehabilitation programs, exercise is no longer just a means for improving health and fitness but becomes a definite therapeutic agent designed to promote a beneficial *clinical* effect. As such, exercise has specific indications and contraindications as well as potential toxic or adverse effects. Therefore the design of the exercise prescription is usually the responsibility of the physician (often with the help of a trained physical educator), and the implementation is carried out by the physical educator under the supervision of the physician.

The American College of Sports Medicine (2) provides recommendations for exercise prescription for inpatient programs (phase I), outpatient programs (phase II), and community exercise programs (phase III).

Phase I Exercise Programs

The goals of inpatient exercise programs are to (2):

1. Provide medical surveillance of patients.
2. Return patients to daily physical activities.
3. Offset the deleterious physiologic and psychologic effects of bed rest.

4. Prepare patients for stages of cardiac rehabilitation that will follow.

Phase I exercise programs are highly supervised with a staff-patient ratio of 1:1. Furthermore, an emergency team should be on the premise and ECG monitoring should be readily available.

The American College of Sports Medicine has provided recommendations regarding contraindications for entry into an exercise program and criteria for ending an inpatient exercise session. These guidelines are a valuable resource for individuals who are responsible for prescribing and monitoring exercise programs for cardiac patients.

The initial phase of the inpatient exercise program usually begins one to three days after surgery or myocardial infarction and involves very low intensity work (2 to 3 METs) (table 15.4 in chapter 15). These activities normally include self-care procedures or arm and leg exercise designed to:

1. Maintain muscle tone.
2. Reduce orthostatic hypotension.
3. Maintain joint mobility.

As early as three to five days after the myocardial infarction or surgery, the patient can begin a walking, treadmill, or cycle ergometer program which, in the beginning, should be performed two to four times per day but last only five to ten minutes per session. The patient's functional capacity is usually not known at this point and therefore should be estimated at approximately 3 to 5 METs.

During this phase of the inpatient program, the intensity of exercise should be approximately 20 to 30 beats per minute above the standing resting heart rate value or an RPE of 12 to 13. As the patient progresses, the duration of the exercise should increase to twenty to thirty minutes performed one to two times per day. The intensity of exercise should be maintained at less than or equal to 5 METs.

Phase II Exercise Programs

Phase II programs are outpatient or home exercise programs designed to continue the progress made during phase I. It is best if phase II programs are administered in hospital settings under close supervision of trained personnel. If this is not possible, however, they can be implemented by patients at home or at a community-based facility. The goals of phase II programs are to

1. Provide physical rehabilitation for resumption of habitual and occupational activities.
2. Promote positive life-style changes.

Phase II programs normally begin within one week of discharge from the hospital and last eight to sixteen weeks. The typical intensity, duration, and frequency prescription for patients in phase II programs who have a functional capacity that is greater than 5 METs is listed below.

1. Intensity = 50% to 85% of functional capacity.
2. Duration = ten to fifteen minutes per session initially and increasing to thirty to sixty minutes as physical fitness improves.
3. Frequency = three to four sessions per week.

For phase II patients with a functional capacity less than or equal to 5 METs, the exercise format for phase I should be used.

Phase III Exercise Programs

Phase III exercise programs are community-based and normally include patients who are six to twelve weeks post-hospital discharge. These programs are ongoing and provide for improvement as well as maintenance of physical fitness. The participants in phase III programs have

1. Clinically stable or decreasing angina.

2. Medically controlled arrhythmias during exercise.
3. A knowledge of symptoms.
4. The ability to self-regulate their exercise.

The prescription for exercise during phase III should be consistent with the recommendation of the ACSM (3) for healthy adults. The gradually increasing program should eventually include a duration of up to sixty minutes per session, an intensity of 50% to 85% of functional capacity, and a frequency of three to five days per week. It is important during phase III to emphasize program adherence and compliance as well as behavior modification. This often requires the use of recreational activities as a supplement to the patient's usual mode of exercise.

Weight Training for Cardiac Rehabilitation

Weight training has not been traditionally prescribed for cardiac rehabilitation because of the potential for transient hypertension and the primary need for improvement in functional aerobic capacity. Recently, however, weight training has been recommended as a supplement to exercise programs that emphasize cardiorespiratory fitness. The American Association of Cardiovascular and Pulmonary Rehabilitation (AACPR) recommends the following guidelines for weight training in cardiac patients (1):

1. To prevent soreness and injury, initially choose a weight that will allow the performance of ten to twelve repetitions comfortably, corresponding to approximately 40% to 60% of the maximum weight load that can be lifted in one repetition. High-risk adults and low-risk cardiac patients should select an initial weight load that can be lifted for twelve to fifteen repetitions.

2. Two to three sets of each exercise is generally recommended.

3. Don't strain! Ratings of perceived exertion (6 to 20 scale) should not exceed "fairly light" to "somewhat hard" during lifting.

4. Avoid breath-holding. Exhale (blow out) on the most strenuous part of an exercise. For example, exhale when lifting a weight stack overhead and inhale when lowering it.

5. Increase weight loads by 5 to 10 pounds when ten to twelve repetitions can be comfortably accomplished; for high-risk adults and cardiacs, weight can be added when twelve to fifteen repetitions can be managed easily.

6. Raise the weight to a count of two and lower the weight gradually to a count of four; emphasize complete extension of the limbs when lifting.

7. Exercise large muscle groups before small muscle groups. Include devices (exercises) for both the upper and lower body.

8. Weight train three times per week.

9. Avoid sustained handgripping when possible, since this may evoke an excessive blood pressure response to lifting.

10. Stop exercise in the event of warning signs or symptoms, especially dizziness, abnormal heart rhythm, unusual shortness of breath, and/or chest pain.

11. Keep moving from one device to another; in other words, don't rest for extended periods between sets.

Program Development

The entire program, including the underlying principles and the methods to be used, must be explained to the patient at the beginning of the program. The collaborative efforts of physician and physical educator probably result in the best communication.

1. *Physiological Basis of the Disease.* The patient needs to be aware of the rudimentary anatomy and physiology underlying the cardiac disease processes. Well-prepared audiovisual aids can help the patient understand the limitations imposed by heart disease and also the potential for rehabilitation.

2. *Physiological Basis for Rehabilitation.* The principles of training and conditioning as presented in chapter 15 can be used to help the patient better understand what the rehabilitation program is all about.

3. *Monitoring Heart Rate.* Since the best single parameter for monitoring the response of the patient to the combined stresses of the exercise plus environment is the exercise heart rate, the patient must be taught how to take his or her own pulse rapidly and accurately. Heart rate can also be easily monitored using a cardiomonitor system.

4. *Precautions to Be Observed.* The patient should be made aware of the various symptoms and their meaning. His or her own sensing of special types of discomfort or distress may signal the presence of an adverse response. The patient should be clearly informed that these are signals to stop or reduce the intensity of effort. Above all, the patient must be impressed with the fact that overdoing is counterproductive, even for normal individuals, as well as hazardous for the cardiac patient.

It must also be pointed out in the clearest terms that there is to be no interindividual competition. Those who have led competitive lives may need frequent admonishment. This point is important not only because of potential overdoing but also because of the doubly hazardous likelihood of undesirable catecholamine responses.

5. *Prevention of Muscle Soreness.* Previous investigators have reported rather large dropout rates due to muscle and joint soreness (43, 55). However, it is possible to minimize this problem, even when working with individuals in their seventh, eighth, and ninth decades in jog-walk training programs (15). The important points here are 1) start at a level well within the individual's capacity; 2) use very gentle progression in increasing the intensity and duration; 3) minimize accelerated and decelerated (jerky) movements; and most important, 4) apply the static stretching principles of chapter 25 following each workout.

6. *Retesting Schedule.* According to the American Heart Association recommendations, the patient should report back to the physician after the first week to discuss heart rate responses, symptomatic responses, and exercise pattern. Within six weeks, the patient should be reevaluated clinically and probably also by tolerance test or simple ECG monitoring to revise the exercise prescription (12).

7. *Is Athletic Competition Possible?* The discussion thus far has dealt only with the program in the early (and probably most hazardous) period in the rehabilitation program. How far can the individual go with respect to picking up old interests in competitive athletics and such physically demanding activities as marathon running? The answer to this question depends to the greatest extent on the severity of the disease processes, and these can be evaluated only by the skilled cardiologist. However, the outer boundaries have been explored, and while the results of investigation in this field cannot be termed conclusive, they do permit some cautious optimism for those with lesser levels of coronary disease.

As early as 1968, Hellerstein, one of our American pioneers in cardiac rehabilitation, reported on 254 CHD patients whose training results were very impressive. Outstanding among his patients was a forty-two-year-old businessman who had suffered a documented myocardial infarct and who trained to the point where he could run 5 miles in thirty-nine minutes without ischemic changes or discomfort (32). This compares favorably with the outstanding results found by Naughton (47) on one patient and reported on earlier in this chapter. Perhaps the most startling evidence of high level performance by CHD patients was furnished by Gottheiner, of Tel Aviv, Israel. deVries had the good fortune to listen to Gottheiner's presentation in Rome at the sports medicine meeting held in conjunction with the 1960 Olympics where he presented movie evidence of his patients performing in competition in sprint running, distance running, and even weight lifting. It was not until some years later that his data were published. They showed that great care in selection of patients and training over periods of several years preceded such performances (29).

Gottheiner used a progressive classification system of seven levels of physical activity groups. Three were preparatory and the upper four were sports classes. Class 1 started with breathing exercises and slow walking for twenty minutes per day. In accordance with their cardiac status, the class 1 participants added warming-up and strength-building exercises to enter classes 2 and 3. Admission to the lowest level sports class (class 4) was usually possible after nine months of preparation. Further progression was slower until qualification for participation in competitive sports teams in class 7 was attained.

Gottheiner's results over the years, involving some 3,000 subjects to the date of his report, showed 55% graduating through all seven classes, 25% reaching classes 5 and 6, and 20% remaining in the lower classes. These data appear overly optimistic, however, in that 910 of the 3,000 were precardiacs with no definite cardiovascular diagnosis. The philosophy is worthy of consideration in that the program for rehabilitation by means of outdoor sports activities, including certain competitive sports, offers more variety and stimulation than most exercise programs, which may result in emotional, environmental, and physical advantages. Whether such a program is feasible in the medicolegal environment of the United States is another question.

More recent evidence regarding high-level performance by CHD patients showed that five patients with recent histories of disease ranging from asymptomatic to severe coronary artery disease were capable, after a training program of long distance running, to compete in the 1974 Honolulu marathon (standard course of over 26 miles) (16). Thus it is possible for at least some carefully selected CHD patients to undergo and benefit by a rigorous aerobic conditioning program, but this requires close medical supervision and careful coaching.

Summary

1. Evidence from autopsies performed on battle casualties of the Korean War suggest that the majority of young people have the beginnings of coronary artery disease.

2. It seems likely that health and physical education professionals can make important contributions to improving the life-style of the American population at all ages through instructing people in the appropriate use of physical conditioning, weight control, improvement of nutrition, and relaxation skills.

3. The myocardium is capable of very little anaerobic metabolism, and since O_2 extraction is already close to maximum at rest, the heart is almost completely dependent on increased coronary blood flow to meet the increased O_2 demand of exercise.

4. Angina pectoris is a severe constricting pain in the chest that results from ischemia in the heart muscle usually caused by coronary artery disease. It is typically transient and reversible when myocardial O_2 demand is decreased to the level of the O_2 supply made available by the coronary arteries.

5. When myocardial ischemia is of sufficient severity and duration to cause cell death, the individual is said to have suffered a myocardial infarction, which the layman calls a heart attack.

6. Sudden death accounts for the majority of deaths from CHD and is due to ischemic changes that affect the rhythm of the heart, causing such potentially lethal effects as ventricular tachycardia and fibrillation with ultimate cardiac standstill and death.

7. Although the major cause of CHD is undoubtedly the occlusion of the coronary arteries by atherosclerotic plaque formation, some cardiologists believe that neurogenic-metabolic factors and hormonal effects contribute.

8. It is also believed by some cardiologists that personality pattern type A, which is typified by aggressive involvement in a chronic, incessant struggle for achievement, is an important determinant of CHD.

9. Epidemiological studies have identified the most important risk factors for CHD as male gender, age over thirty-five, smoking, high blood pressure, high serum cholesterol, glucose intolerance, and ECG abnormalities.

10. While physiological evidence for the therapeutic and prophylactic effects of exercise with respect to CHD is still inconclusive, many physiological changes known to be affected by conditioning can be mustered to support this hypothesis. Important literature reviews are available and cited.

11. It has been estimated that 80% of the survivors of myocardial infarction should be able to return to work and normal levels of physical activity.

12. While many investigators have demonstrated significant improvement in PWC after cardiac rehabilitation, there is as yet no clear evidence for improvement of coronary collateral circulation in humans.

13. Recent evidence suggests that the major effect of exercise training on angina patients is related to a reduction in myocardial O_2 demand.

14. Available evidence suggests that exercise training in CHD results in a considerable reduction in mortality rate.

15. Virtually all investigators seem to find that exercise training results in an increased angina threshold.

16. Most subjects trained after a heart attack can achieve the performance levels of normal, untrained sedentary subjects.

17. Normal and abnormal responses of the CHD patient to exercise testing are defined and discussed.

18. The minimal parameters to be measured and recorded in CHD patient exercise testing are ECG, and HR and BP from which the double product is calculated. Also desirable is the measurement of $\dot{V}O$ with all possible derived parameters.

19. In a survey of seventy-three medical centers that had conducted a total of 170,000 exercise stress tests, the mortality rate among cardiac patients was 0.01%, and the combined mortality and morbidity rate was 0.04%. Successful litigation with an out-of-court settlement was reported in one case.

20. A recent report indicated that for a medically supervised cardiac rehabilitaton program there was one fatality per 783,972 patient-hours of exercise.

21. For CHD patients, exercise intensity must be prescribed by the physician on the basis of maximal limits determined by *symptoms* instead of by performance, as used with normals.

22. The CHD patient should be educated before entering the rehabilitation program about the nature of the limitations imposed by the disease and the potential for improvement as well as about methods of HR monitoring and important precautions to be observed.

References

1. American Association of Cardiovascular and Pulmonary Rehabilitation. *Guidelines for Cardiac Rehabilitation Programs.* Champaign, IL: Human Kinetics Books, 1991.

2. American College of Sports Medicine. *Guidelines for Exercise Testing and Prescription.* Philadelphia: Lea and Febiger, 1986.

3. American College of Sports Medicine. The recommended quantity and quality of exercise for developing and maintaining cardiorespiratory and muscular fitness in healthy adults. *Med. Sci. Sports Exerc.* 22:265–74, 1990.

4. Adams, W. C., McHenry, M. M., and Bernauer, E. M. Long-term physiologic adaptations to exercise with special reference to performance and cardiorespiratory function in health and disease. *Exercise in Cardiovascular Health and Disease,* eds. E. A. Amsterdam, J. H. Wilmore, and A. N. DeMaria. New York: Yorke Medical Books, 1977.

5. Amsterdam, E. A., and Mason, D. T. Coronary artery disease: pathophysiology and clinical correlations. *Exercise in Cardiovascular Health and Disease,* eds. E. A. Amsterdam, J. H. Wilmore, and A. N. DeMaria. New York: Yorke Medical Books, 1977.

6. Blomquist, G., and Atkins, J. M. Repeated exercise testing in patients with angina pectoris: Reproducibility and follow-up results. Abstract of paper to American Heart Association, Anaheim, Calif., 1971.

7. Bonanno, J. A. Coronary risk factor modification by chronic physical exercise. *Exercise in Cardiovascular Health and Disease,* eds. E. A. Amsterdam, J. H. Wilmore, and A. N. DeMaria. New York: Yorke Medical Books, 1977.

8. Bouchard, C., Shephard, R. J., Stephens, T., Sutton, J. R., and McPherson, B. D. *Exercise, Fitness and Health.* Champaign, IL.: Human Kinetics Books, 1990.

9. Brand, R. J., Rosenman, R. H., Shultz, R. I., and Friedman, M. Multivariate prediction of coronary heart disease in the western collaborative group study compared to the findings of the Framingham Study. *Circulation* 53:348–55, 1976.

10. Castelli, W. P., Garrison, R. J., Wilson, P. W. F., Abbott, R. D., Kalousdian, S., and Kannel, W. B. Incidence of coronary heart disease and lipoprotein cholesterol levels: The Framingham Study. J.A.M.A. 256:2835–36, 1986.

11. Clausen, J. P., Larsen, O. A., and Trap-Jensen, J. Physical training in the management of coronary artery disease. *Circulation* 40:143–54, 1969.

12. Committee on Exercise, American Heart Association. *Exercise Testing and Training of Individuals with Heart Disease or at High Risk for Its Development: A Handbook for Physicians.* New York: The Association, 1975.

13. Costill, D. L., Branam, G. E., Moore, J. C., Sparks, K., and Turner, C. Effects of physical training in men with coronary heart disease. *Med. Sci. Sports* 6:95–100, 1974.

14. Cunningham, D. A., Ingram, K. J., and Rechnitzer, P. A. The effect of training: Physiological responses. *Med. Sci. Sports* 11:379–81, 1979.

15. deVries, H. A. Physiological effects of an exercise training regimen upon men aged 52–88. *J. Geront.* 25:325–36, 1970.

16. Dressendorfer, R. H., Scaff, J. H., Wagner, J. O., and Gallup, J. D. Metabolic adjustments to marathon running in coronary patients. *Ann. N.Y. Acad. Sci.* 301:466–83, 1977.

17. Eckstein, R. W. Effect of exercise and coronary artery narrowing on coronary collateral circulation. *Circ. Res.* 5:230–35, 1957.

18. Ellestad, M. H. *Stress Testing, Principles, and Practice.* Philadelphia: F.A. Davis Company, 1975.

19. Enos, W. F., Holmes, R. H., and Beyer, J. Coronary disease among United States soldiers killed in action in Korea. *J.A.M.A.* 152:1090–93, 1953.

20. Ferguson, R. J., Cote, P., Gauthier, P., and Bourassa, M. G. Changes in exercise coronary sinus blood flow with training in patients with angina pectoris. *Circulation* 58:41–47, 1978.

21. Ferguson, R. J., Petitclerc, R., Choquette, G., Chaniotis, G., Gauthier, P., Huot, R., Allard, C., Jankowski, L., and Campeau, L. Effect of physical training on treadmill exercise capacity, collateral circulation, and progression of coronary disease. *Am. J. Cardiol.* 34:764–69, 1974.

22. Folkins, C. H., and Amsterdam, E. A. Control and modification of stress emotions through chronic exercise. *Exercise in Cardiovascular Health and Disease,* eds. E. A. Amsterdam, J. H. Wilmore, and A. N. DeMaria. New York: Yorke Medical Books, 1977.

23. Fox, S. M., Naughton, J. P., and Gorman, P. A. Physical activity and cardiovascular health. *Mod. Concepts Cardiovasc. Dis.* 41:17–20, 1972.

24. Fox, S. M., and Paul, O. Physical activity and coronary heart disease. *Am. J. Cardiol.* 23:298–306, 1969.

25. Frick, M. H., and Katila, M. Haemodynamic consequences of physical training after myocardial infarction. *Circulation* 37:192–202, 1968.

26. Friedman, Meyer. *Pathogenesis of Coronary Artery Disease.* New York: McGraw-Hill Book Co., 1969.

27. Gordon, T., and Kannel, W. B. *Coronary Risk Handbook.* New York: American Heart Association, 1973.

28. Gordon, T., Sorlie, P., and Kannel, W. B. Coronary heart disease, atherothrombotic brain infarction, intermittent claudication—a multivariate analysis of some factors related to their incidence: Framingham Study, 16-year follow up, Section 27. Washington, D.C.: U.S. Government Printing Office, 1971.

29. Gottheiner, V. Long-range strenuous sports training for reconditioning and rehabilitation. *Amer. J. Cardiol.* 22:426–35, 1968.

30. Hartung, G. H. Physical activity and coronary heart disease risk—a review. *Am. Correct. Ther. J.* 31:110–15, 1977.

31. Haskell, W. L. Physical activity after myocardial infarction. *Am. J. Cardiol.* 33:776–83, 1974.

32. Hellerstein, H. K. Exercise therapy in coronary disease. *Bull. N.Y. Acad. Med.* 44:1028–47, 1968.

33. Holman, R. L., McGill, H. C., Strong, J. P., and Geer, J. C. The natural history of atherosclerosis: The early aortic lesions as seen in New Orleans in the middle of the 20th century. *Am. J. Pathol.* 34:209–35, 1958.

34. Hurst, J. W., and Logue, B., eds. *The Heart.* New York: McGraw-Hill, 1974.

35. Kannel, W. B., Castelli, W. P., Verter, J., and McNamara, P. M. Relative importance of factors of risk in the pathogenesis of coronary heart disease: the Framingham Study. *Coronary Heart Disease,* eds. H. I. Russek and B. L. Zohman. Philadelphia: J. B. Lippincott Co., 1971.

36. Kavanagh, T., and Shephard, R. J. Maximum exercise tests on "postcoronary patients." *J. Appl. Physiol.* 40:611–18, 1976.

37. Kitamura, K., et al. Hemodynamic correlates of myocardial oxygen consumption during upright exercise. *J. Appl. Physiol.* 32:516–22, 1972.

38. Klouda, M. A., and Randall, W. C. Subendocardial hemorrhages during stimulation of the sympathetic cardiac nerves. *Prevention of Ischemic Heart Disease,* ed. W. Raab, pp. 49–56. Springfield: Charles C Thomas, 1966.

39. Knight, D. R., and Stone, H. L. Alterations of ischemic cardiac function in normal heart by daily exercise. *J. Appl. Physiol.* 55:52–60, 1983.

40. Kramsch, D. M., Aspen, A. J., Abramowitz, B. M., Kreimendahl, T., and Hood, W. B. Reduction of coronary atherosclerosis by moderate conditioning exercise in monkeys on an atherogenic diet. *New Eng. J. Med.* 305:1483–89, 1981.

41. Lapiccirella, V. Emotion-induced cardiac disturbances and possible benefits from tranquil living. *Prevention of Ischemic Heart Disease,* ed. W. Raab, pp. 212–16. Springfield: Charles C Thomas, 1966.

42. Levi, L. Life stress and urinary excretion of adrenaline and noradrenaline. *Prevention of Ischemic Heart Disease,* ed. W. Raab, pp. 85–95. Springfield: Charles C Thomas, 1966.

43. Mann, G. V., Garrett, H. L., Farhi, A., Murray, H., and Billings, F. T. Exercise to prevent coronary heart disease. *Am. J. Med.* 46:12–27, 1969.

44. Marti, B., Suter, E., Riesen, W. F., Tschopp, A., Wanner, H. U., and Gutzwiller, F. Effects of long-term, self-monitored exercise on the serum lipoprotein and apolipoprotein profile in middle-aged men. *Atherosclerosis* 81:19–31, 1990.

45. Melville, K. I. Cardiac ischemic changes induced by central nervous system stimulation. *Prevention of Ischemic Heart Disease,* ed. W. Raab, pp. 31–38. Springfield: Charles C Thomas, 1966.

46. Mendoza, S. G., Carrasco, H., Zerpa, A., Briceno, Y., Rodrigues, F., Speirs, J., and Gluek, C. J. Effect of physical training on lipids, lipoproteins, apolipoproteins, lipases, and endogenous sex hormones in men with premature myocardial infarction. *Metabolism* 40:368–77, 1991.

47. Naughton, J. Cardiac rehabilitation: Principles, techniques, applications. *Exercise in Cardiovascular Health and Disease,* eds. E. A. Amsterdam, J. H. Wilmore, and A. N. DeMaria. New York: Yorke Medical Books, 1977.

48. Neill, W. A. Coronary and systemic circulatory adaptations to exercise training and their effects on angina pectoris. *Exercise in Cardiovascular Health and Disease,* eds. E. A. Amsterdam, J. H. Wilmore, and A. N. DeMaria. New York: Yorke Medical Books, 1977.

49. Ornish, D., Brown, S. E., Scherwitz, L. W., Billings, J. H., Armstrong, W. T., Ports T. A., McLanahan, S. M., Kirkeeide, R. L., Brand, R. J., and Gould, K. L. Can lifestyle changes reverse coronary heart disease? *Lancet* 336:129–33, 1990.

50. Paffenbarger, R. S., and Hale, W. E. Work activity and coronary heart mortality. *New Eng. J. Med.* 292: 545–50, 1975.

51. Paffenbarger, R. S., Hale, W. E., Brand, R. J., and Hyde, R. T. Work energy level, personal characteristics and fatal heart attack: A birth-cohort effect. *Am. J. Epidemiol.* 105:200–13, 1977.

52. Paffenbarger, R. S., Wing, A. L., and Hyde, R. T. Physical activity as an index of heart attack risk in college alumni. *Am. J. Epidemiol.* 108:161–75, 1978.

53. Perper, J. A., Kuller, L. H., and Cooper, M. Arteriosclerosis of coronary arteries in sudden, unexpected deaths. *Circulation,* suppl. 3, 52:27–33, 1975.

54. Pisa, Z. Programme of the European office of WHO in rehabilitation of cardiac patients. *Acta Cardiol.,* suppl. 14, 1970.

55. Pollock, M. L., Gettman, L. R., Milesis, C. A., Bah, M. D., Durstine, L., and Johnson, R. B. Effects of frequency and duration of training on attrition and incidence of injury. *Med. Sci. Sports* 9:31–36, 1977.

56. Raab, W. Myocardial electrolyte derangement: Crucial feature of pluricausal so-called coronary heart disease. *Ann. N.Y. Acad. Sci.* 147: 627–86, 1969.

57. Robinson, B. F. Relation of heart rate and systolic blood pressure to the onset of pain in angina pectoris. *Circulation* 35:1073–83, 1967.

58. Rochmis, P., and Blackburn, H. Exercise tests—a survey of procedures, safety, and litigation experience in approximately 170,000 tests. *J.A.M.A.* 217:1061–66, 1971.

59. Scheuer, J., and Tipton, C. M. Cardiovascular adaptations to physical training. *Ann. Rev. Physiol.* 39:221–51, 1977.

60. Sim, D. N., and Neill, W. A. Investigation of the physiological basis for increased exercise threshold for angina pectoris after physical conditioning. *J. Clin. Invest.* 54:763–70, 1974.

61. Van Camp, S. P., and Peterson, R. A. Cardiovascular complications of outpatient cardiac rehabilitation programs. J.A.M.A. 256:1160–63, 1986.

62. Verani, M. S., Hartung, G. H., Hoepfel-Harris, J., Welton, D. E., Pratt, C. M., and Miller, R. R. Effects of exercise training on left ventricular performance and myocardial perfusion in patients with coronary artery disease. *Am. J. Cardiol.* 47:797–803, 1981.

63. Wenger, N. K., Hellerstein, H. K., Blackburn, H., et al. Uncomplicated myocardial infarction; current physician practice in patient management. *J.A.M.A.* 224:511–14, 1973.

17

Metabolism and Weight Control

Body Weight and Health

Physiology of Weight Gain and
Weight Loss
*Metabolism of Carbohydrate, Fat,
and Protein*

What Is Normal Weight?

Methods for Estimating Body
Composition
Underwater Weighing
Measurement of Body Volume
Hydrometric Method
*Estimation of Body Fat from
Skinfold Measures*
*Bioelectrical Impedance Analysis
(BIA)*
*Near-Infrared Spectophotometry
(NIR)*

Gaining Weight

Reducing Weight
*Recommendations of the American
College of Sports Medicine
Regarding Weight Loss Programs*
Etiology of Obesity
The Fat Cell Theory
*Feasibility of Weight Loss through
Exercise*
*Misconceptions in Exercise and
Weight Control*
Metabolic Aftereffects of Exercise
What Kind of Exercise Is Best?
Dieting to Lose Weight

Water Retention in Weight Reduction
Programs

Spot Reducing

The Long-Haul Concept of Weight
Control

Weight control is a major component of physical fitness. We immediately recognize the desirability of normal weight in respect to appearance. In physical performance obesity is a distinct disadvantage because a large proportion of the body weight that does not contribute to performance must nevertheless be moved at a definite cost in terms of energy. Thus an athlete who carries an excess twenty pounds of fat would compete on equal terms with athletes of normal weight only if they were forced to carry twenty-pound weights about their middle.

Most important, obesity has been shown to be associated with increased incidence of diabetes, gallstones, high blood pressure, and heart disease. Hubert and colleagues (29) found that obesity was an independent risk factor for cardiovascular disease even when adjusted for the confounding influence of other risk factors including age, cholesterol, systolic blood pressure, cigarette smoking, left ventricular hypertrophy, and glucose intolerance. Our society has learned only very recently to produce food in superabundance, and only in the industrially advanced cultures. Consequently, obesity as an endemic problem is also relatively new. As with most emerging health problems, passage of time is required before the facts can be sifted from the misinformation and conventional wisdom. It is the purpose of this chapter to synthesize the experimentally established facts into a practical approach to the problem of weight control.

Body Weight and Health

Andres (2) has provided some interesting data regarding the concept of an ideal (healthy) body weight. Figure 17.1 describes the relationships for the ratio of actual to expected mortality (percent) versus body mass index (BMI = body weight divided by height squared: kg/m^2) for a variety of diseases and causes of death in forty- to sixty-nine-year-old men.

This figure clearly demonstrates that the relationship between the risk of death and BMI is disease specific. For example, with respect to heart and circulatory diseases, artery disease, and diabetes mellitus, a low body weight (at a given height) is beneficial. For other diseases, however, such as hypertensive heart disease, vascular lesions of the central nervous system, and nephritis, the greatest risk of death is associated with both low and high body weights. Interestingly, death from pneumonia and influenza as well as suicide is more likely to occur with a low body weight. These data should provide much food for thought for professionals who routinely council individuals with respect to body weight goals in an attempt to improve health and increase longevity.

Physiology of Weight Gain and Weight Loss

We must first recognize the fact that the human organism is a heat exchange engine and, although "wondrously and fearfully" constructed, must obey all the physical laws that govern energy exchange. The net energy exchange that expresses the process of metabolism most simply can be written:

Caloric balance =
    kilocalories from food − (kilocalories of basal metabolism + kilocalories of work metabolism + kilocalories lost in excreta)

It can be seen that if the energy intake exceeds the energy outgo, an individual is in positive energy (caloric) balance. Since the law of the conservation of energy tells us that energy can neither be gained nor lost but only changed in form, we must look for this energy to be deposited in the form of body fat, which is indeed what happens. One gram of fat produces (or can be considered equal to) approximately 9.3

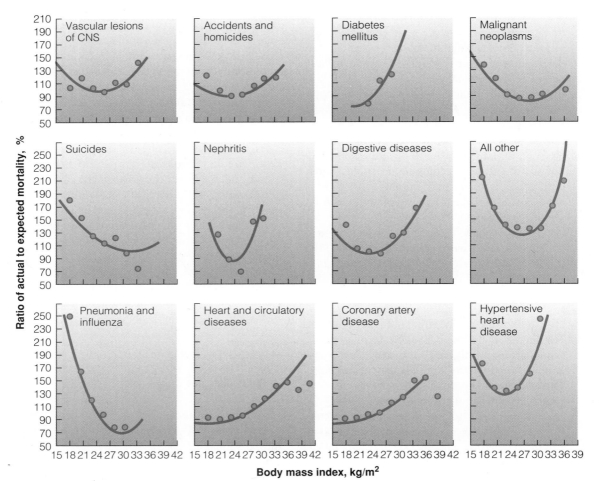

Figure 17.1   Effect of body mass index on specific causes of death. Data for men aged 40 to 69. (Note: From "Discussion: Assessment of Health Status" by R. Andres. In *Exercise, Fitness, and Health* (pp. 135) by C. Bouchard, R. J. Shepard, T. Stephens, J. R. Sutton, and B. D. McPherson (Eds.), 1990. Champaign, IL: Human Kinetics. Copyright 1990 by Human Kinetics Publishers, Inc. Reprinted by permission.)

kcal. Allowing for the water content and connective tissue in fat tissue, one pound of fat will be deposited in the body when an excess of approximately 3,500 kcal has been consumed. That is, one pound of fat equals approximately 3,500 kcal.

Conversely, if the energy expended is greater than the energy consumed, there is a negative caloric balance. For a negative balance of 3,500 kcal, a pound of fat would be lost.

A most important point here is that the metabolism equation does not dictate the *rate* at which weight can be gained or lost. Obviously a pound of weight is lost if we have a negative caloric balance of 3,500 kcals at a rate of 100 kcals per day for thirty-five days or 350 kcals for ten days. In the first case we lose one pound in thirty-five days and in the second case one pound in ten days. Many people have been discouraged from using exercise to reduce weight because of misleading salesmanship that said that one needed to walk for thirty-six hours or perform some other ridiculously heavy work load to lose one pound of weight. It is indeed undesirable, as well as impossible, to lose one pound per day in this fashion. However, by applying only a very low level of salesmanship and *sound physiology,* we might say that walking an extra half hour per day would result in a weight loss of five pounds per year. It is the *long haul* that counts.

Metabolism of Carbohydrate, Fat, and Protein

One may ask how fatty tissue comes to be deposited—in keeping with the energy balance equation—if a person eats a balanced diet that consists of all three basic foodstuffs (carbohydrates, fat, and protein), or even a pure carbohydrate or protein diet. The discussion in chapter 3 and figure 3.2 illustrates the fact that the three different foodstuffs have a common path in the final stages of their metabolic breakdown.

In the case of a negative caloric balance, as exists during dieting, it is easy to understand how stored fat may be used as a source of energy. In fact, the fatty tissues that are found beneath the skin between the muscles and padding the viscera are in a constant state of flux. Neutral fat from the blood constantly replenishes the fat stores of the various fat cells, which release them when they are needed for energy purposes.

When a positive energy balance exists, synthesis of fat (triglycerides) from the excess carbohydrate or protein occurs in the liver and is transported to the fat cells. Some synthesis of fat from glycerol and fatty acids also occurs in the fat tissue cells themselves. In this fashion, weight gain (of fatty tissues) occurs when the food intake (energy) is greater than the energy output.

Although the basic laws of energy balance are always applicable, evidence is accumulating that people vary in the methods by which they metabolize food (21), and because of this there are differences in the efficiency with which food is converted into energy. Differences in the efficiency of food utilization probably account for the fact that some people can "eat like a horse" and remain thin, while others "eat like a bird" and become obese.

What Is Normal Weight?

Overweight and *underweight* are widely used terms and imply that we know what constitutes normal weight for a given individual. Ordinarily, normal weight is predicted from tables that have been developed by insurance actuaries and that provide minimum, average, and maximum weights for any given age, height, and gender. But does such a table really tell us one's proper weight? We could answer yes only if the data from which the tables were calculated were taken from a population of people whose weights were normal. Obviously this situation does not exist.

By the use of such age-height-weight tables, gross errors are not uncommon in assessing normal weight. For example, a man six feet tall, with a very light skeletal framework, might be 30 to 40 pounds overweight at 200 pounds, whereas an extremely muscular man might be at his best weight for athletic competition at 200 pounds.

Furthermore, age-height-weight tables commonly allow small increments in body weight with increasing age, and this concept also is erroneous. U.S. Air Force standards have been recommended that do not allow weight increases with age. These tables essentially retain the current recommended weight for ages twenty-six through thirty as applicable to all ages. This is a more logical approach to the prediction of normal weight because of evidence that during each decade after age twenty-five the body loses about 3% of its metabolically active cells. If this loss of tissue is replaced, it is probably replaced by fat tissue, so that even if an individual maintains constant weight while growing older, that person probably carries an increasing proportion of fat tissue. Obviously, it is the proportion of fat tissue in the body's composition rather than the reading on a scale that is of paramount importance to health and performance.

According to U.S. Air Force standards, 115% of the standard weight is defined as overweight. For young males, *obesity* is frequently defined as the condition in which more than 20% of the body weight is composed of fat tissue. Thirty percent is the cut-off point for females.

When fifty-one male USAF personnel were compared by these two standards (61), it was found that fifteen males who were not 15% over the standard weight were nevertheless obese (more than 20% body fat). Furthermore, six men who would have been considered overweight by the tables were found to have less than 20% body fat, and consequently were not really obese. Thus twenty-one of the fifty-one cases would have been incorrectly classified by use of the age-height-weight tables alone. This clearly illustrates the need for estimation of body composition rather than a complete reliance on tables of averages. It should be obvious that being overweight due to a preponderance of bone and muscle does not have the same significance as being overweight due to fatty tissue. Fortunately, methods have been devised for determining the relative proportions of fat and fat-free tissues of the body.

Methods for Estimating Body Composition

Underwater Weighing

It is common knowledge that fat people float better than thin people. This is because fat tissue is less dense than water as well as other tissues (except lung tissue). Consequently, underwater weighing, which provides measures of body density and specific gravity, can provide reasonably accurate estimates of the proportions of fat-free weight and *body fat tissue* (34). Such estimates are based on measurements of cadaver proportions of lean and fat tissue and their calculated relationship to total body density. This underwater weighing method is highly reliable (8, 33) and has become the standard against which all other methods are compared and evaluated. However, as pointed out by Wilmore (62, 63), this method rests on the following assumptions:

1. The densities of the fat and lean components are known.

2. The densities of the components are relatively constant among individuals.

3. The density of individual tissues of the lean component, for example, bone and muscle, are constant within and among individuals, and their proportional contribution to the density of the lean component remains constant.

4. The individual being assessed differs from the standard "reference person" only in the amount of depot fat.

Obviously these assumptions are not entirely true, particularly for populations such as children (37), adolescents (37), and the elderly (63). Violations of these assumptions can result in errors in the validity of percent body fat estimations from underwater weighing. Lohman (36) has suggested that the total error for a specific population in estimating percent body fat from body density using the underwater weighing technique is $\pm$ 2.5% fat. In spite of the potential error, underwater weighing is presently considered the best technique for estimating body composition (fig. 17.2).

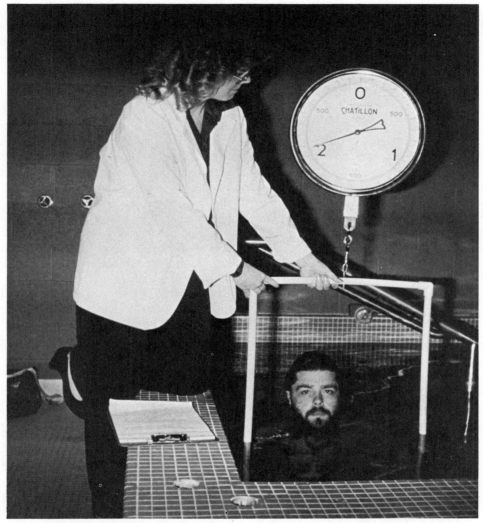

Figure 17.2   Subject being submerged for underwater weighing to determine body density, which allows estimation of body composition (percent of body fat). Courtesy of Fitness Research Center, University of Michigan/Gary Helfand, photographer.

In this procedure the subject is completely submerged. Then, by Archimedes's principle, an individual's specific gravity is calculated:

$$\text{Specific gravity} = \frac{\text{Dry weight}}{\text{Loss of weight in water}}$$

This value must be corrected for residual lung volume, which is determined by a nitrogen washout of the lungs or oxygen dilution technique. With the corrected specific gravity, one may enter tables to arrive at the percent of body fat. The normal body fat percentage for young men has been estimated at 10% to 15% by various investigators; the normal value for young women is slightly higher (15%–20%).

Measurement of Body Volume

Specific gravity of the human body can also be calculated if its volume is known.

$$\text{Specific gravity} = \frac{\text{Weight of body (dry)}}{\text{Weight of equivalent}} \atop {\text{volume of water}}$$

This technique also involves complete submersion of the subject, with measurement of the water displaced by the introduction of the subject's body into a small tank called a *volumeter* whose shape is such that small volume changes make large changes in water level. The measurement must be corrected for residual lung volume.

Hydrometric Method

This method depends on the principle that the proportion of fat-free body weight that is water can be assumed to be constant at approximately 72%. Therefore, any of the chemical methods by which the dilution of a solute by the body water can be calculated can yield data on the total body water and, indirectly, the fat-free body weight. This is usually done by having a subject drink a measured amount of *heavy water,* deuterium oxide. Since this heavy water is handled by the human body in exactly the same way as regular water, the amount of deuterium oxide excreted in the urine can be used as the basis for calculating total body water. The calculation for fat-free body weight is simply:

$$\text{Fat-free weight} = \frac{\text{Total body water}}{0.72}$$

The methods discussed thus far require considerable time and laboratory facilities. Simpler methods have been proposed that depend on skinfold measures to estimate subcutaneous fat tissue or on a combination of anthropometric measures to estimate the size of the bony framework. These methods are less accurate, but are nevertheless far better criteria of the degree of obesity or normality of body weight than age-height-weight tables.

Estimation of Body Fat from Skinfold Measures

Over the past several decades many studies have dealt with the use of skinfold measurements to estimate body fatness. Different investigators have used different body sites at which skinfolds were measured and have developed various regression equations relating the thickness of the various skinfolds to the percentage of fat, measured by underwater weighing as the criterion variable. To add further confusion, until very recently no one had developed a procedure that could be applied to both genders and all ages.

Pollock, Schmidt, and Jackson (54), however, have provided regression equations for both genders and all ages for estimating percent of body fat from the sum of three standard skinfolds. Tables 17.1 and 17.2 provide the data for women and men, respectively. Several different skinfold caliper instruments are available that provide accurate measurements under constant skinfold pressure. The pressure between the caliper jaws should be 10 grams/mm^2 regardless of the width of the jaws. The skinfold is grasped firmly by the thumb and index finger, with the caliper perpendicular to the fold at approximately a point one centimeter (¼ to ½ in) from the thumb and finger. Then the caliper grip is released so that full tension is exerted on the skinfold. In grasping the skinfold, the pads at the tip of thumb and finger are used. The dial is read to the nearest 0.5 mm (Lange) and 0.1 (Harpenden) approximately one to two seconds after the grip has been released. A minimum of two measurements should be taken at each site. If the repeated measurement varies by more than one millimeter, a third should be taken. If consecutive fat measurements become

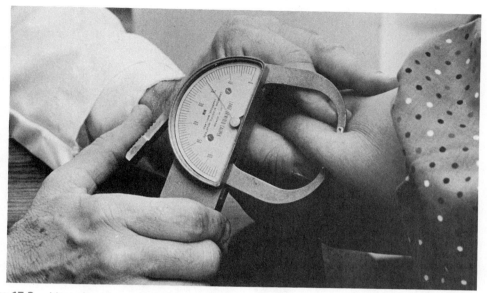

Figure 17.3   Measuring triceps skinfold for estimation of body composition. © John Anderson/Southern Stock

smaller and smaller, the fat is being compressed. This occurs mainly with fleshy people. The tester should go on to the next site and return to the trouble spot after finishing the other measurements. The final value will be the average of the two that seem to best represent the skinfold fat site. It is better to take measurements when the skin is dry because when the skin is moist or wet the tester may grasp extra skin (fat) and get larger values. Practice is necessary to grasp the same size of skinfold consistently at exactly the same location every time. (fig. 17.3.)

For women the sum of skinfolds at the triceps, suprailium, and thigh are used and for men the sum of chest, abdominal, and thigh. The exact locations are as follows:

Chest: a diagonal fold taken one-half of the distance between the anterior axillary line and nipple for men.

Triceps: a vertical fold on the posterior midline of the upper arm (over triceps muscle),

halfway between the acromion and olecranon processes. The elbow should be extended and relaxed.

Abdominal: a vertical fold taken at a lateral distance of approximately two centimeters from the umbilicus.

Suprailium: a diagonal fold above the crest of the ilium at the spot where an imaginary line would come down from the anterior axillary line.

Thigh: a vertical fold on the anterior aspect of the thigh, midway between hip and knee joints.

Having obtained these three skinfold values, one takes the sum and enters the appropriate column in table 17.1 or 17.2 to arrive at the estimated value of fat content as a percentage of body weight (with a standard error of less than 4% body fat). Morbidity and mortality statistics are needed to define the optimal value of percent body fat for good health. In the absence of such data, reasonable values

Table 17.1	Percent Fat Estimates for Women: Sum of Triceps, Suprailium, and Thigh Skinfolds*							
	Age to the Last Year							
Sum of Skinfolds (mm)	**Under 22**	**23 to 27**	**28 to 32**	**33 to 37**	**38 to 42**	**43 to 47**	**48 to 52**	**53 to 57**	**Over 58**
23–25	9.7	9.9	10.2	10.4	10.7	10.9	11.2	11.4	11.7
26–28	11.0	11.2	11.5	11.7	12.0	12.3	12.5	12.7	13.0
29–31	12.3	12.5	12.8	13.0	13.3	13.5	13.8	14.0	14.3
32–34	13.6	13.8	14.0	14.3	14.5	14.8	15.0	15.3	15.5
35–37	14.8	15.0	15.3	15.5	15.8	16.0	16.3	16.5	16.8
38–40	16.0	16.3	16.5	16.7	17.0	17.2	17.5	17.7	18.0
41–43	17.2	17.4	17.7	17.9	18.2	18.4	18.7	18.9	19.2
44–46	18.3	18.6	18.8	19.1	19.3	19.6	19.8	20.1	20.3
47–49	19.5	19.7	20.0	20.2	20.5	20.7	21.0	21.2	21.5
50–52	20.6	20.8	21.1	21.3	21.6	21.8	22.1	22.3	22.6
53–55	21.7	21.9	22.1	22.4	22.6	22.9	23.1	23.4	23.6
56–58	22.7	23.0	23.2	23.4	23.7	23.9	24.2	24.4	24.7
59–61	23.7	24.0	24.2	24.5	24.7	25.0	25.2	25.5	25.7
62–64	24.7	25.0	25.2	25.5	25.7	26.0	26.2	26.4	26.7
65–67	25.7	25.9	26.2	26.4	26.7	26.9	27.2	27.4	27.7
68–70	26.6	26.9	27.1	27.4	27.6	27.9	28.1	28.4	28.6
71–73	27.5	27.8	28.0	28.3	28.5	28.8	29.0	29.3	29.5
74–76	28.4	28.7	28.9	29.2	29.4	29.7	29.9	30.2	30.4
77–79	29.3	29.5	29.8	30.0	30.3	30.5	30.8	31.0	31.3
80–82	30.1	30.4	30.6	30.9	31.1	31.4	31.6	31.9	32.1

are between 10% to 15% body fat for males and 15% to 20% body fat for females. When a male reaches 20% and a female 30%, obesity is at hand.

Bioelectrical Impedance Analysis (BIA)

The concept of BIA for estimating body composition rests on the differences between fat and fat-free tissue in the conduction of an applied electrical current (4, 9, 38). Fat-free weight has a greater electrolyte content than adipose tissue and therefore more readily conducts electrical current (4, 9). The BIA procedure involves placing surface electrodes on the wrist and ankle and applying a pain-free electrical current. The resistance to the flow of the current is then measured. Normally, the resistance (expressed in ohms) is included in

Sum of Skinfolds (mm)	Under 22	23 to 27	28 to 32	33 to 37	38 to 42	43 to 47	48 to 52	53 to 57	Over 58
				Age to the Last Year					
83–85	30.9	31.2	31.4	31.7	31.9	32.2	32.4	32.7	32.9
86–88	31.7	32.0	32.2	32.5	32.7	32.9	33.2	33.4	33.7
89–91	32.5	32.7	33.0	33.2	33.5	33.7	33.9	34.2	34.4
92–94	33.2	33.4	33.7	33.9	34.2	34.4	34.7	34.9	35.2
95–97	33.9	34.1	34.4	34.6	34.9	35.1	35.4	35.6	35.9
98–100	34.6	34.8	35.1	35.3	35.5	35.8	36.0	36.3	36.5
101–103	35.3	35.4	35.7	35.9	36.2	36.4	36.7	36.9	37.2
104–106	35.8	36.1	36.3	36.6	36.8	37.1	37.3	37.5	37.8
107–109	36.4	36.7	36.9	37.1	37.4	37.6	37.9	38.1	38.4
110–112	37.0	37.2	37.5	37.7	38.0	38.2	38.5	38.7	38.9
113–115	37.5	37.8	38.0	38.2	38.5	38.7	39.0	39.2	39.5
116–118	38.0	38.3	38.5	38.8	39.0	39.3	39.5	39.7	40.0
119–121	38.5	38.7	39.0	39.2	39.5	39.7	40.0	40.2	40.5
122–124	39.0	39.2	39.4	39.7	39.9	40.2	40.4	40.7	40.9
125–127	39.4	39.6	39.9	40.1	40.4	40.6	40.9	41.1	41.4
128–130	39.8	40.0	40.3	40.5	40.8	41.0	41.3	41.5	41.8

*Percent fat calculated by the formula of Siri. Percent fat = $[(4.95/BD) - 4.5] \times 100$, where BD = body density.

From M.L. Pollock, D.H. Schmidt, and A.S. Jackson. Compr. Ther. 6:12–27, 1980.

a regression equation with height and body weight to estimate body density, percent body fat, or fat-free weight.

Lukaski (40) and Jackson (31) and their coworkers have reported reliability coefficients of $r > 0.95$ for test-retest BIA measurements. The validity coefficients for body composition determined from BIA versus underwater weighing are normally $r > 0.70$ with standard error of estimate values that range from approximately 1.9 to 3.8 kg of fat-free weight and 2.7 to 4.4 percent body fat (9, 31, 39, 40, 49, 56, 57, 60). Recent studies, however, have questioned the utility of BIA (31, 53). It has been suggested that the accuracy with which BIA equations estimate body composition is a function of the variance accounted for by height and body weight. Jackson and coworkers (31) reported that body mass

Table 17.2 Percent Fat Estimates for Men: Sum of Chest, Abdominal, and Thigh Skinfolds*

Sum of Skinfolds (mm)	Age to the Last Year								
	Under 22	23 to 27	28 to 32	33 to 37	38 to 42	43 to 47	48 to 52	53 to 57	Over 58
8–10	1.3	1.8	2.3	2.9	3.4	3.9	4.5	5.0	5.5
11–13	2.2	2.8	3.3	3.9	4.4	4.9	5.5	6.0	6.5
14–16	3.2	3.8	4.3	4.8	5.4	5.9	6.4	7.0	7.5
17–19	4.2	4.7	5.3	5.8	6.3	6.9	7.4	8.0	8.5
20–22	5.1	5.7	6.2	6.8	7.3	7.9	8.4	8.9	9.5
23–25	6.1	6.6	7.2	7.7	8.3	8.8	9.4	9.9	10.5
26–28	7.0	7.6	8.1	8.7	9.2	9.8	10.3	10.9	11.4
29–31	8.0	8.5	9.1	9.6	10.2	10.7	11.3	11.8	12.4
32–34	8.9	9.4	10.0	10.5	11.1	11.6	12.2	12.8	13.3
35–37	9.8	10.4	10.9	11.5	12.0	12.6	13.1	13.7	14.3
38–40	10.7	11.3	11.8	12.4	12.9	13.5	14.1	14.6	15.2
41–43	11.6	12.2	12.7	13.3	13.8	14.4	15.0	15.5	16.1
44–46	12.5	13.1	13.6	14.2	14.7	15.3	15.9	16.4	17.0
47–49	13.4	13.9	14.5	15.1	15.6	16.2	16.8	17.3	17.9
50–52	14.3	14.8	15.4	15.9	16.5	17.1	17.6	18.2	18.8
53–55	15.1	15.7	16.2	16.8	17.4	17.9	18.5	19.1	19.7
56–58	16.0	16.5	17.1	17.7	18.2	18.8	19.4	20.0	20.5
59–61	16.9	17.4	17.9	18.5	19.1	19.7	20.2	20.8	21.4
62–64	17.6	18.2	18.8	19.4	19.9	20.5	21.1	21.7	22.2
65–67	18.5	19.0	19.6	20.2	20.8	21.3	21.9	22.5	23.1
68–70	19.3	19.9	20.4	21.0	21.6	22.2	22.7	23.3	23.9
71–73	20.1	20.7	21.2	21.8	22.4	23.0	23.6	24.1	24.7

index (body weight divided by height squared) was more highly correlated with percent body fat than a BIA equation that used height, body weight, and resistance. Pennock (53) has also questioned the accuracy of BIA for estimating change in body composition.

Further research is necessary to examine the accuracy of BIA for estimating body composition in various athletic and nonathletic populations. Presently, it is questionable if the expense of a bioelectrical impedance analyzer is justified given the comparable accuracy of skinfold procedures.

Near-Infrared Spectophotometry (NIR)

The estimation of body composition using NIR procedures is based on the principles of light

Sum of Skinfolds (mm)	Age to the Last Year								
	Under 22	23 to 27	28 to 32	33 to 37	38 to 42	43 to 47	48 to 52	53 to 57	Over 58
74–76	20.9	21.5	22.0	22.6	23.2	23.8	24.4	25.0	25.5
77–79	21.7	22.2	22.8	23.4	24.0	24.6	25.2	25.8	26.3
80–82	22.4	23.0	23.6	24.2	24.8	25.4	25.9	26.5	27.1
83–85	23.2	23.8	24.4	25.0	25.5	26.1	26.7	27.3	27.9
86–88	24.0	24.5	25.1	25.7	26.3	26.9	27.5	28.1	28.7
89–91	24.7	25.3	25.9	26.5	27.1	27.6	28.2	28.8	29.4
92–94	25.4	26.0	26.6	27.2	27.8	28.4	29.0	29.6	30.2
95–97	26.1	26.7	27.3	27.9	28.5	29.1	29.7	30.3	30.9
98–100	26.9	27.4	28.0	28.6	29.2	29.8	30.4	31.0	31.6
101–103	27.5	28.1	28.7	29.3	29.9	30.5	31.1	31.7	32.3
104–106	28.2	28.8	29.4	30.0	30.6	31.2	31.8	32.4	33.0
107–109	28.9	29.5	30.1	30.7	31.3	31.9	32.5	33.1	33.7
110–112	29.6	30.2	30.8	31.4	32.0	32.6	33.2	33.8	34.4
113–115	30.2	30.8	31.4	32.0	32.6	33.2	33.8	34.5	35.1
116–118	30.9	31.5	32.1	32.7	33.3	33.9	34.5	35.1	35.7
119–121	31.5	32.1	32.7	33.3	33.9	34.5	35.1	35.7	36.4
122–124	32.1	32.7	33.3	33.9	34.5	35.1	35.8	36.4	37.0
125–127	32.7	33.3	33.9	34.5	35.1	35.8	36.4	37.0	37.6

*Percent fat calculated by the formula by Siri. Percent fat $= [(4.95/BD) - 4.5] \times 100$, where BD = body density.

From M. L. Pollock, O. H. Schmidt, and A. S. Jackson. Compr. Ther. 6:12–27, 1980.

absorption and reflection (38). The NIR instrumentation includes a fiber-optic probe or "light wand," which emits low level electromagnetic radiation light waves at approximately 940 and 950nm (nonionizing and nondamaging) to a selected site on the body such as the biceps, triceps, subscapular, suprailiac, or thigh (10, 18, 38). A detector then measures the intensity of the light (optical density = OD) that is re-emitted from the measurement site for both wavelengths. The amount of light energy reflected back to the probe by the tissue contains information about the chemical composition of the sample (38). The OD values are then used in an equation with other variables such as gender, body weight, height, and exercise level to estimate percent body fat (18).

Davis and others (12) reported a test-retest intraclass reliability coefficient for NIR measurements of body composition of R = 0.94. Recent studies have also examined the validity of NIR. Conway and others (10) reported a validity coefficient of $r = 0.94$ for percent body fat estimates from NIR versus deuterium oxide dilution for a combined sample of males and females that was heterogeneous in terms of age (range = 23 to 65 years) and percent body fat (mean ± SD = 29.1 ± 8.7%). Houmard (28) and Israel and their coworkers (30) compared percent body fat estimates from NIR to those from underwater weighing in college football players and healthy active males, respectively. In both studies, NIR significantly underestimated percent body fat. For white males, the underestimation averaged approximately 3% body fat. For black football players in Houmard's study, the underestimation exceeded a mean of 7% body fat. Thus, in young, athletic males the error associated with body composition estimates from NIR are too large to be of practical value. Houmard has suggested that the magnitude of the error "may involve application of a generalized prediction equation to a specific population or use of an inappropriate body site (bicep) as an index of whole-body fat content." Although it is not possible to derive definitive conclusions from the limited available research, the utility of NIR for estimating body composition in various populations is not presently supported.

Gaining Weight

The purposeful gaining of weight is a problem for a relatively small segment of our population. However, some persons desire to pad a slender or frail frame for purposes of appearance, and sometimes to provide a greater mass for body contact sports, such as football. It is obvious from the foregoing that this can be accomplished simply by ingesting more calories (in the form of food) than are spent in energy every day. For some individuals this constitutes a problem because they have a prodigious energy output due to a restless (nervous) temperament. Furthermore, this approach to the problem results in deposition of fat tissue that—beyond the normal values mentioned earlier—is not desirable.

The best method for gaining weight for any normal, healthy young individual consists of an exercise program designed to provide muscular hypertrophy with a minimum of energy expenditure. This type of exercise is best provided by professionally directed weight training and almost invariably results in weight gains—of muscle tissue, not fat. This approach is suitable for females as well as males.

Females frequently express concern about becoming muscular, but gender differences prevent this from happening in all but the most extreme exercise programs. Even in extremely heavy resistance exercise programs, there is little evidence to support the belief that females can develop large muscles. It is more likely that excessively muscular females are seen in heavy resistance sports because of a selective process: they choose to participate in sports in which they will excel.

Reducing Weight

Although the theory underlying weight reduction is beautifully simple, the practice for many millions of Americans is definitely not a simple process after obesity has set in. This is probably due to the interaction of psychological (emotional) and social problems with the physiology underlying the obesity (59).

From the standpoint of energy metabolism, obesity is necessarily the end result of a *positive energy balance*. Although this is a great oversimplification, it will aid temporarily in understanding the problem. From this point of view, only three alternative methods are available for the reduction of weight:

1. Increased energy expenditure and constant food intake.

2. Decreased food intake and constant energy expenditure.

3. A combination of methods 1 and 2.

The first method can be accomplished by exercise programs, the second by diet.

Recommendations of the American College of Sports Medicine Regarding Weight Loss Programs

Based on the existing evidence concerning the effects of weight loss on health status, physiologic processes, and body composition parameters, the American College of Sports Medicine makes the following statements and recommendations for weight-loss programs (1).

For the purposes of this position statement, body weight will be represented by two components, fat and fat-free (water, electrolytes, minerals, glycogen stores, muscular tissue, bone, etc.):

1. Prolonged fasting and diet programs that severely restrict caloric intake are scientifically undesirable and can be medically dangerous.

2. Fasting and diet programs that severely restrict caloric intake result in the loss of large amounts of water, electrolytes, minerals, glycogen stores, and other fat-free tissue (including proteins within fat-free tissues), with minimal amounts of fat loss.

3. Mild calorie restriction (500–1,000 kcal less than the usual daily intake) results in a smaller loss of water, electrolytes, minerals, and other fat-free tissue, and is less likely to cause malnutrition.

4. Dynamic exercise of large muscles helps to maintain fat-free tissue, including muscle mass and bone density, and results in losses of body weight. Weight loss resulting from an increase in energy expenditure is primarily in the form of fat weight.

5. A nutritionally sound diet resulting in mild calorie restriction coupled with an endurance exercise program along with behavioral modification of existing eating habits is recommended for weight reduction. The rate of sustained weight loss should not exceed 1 kg (2 lb) per week.

6. To maintain proper weight control and optimal body fat levels, a lifetime commitment to proper eating habits and regular physical activity is required.

Therefore, a desirable weight loss program is one that (1):

1. Provides a caloric intake not lower than 1,200 kcal/day for normal adults in order to get a proper blend of foods to meet nutritional requirements. (Note: this requirement may change for children, older individuals, athletes, etc.)

2. Includes foods acceptable to the dieter from viewpoints of socio-cultural background, usual habits, taste, cost, and ease in acquisition and preparation.

3. Provides a negative caloric balance (not to exceed 500–1,000 kcal/day^{-1} lower than recommended), resulting in gradual weight loss without metabolic derangements. Maximal weight loss should be 1 kg/week.

4. Includes the use of behavior modification techniques to identify and eliminate dieting habits that contribute to improper nutrition.

5. Includes an endurance exercise program of at least three days a week, 20–30 minutes in duration, at a minimum intensity of 60% of maximum heart rate (refer to ACSM Position Statement on the Recommended Quantity and Quality of Exercise for Developing and Maintaining Cardiorespiratory and Muscular Fitness in Healthy Adults, *Med. Sci. Sports Exerc.* 22:265–274, 1990).

6. Provides that the new eating and physical activity habits can be continued for life in order to maintain the achieved lower body weight.

Etiology of Obesity

Since the easiest *cure* for obesity is prevention, let us consider the etiology of this health problem. A few years back it was fashionable to place the blame for obesity on endocrine malfunction. This was a popular theory because obese people could absolve themselves of blame. Medical research, however, has not substantiated this theory; on the contrary, evidence is accumulating that indicts our sedentary way of life as the real culprit.

Greene (22), who studied 350 cases of obesity, found inactivity was associated with the onset of obesity in 67.5% of the cases and that a history of increased food intake was found in only 3.2%. Pariskova (52), who analyzed the body composition of 1,460 individuals of all ages, concluded: "One of the most important factors influencing body composition is the intensity of physical activity, and this is true in youth, adulthood, and old age." In a study by Corbin and Pletcher (11), using 16 mm movie films to evaluate the activity level of elementary school children, it was shown that body fatness was significantly correlated

($r = -.520$) with lack of physical activity but not with caloric intake ($r = .155$). Many other investigations, too numerous to cite, provide indirect support for the belief that lack of physical activity is the most common cause of obesity. Thus a compelling case can be made for the importance of habitual, lifelong, vigorous physical activity as a preventive measure against obesity.

The Fat Cell Theory

In the past decade much interesting research has been done to elucidate the relationships of fat cell size and number to obesity. Hirsch and Knittle (26) developed a painless method of needle aspiration of adipose tissue from subcutaneous fat depots such as the arm, abdomen, or buttock. From these tissue samples, it is possible to estimate both cell size and number. The results of such research suggest the following:

1. The number of fat cells in the human body is established during periods of rapid growth: (a) the latter part of gestation, (b) the first year of infancy, and (c) adolescence (25).

2. Once established, the number of fat cells appears to be fixed in spite of experimental weight gain or weight loss (7, 23, 58).

3. Nonobese human adults have about 27 billion fat cells, while the obese have from 42 to 106 billion (24).

4. Fat cell size is labile and varies with experimental weight gain or loss.

5. Comparing obese and nonobese human adults, cell size is only some 40% greater, while cell number is about 190% higher in the obese (24).

6. Comparing individuals with varying percentages of ideal weight shows that there is a high correlation between cell number and percent ideal weight ($r = .8117$) but no significant

correlation with cell size (24). Others have found moderate relationships between cell size and percent ideal weight but only up through the range of relatively normal fat levels beyond which cell size no longer relates to total body fat (5, 6).

The sum total of this very interesting research permits a cautious conclusion that gross obesity (typically of childhood-onset) is the result of an abnormally large number of fat cells laid down during growth. Lesser levels of obesity (possibly up to 150% ideal weight and typically adult-onset obesity) appear to be due to enhanced cell size. The latter conclusion is supported by the work of Sims (58), who induced normally nonobese volunteers to greatly increase their body fat by overeating. The size of the adipose cells correlated closely with the increase in body fat, thus suggesting no change in number. Furthermore, Sims saw considerable variability in the ease with which these volunteers could gain weight. There appeared to be a correlation between the ease of weight gain and the fat cell number, thus validating to some extent the complaint of the obese individual that is so commonly heard, "My friend eats like a horse and stays thin, while I eat like a canary and gain weight."

The important question remaining is: To what extent can gross obesity (the increase in cell *number*) be prevented by exercise and/or food restriction? Although we do not yet have data on human subjects, well-controlled studies have been performed by Oscai and his colleagues on rats (50, 51). Their data show quite clearly that significant differences in future weight gain can be brought about by both exercise and dietary restriction during the growth period of rats. To the extent that these data may be extrapolated to the human, it would seem possible to prevent the laying down of excess numbers of adipose cells by providing adequate physical activity for young children and adolescents. Physical activity appears to be even more important than eating habits.

Feasibility of Weight Loss through Exercise

Planned exercise such as jog-walk combinations as a feasible method of weight reduction in the obese, even in the absence of any dietary restriction, has been well demonstrated by Moody, Kollias, and Buskirk (45). Obese college-age women lost on the average 5.3 pounds over an eight-week period in which they participated in about an hour of jogging-walking for an average of four times per week. Skinfold measurements suggested the weight loss was the result of a much larger loss of fatty tissue with a concomitant gain of solid tissue (fat-free weight). This latter observation is very important because the converse is true when weight is lost by fasting. Fasting has been shown to result in weight losses that are, to a large extent, losses in lean body tissue, which is undesirable. Under total fasting conditions, the weight loss due to losses in lean body mass appears to be from 8% (3) to between 30% and 45% (16, 19) of the total weight loss. Zuti and Golding (64) have shown clearly the advantages of including exercise in weight reduction programs. Twenty-five women were randomly assigned to a diet group, an exercise group, or a combination of the two. In each case, a negative caloric balance of 500 kcal/day was established. All the women lost similar amounts of weight, but those who exercised lost more fat and gained lean tissue, while those on diet alone lost lean body mass and lesser amounts of fat.

Can we infer from the above that exercise is also the best means for treating the severely obese? Not necessarily. Although exercise can certainly make a contribution, medical supervision is necessary to protect the severely obese person from overstraining the cardiovascular system, the connective tissues, and so on. For the moderately obese (10% to 30% above predicted normal weight), a combination of diet and exercise is probably the optimal procedure.

Misconceptions in Exercise and Weight Control

Despite the evidence that has been cited in favor of exercise as a means of weight control, in recent years it has been popular to ridicule this practice. Data are sometimes presented that suggest that one needs to run for thirty-five miles or walk for thirty-six hours—or some other ridiculous amount of physical activity—to lose one pound of weight. Two outstanding authorities in the area of nutrition, Mayer and Stare (43), have provided experimental evidence to rectify this and other misconceptions. They have pointed out that it is neither necessary nor desirable to expend the energy required to lose one pound in one exercise bout. Further, "a half hour of handball or squash a day would be equivalent to 19 pounds per year."

Another general misconception is that exercise is not effective in weight reduction because appetite automatically increases in direct proportion to the increased activity. Mayer and colleagues (42) have shown that while appetite follows activity in the range of normal activity in animals, this is not so in the low levels of activity. Figure 17.4 illustrates their work and shows that sedentary animals (those most apt to be obese) actually display a decrease in appetite with an increase of up to one hour of daily exercise. This was corroborated more recently by Dohm and colleagues (15). Mayer and his collaborators have also shown that this principle applies to humans.

Metabolic Aftereffects of Exercise

The increase in metabolic rate incurred during physical activity is the main cause of energy loss. As long ago as 1933, the work of Margaria, Edwards, and Dill (41) mentioned an increased *resting* metabolic rate that lasted for several hours after completion of exercise and that could not be attributed to repayment of oxygen debt.

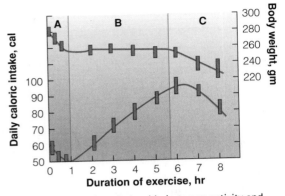

Figure 17.4   The relationship between activity and appetite and the effects upon body weight in animals. (From Mayer, J. et al. Exercise, Food Intake, and Body Weight in Normal Rats and Genetically Obese Adult Mice, in *American Journal of Physiology* 177:546. © 1954 American Physiological Association. Reprinted by permission of the publisher and author.)

This increased metabolic rate was further investigated in deVries's laboratory (14). In a controlled experiment it was found that the resting metabolic rate was from 7.5% to 28% higher four hours after a vigorous workout than it was at the same time of day on *nonexercise* control days. This higher metabolic rate was shown to persist for at least six hours after exercise, and this effect of exercise—over and above the energy cost of the exercise itself—would have resulted in a weight loss of four or five pounds per year if the individuals tested had exercised daily. Figure 17.5 illustrates the results of the experiment.

What Kind of Exercise Is Best?

To be effective in reducing weight, exercise must be of the vigorous, endurance type so that energy expenditure is maximized. In designing such an exercise program, the following seven factors must be considered.

1. The exercise must allow *gradual progression* from low levels to higher levels of energy expenditure.

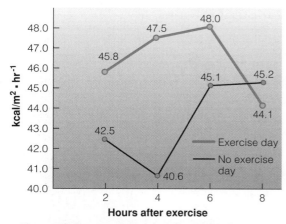

Figure 17.5 Metabolic aftereffects of a vigorous workout compared with a similar day in which no workout was taken. Each experimental point represents the mean of at least six observations for each of two middle-aged male subjects.

2. Participants must be protected from injury to bony and connective tissues in the early stages.

3. The exercise must be vigorous enough to result in increased body heat, as evidenced by sweating.

4. Intensity of the exercise should be as high as possible, consistent with a duration of thirty to sixty minutes. Maximal total energy output cannot be obtained if the musculature is quickly exhausted by a few quick maximal repetitions, as in weight lifting or sprint workouts.

5. Exercise involving large components of anaerobic work does not appear to be as effective as aerobic exercise (20).

6. Soreness should be prevented, or relieved, by the procedures described in chapter 26.

7. After a minimum level of fitness is achieved, the program should be built around activities that are enjoyable and thus self-motivating.

Table 17.3 provides a rather complete survey of the energy requirements of various activities.

For jogging or running, the energy expenditure can be estimated as 1 kcal per kilogram of body weight per kilometer covered (44). Table 17.3 shows the energy costs for various rates of walking. The data for running and walking can be applied to both males and females (17).

Dieting to Lose Weight

Severe dietary restriction is a procedure that requires medical supervision and cannot be properly treated in this text. Moderate dietary restriction, which results in weight losses of one or two pounds per week, can be accomplished by estimating the daily energy expenditure and maintaining a daily food intake of 500 to 1,000 kcals per day below the expenditure level. These figures are readily available in various texts on health and nutrition (13).

Some interesting concepts about the physiology of weight reduction deserve comment here. It has been shown (27) that rats trained to eat their entire daily food ration in one to two hours gain more weight than animals eating ad libitum. It was further demonstrated that the trained rats increased the rate at which their adipose tissue incorporated food breakdown products into lipids (fats) by twenty-five times.

This work was extended and applied to the medical treatment of obesity in humans by Gordon, Goldberg, and Chosy (21). They initiated treatment in obese patients with a forty-eight-hour fast (to break the metabolic pattern of augmented lipogenesis), then instituted a 1,320-kcal diet that consisted of 400 kcals of protein, 720 kcals of fat, and 200 kcals of carbohydrate. This diet was given in six feedings daily, corresponding to breakfast, midmorning, lunch, midafternoon, supper, and bedtime. All feedings were approximately similar in size. They report that results have

Table 17.3   Energy Requirements of Various Activities

Activity or Exercise	METs[1]	Kcal per hr[2]	Activity or Exercise	METs[1]	Kcal per hr[2]
Archery	2–3	150–250	Football (while		
Backpacking	3–8	250–600	active)	6–9	450–700
Badminton			Gardening	2–8	150–600
Social doubles	3–4	250–300	Golf	2–4	150–300
Social singles	6	450	Gymnastics	3–5	250–400
Compet. singles	8–10	600–750	Handball	6–10	450–750
Baseball or softball			Handsawing		
Except pitcher	2–3	150–250	hardwood	6–8	450–600
Pitcher	6	450	Hockey		
Basketball	4–10	300–750	Field	8–10	600–750
Bicycling (on level)			Ice	8–10	600–750
5 mph	3	250	Horseback riding	6–8	480–600
10 mph	6	450	Isometrics	2–5	150–400
13 mph	9	650	Isotonics	2–10+	150–800
Boardsailing	3–8	250–600	Fencing	6–9	450–700
Bowling	1.5–3	100–225	Jogging (see running)		
Calisthenics	2–8	150–600	Karate/Judo	6–10+	450–800+
Canoeing			Kayaking (see		
Flat water	2–8	150–600	canoeing)		
White water	5–10	400–750	Mountain climbing	6–8	450–800
Dancing			Mowing		
Ballet and modern	4–9+	300–700+	Pushing power	3–4	250–300
Vigorous ballroom	3–8+	250–600	Pushing hand	6–8	450–600
Folk and square	3–8+	250–600+	Paddleball/Platform		
"Aerobic"	5–9	300–700	tennis	4–8	300–600
Driving car		170–200			
Fishing					
Casting	2–3	150–250			
Walking with					
waders	4–6	300–500			

been encouraging, and they have been surprised that no patient has complained of hunger at any time, although some have lost as much as 100 pounds.

If these results can be generalized, it would seem that concentrating a large part of the daily food intake into one large meal has unfavorable metabolic consequences (increased lipogenesis, or fat deposition). Furthermore, skipping breakfast seems undesirable. Indeed, if these data are substantiated by other investigators, it suggests that Americans should change their eating patterns.

Water Retention in Weight Reduction Programs

Obese people are very frequently discouraged by the results of their dieting. After one, two, or even three weeks of semistarvation the scale still reads the same. If they have honestly adhered to a negative caloric balance, the reason for this phenomenon is probably water retention. It has been shown that even though body

Activity or Exercise	METs[1]	Kcal per hr[2]	Activity or Exercise	METs[1]	Kcal per hr[2]
Ping-Pong (Table tennis)	4–6	300–450	Skin diving	6–10	450–750
Racquetball	6–10	450–750	Soccer	8–10+	600–750+
Raking leaves	3–5	250–400	Squash	8–10+	600–750
Rope skipping	8–12	600–900	Surfing	4–7	300–500
Rowing			Swimming	4–10+	300–750
2 mph	3	250	Tennis	4–10	300–750
4 mph	7	500	Volleyball	4–7	300–500
6 mph	12	900	Walking (on level)		
Rugby	6–8	450–600	2 mph		
Running and jogging			3 kph	2	150
5 mph	7–8	500–600	3 mph		
7 mph	12	800	5 kph	3+	250
9 mph	15	1100	4 mph		
Sailing			6.5 kph	5–6	400–500
Crew	2–4	150–300	(stairs/hills)	7–12+	500–900
Skipper	1–3	75–200	Waterskiing	4–8	300–600
Sexual intercourse	5–8	400–600	Weight lifting	3–6	250–450
Shovelling	5–9	400–700	Woodsplitting	2–6+	150–500
Skating	4–10+	300–800+	Yoga	1–4	75–300
Skiing					
Cross-country	5–12+	400–900+			
Downhill	4–10+	300–800+			

1. METs = Multiples of resting metabolic rate—when sitting. The range reflects the varying intensity, from the leisurely or recreational pace to the competitive or frenetic.

2. Kilocalories per hour—based on a weight of 70 kg (154 lbs). A 10% increase or decrease can be applied for each 7 kg (15 lbs) over or under 70 kg, respectively.

Data based largely on a paper by Samuel M. Fox, M.D., Preventive Cardiology Program, Georgetown University Medical Center, and presented by W.L. Haskell at N.I.M.H. meeting, Washington, D.C., April 1984.

tissues are being oxidized and the end products excreted, the loss may not be shown by weight because sufficient water is retained by the tissues to offset the weight of the oxidized tissues. This water retention cannot continue indefinitely, however, so the predicted weight change eventually occurs although it may not follow the day-to-day caloric deficit (46). Figure 17.6 illustrates the phenomenon.

The physiology of this water retention can be explained by the fact that the water formed as a by-product of the metabolism of the body's fat stores is not excreted immediately via the kidney in obese subjects because of an increased level of antidiuretic hormones.

Gordon, Goldberg, and Chosy (21) have also demonstrated the *water-binding effect* of consuming an appreciable quantity of concentrated carbohydrate food. A severely obese man, who had been losing weight successfully, was given an 800-gm carbohydrate, 4,000-kcals per day diet for two days. He promptly gained eighteen pounds, which required three weeks to lose. The weight gained was shown to be water.

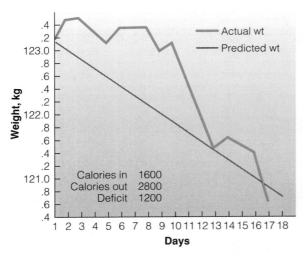

Figure 17.6   Water retention in weight reduction programs. (From Newburgh, L. H. *Physiological Reviews* 28:18. © 1944 American Physiological Association. Reprinted by permission.)

It is extremely important that anyone embarking on a diet to lose weight be aware of these facts so as not to be discouraged when results are delayed by water retention.

Spot Reducing

Women are frequently encouraged to use localized exercises to reduce fatty stores in the areas of greatest fat deposition, usually buttocks, hips, and thighs. Schade and associates (55) conducted an experiment on twenty-two overweight college women in which one group used *spot reducing exercises* and the other general exercise. They concluded there was no significant difference in the effect of spot and generalized exercise on fat distribution in their subjects. Conflicting evidence was reported by Olsen and Edelstein (48). The most convincing evidence against the spot reducing concept is that tennis players whose playing arm showed a mean difference of 2.25 cm in girth (hypertrophy) compared with the non-playing arm nevertheless showed no significant difference in skinfold dimensions (23). A

study by Noland and Kearney (47) supports this position and provides an excellent review of the literature on this subject. Work at the cellular level confirms the ineffectiveness of spot reducing (32, 35).

The best evidence available seems to indicate that in negative caloric balance situations the fat comes off the area of greatest concentration, regardless of how the exercise is performed.

The Long-Haul Concept of Weight Control

It should be emphasized that weight is best controlled as a matter of childhood habit formation, which then automatically takes care of the *long haul*. This habit formation should include the development of physical skills that will permit, indeed encourage and motivate, regular participation in a vigorous activity. Such sports as tennis, badminton, handball, skiing, and horseback riding are ideally suited to lifetime needs since they are vigorous, enjoyable, and can be performed with a minimum of cooperation by other persons. Individuals who develop these skills and participate in them regularly—at least twice and preferably three or four times a week—will seldom have to be unduly concerned about their diet. With normal moderation in eating, including a gradual decrease in caloric intake with age above twenty-five years, they will in all likelihood have no problem with obesity.

When obesity gets a start due to inactivity or overeating, it is wise to apply corrective efforts as early as possible. The corrective measures, exercise and diet, should be set up with habit formation in mind. Thus one cannot set up a habit pattern that involves any of the many popular. *crash diets*. When normal weight is regained, a change is necessary, and all too often the change is a reversion to the pre-diet obesity-causing regimen. A series of cycles of weight gain and loss is then set up, causing discouragement and complete loss of control.

On the other hand, a sensible approach involves a dietary restriction of only 300 to 500 kcals per day, with a progressive buildup of exercise such as an hour of tennis or horseback riding (another loss of 400 to 600 kcals). In this fashion, pleasurable habits can be formed that require no changes and that do not cause the distress of semistarvation on a crash diet. The process may take a little longer, but it will be infinitely more successful.

If the effectiveness of exercise for losing weight is questioned, the layperson can most readily see the answer not in research but in the empirical wisdom of the experience of humankind. Obesity is practically unknown among vigorous, healthy athletes, ditchdiggers, and heavy laborers, many of whom daily consume prodigious amounts of food.

Summary

1. Besides the aesthetic disadvantages, obesity has been shown to be associated with many degenerative diseases.

2. Weight gain and loss follow the laws of thermodynamics. A positive energy balance results in a gain in weight, and a negative energy balance results in a loss.

3. Carbohydrate, fat, and protein follow the same final pathway in their metabolism, and thus fat and protein can substitute for carbohydrate in furnishing energy. All three foodstuffs, if eaten in excess, can result in deposition of fat tissue.

4. Estimation of what constitutes normal or proper body weight is subject to great inaccuracy unless body composition is measured. Scale readings are relatively meaningless unless we know the proportion of the reading that is due to fatty tissues.

5. A gain in weight is best accomplished by heavy resistance, low repetition-type exercise (such as weight training), in which weight gain is brought about through muscular hypertrophy.

6. Weight loss can be accomplished by increased activity (exercise) or dietary restriction. If the weight is not grossly abnormal, a progressive exercise program, although slower, is the sounder approach.

7. Recent biopsy data have shown that the *number* of fat cells is established in early life and does not vary significantly in later life even with gross changes in body fat.

8. The number of fat cells in the nonobese is about 25–30 billion. Grossly obese individuals may have three times as many fat cells as nonobese individuals.

9. Fat cell *size* varies proportionately with body fat changes in a given individual.

10. In rats, the laying down of fat cells and the level of fatness in later life can be influenced by both exercise and diet in the adolescent growth period.

11. Moderate increases in activity level, contrary to popular opinion, do not result in increased food intake if the individual has been sedentary previously.

12. Vigorous exercise not only creates an immediate increase in metabolism, it also brings about a longer lasting (six- to eight-hour) rise in resting metabolism, which further contributes to weight loss.

13. Considerable evidence indicates that concentrating the daily food consumption into one or two large meals results in a greater tendency toward obesity.

14. In dieting to lose weight, a temporary water retention (up to three weeks) may obscure the true fat-tissue loss that is occurring.

15. *Spot reducing* rests on no sound physiological basis. Rather, the best available evidence indicates that regardless of the part of the anatomy exercised, weight loss first occurs in the largest fat deposits.

16. Maintaining normal weight should be a long-term process that involves hygienic habit formation. *Crash diets* are usually foredoomed to failure because they do not accomplish habit formation.

References

1. American College Sports Medicine. Position statement on: Proper and improper weight loss programs. *Med. Sci. Sports Exer.* 15:ix–xi, 1983.

2. Andres, R. Discussion: Assessment of health status. Chap. 12 in *Exercise, Fitness, and Health, A consensus of current knowledge,* ed. C. Bouchard et al., pp. 133–36. Champaign: Human Kinetics Books, 1990.

3. Ashley, B. C. E. Drastic dietary reduction of obesity. *Med. J. Aust.* 1:593–96, 1964.

4. Baumgartner, R. N., Chumlea, W. C., and Roche, A. F. Bioelectric impedance for body composition. Chap. 6 in *Exercise and Sport Sciences Reviews,* ed. K. B. Pandolf and J. O. Holloszy, pp. 193–224. Baltimore: Williams and Wilkins, 1990.

5. Bjorntorp, P., and Sjostrom, L. Fat cell size and number in adipose tissue in relation to metabolism. *Isr. J. Med. Sci.* 8:320–24, 1972.

6. Bonnet, F., Gosselin, L., Chantraine, J., and Senterre, J. Adipose cell number and size in normal and obese children. *Rev. Eur. Etudes Clin. Biol.* 15:1101–4, 1970.

7. Booth, M. A., Booth, M. J., and Taylor, A. W. Rat fat cell size and number with exercise training, detraining and weight loss. *Fed. Proc.* 33:1959–63, 1974.

8. Bouchard, C. Reproducibility of body composition and adipose-tissue measurements in humans. In *Body-Composition Assessments in Youth and Adults,* ed. A. F. Roche, pp. 9–13. Columbus: Ross Laboratories, 1985.

9. Chumlea, W. C., and Baumgartner, R. N. Bioelectric impedance methods for the estimation of body composition. *Can. J. Spt. Sci.* 15:172–79, 1990.

10. Conway, J. M., Norris, K. H., and Bodwell, C. E. A new approach for the estimation of body composition: Infrared interactance. *Am. J. Clin. Nutr.* 40:1123–30, 1984.

11. Corbin, C. B., and Pletcher, P. Diet and physical activity patterns of obese and nonobese elementary school children. *Res. Q.* 39:922–28, 1968.

12. Davis, P. O., Dotson, C. O., and Manny, P. D. NIR evaluation for body composition analysis. *Med. Sci. Sports Exerc.* 20:S8, 1988.

13. deVries, H. A. *Health Science: The Positive Approach.* Glenview, IL: Scott, Foresman, 1979.

14. deVries, H. A., and Gray, D. E. Aftereffects of exercise upon resting metabolic rate. *Res. Q.* 34:314–21, 1963.

15. Dohm, G. L., Beecher, G. R., Stephenson, T. P., and Womack, M. Adaptations to endurance training at three intensities of exercise. *J. Appl. Physiol.* 42:753–57, 1977.

16. Drenick, E. J. The effects of acute and prolonged fasting and refeeding on water, electrolyte and acid-base metabolism. Chap. 32 in *Clinical Disorders of Fluid and Electrolyte*

Metabolism, eds. M. H. Maxwell and C. R. Kleeman. New York: McGraw-Hill, 1972.

17. Falls, H. B., and Humphrey, L. D. Energy cost of running and walking in young women. *Med. Sci. Sports* 8:9–13, 1976.

18. Futrex-5000 Research Manual. Gaithersburg, MD: Futrex Inc., 1991.

19. Gilder, H., et al. Components of weight loss in obese patients subjected to prolonged starvation. *J. Appl. Physiol.* 23:304–10, 1967.

20. Girandola, R. N. Body composition changes in women: effects of high and low exercise intensity. *Arch. Phys. Med. Rehabil.* 57:297–300, 1976.

21. Gordon, E. S., Goldberg, M., and Chosy, G. J. A new concept in the treatment of obesity. *J.A.M.A.* 186:50–60, 1963.

22. Greene, J. A. A clinical study of the etiology of obesity. *Ann. Intern. Med.* 12:1797–1803, 1939.

23. Gwinup, G., Chelvam, R., and Steinberg, T. Thickness of subcutaneous fat and activity of underlying muscles. *Ann. Intern. Med.* 74:408–11, 1971.

24. Hirsch, J. Adipose cellularity in relation to human obesity. *Adv. Intern. Med.* 17:289–300, 1971.

25. Hirsch, J. Can we modify the number of adipose cells? *Postgrad. Med.* 51:83–86, 1972.

26. Hirsch, J., and Knittle, J. Cellularity of obese and nonobese human adipose tissue. *Fed. Proc.* 29:1516–21, 1970.

27. Hollifield, G., and Parson, W. Metabolic adaptations to a "stuff and starve" feeding program. *J. Clin. Invest.* 41:250–53, 1962.

28. Houmard, J. A., Israel, R. G., McCammon, M. R., O'Brein, K. F., Omer, J., and Zamora, B. S. Validity of a near-infrared device for estimating body composition in a college football team. *J. Appl. Sport Sci. Res.* 5:53–59, 1991.

29. Hubert, H. B., Feinleib, M., McNamara, P. M., Castelli, W. P. Obesity as an independent risk factor for cardiovascular disease: A 26-year follow-up of participants in the Framingham Heart Study. *Circulation* 67:968–77, 1983.

30. Israel, R. G., Houmard, J. A., O'Brien, K. F., McCammon, M. R., Zamora, B. S., and Eaton, A. W. Validity of a near-infrared spectrophotometry device for estimating human body composition. *Res. Quart. Exerc. Sport* 60:379–82, 1989.

31. Jackson, A. S., Pollock, M. L., Graves, J. E., and Mahar, M. T. Reliability and validity of bioelectrical impedance in determining body composition. *J. Appl. Physiol.* 64:529–34, 1988.

32. Katch, F. I., Clarkson, P. M., Kroll, W., McBride, T., and Wilcox, A. Effects of sit-ups exercise training on adipose cell size and adiposity. *Res. Q. Exer. Sports* 55:242–47, 1984.

33. Katch, F., Michael, E. D., and Horvath, S. M. Estimation of body volume by underwater weighing: Description of a simple method. *J. Appl. Physiol.* 23:811–13, 1967.

34. Keys, A., and Brozek, J. Body fat in adult man. *Physiol. Rev.* 33:245–325, 1953.

35. Krotkiewski, M., Aniansson, A., Grimby, G., Bjorntorp, P., and Sjostrom, L. The effect of unilateral isokinetic strength training on local adipose and muscle tissue morphology, thickness and enzymes. *Eur. J. Appl. Physiol. Occup. Physiol.* 42:271–81, 1979.

36. Lohman, T. G. Skinfolds and body density and their relation to body fatness: A review. *Human Biol.* 53: 181–225, 1981.

37. Lohman, T. G. Applicability of body composition techniques and constants for children and youths. Chap. 11 in *Exercise and Sports Sciences Reviews,* ed. K. B. Pandolf, pp. 325–57. New York: MacMillan Publishing Co., 1987.

38. Lukaski, H. C. Methods for the assessment of human body composition: Traditional and new. *Am. J. Clin. Nutr.* 46:537–56, 1987.

39. Lukaski, H. C., Bolonchuk, W. W., Hall, C. B., and Siders, W. A. Validation of tetrapolar bioelectrical impedance method to assess human body composition. *J. Appl. Physiol.* 60: 1327–32, 1986.

40. Lukaski, H. C., Johnson, P. E., Bolonchak, W. W., and Lykken, G. I. Assessment of fat-free mass using bioelectrical impedance measurements of the human body. *Am. J. Clin. Nutr.* 41:810–17, 1985.

41. Margaria, R., Edwards, H. T., and Dill, D. B. The possible mechanisms of contracting and paying the O_2 debt, and the role of lactic acid in muscular contraction. *Am. J. Physiol.* 106: 689–715, 1933.

42. Mayer, J., Marshall, N. B., Vitale, J. J., Christensen, J. H., Mashayek, M. B., and Stare, F. J. Exercise, food intake and body weight in normal rats and genetically obese adult mice. *Am. J. Physiol.* 177:544, 1954.

43. Mayer, J., and Stare, F. J. Exercise and weight control: Frequent misconceptions. *J. Am. Diet. Assoc.* 29:340–43, 1953.

44. McMiken, D. F., and Daniels, J. T. Aerobic requirements and maximum aerobic power in treadmill and track running. *Med. Sci. Sports* 8:14–17, 1976.

45. Moody, D. L., Kollias, J., and Buskirk, E. R. The effect of a moderate exercise program on body weight and skinfold thickness in overweight college women. *Med. Sci. Sports* 17:75–80, 1969.

46. Newburgh, L. H. Obesity and energy metabolism. *Physiol. Rev.* 24:18, 1944.

47. Noland, M., and Kearney, J. T. Anthropometric and densitometric responses of women to specific and general exercise. *Res. Q.* 49:322–28, 1978.

48. Olson, A. L., and Edelstein, E. Spot reduction of subcutaneous adipose tissue. *Res. Q.* 39:647–52, 1968.

49. Oppliger, R. A., Nielsen, D. H., Heogh, J. E., and Vance, C. T. Bioelectrical impedance prediction of fat free mass for high school wrestlers validated. *Med. Sci. Sports Exerc.* 23 (suppl.):S73, 1991.

50. Oscai, L. B., Babirak, S. P., Dubach, F. B., McGarr, J. A., and Spirakis, C. N. Exercise or food restriction: Effect on adipose tissue cellularity. *Am. J. Physiol.* 227:901–4, 1974.

51. Oscai, L. B., Babirak, S. P., McGarr, J. A., and Spirakis, C. N. Effect of exercise on adipose tissue cellularity. *Fed. Proc.* 33:1956–58, 1974.

52. Pariskova, J. Impact of age, diet and exercise on man's body composition. In *International Research in Sport and Physical Education,* eds. E. Jokl and E. Simon. Springfield, IL: Charles C Thomas, 1964.

53. Pennock, B. E. Letter to the editor. Sensitivity of bioelectrical impedance to detect changes in human body composition. *J. Appl. Physiol.* 68:2246, 1990.

54. Pollock, M. L., Schmidt, D. H., and Jackson, A. S. Measurement of cardiorespiratory fitness and body composition in the clinical setting. *Compr. Ther.* 6:12–27, 1980.

55. Schade, M., Hellebrandt, F. A., Waterland, J. C., and Carns, M. L. Spot reducing in overweight college women. *Res. Q.* 33:461–71, 1962.

56. Segal, K. R., Gutin, B., Priesta, E., Wang, J., and Van Itallie, T. B. Estimation of human body composition by electrical impedance methods: A comparative study. *J. Appl. Physiol.* 58:1565–71, 1985.

57. Segal, K. R., Van Loan, M., Fitzgerald, P. I., Hodgdon, J. A., and Van Itallie, T. B. Lean body mass estimation by bioelectrical impedance analysis: A four-site cross-validation study. *Am. J. Clin. Nutr.* 47:7–14, 1988.

58. Sims, E. A. H. Studies in human hyperphagia. In *Treatment and Management of Obesity,* eds. G. A. Bray and J. E. Bethune. New York: Harper & Row, 1974.

59. Stunkard, A. J. Obesity and the social environment: current status, future prospects. *Ann. N.Y. Acad. Sci.* 300:298–319, 1976.

60. Van Loan, M., and Mayclin, P. Bioelectrical impedance analysis: Is it a reliable estimator of lean body mass and total body water? *Human Biol.* 59: 299–309, 1987.

61. Wamsley, J. R., and Roberts, J. E. Body composition of USAF flying personnel. *Aerospace Med.* 34:403–5, 1963.

62. Wilmore, J. H. Appetite and body composition consequent to physical activity. *Res. Q.* 54:415–25, 1983.

63. Wilmore, J. H. Body composition in sport and exercise: Directions for future research. *Med. Sci. Sports Exerc.* 15:21–31, 1983.

64. Zuti, W. B., and Golding, L. A. Comparing diet and exercise as weight reduction tools. *Physician and Sportsmed.* 4:49–53, 1976.

18

Growth, Development, and Exercise in Children and Adolescents

Growth, Development, and Maturation
  Infancy, Childhood, and Adolescence
  Puberty
Normal Growth Patterns
  Height and Body Weight
  Body Composition
"Making Weight" in Athletics
Exercise and Aerobic Fitness
  Aerobic Fitness and Endurance
    Performance
  Endurance Training and Aerobic
    Fitness
  Long-Distance Running
Exercise and Anaerobic Fitness
  The Effect of Anaerobic Training

Strength
Weight Training versus Weight Lifting
  versus Body Building
Weight Training during Prepubescence
  and Postpubescence
  Mechanisms of Strength Increases in
    Prepubescent Children
Potential Hazards of Weight Training
  Acute Musculoskeletal Injuries
  Chronic Musculoskeletal Injuries
  Hypertension and Weight Lifter's
    Blackout
Characteristics of a Weight Training
  Program

Many physical educators and coaches work with individuals between the ages of five and eighteen years, especially in public and private schools. Because children's interest and participation in competitive sports has increased dramatically in recent years, professionals must be knowledgeable in the areas of normal growth and development as well as the effects of exercise on young competitors. Athletes, parents, and the community at large frequently ask physical educators and coaches to answer questions regarding the potential benefits and hazards of certain types of exercise for young populations. If a coach or physical educator can answer these questions with scientifically based information he or she can dispel popular but inaccurate myths and make a positive impact on the health and performance of children and adolescents.

Growth, Development, and Maturation

Malina and Bouchard (29) have defined growth, development, and maturation as follows:

1. Growth is an increase in the size of the body as a whole or the size attained by specific parts of the body.

2. Development is often used in two distinct contexts. In a biological context development is the differentiation of cells along specialized lines of function. In a behavioral context it relates to the development of competence in a variety of interrelated domains as the child adjusts to his or her cultural milieu— the amalgam of symbols, values, and behaviors that characterize a population.

3. Maturation refers to the tempo and timing of progress toward the mature biological state.

Clearly, growth, development, and maturation are related concepts and commonly (but incorrectly) used interchangeably. Growth is usually expressed in absolute terms such as the change in height in centimeters (cm) and body weight in kilograms (kg) or as a rate such as change in height or body weight per year (cm per year or kg per year), while maturation reflects the percentage of height or body weight attained compared to adult expectations. For example, increases in height from 138 to 142 centimeters between ten and eleven years of age for a male and female would reflect a similar growth rate (4 cm per year) but it is likely that the male would be less mature since adult males on the average tend to be approximately 12 centimeters taller than adult females. Thus, in this example, at eleven years of age, the female would have attained 87% of her expected adult stature (approximately 163 cm), while the male would have attained only 81% of his expected adult stature (approximately 175 cm). The term development is often used in a broad sense to include both growth and maturation as they relate to the functions of the systems of the body or to the behavior of the child.

Infancy, Childhood, and Adolescence

1. Infancy is defined as the first year of life and is a time of rapid growth in almost all bodily functions and physical characteristics (29).

2. Childhood is defined as the time between the first birthday and puberty and is characterized by steady growth and maturation with particularly rapid progress in motor development (29). The relatively stable rate of growth makes childhood a good time for the introduction and development of motor skills (14).

3. The beginning of adolescence is usually defined by the adolescent growth spurt and the onset of puberty. The adolescent growth spurt normally occurs between 10.5 to 13 years of age in females and 12.5 to 15 years of age in males (14). Malina and Bouchard (29), however, have indicated that the age of adolescence ranges from eight to nineteen and ten to twenty-two years for females and males, respectively. The difference in the age ranges used to define adolescence reflects the high degree of interindividual variability in the maturational status of this age group. Clearly some children are late maturers while others mature much earlier. Differences in maturity are manifested in dramatic differences in strength, sports skill, and performance.

Puberty

The term puberty is derived from the Latin word *pubertas,* which means the period of life at which the ability to reproduce begins or the time of sexual maturation. It is important to be able to identify the onset of puberty because normal growth patterns as well as the responses to exercise training are substantially different in children than they are in adolescents. Coaches, athletes, and physical educators should have very different expectations for a training program depending on the level of maturation of the individuals involved.

In females, the beginning of puberty is the period when breasts normally begin to develop and pubic hair first appears. This is followed by the first menstruation (14). The onset of menarche provides a definitive landmark for the assessment of maturation in females (14). In males, the circulating level of testosterone is an indicator of puberty. During adolescence the testosterone concentration increases 10 to 20 fold from the childhood value of 20 to 60 ng/dl to the adult value of approximately 600 ng/dl (14). In contrast, females exhibit low (prepubescent) testosterone levels throughout life. The measurement of blood testosterone as an indicator of maturational development in males requires invasive procedures, however, which limits its common usage.

Puberty, in both genders, can also be indirectly assessed based on the level of development of secondary sex traits such as the breasts, pubic hair, and genitals. Tanner (29) developed a commonly used technique to assess maturity that uses a 1 to 5 scale based on direct visual observation or nude photographs. Stage 1 is characterized by an absence of development of the secondary sex traits and is clearly prepubertal, while Stage 5 indicates adult standards of maturity. Stages 2, 3, and 4 represent varying levels of development with defined characteristics. Although the stages overlap to some degree, making the judgement somewhat arbitrary, the determination of Tanner stages can be very useful for identifying an individual's approximate level of maturity.

Additional procedures for assessing the timing of the adolescent growth spurt are called peak height velocity and peak weight velocity (figs. 18.1 and 18.2). If longitudinal height and body weight data are available for an individual, it is possible to identify the adolescent growth spurt by examining the yearly change in height or body weight as a function of age. The dramatic increases in height and body weight coincide with the onset of puberty and are reflected in increases in the rate of height and body weight changes from approximately 5 cm per year to 10 cm per year and 3 kg per year to 10 kg per year, respectively (29).

Normal Growth Patterns

Height and Body Weight

Normal growth in height and body weight develop along an S-shaped curve from birth

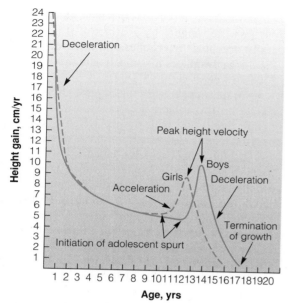

Figure 18.1   Peak height velocity curves (cm/yr) for boys and girls. (From Tanner, J. M., Whitehouse, R. H., and Takaishi, M. "Standards from Birth to Maturity for Height, Weight, Height Velocity, and Weight Velocity: British Children 1965–1" in *Archives of Diseases of Childhood* 41:454–471, 1966. Reprinted by permission.)

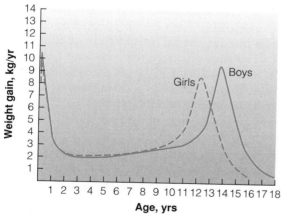

Figure 18.2   Peak weight velocity curves (kg/yr) for boys and girls. (From Tanner, J. M., Whitehouse, R. H., and Takaishi, M. "Standards from Birth to Maturity for Height, Weight, Height Velocity, and Weight Velocity: British Children 1965–1" in *Archives of Diseases of Childhood* 41:454–471, 1966. Reprinted by permission.)

through adolescence (fig. 18.3) (14). During infancy there are rapid increases in both parameters, which are greater than those during childhood. At the time of the adolescent growth spurt, males exhibit a dramatic increase in height and body weight while the growth curves for females begin to level off as they approach adult standards of maturity.

Of interest to coaches, parents, and athletes is the effect of exercise and competitive sports on normal growth and development patterns. That is, does athletic participation have any beneficial or detrimental effect on body size? Malina and Bouchard (29) have answered this question by stating "the experience of athletic training and competition does not appear to accelerate or decelerate the growth and maturation of young athletes. Regular training has no apparent effects on stature, body proportions, physique, or biological maturation."

Body Composition

Figure 18.4 describes the normal growth patterns for percent body fat, fat weight, and fat-free weight from birth to twenty years of age. Fat weight and fat-free weight increase gradually throughout childhood in both males and females. At the adolescent growth spurt, males exhibit an increased rate of development in fat-free weight while females tend to maintain a constant level from approximately fourteen to twenty years of age. Percent body fat increases dramatically during infancy for both genders. Throughout childhood and adolescence, however, females remain stable or increase slightly in percent body fat while males decrease gradually.

Physical activity has beneficial effects on body composition characteristics. In general, active children and adolescents have lower levels of percent body fat and fat weight but more fat-free weight than their inactive peers. Thus, exercise can positively impact athletic performance by aiding in the development of

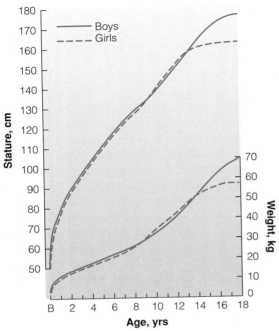

Figure 18.3   Height (cm) and body weight (kg) across age for boys and girls. (Note: From *Growth, Maturation, and Physical Activity* (p. 46) by R. M. Malina and C. Bouchard, 1991. Champaign, IL: Human Kinetics. Copyright 1991 by Robert M. Malina and Claude Bouchard. Reprinted by permission.)

optimal sport-specific body composition characteristics as well as potentially decreasing the health risks associated with obesity.

"Making Weight" in Athletics

Although physical activity and sports participation, per se, do not adversely affect normal growth and development patterns, it is possible that the excessive intentional weight loss called "making weight" associated with such sports as wrestling, boxing, and gymnastics may have detrimental effects. In many sports, competition is organized into divisions by body weight. Also, some states set up high school and junior high school athletics on the basis of

a classification system that depends, at least in part, on the weight of the athletes. It is generally accepted by coaches and athletes that there are advantages to competing in the lowest possible weight class.

For mature athletes, making weight is not a large health problem because experience has taught them what their normal weight should be. However, there are extreme cases of weight loss by high school athletes: on occasion 15 or more pounds in an athlete whose normal weight is 150 to 160 pounds. This practice should be condemned in the strongest terms, for these short-term weight losses are often obtained by drastic changes in caloric intake and water metabolism (sweating, water restriction, starvation, and purging), causing attendant changes in kidney and cardiovascular function (whose consequences are still difficult to evaluate). In secondary school and college athletes, a 5% weight loss should certainly be the outside limit of prudence, and it is quite likely that even this amount (without medical supervision) is too great for some of the leaner athletes.

Recent evidence has shown that not only many high school wrestlers but many NCAA championship team members enter competition in a dehydrated state (50). In an effort to correct such practices, the American College of Sports Medicine (6) issued the following instructions as part of its position stand with respect to weight loss in wrestlers.

1. Assess the body composition of each wrestler several weeks in advance of the competitive season. Individuals with a fat content less than 5% of their certified body weight should receive medical clearance before being allowed to compete.

2. Emphasize the fact that the daily caloric requirements of wrestlers should be obtained from a balanced diet and determined on the basis of age, body surface area, growth, and physical

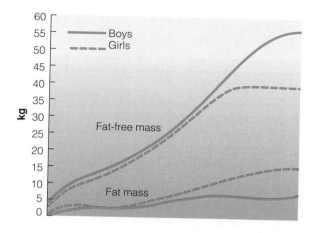

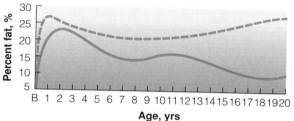

Figure 18.4 Body composition across age for boys and girls. (Note: From *Growth, Maturation, and Physical Activity* (p. 97) by R. M. Malina and C. Bouchard, 1991, Champaign, IL: Human Kinetics. Copyright 1991 by Robert M. Malina and Claude Bouchard. Reprinted by permission.)

activity levels. The minimal caloric needs of wrestlers in high schools and colleges will range from 1,200 to 2,400 kcals/day. Therefore, it is the responsibility of coaches, school officials, physicians, and parents to discourage wrestlers from securing less than their minimal needs without prior medical approval.

3. Discourage the practice of fluid deprivation and dehydration. This can be accomplished by:

   a. Educating the coaches and wrestlers on the physiological consequences and medical complications that can occur as a result of these practices.

   b. Prohibiting the single or combined use of rubber suits, steam rooms, hot-boxes, saunas, laxatives, and diuretics to "make weight."

   c. Scheduling weigh-ins just prior to competition.

   d. Scheduling more official weigh-ins between team matches.

4. Permit more participants per team to compete in those weight classes (119–145 pounds) that have the highest percentages of wrestlers certified for competition.

5. Standardize regulations concerning the eligibility rules at championship tournaments so that individuals can participate only in those weight classes in which they had the highest frequencies of matches throughout the season.

6. Encourage local and county organizations to systematically collect data on the hydration state of wrestlers and its relationship to growth and development.

Exercise and Aerobic Fitness

Maximal O_2 uptake is often used as an indicator of aerobic fitness because it reflects the efficiency of the cardiorespiratory system as well as the effectiveness with which the active muscles are able to utilize O_2. Figure 18.5 describes the normal developmental patterns of absolute (l/min) maximal O_2 uptake during childhood and adolescence for both genders. In general, males and females increase in absolute maximal O_2 uptake through childhood. During adolescence, however, males tend to continue to increase while females level off at about fourteen years of age.

The increase in maximal oxygen uptake that occurs throughout childhood is, in part, a function of growth in the lungs, circulatory

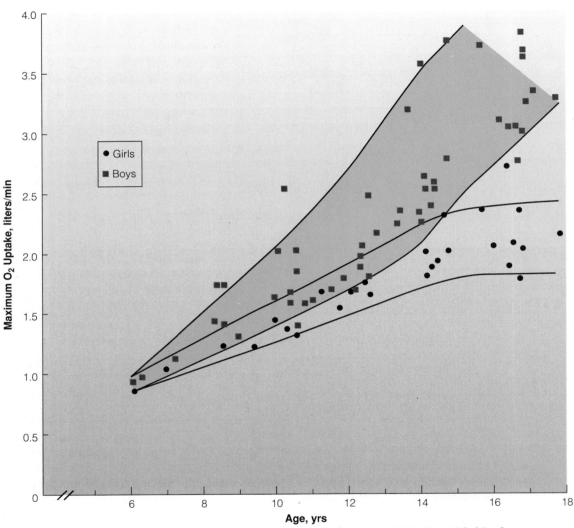

Figure 18.5   Absolute maximal oxygen uptake (l/min) across age for boys and girls. (From Oded Bar-Or, *Pediatric Sports Medicine for the Practitioner: From Physiologic Principles to Clinical Applications*. Copyright © 1983 Springer-Verlag, New York. Reprinted by permission.)

system, and musculature (39). Therefore, to validly compare children of different ages and body sizes or to examine the effect of growth on maximal oxygen uptake it is necessary to normalize the values based on a parameter that will account for maturational differences. The most common way to normalize maximal oxygen uptake values is to express them relative to body weight (ml/kg·min⁻¹). Figure

18.6 describes the changes in maximal oxygen uptake expressed in ml/kg· min⁻¹ for both genders between approximately six and eighteen years of age. The trends indicate that the relative maximal oxygen uptake of males remains stable across these ages while females tend to decrease gradually. In females, this pattern may reflect the increase in fat weight

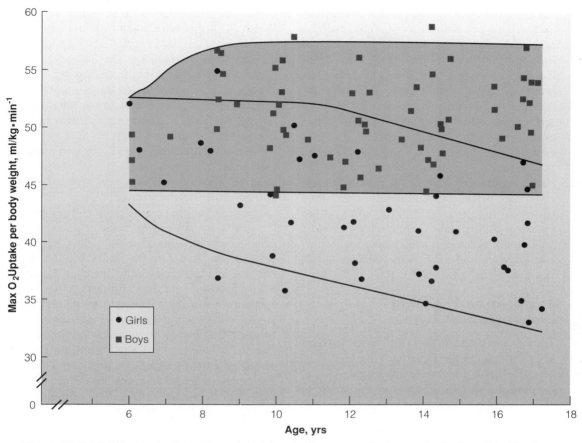

Figure 18.6   Relative maximal oxygen uptake (ml/kg·min⁻¹) across age for boys and girls. (From Oded Bar-Or, *Pediatric Sports Medicine for the Practitioner: From Physiologic Principles to Clinical Applications.* Copyright © 1983 Springer-Verlag, New York. Reprinted by permission.)

that normally occurs throughout childhood and adolescence (10).

It should be noted at this point that there is much controversy regarding the appropriateness of normalizing maximal oxygen uptake by expressing it relative to body weight (37, 39). Other potential normalizing parameters have been suggested such as body surface area, fat-free weight, skeletal age, and height (9, 24, 39). Rowland (39) has stated that "It appears prudent to investigate means of normalizing $\dot{V}O_2$ max independently of body dimension." Presently, however, there is no concensus regarding the most valid method

for normalizing maximal oxygen uptake values in children and adolescents.

Aerobic Fitness and Endurance Performance

In adults, maximal oxygen uptake is a valuable determinant of endurance performance. In children, however, the relationship between maximal oxygen uptake and age-related changes in endurance performance is less clear because of the confounding influences of normal growth and development. The multifactorial nature of endurance performance requires an examination of the interactions among many contributing parameters such as maximal oxygen uptake, submaximal exercise economy, qualitative changes in oxygen delivery not indicated by $\dot{V}O_2$ max, biomechanical factors, speed, and strength (37). The interrelationships are clearly evidenced by the fact that while relative maximal oxygen consumption (ml/kg$\cdot$ min^{-1}) remains stable or declines during childhood and adolescence, endurance performance on tests such as timed runs steadily improves. Thus, factors other than maximal oxygen uptake must influence endurance performance in children. Rowland (37) has suggested that "Maximal oxygen uptake in children may therefore be a less valid indicator of cardiopulmonary function, endurance capacity and response to training than in adult subjects."

Endurance Training and Aerobic Fitness

There is some controversy regarding the trainability of children with respect to aerobic fitness. Rowland (38) reviewed the results of longitudinal studies of endurance training in children and concluded that when the exercise protocol was consistent with that which has been shown to improve aerobic fitness in adults (7), most of the studies with children demonstrated increases of 7% to 26% in maximal oxygen uptake. Thus, it appears that adult standards such as those recommended by the American College of Sports Medicine (7) should be utilized for improving maximal oxygen uptake in children.

Long-Distance Running

The popularity of running for adults has led to an increase in the participation of children in long-distance running. The American Academy of Pediatrics (4) has identified many of the potential hazards associated with long-distance running in children, which include heel cord injuries, epiphyseal growth plate injuries, chronic joint trauma, thermal intolerance, and psychological problems as result of

unrealistic goals. In addition, Rowland and Walsh (41) reported that shin splints was the most common injury reported among runners eight to fifteen years of age. Do these potential hazards preclude children from running? The answer to this question is clearly no. Thousands of children, some as young as four years of age, run safely in recreational as well as competitive situations (40, 41).

Several authorities (4, 30, 40) have made recommendations regarding the distances children should run. The American Academy of Pediatrics (4) has stated "Long-distance competitive running events primarily designed for adults are not recommended for children prior to physical maturation. Under no circumstances should a full marathon be attempted by immature youths (less than Tanner Stage 5 sexual maturity rating). After pubertal development is complete, guidelines for adult distance running are appropriate." Micheli (30) has recommended that children under fourteen years of age should not train or compete at distances greater than 10 km. Furthermore, Rowland and Hoontis (40) have suggested that a 2-mile race over a flat course is appropriate for children aged 12 and younger.

There is a substantial difference between high-pressure competitive racing and recreational or health-related training. It is important that children participate without excessive parental and peer pressure to succeed. Children should engage in regular physical activity because it is enjoyable and because it encourages a lifelong commitment to a healthy life-style. The recommendations above should be used as guidelines for organizing competitive and recreational races for children.

Exercise and Anaerobic Fitness

Children have a substantially lower capacity for performing anaerobic exercise than adolescents and adults (10, 11, 25, 51). This is clearly evidenced by examining the age-related changes in mean power (total work performed during a maximal 30-second cycle ergometer test) and peak power (highest amount of work performed during a 5-second period) from the Wingate Anaerobic Test. It is generally assumed that mean power represents principally the capacity of the glycolytic energy production pathway while peak power reflects the efficiency of the phosphagen system (ATP and CP breakdown). Figures 18.7 and 18.8 describe the positive relationships (males and females) for absolute mean and peak power (expressed in watts) versus age. As illustrated in figures 18.9 and 18.10, the same general trend, although less pronounced, is true when mean and peak power are expressed relative to body weight (watt/kg). These findings have also been confirmed using the Margaria step-running anaerobic power test (fig. 18.11). Thus, as children develop throughout childhood, their performance capacity in anaerobic sports and activities increases.

The ability to perform anaerobic activities is limited by the availability of stored energy sources (ATP, CP, and glycogen) and the enzyme activity of the anaerobic energy systems. Children have a diminished capacity for anaerobic activity, in part because of smaller CP stores and lower concentrations of phosphofructokinase than adults (10, 18). Thus, compared to adults, the anaerobic metabolic systems of children are less effective at energy production, which translates into poorer performance in high-intensity, short-duration activities.

The Effect of Anaerobic Training

Children and adolescents respond favorably to anaerobic training (11). The metabolic adaptations associated with anaerobic training include increased phosphofructokinase (17, 19), myosin ATPase, creatine phosphokinase, and myokinase activity (10) as well as increased stores and rate of utilization of ATP, CP, and

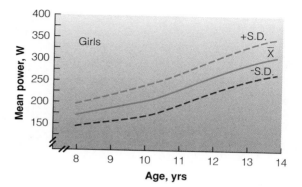

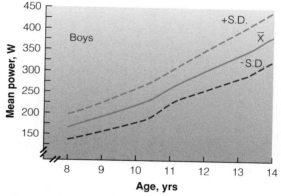

Figure 18.7   Absolute mean power (watt) from the Wingate Anaerobic Test across age for boys and girls. (From Oded Bar-Or, *Pediatric Sports Medicine for the Practitioner: From Physiologic Principles to Clinical Applications.* Copyright © 1983 Springer-Verlag, New York. Reprinted by permission.)

glycogen (10, 17, 19). These metabolic changes are manifested as improvements in the performance of anaerobic activities (10).

Unlike aerobic exercise, there has been limited research designed to identify the optimal protocol for improving anaerobic capabilities. In general, the studies that have reported improved anaerobic capacity following training in children and adolescents have used sprint running (19, 23, 36) or stationary cycling (17, 18, 23); submaximal (2) to supramaximal exercise intensities (23); three (36) to six (22) exercise sessions per week; for six (23) to sixteen weeks (18).

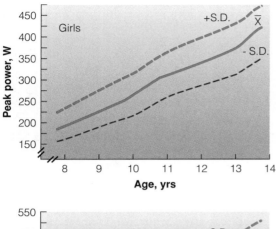

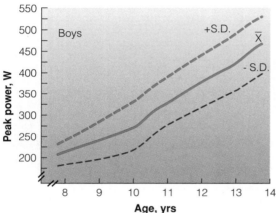

Figure 18.8 Absolute peak power (watt) from the Wingate Anaerobic Test across age for boys and girls. (From Oded Bar-Or, *Pediatric Sports Medicine for the Practitioner: From Physiologic Principles to Clinical Applications.* Copyright © 1983 Springer-Verlag, New York. Reprinted by permission.)

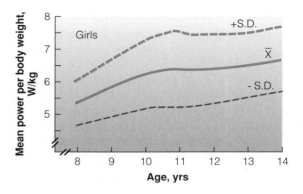

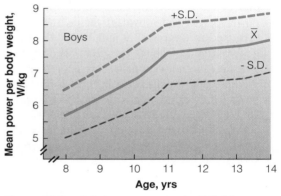

Figure 18.9 Relative mean power (watt/kg) from the Wingate Anaerobic Test across age for boys and girls. (From Oded Bar-Or, *Pediatric Sports Medicine for the Practitioner: From Physiologic Principles to Clinical Applications.* Copyright © 1983 Springer-Verlag, New York. Reprinted by permission.)

Studies (20, 49) have recommended sprint training protocols for adults, but it is not clear if these standards are appropriate for children. For example, Wilt (49) has recommended repeated maximal sprints of 60 to 70 yards with full recovery between repetitions. Fox (20) has suggested multiple sprints of approximately 100 to 220 yards with a ratio of work to rest (walking) of 1:3. That is, if the 110-yard sprint is performed in 15 seconds, it should be followed by 45 seconds of walking.

Although the applicability of these recommended adult protocols to children is uncertain, it is appropriate to use a training program that closely mimics the intended sporting activity with respect to the mode (type) of exercise as well as the metabolic demands. That is, if the training is designed to improve 100-meter sprint running performance, the exercise should consist of running as opposed to stationary cycling or other modes of activity. Furthermore, it is important to identify which anaerobic metabolic system (phosphagen or glycolysis) is most responsible for the energy production for the intended sporting activity.

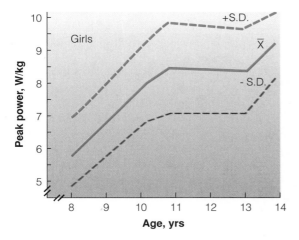

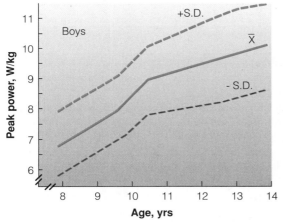

Figure 18.10 Relative peak power (watt/kg) from the Wingate Anaerobic Test across age for boys and girls. (From Oded Bar-Or, *Pediatric Sports Medicine for the Practitioner: From Physiologic Principles to Clinical Applications.* Copyright © 1983 Springer-Verlag, New York. Reprinted by permission.)

To use the example of the 100-meter sprint, which utilizes primarily the phosphagen system, the training protocol should include repeated repetitions that tax the phosphagen system to a high degree such as 100-meter sprints as opposed to longer sprints (200 to 400 meters), which rely heavily on anaerobic glycolysis for energy production. This level of specificity of training will help to insure favorable physiological adaptations and improved performance.

Strength

Figure 18.12 describes the changes in strength during childhood and adolescence for both genders. In general, there is an increase in strength across age for both genders with males only slightly stronger than females throughout childhood (29). At approximately thirteen to fourteen years of age (corresponding to the adolescent growth spurt), males begin to increase in strength at a greater rate than females. The changes in strength during childhood and adolescence coincide with increases in body weight (fig. 18.3) and muscle mass (fig. 18.13). It is likely that the accelerated increase in strength during puberty in males reflects the anabolic effect of circulating testosterone as well as neural maturation (1, 14, 29).

Weight Training versus Weight Lifting versus Body Building

The American Academy of Pediatrics (5) has recommended the following definitions to differentiate among weight training, weight lifting, and body building.

1. Weight training (also called strength or resistance training) is the use of a variety of methods, including exercises with free weights and weight machines, to increase muscular strength, endurance, and/or power for sports participation or fitness enhancement.

2. Weight lifting and power lifting are competitive sports in which an athlete attempts to lift a maximal amount of free weight in specific lifts. In weight

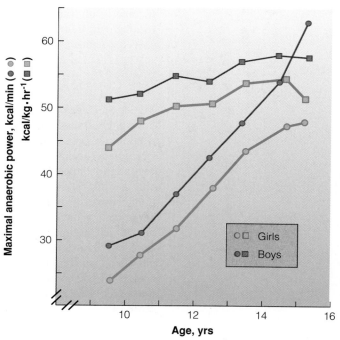

Figure 18.11   Absolute (kcal/min) and relative (kcal/kg·hr⁻¹) maximal anaerobic power from the Margaria Step-Running Anaerobic Power Test across age for boys and girls. (From Oded Bar-Or, *Pediatric Sports Medicine for the Practitioner: From Physiologic Principles to Clinical Applications.* Copyright © 1983 Springer-Verlag, New York. Reprinted by permission.)

lifting, the lifts performed are the clean and jerk and the snatch. In power lifting, they are the squat lift, dead lift, and bench press.

3. Body building is a competitive sport in which the participant uses several resistance training methods, including free weights, to develop muscle size, symmetry, and definition.

Weight Training during Prepubescence and Postpubescense

It has long been known that after puberty, weight training results in increased strength (21, 45, 46). For many years, however, a controversy existed regarding the effectiveness of weight training in prepubescent children (16, 26, 28). Conventional wisdom held that prepubescent children should not perform weight training for three primary reasons: 1) low levels of circulating androgens make significant increases in strength impossible; 2) strength gains do not improve motor performance or reduce the risk of sports-related injuries in children; and 3) the potential hazards associated with weight training in children outweigh the benefits (16, 28). Recent studies, however, have shown these ideas to be in error.

A number of studies have shown that weight training results in increased strength in prepubescent children (33, 34, 43, 44, 47). These increases normally range from approximately 5% to 40% depending on the characteristic of the training program and are substantially larger than the small increases

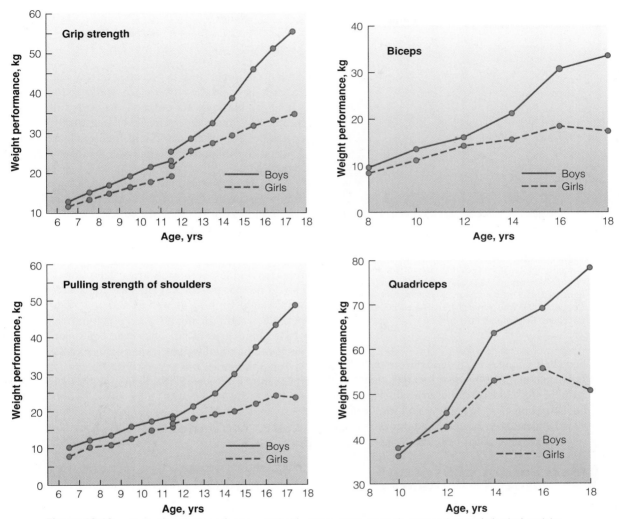

Figure 18.12   Strength across age for boys and girls. (Note. From *Growth, Maturation, and Physical Activity* (p. 191) by R. M. Malina and C. Bouchard, 1991, Champaign, IL: Human Kinetics. Copyright 1991 by Robert Malina and Claude Bouchard. Reprinted by permission.)

exhibited in short term studies (five to twenty weeks) by age-matched control groups (27). Thus, the increases in strength as a result of weight training are greater than those attributable to normal growth and development. Strength increases in prepubertal children have been shown to result from weight training that involved hydraulic resistance (47), isotonic exercise (33, 34), weight bearing activ-

ities (44), and variable resistance (Nautilus and CAM II) training (43). These investigations indicate that prepubescent children respond favorably to a variety of weight training modalities. In addition to the increases in strength associated with weight training, other potential benefits for prepubescent children include improved flexibility (47), favorable changes in blood lipid profiles (48), enhanced

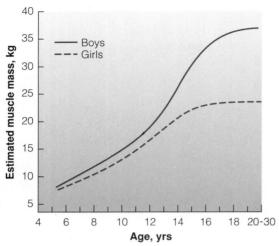

Figure 18.13   Muscle mass (kg) across age for boys and girls. (Note. From *Growth, Maturation, and Physical Activity* (p. 127) by R. M. Malina and C. Bouchard, 1991, Champaign, IL: Human Kinetics. Copyright 1991 by Robert M. Malina and Claude Bouchard. Reprinted by permission.)

bone and connective tissue development (27), favorable changes in body composition (44), reduced musculoskeletal injuries during sports participation (27, 42), improved motor skills (8, 47), increased muscular endurance (8), and positive psychological benefits (8, 42).

Mechanisms of Strength Increases in Prepubescent Children

It is likely that the strength increases in response to weight training in prepubescent children are a result of neural adaptations (27, 34). The neural factors that contribute to strength gains are primarily associated with increased neural drive and synchronization of motor unit firing (38). Furthermore, part of the strength increase is probably a function of improved lifting technique (34). The presently available evidence suggests that hypertrophy does not contribute significantly to the increases in strength that result from weight training in prepubertal children (27, 34, 47).

Potential Hazards of Weight Training

An issue of importance to parents, athletes, and coaches is the safety of weight training for young populations. Its potential hazards fall into three primary categories (31): acute musculoskeletal injuries, chronic musculoskeletal injuries, and hypertension and weight lifter's blackout.

In 1979 it was estimated that competitive maximal weight lifting in individuals between ten and nineteen years of age resulted in over 17,000 injuries that required emergency treatment (3). In addition, it is likely that each year submaximal weight training causes many unreported and less serious injuries. Therefore it should be recognized that risks are associated with weight training as well as maximal competitive weight lifting in young populations (15). The degree of risk, however, for supervised submaximal weight training programs is low, and therefore, it is generally accepted that the benefits outweigh the potential hazards (5, 8, 13, 27, 31, 35, 42).

Acute Musculoskeletal Injuries

Acute musculoskeletal injuries result from trauma experienced during a single episode of weight training (31). Examples of this type of injury include epiphyseal fractures, ruptured intervertebral disks, and low back bony disruption (5). Of these, damage to the epiphyseal growth plate at the end of long bones has received the most attention. The epiphyseal growth plate contributes to the normal development of long bones and premature closure due to trauma may result in long-term deformity of the limb.

Lifting excessive amounts of weight or using improper technique can result in epiphyseal fractures in children and adolescents (12). The number of epiphyseal fractures as a result of weight training, however, is small compared to contact sports such as football, hockey, and basketball (12). In addition, it has been estimated that 5% or fewer of all epiphyseal injuries result in a measurable variation in growth (32). Therefore, although the risk of epiphyseal damage as a result of weight training in children and adolescents is small, and long-term deformity is unlikely, it is important that those individuals responsible for supervision of the training sessions teach proper lifting techniques and take steps to prevent such injuries from occurring (5, 8, 31).

Chronic Musculoskeletal Injuries

Chronic injuries are generally a result of repeated microtrauma due to overuse. Examples of these injuries include stress fractures, musculotendinous strains, and osteochondrites dissecans of the knee and elbow. With respect to weight training, the risk of these injuries can be reduced by a properly supervised program that avoids an excessive frequency and number of repetitions. If weight training is conducted properly by children and adolescents, the risk of developing severe chronic musculoskeletal injuries is considered small (8, 31).

Hypertension and Weight Lifter's Blackout

Maximal weight lifting can result in weight lifter's blackout. This involves a loss of consciousness due to hypertension, transient diminution of cardiac output, and/or an arrhythmia (3, 31). It is often the result of a valsalva maneuver where there is a voluntary increase in abdominal pressure while struggling to overcome the resistance (31). If unconsciousness occurs, there is a considerable risk of injury due to the falling weights. The possibility of injury from weight lifter's blackout can be reduced by the mandatory presence of spotters during the lifting of free weights (3).

Weight lifting and weight training should not be performed by children, adolescents, or adults who have a compromised cardiovascular system or hypertension without a physician's approval (3). Small increases in resting blood pressure have been reported as a result of chronic weight training but this trend has not been consistently demonstrated (31). At the present time, it is generally accepted that a properly executed weight training program does not lead to a chronic elevation in blood pressure in normotensive individuals. Therefore, in healthy young populations, it is not necessary to avoid weight training because of a fear of developing hypertension.

Characteristics of a Weight Training Program

The American Academy of Pediatrics (5) has made the following recommendations:

1. Strength training programs for prepubescent, pubescent, and postpubescent athletes should be permitted only if conducted by well-trained adults. The adults should be qualified to plan programs appropriate to the athlete's stage of maturation, which should be assessed objectively by medical personnel.

2. Unless good data become available that demonstrate safety, children and adolescents should avoid the practice of weight lifting, power lifting, and body building as well as the repetitive use of maximal amounts of weight in strength training programs, until they have reached Tanner Stage 5 level of developmental maturity.

Tanner Stage 5 indicates the adult level of maturity for pubic hair, breasts, and genitals (29) and is usually reached at a mean of approximately fifteen years of age for both males

Table 18.1	Weight Training Progression for Children		
	Base Program	**Intermediate Program**	**Advanced Program**
1. Intensity	low (12–15 RM*)	moderate (10–12 RM)	high (8–10 RM)
2. Duration	2 to 6 weeks	8 to 24 weeks	ongoing
3. Number of sets	1 to 2	2 to 3	3 to 4
4. Rest periods between sets	2 to 3 minutes or more	2 minutes	2 minutes
5. Frequency	2 to 3 times per week	3 times per week	3 times per week
6. Metabolic stress	low	low to moderate	moderate

*RM (repetition maximum) = the maximal amount of weight that can be lifted for a specific number of repetitions. For example, a 1 RM load is the maximal amount of weight that can be lifted only one time. A 10 RM load is the maximal amount of weight that can be lifted ten times but not eleven.

and females. It must be noted, however, that there is a great deal of interindividual variability in sexual development and therefore, chronological age is not a precise indicator of the level of maturity.

Several authorities have recommended weight training programs for children (8, 27, 31). While they are all similar in philosophy, the recommendations of Kraemer and colleagues (27) are the most extensive and provide specifics for the progression from a base program for beginners to an advanced program. Table 18.1 provides a weight training progression for children based on Kraemer's recommendations and the American Orthopaedic Society for Sports Medicine (8). The exercises suggested by Kraemer and colleagues include single leg extensions, single leg curls, calf raisers, bench press, bent leg sit-ups, reverse sit-ups, arm curls, tricep extensions, leg presses or squats, military presses, upright rows, lateral pull-downs, and seated rows. Typically, the order of exercises involves a progression from arm to leg or non-arm exercise.

Summary

1. The term "growth" refers to an increase in the size of the body.

2. The term "development" refers to the differentiation of cells along specialized lines of function.

3. The term "maturation" refers to the tempo and timing of progress toward the mature biological state.

4. Infancy is the first year of life.

5. Childhood is the time between the first birthday and the onset of puberty.

6. Adolescence is the time between the onset of puberty and the attainment of adult status.

7. Puberty is the time of sexual maturation.

8. Height and body weight increase along an S-shaped curve from birth through adolescence.

9. The American College of Sports Medicine (6) has recommended that individuals with less than 5% body fat receive medical clearance before being allowed to compete in wrestling.

10. Males and females increase in absolute maximal oxygen uptake (l/min) during childhood and adolescence.

11. Endurance performance improves steadily throughout childhood and adolescence while relative maximal oxygen uptake (ml/kg · min^{-1}) remains stable or declines.

12. The adult standards recommended by the American College of Sports Medicine (7) should be used for improving maximal oxygen uptake in children.

13. The American Academy of Pediatrics (4) has stated "Under no circumstances should a full marathon be attempted by immature youths."

14. Children have a substantially lower capacity for anaerobic exercise than adolescents and adults.

15. Children and adolescents respond favorably to anaerobic training.

16. There is an increase in strength across age for both genders throughout childhood.

17. Children's strength increases as a result of weight training.

18. The American Academy of Pediatrics (5) supports supervised weight training but not maximal competitive weight lifting, power lifting, or body building for children prior to Tanner Stage 5.

References

1. Adams, R. D., and Victor, M. *Principles of Neurology*. St. Louis: McGraw-Hill Book Co., 1985.

2. Adeniran, S. A., and Toriola, M. A. Effects of continuous and interval running programmes on aerobic and anaerobic capacities in schoolgirls aged 13 to 17 years. *J. Sports Med. Phys. Fitness* 28:260–66, 1988.

3. American Academy of Pediatrics. Policy statement on weight training and weight lifting: Information for the pediatrician. *News and Comments:* 33:7–8, 1982.

4. American Academy of Pediatrics. Risks in long-distance running for children. *Phys. Sportsmed.* 10:82–86, 1982.

5. American Academy of Pediatrics. Strength training, weight and power lifting, and body building by children and adolescents. *Pediatrics* 86:801–3, 1990.

6. American College of Sports Medicine. Position stand on: Weight loss in wrestlers. *Med. Sci. Sports* 8:xi, 1976.

7. American College of Sports Medicine. Position stand on: The recommended quantity and quality of exercise for developing and maintaining cardiorespiratory and muscular fitness in healthy adults. *Med. Sci. Sports Exerc.* 22:265–74, 1990.

8. American Orthopaedic Society for Sports Medicine. *Proceedings of the Conference on Strength Training and the Prepubescent,* ed. B. R. Cahill. Chicago: AOSSM, 1988.

9. Bailey, D. A., Ross, W. D., Mirwald, R. L., and Weese, C. Size dissociation of maximal aerobic power during growth in boys. *Med. Sport* 11:140–51, 1978.

10. Bar-Or, O. *Pediatric Sports Medicine for the Practitioner: From Physiologic Principles of Clinical Applications.* New York: Springer-Verlag, 1983.

11. Bar-Or, O. Trainability of the prepubescent child. *Phys. Sportsmed.* 17:65–82, 1989.

12. Benton, J. W. Epiphyseal fracture in sports. *Phys. Sportsmed.* 10:63–71, 1982.

13. Brady, T. A., Cahill, B. R., and Bodnar, L. M. Weight training-related injuries in the high school athlete. *Am. J. Sports Med.* 10:1–5, 1982.

14. Brooks, G. A., and Fahey, T. D. *Exercise Physiology: Human Bioenergetics and its Applications.* New York: Macmillian Publishing Co., 1985.

15. Brown, E. W., and Kimball, R. G. Medical history associated with adolescent powerlifting. *Pediatrics* 72:636–44, 1983.

16. Duda, M. Prepubescent strength training gains support. *Phys. Sportsmed.* 14:157–61, 1986.

17. Eriksson, B. O. Physical training, oxygen supply and muscle metabolism in 11–13 year old boys. *Acta Physiol. Scand.* (Suppl.) 384:1–48, 1972.

18. Eriksson, B. O., Gollnick, P. D., and Saltin, B. Muscle metabolism and enzyme activities after training in boys 11–13 years old. *Acta Physiol. Scand.* 87:485–97, 1973.

19. Fournier, M., Ricci, J., Taylor, A. W., Ferguson, R. J., Montpetit, R. R., and Chaitman, B. R. Skeletal muscle adaptation in adolescent boys: Sprint and endurance training and detraining. *Med. Sci. Sports Exerc.* 14:453–56, 1982.

20. Fox, E. L. Physical training: Methods and effects. *Ortho. Clin. North Amer.* 8:533–48, 1977.

21. Gillam, G. M. Effects of frequency of weight training on muscle strength enhancement. *J. Sports Med. Phys. Fitness* 21:432–36, 1981.

22. Grodjinovsky, A., and Bar-Or, O. Influence of added physical education hours upon anaerobic capacity, adiposity, and grip strength in 12–13-year-old children enrolled in a sports class. In *Children and Sport,* eds. J. Ilmarinen and I. Valimaki. Berlin: Springer Verlag, 1984.

23. Grodjinovsky, A., Bar-Or, O., Dotan, R., and Inbar, O. Training effect on the anaerobic performance of children as measured by the Wingate anaerobic test. In *Children and Exercise,* eds. K. Berg and B. O. Eriksson. Baltimore: University Park Press, 1980.

24. Holliday, M. A., Potter, D., Jarrah, A., and Bearg, S. The relation of metabolic rate to body weight and organ size. *Pediatr. Res.* 1:185–95, 1967.

25. Inbar, O., and Bar-Or, O. Anaerobic characteristics in male children and adolescents. *Med. Sci. Sports Exerc.* 18:264–69, 1986.

26. Jacobson, B. H., and Kulling, F. A. Effect of resistive weight training in prepubescents. *J. Orthop. Sports Phys. Ther.* 11:96–99, 1989.

27. Kraemer, W. J., Fry, A. C., Frykman, P. N., Conroy, B., and Hoffman, J. Resistance training and youth. *Ped. Exer. Sci.* 1:336–50, 1989.

28. Legwold, G. Does lifting weights harm a prepubescent athlete? *Phys. Sportsmed.* 10:141–44, 1982.

29. Malina, R. M., and Bouchard, C. *Growth, Maturation, and Physical Activity.* Champaign: Human Kinetics Books, 1991.

30. Micheli, L. J. Complications of recreational running. *Ped. Alert* 6:1–2, 1981.

31. *National Strength and Conditioning Association.* Position paper on prepubescent strength training. *Nat. Strength Cond. Assoc.* 7:27–31, 1985.

32. Pappas, A. M. Epiphyseal injuries in sports. *Phys. Sportsmed.* 11:140–48, 1983.

33. Pfeiffer, R. D., and Francis, R. S. Effects of strength training on muscle development in prepubescent, pubescent and postpubescent males. *Phys. Sportsmed.* 14:134–43, 1986.

34. Ramsay, J. A., Blimkie, C. J. R., Smith, K., Garner, S., MacDougall, J. D., and Sale, D. G. Strength training effects in prepubescent boys. *Med. Sci. Sports Exerc.* 22:605–14, 1990.

35. Rians, C. B., Weltman, A., Cahill, B. R., Janney, C. A., Tippett, S. R., and Katch, F. I. Strength training for prepubescent males: Is it safe? *Am. J. Sports Med.* 15:483–89, 1987.

36. Rotstein, A., Dotan, R., Bar-Or, O., and Tenenbaum, G. Effect of training on anaerobic threshold, maximal aerobic power, and anaerobic performance of preadolescent boys. *Int. J. Sports Med.* 7:281–86, 1986.

37. Rowland, T. W. Oxygen uptake and endurance fitness in children: A developmental perspective. *Ped. Exer. Sci.* 1:313–28, 1989.

38. Rowland, T. W. *Exercise and Children's Health.* Champaign: Human Kinetics Books, 1990.

39. Rowland, T. W. "Normalizing" maximal oxygen uptake, or the search for the holy grail (per kg). *Ped. Exer. Sci.* 3:95–102, 1991.

40. Rowland, T. W., and Hoontis, P. P. Organizing road races for children: Special concerns. *Phys. Sportsmed.* 13:126–32, 1985.

41. Rowland, T. W., and Walsh, C. A. Characteristics of child distance runners. *Phys. Sportsmed.* 13:45–53, 1985.

42. Schafer, J. Prepubescent and adolescent weight training: Is it safe? Is it beneficial? *Nat. Strength Cond. Assoc.* 13:39–46, 1991.

43. Sewall, L., and Micheli, L. J. Strength training for children. *J. Ped. Ortho.* 6:143–46, 1986.

44. Siegel, J. A., Camaione, D. N., and Manfredi, T. G. The effects of upper body resistance training on prepubescent children. *Ped. Exer. Sci.* 1:145–54, 1989.

45. Smith, M. J., and Melton, P. Isokinetic versus isotonic variable-resistance training. *Am. J. Sports Med.* 9:275–79, 1981.

46. Vrijens, J. Muscle strength development in the pre- and post-pubescent age. *Med. Sport* 11:152–58, 1978.

47. Weltman, A., Janney, C., Rians, C. B., Strand, K., Berg, B., Tippitt, S., Wise, J., Cahill, B. R., and Katch, F. I. The effects of hydraulic resistance strength training in pre-pubertal males. *Med. Sci. Sports Exerc.* 18:629–38, 1986.

48. Weltman, A., Janney, C., Rians, C. B., Strand, K., and Katch, F. I. The effects of hydraulic-resistance strength training on serum lipid levels in prepubertal boys. *Am. J. Dis. Child.* 141:777–80, 1987.

49. Wilt, F. Training for competitive running. In *Exercise Physiology,* ed. H. Falls. New York: Academic Press, 1968.

50. Zambraski, E. J., Foster, D. T., Gross, P. M., and Tipton, C. M. Iowa wrestling study: Weight loss and urinary profiles of collegiate wrestlers. *Med. Sci. Sports* 8:105–8, 1976.

51. Zwiren, L. D. Anaerobic and aerobic capacities of children. *Ped. Exer. Sci.* 1:31–44, 1989.

19

Age and Exercise

Age Changes in Muscle Function
  Strength
  Muscular Endurance
  Force-Velocity Curve
  Capacity for Hypertrophy
  Changes at the Cellular Level
Age and the Cardiovascular System
  Maximum Heart Rate
  Cardiac Output
  Coronary Artery Changes
  Circulatory Changes
Changes in Pulmonary Function
  Lung Volumes and Capacities
  Thoracic Wall Compliance
  Pulmonary Diffusion
  Ventilatory Mechanics in Exercise
Age and Physical Working Capacity
  (PWC)
  Maximal O_2 Consumption
  Muscular Efficiency
Age and the Nervous System
Age and Body Composition
  Stature
Effects of Physical Conditioning on Losses
  in Functional Capacities Caused
  by Aging

Principles for Conduct of Conditioning
  Programs for Older Men and
  Women (over Sixty)
  Medical Examination
  *Physiological Monitoring (in the
    Laboratory)*
  *Physiological Monitoring (Gym or
    Field)*
  *Prescription of Exercise (Dose-
    Response Data)*
  Progression
  *Type of Exercise as a Determinant of
    Heart Stress in Older People*
  *Musculoskeletal Injuries and
    Physical Activity*
Implications for Physical Education and
  Athletics
  Maturity
  Old Age
  The Very Old and the Frail Elderly

In terms of the biblical concept of three score and ten, we have a lifetime of seventy years. However, if we judge the interest of the physical education profession by the nature of the curricula offered in teacher training institutions, virtually all of our efforts seem to be directed to ten years of that life span, the years involved in secondary and college education. Should physical education start in junior high school and end after two or four years of college? This seeming preoccupation of physical education with only 14% of the total life span is certainly undesirable.

That the need for physical education exists at all ages is amply demonstrated by the success of various athletic programs for children (Little League, Pop Warner League, and age-group swimming) and by weight training and conditioning gyms for adults. It seems inevitable that the scope of physical education must somehow grow to include programs that are organized and administered by professional people for *all ages* and not just for high school and college students who need the attention least. It behooves us, then, to consider the physiological changes that occur as a function of the aging process.

With respect to the entire age range of human life, physical performance measures and physiological function in general improve rapidly from early childhood to a maximum somewhere between the late teens and about thirty years of age. In most cases a slow decline occurs during maturity and becomes more rapid with increasing age. The decline in function with age deserves a great deal more emphasis by scientific investigators than it has been accorded in the past.

Indeed the entire body of knowledge regarding the loss of function with increasing age must be viewed with caution since in very few cases has the effect of habitual physical activity been controlled or ruled out. Wessel and Van Huss (93) have shown that physical activity decreases significantly with increasing age. This is not surprising news but does provide scientific validation of the need for considering this variable in all investigations directed toward aging changes in performance. To support this contention further they showed that losses in physiological variables important to human performance resulting from age were more highly related to the *decreased habitual activity* level than they were to *age itself*.

Statistics on population trends for the United States indicate that we are rapidly becoming a nation of older people. The absolute number, as well as the proportion of our older population segments, is increasing rapidly. In evaluating the effects of the aging process on human function, several problems arise. First, it is difficult to separate the effects of aging per se from those of concomitant disease processes (particularly cardiovascular problems) that become more numerous as age progresses. Second, the sedentary nature of adult life in the United States makes it very difficult to find *old* populations for comparisons with *young* populations at equal activity levels. Third, very little work has been done on longitudinal studies of the same population over a period of time. Conclusions drawn from cross-sectional studies in which various age groups are compared must be accepted with reservations because the weaker biological specimens are not likely to be represented in as great numbers in the older populations tested as in the younger (due to a higher mortality rate).

Just as individuals age at different rates, various physiological functions seem to have their own rates of decline with increasing age (fig. 19.1). Indeed, some functions do not seem to degenerate with age (78). Under resting conditions, there seem to be no changes in blood sugar, blood pH, or total blood volume. In general, the functions that involve the coordinated activity of more than one organ system decline most with age, and, as might be expected, changes due to the aging process

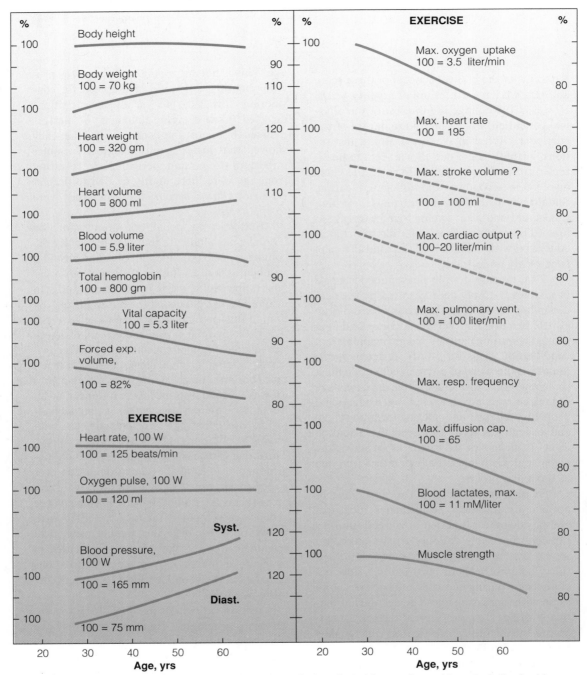

Figure 19.1 Functional variables with age. Data have been collected from various subjects, including healthy men. For data on the same function, only one study has been consulted. The values for the twenty-five-year-old subjects = 100%. For the older ages the mean values are expressed in percentage of the twenty-five-year-old individuals' values. The values should not be considered normal values but values that illustrate the effect of aging. Note that heart rate and oxygen pulse at a given work load (100 W or 600 kgm/min, oxygen uptake about 1.5 liters/min) are identical throughout the age range covered, but the maximal oxygen uptake, heart rate, cardiac output, etc., decline with age. The data on cardiac output and stroke volume are based on few observations and are therefore uncertain. (From *Textbook of Work Physiology* by Astrand, P.–O., and Rodahl, K. Copyright © 1977 McGraw-Hill, Inc. Used with permission of McGraw-Hill Book Company.)

are most readily observed when the organism is stressed. Homeostatic readjustment is considerably slower with increasing age.

Age Changes in Muscle Function

Strength

All investigators have found that rapid improvement in strength accompanies the growth of children, and maximal strength is found to occur for most muscle groups between the ages of twenty-five and thirty. This increase in strength is almost entirely accounted for by the increased size of the muscle. Even differences in muscle quality between the genders are not very large. When strength is expressed per unit of cross-sectional area (kilograms per square centimeters), differences due to age and gender are very small.

Strength decreases very slowly during maturity. After the fifth decade, strength decreases at a greater rate, but even at age sixty the loss does not usually exceed 10% to 20% of the maximum, with women's losses being somewhat greater than those of men.

Figures 19.2 and 19.3 show the changes with age in arm strength and grip strength found by Montoye and Lamphiear (59) in the Tecumseh, Michigan, study in which they studied the entire community. These data probably represent the best controlled study to date. Interestingly, in another study where maximal grip strength was investigated in 100 men who all did similar work in a machine shop, no change in either grip strength or endurance was found from age twenty-two to sixty-two (69). These data suggest that in this age bracket the more typical finding of small losses with age may be due largely to disuse phenomena rather than a true age effect. However, in old age there is little question that sizable decrements in strength do occur.

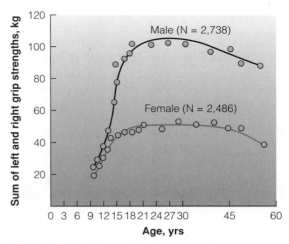

Figure 19.2   Changes in grip strength with age. (From Montoye, H. J., and D. E. Lamphiear in *Research Quarterly* 48:109 (Tecumseh Study). © 1977 American Alliance for Health, Physical Education and Recreation. Reprinted by permission.)

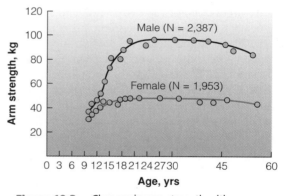

Figure 19.3   Changes in arm strength with age. (From Montoye, H. J., and D. E. Lamphiear in *Research Quarterly* 48:109 (Tecumseh Study). © 1977 American Alliance for Health, Physical Education and Recreation. Reprinted by permission.)

Muscular Endurance

Larsson (51), who did a careful and comprehensive study on the functional changes in skeletal muscle with age, found that isometric endurance measured as the ability to maintain 50% of a maximal voluntary contraction (MVC) and also dynamic endurance measured as the rate of force decline during repeated isokinetic contractions of knee extension showed a small improvement with age, although the improvement was not significant. Petrofsky and Lind (69), who reported similar findings with respect to handgrip endurance, suggested that these results might be explained by the increasing proportion of slow twitch (ST) fibers in the muscles of the older subjects (see below). It has also been suggested that this greater endurance might be explained by the hypothesis that ST fibers serve as a lactate recipient for the greater lactate production of the fast twitch (FT) fibers during a fatiguing contraction.

These findings are somewhat surprising and conflict with earlier data from deVries's laboratory. Evans (33) has shown with the EMG curve technique that fatigue rate is significantly greater in the old than the young when isometric contractions are held to 20%, 25%, 30%, 35%, 40%, and 45% of MVC. Since the observations by EMG are relatively free of confounding subjective factors, further investigation is needed before we can conclude that muscular endurance improves with age.

Force-Velocity Curve

Damon (19) has shown that the maximum velocity produced against any given mass is less for the old than the young, although the shape of the force-velocity curve is similar (fig. 19.4). His work also showed that age decrements in strength at ages fifty-five to seventy-one exist whether measured in isometric, concentric, or eccentric muscle contraction and whether measured as maximal instantaneous force

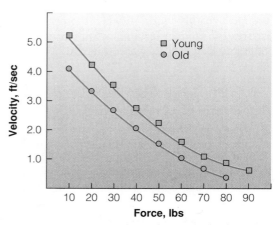

Figure 19.4   Comparison of young and old groups on force-velocity relationships. (From Damon, E. L., *An Experimental Investigation of the Relationship of Age to Various Parameters of Muscle Strength*. Ph.D. diss. Reprinted by permission.)

achieved or as a mean value over a finite time period. However, his work showed isotonic strength to be affected to a greater extent than isometric. The more recent work of Aniansson and colleagues (2) with respect to force-velocity relationship is in good agreement with that of Damon (19). A loss of maximum knee extension velocity of 7% from age in the twenties to age in the sixties was also reported by Larsson (51). To summarize, the loss of strength with age is greatest at the higher velocities of movement, as is shown in figure 19.4.

Capacity for Hypertrophy

With respect to human strength gain, Moritani and deVries (60) investigated the time course of strength gain through weight training in old and young men to define the contribution of hypertrophy and such neural factors as disinhibition to the total change in strength over a period of eight weeks. Young and old men showed similar and significant percentage increases in strength, although the young made greater absolute gains, of course. However, the physiological adaptations of the two groups were quite different, as shown in figure 19.5. While young subjects showed highly significant hypertrophy, the strength gained by the old men was almost entirely due to learning to achieve higher activation levels as measured by EMG methods.

Although Moritani and deVries found only small and statistically nonsignificant levels of hypertrophy in their subjects, more recent studies using more sensitive techniques such as computer tomography and magnetic resonance imaging have found considerably larger and statistically significant levels of hypertrophy to occur in elderly populations using weight training methods (12, 18, 35, 37). It is now clear that heavy resistance training can bring about not only statistically significant but also physiologically significant hypertrophy in the musculature of the elderly. This is true for both men and women and has even been demonstrated in the very old up to age 96 (35). Meredith and colleagues (57) have suggested that muscle hypertrophy in the elderly after weight training can be enhanced by the addition of a complete nutritional supplement.

Changes at the Cellular Level

Animal studies have shown that important changes occur at the cellular level with increasing age. First there is a loss of contractile elements, which accounts for the decrement in strength. While this loss could be the result of losses in motor nerve fibers, this explanation has been ruled out by studies on rats, which have shown that while muscle fiber numbers may be down by about 25% in old rats, no change occurs in nerve fibers (39). The loss of contractile elements appears to be largely due to a loss of FT fibers, so that the proportion of ST fibers represents an ever-increasing proportion of the total (51). This seems to explain the changes in the force-velocity curve and the losses in high-speed movements noted above. The loss of muscle tissue with age also accounts for the downward trend in basal metabolism that accompanies the aging process (89).

Fiber Atrophy

In addition to the loss of contractile elements, there is also a progressive atrophy of the remaining muscle fibers, and again this seems to involve mainly the FT fiber population (52). Larsson's work, however, suggests that fiber atrophy is not the major cause of the loss of strength in old age. The most plausible mechanisms seem to be the decrease in the total number of muscle fibers noted above, or impaired excitation contraction coupling, or even possibly a decreased ability to activate the remaining high threshold (FT) motor units.

Fiber Hypertrophy

Goldspink and Howells (38) taught hamsters to lift weights to evaluate cellular hypertrophy. After weight training for five weeks, the mean fiber area of the biceps in the young animals increased by a significant 35.6%. Fiber area in the old animals increased by 17.7%, which was of marginal significance. All signs of hypertrophy were lost in fifteen weeks.

More recently, research on humans by muscle biopsy technique (52) has also shown the capacity for *fiber* hypertrophy in older men (age fifty-six to sixty-five). ST fiber area was increased by 38% and FT fiber area by 52%, but these changes were not accompanied by any increase in strength.

Effect of Aerobic Training

Kiessling and colleagues (50) compared the volume fraction of mitochondria in leg muscle of young and old healthy men, physically trained and untrained. They found that training caused a considerable increase of approximately 100% in young men but only a small increase of 20% in old men. The increased volume fraction in the young resulted

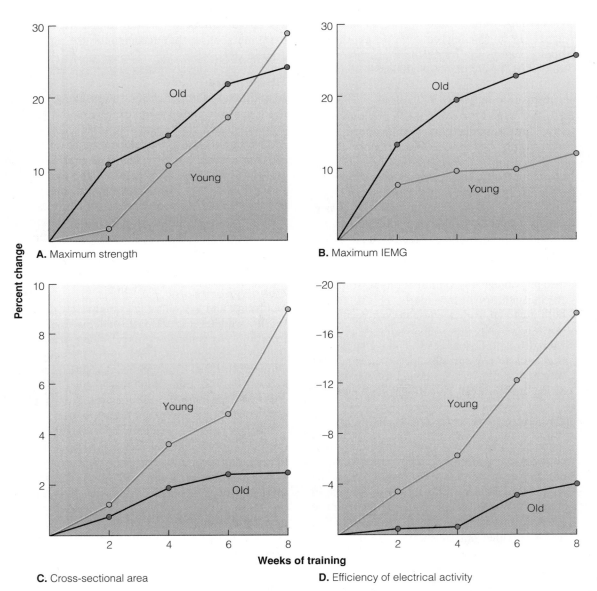

Figure 19.5   Changes occurring in the elbow flexor muscles of young and old men during weight training. (By permission of the *Journal of Gerontology* Moritani, T., and deVries, H. A., 36:294–97, 1981.)

from an increase in the number of mitochondria, but the increase in old men was due to an increased size.

Larsson (51) reported that there is no overall decrease in enzyme activity of skeletal muscle energy metabolism up to the age of sixty-five in healthy sedentary men. Recent work with rats (95) also suggests that the adaptive response of the mitochondria to aerobic training is maintained in old age. These findings suggest that the declining physical work capacity in old age is not due to losses in muscle respiratory capacity but more likely to the gradual decline in maximal cardiac output.

Age and the Cardiovascular System

The effects of a lifetime of vigorous exercise on the cardiovascular system have not yet been investigated extensively by scientific methods. Evidence, however, has been presented from observations on isolated individuals who have trained very hard into old age. Clarence DeMar, the famous marathon runner, made it a habit to run twelve miles every day and maintained this level of training throughout his lifetime. He was still competing in twenty-five- and twenty-six-mile marathons at age sixty-five, and he ran his last fifteen-kilometer race at sixty-eight—two years before his death (from cancer). At the autopsy it was found that this unusually strenuous exercise had not only *not* hurt his heart but had left him with a myocardium that was unusually well developed, valves that were normal, and coronary arteries estimated to be two or three times normal size (10).

Maximum Heart Rate

As was discussed in chapter 6, the maximum heart rate attainable during exercise decreases with age. Maximum heart rate for young adults is usually between 190 and 200 bpm; in old age this value decreases gradually. The maximum heart rate in older adults can be estimated as follows: MHR = 220 − age.

Recently Londeree and Moeschberger (54) have provided more scientifically derived equations based on over 23,000 subjects from five to eighty-one years of age. They showed that MHR differs not only with age but is higher when measured on a treadmill than on a bicycle. Young, fit subjects have a slightly lower MHR, but the values are higher in the older data. The two most important facts to emerge were: 1) there is no gender difference with respect to MHR, and 2) the error in predicting MHR is large, plus or minus 22 bpm at the 95% confidence level. This potential error must be considered when prescribing exercise as discussed in chapter 15.

Data from animal studies suggest that the reduction in MHR with age is due to intrinsic changes in the myocardium itself rather than to changes in neural influences (17).

Cardiac Output

The at-rest cardiac output declines approximately 1% per year after maturity (10). This evidence is supported by the fact that the strength of the myocardium measured by ballistocardiography declines at a similar rate (85). The most important parameter is the capacity for cardiac output at maximal exercise, which appears to decrease at a similar rate to that of resting cardiac output (44, 47).

Coronary Artery Changes

Simonson (81) has shown that in normal hearts, the cross-sectional area of the lumen of coronary arteries is reduced with age. The percentage of the total arterial cross section that is open to blood flow is 29% less in age group forty to fifty-nine than it is in the age group ten to twenty-nine.

Circulatory Changes

One method for assessing vasomotor responsiveness to stress is strapping a subject to a tiltboard so that orientation in space can be changed quickly from supine to vertical posture as well as to intermediate postures, thus bringing about quick changes in hydrostatic pressures within the circulatory system. After a tilt to 45 degrees, older subjects showed larger decreases in and slower recovery of systolic blood pressure than the younger group. When tilted to standing, the older group had larger decreases in and slower recovery of diastolic blood pressure. In both cases, the younger group had a greater increase in heart rate (a desirable response), which increased the blood pressure available to compensate for the increased hydrostatic pressure (64).

There appear to be no significant differences in the blood flow to the extremities at rest or in the vasomotor reflex responses to warming and cooling between healthy young and old adults. However, the response of blood flow to the stimulus of exercise is markedly less in the old than in the young subjects (92), although blood pressure shows a greater response in the old than in the young (65). Lower flow with greater pressure would be the logical result of increased peripheral resistance (chap. 7).

Circulation time from arm to thigh was measured in 237 normal subjects and found to be 30% to 40% slower in older subjects (over sixty) compared with the values for the young (9).

Capillary density does not appear to change with age, but the ratio of capillary to muscle fibers decreases because of the greater number of fibers per unit cross section due to atrophic processes (66).

A more hopeful note is sounded by Russian workers who have reported that the hardening of the arteries associated with aging may be reversible through systematic physical conditioning. They found a 14% slowing of pulse wave velocity after six to seven months of

training in a group whose age averaged fifty-four years (90). A slower pulse wave propagation is associated with better elasticity in the arterial wall.

Recent research (75) also suggests that lifelong regular exercise may alter the known biochemical changes in the heart muscle related to declining cardiac function with age. While sedentary rats show a steady decline in the ATPase activity of the heart's contractile proteins, this loss did not occur in rats that were exercised five times weekly by fifteen minutes of swimming throughout their life span.

Changes in Pulmonary Function

Lung Volumes and Capacities

It has been firmly established that vital capacity declines with age. There appears to be no very good evidence for any change in total lung capacity, and consequently residual volume increases with age (62, 63). Aging increases the ratio of residual volume (RV) to total lung capacity (TLC), and anatomic dead space also increases with age (16).

Thoracic Wall Compliance

Some tissues of the lungs and chest wall have the property of elasticity. Thus, in inspiration, the muscles must work against this elasticity, which then aids the expiration phase through elastic recoil. This relationship between force required (elastic force) per unit stretch of the thorax is called *compliance*. It is measured by the size of the ratio of volume change per unit pressure change. It may be thought of as the elastic resistance to breathing. That is to say, the less compliant the tissues, the more elastic force must be overcome in breathing. Two tissues offer elastic resistance to breathing: the lung tissue itself and the wall of the thoracic cage. The evidence suggests that lung compliance increases with age (88), but more important, thoracic wall compliance decreases

(58, 73, 88). Thus the older individual may do as much as 20% more elastic work at a given level of ventilation than the young, and most of the additional work is performed in moving the chest wall (88).

It seems entirely likely that the age differences in lung volumes and capacities noted before can be explained largely on the basis of this lessening mobility of the chest wall with age.

Pulmonary Diffusion

A significant decrease in the capacity for pulmonary diffusion both at rest and at any given work load accompanies the aging process (29).

Ventilatory Mechanics in Exercise

In view of the changes in pulmonary function already cited, it is not surprising to find that the process of breathing becomes less efficient with age. Figure 19.6 presents data from deVries's laboratory that shows clearly the need for greater ventilation in old men compared with young men at any given level of work or O_2 consumption (25). Interestingly, there is a difference in the mechanics by which the old subjects met the increased ventilatory demand. While the young first increased breathing frequency, the older men increased their tidal volume (the more efficient mechanism), thus reaching their maximal tidal volume (TV) early at work loads where the young still had large reserves of TV for work at higher loads.

Age and Physical Working Capacity (PWC)

Maximal O_2 Consumption

As was mentioned earlier, the best single measure of physical working capacity (PWC) is

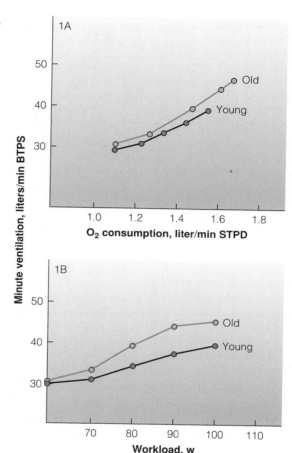

Figure 19.6   *Top:* expiratory minute volume (liters/min BTPS) as a function of O_2 consumption (liters/min STPD). *Bottom:* expiratory minute volume as a function of work load in watts. (From deVries, H. A., and Adams, G. M., in *Journal of Gerontology* 27:350. © 1972 Gerontological Society of America. Reprinted by permission.)

maximal oxygen consumption, and two excellent studies have related this variable to age. Robinson (74) tested a total of seventy-nine male subjects, ranging in age from six to seventy-five. The results are shown in table 19.1. Astrand (3) tested forty-four women, ranging in age from twenty to sixty-five, and these results are tabulated in table 14.5.

For adults of both genders, there is a gradual decline in maximal O_2 consumption

| Table 19.1 | | Highest Oxygen Intake Attained in Maximal Work as Related to Body Weight and Age | | | | | | |

Age Group	No. of Subjects	Age in Years (Mean)	Weight in kg (Mean)	Maximal O_2 Intake*				
				Liters/min		ml/kg·min^{-1}		
				(Mean)	(Extremes)	(Mean)	(Extremes)	
I	4	6.1	21.0	0.98	0.80–1.30	46.7	42.8–49.5	
II	9	10.4	30.0	1.56	1.24–2.00	52.1	49.0–56.1	
III	9	14.1	55.8	2.63	1.89–3.41	47.1	36.4–55.4	
IV	11	17.4	68.5	3.61	2.96–4.20	52.8	44.6–62.5	
V	11	24.5	72.5	3.53	2.56–4.50	48.7	41.9–55.6	
VI	10	35.1	79.3	3.42	2.76–3.97	43.1	37.6–52.8	
VII	9	44.3	74.1	2.92	2.30–3.62	39.5	33.7–46.5	
VIII	7	51.0	68.7	2.63	2.24–3.35	38.4	33.7–43.2	
IX	8	63.1	67.4	2.35	1.64–3.15	34.5	30.2–41.7	
X	3	75.0	67.4	1.71	1.43–1.90	25.5	21.8–29.6	

*Dry gas at 0° C and 760 mm Hg

From S. Robinson. *Arbeitsphysiologie* 10:279, 1938. Verlag Julius Springer, Berlin.

with age. For men, the maximal values were found at mean age 17.4 years, and they declined to less than half those values at mean age 75. For women, the maximal values were found in the age group twenty to twenty-nine, and they fell off by 29% in the age group fifty to sixty-five.

More recent data suggest that for both men (20) and women (30) the rate of decline may be slower in those who are physically active. Indeed, Kasch and Wallace (48) have provided longitudinal data suggesting that the usual 9% to 15% decline in $\dot{V}O_2$ max from age forty-five to fifty-five can be forestalled by regular endurance exercise. Hodgson and Buskirk (43) have summarized the data from many cross-sectional studies (fig. 19.7), which suggests that active male athletic subjects start at higher values and at age sixty are still at or above the level of the sedentary twenty-year-old men, although the rate of decline is similar.

Another parameter related to physical work capacity is the O_2 kinetics in response to an imposed workload. In other words, the time delay during which the $\dot{V}O_2$ is adjusted to meet the demands of the imposed demand is shorter in the well trained. Robinson in his classic study of 1938 (74) observed that the older men required more time to adjust than the young, but his subjects were not selected for equal fitness level. deVries and colleagues (27) compared the O_2 kinetics of equally well-trained old and young men and found no significant differences.

It is of interest to consider the physiological functions whose decline with increasing age might contribute to this loss of ability to transport and utilize O_2. The following functions are probably the most important in achieving maximal O_2 consumption: 1) lung ventilation, 2) lung diffusion capacity for O_2, 3) heart rate, 4) stroke volume, and 5) O_2 utilization by the tissues. The implication of

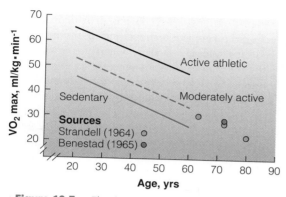

Figure 19.7 The decrease of maximum oxygen consumption with age in men twenty to sixty from a review of cross-sectional studies.

Sedentary men $\dot{V}O_2max = 54.1-0.41$ (age)
Moderately active men $\dot{V}O_2max = 61.6-0.44$ (age)
Active athletic men $\dot{V}O_2max = 76.1-0.48$ (age)

(Reprinted from the *Journal of the American Geriatrics Society*, Vol. 25, 1977, page 386, with the permission of the publisher and authors.)

direct or indirect evidence is that all of these functions decline with age. Recent evidence showed that O_2 pulse (O_2 consumption per heart beat) was identical in well-trained old and young athletes in spite of a 15% lower $\dot{V}O_2$ max in the old. This suggests that the decline in $\dot{V}O_2$ max with age is due largely to the decline in max HR (40, 42).

Muscular Efficiency

According to the data of Robinson (74), adult males tend to be more economical in their adjustment to work than boys. He found no clear-cut differences with increasing age during maturity. Astrand (3) found significant decreases in efficiency with age in women. These differences were very small, however: 21.9% for the twenty to twenty-nine age group and 19.6% for the fifty to sixty-five age group. In their comparison of equally well-trained old and young men, deVries and colleagues (27) found no significant difference in efficiency (20.5% for the young versus 19.8% for the old).

The only longitudinal data available on muscular efficiency were gathered from D.B. Dill. Dill and his associates (28) found that his efficiency in running on a treadmill declined greatly between ages forty-one and sixty-six. However, two confounding factors operated in this comparison. First, Dill had gained 16.5 pounds in the interim. Second, although the same work load was used in both instances, it represented his maximum effort at age sixty-six but only some 66% of his maximal effort at forty-one. Consequently, considerably more energy utilized at age sixty-six came from anaerobic sources, which may be less efficient. In summarizing this data, it would appear that muscular efficiency decreases with age but probably to a very slight degree.

Age and the Nervous System

Age changes (slowing) in reaction time and speed of movement have been verified. Birren and his coworkers (7, 8), who have done extensive investigation in this area, have reached the conclusion that this psychomotor slowing is probably an effect of the aging of the central nervous system because the slowing is common to several sensory modalities and to several motor pathways. The decreases in conduction time, both afferent and efferent, are insufficient to account for the total slowing.

Considerable recent work suggests that a life-style of vigorous physical activity has a beneficial effect in lessening the decline in reaction and movement times (15, 26, 77, 83, 84). Spirduso (84) has postulated a mechanism to explain this effect of exercise on the aging motor system based on the observation of similarities between age effects and Parkinsonism. A loss of brain cells that produce the neurotransmitter dopamine occurs both in normal aging and at an accelerated rate in Parkinsonism. Spirduso provided evidence that suggests that exercise may postpone the deterioration in response speed—generally observed in the aged motor system—by maintaining the nigrostriatal dopamine system. On the basis of her data she suggests that optimizing physical fitness may postpone the symptoms of aging in the nervous system. Others have found similar results (31).

Cerebral function is much more vulnerable to circulatory deficits than most tissues. It must have a constant source of O_2, and it cannot function anaerobically (as can muscle tissue, for instance). For this reason it is tempting to associate the effects of aging with a decreased cerebral blood flow and with the resulting hypoxia. However, when the effects of aging per se have been separated from the effects of arteriosclerosis, which frequently accompanies the aging process, it appears to be arteriosclerosis that is at fault. Aging per se, in the absence of arteriosclerotic changes, probably does not result in circulatory or metabolic changes in cerebral function (7, 8).

The German neurophysiologists C. and O. Vogt have made the extremely interesting observation that the degree of activity of a particular type of nerve cell has a great effect on its aging process. They have found that involution (part of the aging process) "is delayed not only by normal but also by such excessive activity of nerve cells as results in their hypertrophy" (91). This suggests that physical activity involving overuse of neural pathways of the central nervous system may have beneficial effects, such as we know occur in the case of muscle tissue. Their work has received support from the work of Retzlaff and Fontaine (71), who also found improved spinal motor neuron function as the result of conditioning in rats. Much more scientific research is needed into the possible benefits of vigorous exercise for aging populations.

Age and Body Composition

As has been discussed in earlier chapters, it is typical for aging humans to increase their weight, and Brozek (13) has provided interesting data on the composition of the human body as it ages (table 19.2). Clearly, this weight gain represents a mean increase in Brozek's sample of 12.24 kg (27 lb) of fat, while the fat-free body weight has actually decreased from age twenty to age fifty-five. It is obvious that, to maintain a constant proportion of body fat as one ages, weight must not merely be maintained at a constant level, it must be decreased. It is conceivable, however, that the loss in fat-free weight represents disuse atrophy of muscle tissue and, if vigorous exercise is maintained, does not have to be a necessary component of the aging changes.

Shock and his coworkers (79) have furnished compelling evidence that this loss of active tissue is the cause of the well-known decline in the basal metabolic rate (BMR) with age. When they computed BMR on the basis of body water (which reflects the amount of active tissue cells in the body), no significant changes were observed in relation to age. The customary method of calculating BMR (per unit of surface area) does not differentiate between fat and active tissue. Thus we find that the aging body contains fewer and fewer cells, although the activity of individual cells probably does not change significantly. Again, we would like to know the effects vigorous exercise programs might have on this process.

Stature

It has been shown that, on the average, we also grow shorter as we grow older and fatter. DeQueker, Baeyens, and Claessens showed the loss rate to average about one-half inch per decade after age thirty (21).

Effects of Physical Conditioning on Losses in Functional Capacities Caused by Aging

All of the aging changes described thus far can only be said to *accompany* the aging process.

Table 19.2	Average Estimated Changes in Body Composition during Maturity (20–55 Years) (Standard Weights Refer to Men 176 cm Tall)			
Age	Standard Weight (kg)	Standard Fat (%)	Fat (kg)	Fat-free Weight (kg)
20	67.6	10.30	6.96	60.6
25	69.9	13.42	9.38	60.5
30	71.3	16.20	11.55	59.8
35	72.9	18.64	13.59	59.3
40	74.1	20.74	15.37	58.7
45	75.5	22.50	16.99	58.5
50	76.0	23.92	18.18	57.8
55	76.8	25.01	19.20	57.6

From J. Brozek. Changes of body composition in man during maturity and their nutritional implications in *Federation Proceedings* 11:787. © 1952 Federation of American Societies for Experimental Biology. Reprinted by permission.

Causal relationships have not been established. We can infer that changes in these various functional capacities observed in different groups of subjects at increasing age levels may result from a combination of at least three factors: 1) true aging phenomena, 2) unrecognized disease processes whose incidence and severity increase with age, and 3) *disuse phenomena,* or the increasing sedentariness of our life-style as we grow older. Since we can do little to modify the first two factors, and since the third factor offers the potential for being modified by the methods of conditioning and training already well known to our profession, deVries and other investigators have addressed themselves to the question of how trainable the older human organism is.

The capacity for improvement of performance by training in children and young adults has long been established. The results of investigations over the last two decades that demonstrate the beneficial effects of physical conditioning for middle-age adults are also too numerous to cite. However, only recently have we turned our attention to the problem of maintaining and improving physical fitness and associated functional capacities in the elderly male and female, arbitrarily defined here as those persons over sixty. Table 19.3 shows the results of recent research in this area.

There seems little doubt that the PWC of the older individual can be improved by significant increments. While improved PWC may not add years to our life, it most certainly does add "life to our years." The improvement of PWC is tantamount to increasing the *vigor* of the older individual, and this can make a very important contribution to the later years of life, certainly in terms of life-style and possibly even in terms of *health*. Kasch and colleagues (49) followed a group of men over twenty years and found that physical conditioning slowed the usual losses in aerobic power.

The physiological basis for the improvement in PWC is still very much in question. All of the data reported seem to agree that the

Table 19.3 Effects of Physical Conditioning on the Functional Capacities of Older Men and Women (Mean Age over Sixty)

Measurement	Gender	N	% Improvement	Source
Cardiovascular system				
1. Decrease in HR at submaximal work	M	5	19	Barry et al. (5)
	F	3		
	M	8	3–5	Niinimaa and Shephard (61)
	F	7	3	Niinimaa and Shephard (61)
2. O_2 pulse	M	13	11	Benestad (6)
	M	48	4 (6 weeks)	deVries (22)
	M	5	29 (42 weeks)	deVries (22)
	F	17	7 (12 weeks)	Adams and deVries (1)
	M	8	1–5 (11 weeks)	Niinimaa and Shephard (61)
	F	7	0–3 (11 weeks)	Niinimaa and Shephard (61)
3. Increased blood volume	M	13	9	Benestad (6)
4. Increased total Hb	M	13	7	Benestad (6)
5. Cardiac output at submaximal work	M	34	0	deVries (22)
	M	8	−9	Niinimaa and Shephard (61)
	F	7	0	Niinimaa and Shephard (61)
6. Stroke volume at submaximal work	M	34	6	deVries (22)
	M	8	0	Niinimaa and Shephard (61)
				Niinimaa and Shephard (61)
	F	7	0	
7. Resting systolic BP	M	5		Barry et al. (5)
	F	3	13	
	M	66	2	deVries (22)
	F	17	0	Adams and deVries (1)
8. Resting diastolic BP	M	5		Barry et al. (5)
	F	3	6	
	M	66	4	deVries (22)
	F	17	0	Adams and deVries (1)
9. Regression of ECG abnormalities	M	5	50% of abnormalities definitely improved	Barry et al. (5)
	F	3		
Respiratory system				
1. Vital capacity	M	5	0	Barry et al. (5)
	F	3		
	M	66	5 (6 weeks)	deVries (22)
	M	8	20 (42 weeks)	deVries (22)
	F	17	0	Adams and deVries (1)

Measurement	Gender	N	% Improvement	Source
Respiratory system				
2. Maximum ventilation during exercise	M	47	12 (6 weeks)	deVries (22)
	M	7	35 (42 weeks)	deVries (22)
	M	5		Barry et al. (5)
	F	3	50	
	M	13	0	Benestad (6)
	F	17	0	Adams and deVries (1)
				Badenhop et al. (4)
	M	7	26 (low intensity)	
	F	21	19 (high intensity)	

Physical work capacity, $\dot{V}O_2$ max	Gender	N	% Improvement	Source
	M	61	9 (6 wks)	deVries (22)
	F	8	16 (42 wks)	
	M	5	76	Barry et al. (5)
	F	3		
	M	14	29	Sidney and Shephard (80)
	F	28	29	Sidney and Shephard (80)
	M	14	11	Suominen et al. (86)
	F	12	12	Suominen et al. (86)
	M	7	16 (low intensity)	Badenhop et al. (4)
	F	21	15 (high intensity)	

Muscular strength				
	M	68	6 (6 weeks)	deVries (22)
	M	8	12 (42 weeks)	deVries (22)
	M	5	50	Perkins and Kaiser (68)
	F	15		

Muscle hypertrophy				
	M	14	17 arm	Brown et al. (12)
	M	10	9 leg	Fiatarone et al. (35)
	M	12	11 leg	Frontera et al. (37)

Neuropsychological function				
	M	15	10	Dustman et al. (31)
	F	31	4–10	Rikli and Edwards (72)

Complete source data are given in the references section at the end of the chapter.

older organism is trainable and that the capacity for improvement percentagewise is probably not greatly different from that of the young. The capacity for maximum achievement is, of course, severely compromised since the older subject starts from a lower level. As to the mechanism by which improved PWC is brought about, the results reported by Saltin and colleagues (76) and Hartley and co-workers (41) suggest a difference in the mechanisms of adaptation from young adulthood to middle age (thirty-four to fifty-five years) in that the young respond with increases of 1) cardiovascular dimensions (heart size), 2) better redistribution of blood flow to the active tissues, and 3) increased cardiac output and other functional improvements. In middle-age men the third factor alone seems to account for the improvement of aerobic capacity. Whether this is also true for the older population (sixty and over) remains unanswered at this time. The data in table 19.3 suggest that improvement of respiratory function may be another important factor in improvement of PWC in the older male.

Important effects of physical conditioning on bone and connective tissues have also been reported. One of the very serious problems for older people, especially older women, is the loss of bony tissue (osteoporosis). Smith and Reddan (82) showed that twenty women with a mean age of eighty-two *gained* 4.2% in bone mineral composition as the result of exercise compared with controls who lost 2.5% over the thirty-six-month experimental period. More recent data support these findings (87).

Losses of joint mobility constitute another serious problem for the elderly. Here again, appropriate exercise can result in significant improvement (14).

Principles for Conduct of Conditioning Programs for Older Men and Women (over Sixty)

The principles set forth in this section have been developed specifically around programs for the elderly and constitute an extension of the discussion in chapter 15.

Medical Examination

It is absolutely essential that every individual over sixty be examined and have the approval of a physician before entering any physical conditioning program. In recent years, many cardiologists have added stress tests to their examinations in which the individual's ECG is monitored *during* the stress of progressively increasing exercise work loads. Such data are invaluable in conducting conditioning programs for middle-age and older people.

Physiological Monitoring (in the Laboratory)

Ideally, the individual's initial condition and progress in the program would be evaluated in depth, including responses with respect to O_2 consumption, cardiovascular function (blood pressure, cardiac output, ECG), respiratory function, muscular status, and anthropometric measurements. This is seldom feasible, and it is fortunate that simple measures can provide considerable insight into the individual's status (assuming prior medical clearance). At a minimum expenditure of money, time, and effort, at least the following parameters can and should be measured: 1) HR and BP response to submaximal exercise (Astrand test), 2) resting BP, 3) strength of selected muscle groups, 4) body weight, and 5) percentage of body fat estimated from skinfolds. Such measurements form the basis for a scientific approach to the use of exercise in conditioning older people in that they 1) allow prescription of exercise on a dose-response basis, and 2) provide considerable motivation for the participants who can thus see their own progress with respect to health benefits they can understand. When the interest is less in the physiology involved and an approximation of status and improvement is all that is required, Jackson and coworkers (45) have devised a method by which surprisingly good estimates can be made of aerobic power from gender, age, body composition, and self-report of activity, with no exercise testing required.

Physiological Monitoring (Gym or Field)

Participants should be taught to take their own heart rate, usually at the radial artery. They should be taught to find the artery quickly (in five to ten seconds) and to count pulse beats accurately over a fifteen-second period immediately following exercise. While such a count immediately after exercise in the young may involve considerable error because of the very rapid exponential decline in rate, the rate of decline in older people is much slower, and the rate counted is a valuable criterion of the adequacy of response to any given exercise workout in the middle-aged and elderly.

Prescription of Exercise (Dose-Response Data)

Figure 19.8 shows that the threshold for a training effect in older people requires that they work above that percentage of their heart rate range (HRR) represented by their Astrand score for estimated maximal O_2 consumption in milliliters per kilogram per minute. For example, an estimated maximal O_2 of 30 ml/kg·min^{-1} would require exercising at levels

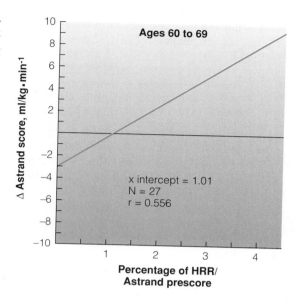

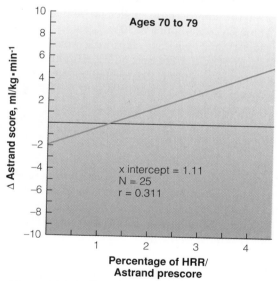

Figure 19.8   Change in Astrand test score after six weeks of training as a function of percentage of heart rate range/Astrand prescore. (From deVries, H. A. *Geriatrics* 26:94. Copyright © 1971 Modern Medicine Publications, Inc. Reprinted by permission.)

that bring HR at least 30% of the way from resting toward maximal (23). Thus a sedentary man seventy years old with a resting rate of seventy and a maximal rate of 155 (table 19.4) would need to work at an HR above

$$70 + .30 (155 - 70) = 70 + 25 = 95.$$

Since 95 represents the *threshold* for a training effect and since there are errors in our calculations, one might raise that value by 15% to 20% and estimate the desirable working HR as approximately 109 to 114, which would be a safe load for the healthy normotensive older individual. Indeed, Sidney and Shephard (80) have reported the use of HR values as high as 130 to 140.

Now, using those figures as a target HR, we enter the nomogram of figure 19.9 (24) to find what combination of jog-walk would furnish the appropriate challenge. For a maximum O_2 consumption of 30 ml/kg·min^{-1}, even the fifty steps jog–fifty steps walk would raise HR to 118 after five sets of 50–50. Therefore the subject would be instructed to start with only two to three sets of fifty jog–fifty walk and to monitor HR carefully.

Progression

The system of gradual progressing exercise work load used in deVries's laboratory and geriatric exercise program is shown in table 19.5. The warm-up is accomplished by calisthenics, the cardiovascular-respiratory challenge is provided by the run-walk program, and static stretching is used to improve joint mobility and to prevent muscle problems (22). The run or jog phase of the run-walk is done at the cadence and stride length normal and comfortable to the individual with no attempt at regulating time at this age level. This program has been shown to be both safe and effective (on a three times per week basis) for a

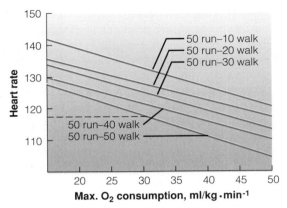

Figure 19.9   Nomogram for the estimation of heart rate response to a given dose of jogging for men sixty to seventy-nine. Example: For a man in this age bracket with a measured (or estimated from Astrand test) maximal oxygen consumption of 30 ml/kg/min, go vertically from 30 on the horizontal axis to the intersection with the 50 run-50 walk regression line. Now go horizontally to the heart rate axis to read 118, which represents the mean response to this dose. The standard error for the 5 regression lines is 8 to 10 beats. (From deVries, H. A., in *Geriatrics* 26:110. Copyright © 1971 Modern Medicine Publications, Inc. Reprinted by permission.)

normal population of older men (22) and women (1) in the presence of medical and physiological monitoring.

Type of Exercise as a Determinant of Heart Stress in Older People

DeVries and Adams conducted an experiment on twelve older men (mean age, sixty-nine) in which the work of the heart in relation to total body work was explored for exercises involving 1) heavy but rhythmic arm and leg work (crawling), 2) heavy rhythmic leg work with moderate static contraction of the upper limbs (cycling), and 3) heavy rhythmic leg

Table 19.4   Maximal Heart Rates Estimated from Age

Age	Sedentary	Active	Moderately Trained
20	193	196	192
25	190	193	190
30	188	191	188
35	185	188	186
40	182	185	183
45	179	181	181
50	175	178	177
55	171	174	174
60	166	169	170
65	161	164	165
70	155	157	159

From B. R. Londeree and M. L. Moeschberger. *Research Quarterly for Exercise and Sports* 53:297–304, 1982.

work without any static muscular activity (walking). The data indicated that the cardiac effort rises more slowly in walking (rhythmic) exercise with increasing loads of total body work than it does in either cycling or crawling effort, which involve static muscular contractions (fig. 15.3). It is important in exercising older people to reduce the sympathetic adrenergic vasoconstrictor reflex to a minimum by maximizing the rhythmic activity of large muscle masses and by minimizing 1) high activation levels of small muscles and 2) static muscle contraction of any kind. The natural activities of walking and running (jogging) are well suited to this purpose.

Musculoskeletal Injuries and Physical Activity

Despite the well-recognized benefits of physical conditioning discussed throughout this text, more and more exercise physiologists have become concerned about the incidence of injury, especially in the aged. Matheson and colleagues (56) have shown that foot and ankle joint injuries are more common in the elderly and the incidence of osteoarthritis is 2.5 times more common in the elderly. Pollock and colleagues (70) also urge caution in the use of strength testing and jogging for the elderly. Manfredi and coworkers (55) suggest that eccentric exercise is even more damaging to the muscles of the elderly. Thus, for the unconditioned elderly, for the older elderly, and certainly for the frail elderly, walking would seem to be the method of choice. Much evidence supports the efficacy of walking in improving physiological function.

Implications for Physical Education and Athletics

After the foregoing review of the effects of aging on physical performance and related physiological functions, the future for the

Table 19.5	Exercise Regimen (Three Times a Week)

A. Calisthenics (15–20 min)
  1. 5BX
  2. President's Council & Administration on Aging Series (1968)
  3. Others
B. Run-walk program (15–20 min)
  1. 50 steps run, 50 steps walk
     a. 5 sets the first day
     b. Each day increase the number of sets by one until 10 sets have been completed
     c. Use the same set procedure for each new series of run-walk
  2. 50 steps run, 40 steps walk
  3. 50 steps run, 30 steps walk
  4. 50 steps run, 20 steps walk
  5. 50 steps run, 10 steps walk
  6. 75 steps run, 10 steps walk
  7. 100 steps run, 10 steps walk
  8. 125 steps run, 10 steps walk
  9. 150 steps run, 10 steps walk
  10. 175 steps run, 10 steps walk
  11. 200 steps run, 10 steps walk
  12. Individual program
C. Static stretching to prevent soreness and to improve joint mobility (15–20 min)

college-age student using this text must seem unattractive indeed. However, two important mitigating factors must be considered.

First, each performance measure discussed has wide variability in its measurement. Since all of the discussion has centered about comparisons of *means* for various age groups, it is extremely important to recognize that, in all of the measurements, it is possible for a superior individual in an older age bracket to surpass the performance of an inferior young individual (superior or inferior in respect to his age group).

Second, for many of the measurements discussed in this chapter, we have no way of knowing how much of the age decrement can be attributed to aging per se and how much to increasingly sedentary habits or increasing degrees of unrecognized disease processes such as arteriosclerosis.

That some decline in physical performance must occur with advanced age is certainly undeniable, but that the ravages of old age can be slowed down by a sensibly vigorous regimen of physical exercise is supported by the available scientific evidence.

Maturity

It is the authors' conviction that limitations on exercise in the adult years are self-imposed by a lack of consistency and continuity in an individual's exercise habits. Probably every activity that is mastered during adolescence or young adulthood can be continued by a healthy individual well into old age. This is true, however, only if participation occurs a minimum of three times weekly. If occupational obligations prevent this degree of participation, calisthenics or weight training programs can be designed to provide the midweek conditioning necessary to prevent the weekend's activity from becoming a strain instead of an exhilarating experience.

For example, skiing, especially cross-country skiing, can be one of the most demanding of all sports. Few adults can ski every weekend, let alone three times per week, but it is a simple matter for a trained physical educator to provide midweek exercise programs for maintaining the physical capacities needed for successful weekend skiing. Suitable calisthenic or weight-training exercises can maintain the muscular strength and range of movement needed, while simple application of interval-training principles to bench-stepping or stair-climbing can maintain the requisite cardiorespiratory fitness. Indeed there are now available cross-country ski machines to be used in the home.

From the standpoint of *preventive medicine,* it is most important that every healthy adult be skilled in one or several sports that are vigorous enough to maintain optimum levels of cardiorespiratory fitness. Such activity will also provide the benefits of maintaining body weight and relieving nervous tension (chap. 13). Ideally, this activity should be so enjoyable and challenging that it is self-motivating. Activities that are interpreted as drudgery are not likely to be continued long,

no matter how rewarding. Excellent activities that meet the above criteria are tennis, handball, volleyball (if played correctly), badminton, skiing, surfing, and so on. It will be noted that some excellent activities, from a standpoint of enjoyment, have been omitted. Golf, for instance, is not vigorous enough for young adults to form the *only* physical recreation, if maximum benefits in physical condition are desired.

It should also be emphasized that any layoff from vigorous activities must be followed by a period of progressive rebuilding to the former level of competency. In general, the older the individual, the lower the first work load should be and the longer the period of progressive rebuilding of condition.

Old Age

Depending on the health of the individual, a greater or lesser reduction in work load (both intensity and duration) is needed. Most activities allow for such adjustment without complete cessation. In tennis and badminton one plays doubles instead of singles; in skiing one skis for shorter periods of time with rest intervals of increasing length. Obviously, in all competitive dual sports, one modification is simply to play opponents of roughly equivalent age.

There is no evidence that appropriate exercise can in any way injure a *healthy* individual in the older age brackets. However, frequent physical examinations, at least yearly, are necessary to protect the individual from overstrain during an incipient illness.

Indeed, a growing body of experimental evidence shows that healthy old individuals improve their functional capacities through physical conditioning much as do young people. In percentage, their improvement is comparable to that in the young, although they start

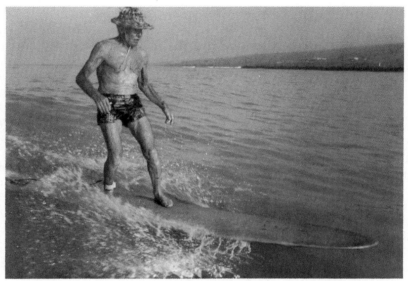

Lorrin "Whitey" Harrison of San Juan Capistrano, California at age 79 still surfs regularly at San Onofre, California and occasionally in Hawaii where this picture was taken. He was a pioneer of West Coast surfing and won the first surfing championship at San Onofre. © Bob Simms.

at and progress to lower achievement levels and probably require less training stimulus to bring about the desired response. In general, it can be said that the effects of physical conditioning on middle-age and older individuals are opposite to those commonly associated with the aging process.

The Very Old and the Frail Elderly

Data from the Framingham Study indicate that 40% of women aged fifty-five to sixty-four, almost 45% of women aged sixty-five to seventy-four, and 65% of women between seventy-five to eighty-four years were unable to lift a 10 lb weight (46). Of even greater concern is that studies of free living aged show that while rising from a chair unassisted requires only 50% of the knee extensor strength of a young adult, it often exceeds 100% of the

strength of an eighty-year-old (94). Until recently, there has been very little interest by exercise physiologists in the very old and the frail elderly, probably because the potential for improvement had not been recognized in such functions as muscular strength and aerobic capacity. However, Fiatarone and Evans reported surprising potential for improvement in the "oldest old" with respect to strength and aerobic capacity. In an excellent review of this work (34) they concluded that "This population may stand to gain more than any other group from the clinical application of exercise physiology."

Summary

1. The entire body of knowledge concerning the loss of function with increasing age must be viewed with caution, since in very few cases has the effect of decreasing levels of physical activity been controlled or ruled out.

2. Various physiological functions seem to have differing rates of decline with increasing age, with some functions being relatively unaffected.

3. Muscular strength decreases very slowly during maturity, with an increasing rate of loss in old age.

4. The capacity for muscular hypertrophy and strength gains are still possible. Such gains in strength appear to result from a "learning" to innervate a larger portion of the motor neuron pool plus hypertrophy.

5. Cardiac output decreases after early maturity by a little less than 1% per year. This seems to be true both at rest and at maximal effort.

6. Peripheral blood flow in general is slowed down with typically increasing resistance to flow and concomitant increases in blood pressure.

7. Pulmonary function declines with age, with the most important changes being seen in vital capacity, lung diffusion, and thoracic wall compliance.

8. During adulthood, there is a gradual decline in aerobic power with age for both genders. Some recent evidence suggests the decline may be slower in those who are physically active.

9. In our culture, it is typical (though not desirable) to gain weight as we grow older, although the lean body mass decreases. Therefore, the typical gain in weight is due to increasing levels of body fat.

10. As we grow older, our reaction and movement times are slower. This is probably due to changes in the central nervous system (CNS) with age.

11. The trainability of the older individual is roughly equal to that of the young adult, when expressed on a relative basis.

12. Important health benefits have been reported from the physical conditioning of the previously sedentary elderly. Such benefits include: (a) improved O_2 transport and aerobic capacity, (b) lowered blood pressure, (c) improved breathing capacity, (d) reduction in osteoporotic changes, (e) improved joint mobility, and (f) a tranquilizer effect that reduces neuromuscular tension (anxiety).

13. Many principles of exercise physiology can be brought to bear on the development of conditioning programs for the elderly are discussed in detail.

References

1. Adams, G. M., and deVries, H. A. Physiological effects of an exercise training regimen upon women aged 52–79. *J. Geront.* 28:50–55, 1973.

2. Aniansson, A., Grimby, G., Hedberg, M., Rungren, A., and Sperling, L. Muscle function in old age. *Scand. J. Rehab. Med.,* suppl. 6:43–49, 1978.

3. Astrand, I. Aerobic work capacity in men and women with special reference to age. *Acta Physiol. Scand.* 49 (suppl. 169), 1960.

4. Badenhop, D. J., Cleary, P. A., Schal, S. F., Fox, E. L., and Bartels, R. L. Physiological adjustments to higher or lower intensity exercise in elders. *Med. Sci. Sports Exer.* 15:496–502, 1983.

5. Barry, A. J., Daly, J. W., Pruett, E. D. R., Steinmetz, J. R., Page, H. F., Birkhead, N. C., and Rodahl, K. The effects of physical conditioning on older individuals. *J. Geront.* 21:182–91, 1966.

6. Benestad, A. M. Trainability of old men. *Acta Med. Scand.* 178:321–27, 1965.

7. Birren, J. E., Butler, R. N., Greenhouse, S. W., Sokoloff, L., and Yarrow, M. R., eds. *Human Aging, a Biological Behavioral Study.* Washington, D.C.: Public Health Service Publication no. 986, 1963.

8. Birren, J. E., Imus, H. A., and Windle, W. F., eds. *The Process of Aging in the Nervous System.* Springfield, IL: Charles C Thomas, 1959.

9. Boerner, W., Moll, E., Schroder, J., and Rau, F. P. Abhangigkeit der kreislaufzeit von alter geschlecht und korperlange. *Archiv fur Kreislaufforschung.* 43:221–35, 1964.

10. Brandfonbrener, M. Landowne, M., and Shock, N. W. Changes in cardiac output with age. *Circulation* 12:557–66, 1955.

11. Brewer, V., Meyer, B. M., Keele, M. S., Upton, S. J., and Hagan, R. D. Role of exercise in prevention of involutional bone loss. *Med. Sci. Sports Exer.* 15:445–49, 1983.

12. Brown, A. B., McCartney, N., and Sale, D. G. Positive adaptations to weight-lifting training in the elderly. *J. Appl. Physiol.* 69:1725–33, 1990.

13. Brozek, J. Changes of body composition in man during maturity and their nutritional implications. *Fed. Proc.* 11:784–93, 1952.

14. Chapman, E. A., deVries, H. A., and Swezey, R. Joint stiffness: Effects of exercise on old and young men. *J. Geront.* 27:218–21, 1972.

15. Clarkson, P. M. The effect of age and activity level on fractionated response time. *Med. Sci. Sports* 10:66, 1978.

16. Comroe, J. H., Forster, R. E., Dubois, A. B., Briscoe, W. A., and Carlsen, E. *The Lung.* Chicago: Year Book Medical Publishers, 1962.

17. Corre, K. A., Cho, H., and Barnard, R. J. Maximum exercise heart rate reduction with maturation in the rat. *J. Appl. Physiol.* 40:741–44, 1976.

18. Craig, B. W., Brown, R., and Everhart, J. The effects of progressive resistance training on growth hormone and testosterone levels in young and elderly subjects. *Mechanisms of Aging and Development* 49:159–69, 1989.

19. Damon, E. L. An experimental investigation of the relationship of age to various parameters of muscle strength. Ph.D. diss. Physical Education, University of Southern California, 1971.

20. Dehn, M. M., and Bruce, R. A. Longitudinal variations in maximum oxygen intake with age and activity. *J. Appl. Physiol.* 33:805–7, 1972.

21. DeQueker, J. V., Baeyens, J. P., and Claessens, J. The significance of stature as a clinical measurement of aging. *J. Am. Geriatr. Soci.* 17:169–79, 1969.

22. deVries, H. A. Physiological effects of an exercise training regimen upon men aged 52–88. *J. Geront.* 25:325–36, 1970.

23. ———. Exercise intensity threshold for improvement of cardiovascular-respiratory function in older men. *Geriatrics* 26:94–101, 1971.

24. ———. Prescription of exercise for older men from telemetered exercise heart rate data. *Geriatrics* 26:102–11, 1971.

25. deVries, H. A., and Adams, G. M. Comparison of exercise responses in old and young men: II. Ventilatory mechanics. *J. Geront.* 27:349–52, 1972.

26. deVries, H. A., Wiswell, R. A., Romero, G. T., and Heckathorne, E. Changes with age in monosynaptic reflexes elicited by mechanical and electrical stimulation. *Am. J. Phy. Med.* 64:71–81, 1985.

27. deVries, H. A.,Wiswell, R. A., Romero, G. T., Moritani, T., and Bulbulian, R. Comparison of oxygen kinetics in young and old subjects. *Eur. J. Appl. Physiol.* 49:277–86, 1982.

28. Dill, D. B., Horvath, S. M., and Craig, F. N. Responses to exercise as related to age. *J. Appl. Physiol.* 12:195–96, 1958.

29. Donevan, R. E., Palmer, W. H., Varvis, C. J., and Bates, D. V. Influence of age on pulmonary diffusing capacity. *J. Appl. Physiol.* 14:483–92, 1959.

30. Drinkwater, B. L., Horvath, S. M., and Wells, C. L. Aerobic power of females, age 10–68. *J. Geront.* 30:385–94, 1975.

31. Dustman, R. E., Ruhling, R. O., Russell, E. M., et al. Aerobic exercise training and improved neuropsychological function of older individuals. *Neurobiology of Aging* 5:35–42, 1984.

32. Ermini, M. Aging changes in mammalian skeletal muscle. *Gerontology* (Basel) 22:301–16, 1976.

33. Evans, S. J. An electromyographic analysis of skeletal neuromuscular fatigue with special reference to age. Ph.D. diss., Physical Education, University of Southern California, 1971.

34. Fiatarone, M. A., and Evans, W. J. Exercise in the oldest old. *Topics in Geriatric Rehabilitation* 5:63–77, 1990.

35. Fiatarone, M. A., Marks, E. C., Ryan, N. D., Meredith, C. N., Lipsitz, L. A., and Evans, W. J. High intensity strength training in nonagenarians. *J.A.M.A.* 263:3029–34, 1990.

36. Fisher, M. B., and Birren, J. E. Age and strength. *J. Appl. Psychol.* 31:490–97, 1947.

37. Frontera, W. R., Meredith, C. N., O'Reilly, K. P., Knuttgen, H. G., and Evans, W. J. Strength conditioning in older men: Skeletal muscle hypertrophy and improved function. *J. Appl. Physiol.* 64:1038–44, 1988.

38. Goldspink, G., and Howells, K. F. Work-induced hypertrophy in exercised normal muscles of different ages and the reversibility of hypertrophy after cessation of exercise. *J. Physiol.* 239:179–93, 1974.

39. Gutman, E., Hanzlikova, V., and Jakoubek, B. Changes in the neuromuscular system during old age. *Exp. Gerontol.* 3:141–46, 1968.

40. Hagberg, J. M., Allen, W. K., Seals, D. R., et al. A hemodynamic comparison of young and older endurance athletes during exercise. *J. Appl. Physiol.* 58:2041–46, 1985.

41. Hartley, L. H., Grimby, G., Kilbom, A., Nilsson, N. J., Astrand, I., Bjure, J., Ekblom, B., and Saltin, B. Physical training in sedentary middle aged and older men: III. Cardiac output and gas exchange at submaximal and maximal exercise. *Scand. J. Clin. Lab. Invest.* 24:335–49, 1969.

42. Heath, G. W., Hagberg, J. M., Ehsani, A. A., and Holloszy, J. O. A physiological comparison of young and old endurance athletes. *J. Appl. Physiol.* 51:634–40, 1981.

43. Hodgson, J. L., and Buskirk, E. R. Physical fitness and age: with emphasis on cardiovascular function in the elderly. *J. Am. Geriatr. Soc.* 25:385–92, 1977.

44. Hossack, K. F., and Bruce, R. A. Maximal cardiac function in sedentary normal men and women: Comparison of age-related changes. *J. Appl. Physiol.* 53:799–804, 1982.

45. Jackson, A. S., Blair, S. N., Mahar, M. T., Russ, R. M., and Stuteville, J. E. Prediction of functional aerobic capacity without exercise testing. *Med. Sci. Sport Exerc.* 22:863–70, 1990.

46. Jette, A. M., and Branch, L. G. The Framingham Disability Study II: Physical disability in the aging. *Am. J. Public Health* 71:1211–16, 1981.

47. Julius, S., Amery, A., Whitlock, L. S., and Conway, J. Influence of age on the hemodynamic response to exercise. *Circulation* 36:222–30, 1967.

48. Kasch, F. W., and Wallace, J. P. Physiological variables during 10 years of endurance exercise. *Med. Sci. Sports* 8:5–8, 1976.

49. Kasch, F. W., Wallace, J. P., VanCamp, S. P., and Verity, L. A longitudinal study of cardiovascular stability in active men aged 45–65 years. *Phys. Sportsmed.* 16:117–26, 1988.

50. Kiessling, K. H., Pilstrom, L., Karlsson, J., and Piehl, K. Mitochondrial volume in skeletal muscle from young and old physically trained healthy men and from alcoholics. *Clin. Sci.* 44:547–54, 1973.

51. Larsson, L. Morphological and functional characteristics of aging skeletal muscle in man. *Acta Physiol. Scand. Suppl.* 457, 1978.

52. ———. Physical training effects on muscle morphology in sedentary males at different ages. *Med. Sci. Sports Exer.* 14:203–6, 1982.

53. ———. Histochemical characteristics of human skeletal muscle during aging. *Acta Physiol. Scand.* 117:469–71, 1983.

54. Londeree, B. R., and Moeschberger, M. L. Effect of age and other factors on maximal heart rate. *Res. Q. Exer. Sports* 53:297–304, 1982.

55. Manfredi, G., Fielding, R. A., O'Reilly, K. P., Meredith, C. N., Lee, H. Y., and Evans, W. J. Plasma creatine kinase activity and exercise induced muscle damage in older men. *Med. Sci. Sports Exerc.* 23:1028–34, 1991.

56. Matheson, G. O., McIntyre, J. G., Taunton, J. E., Clement, D. B., and Lloyd-Smith, R. Musculoskeletal injuries associated with physical activity in older adults. *Med. Sci. Sports Exerc.* 21:379–85, 1989.

57. Meredith, C. N., Frontera, W. R., and Evans, W. J. Effects of diet on body composition change during strength training in elderly men. *Am. J. Clin. Nutr.* 47:767, 1988.

58. Mittman, C., Edelman, N. H., Norris, A. H., and Shock, N. W. Relationship between chest wall and pulmonary compliance and age. *J. Appl. Physiol.* 20:1211–16, 1965.

59. Montoye, H. J., and Lamphiear, D. E. Grip and arm strength in males and females, age 10 to 69. *Res. Q.* 48:109–20, 1977.

60. Moritani, T., and deVries, H. A. Neural factors versus hypertrophy in the time course of muscle strength gain in young and old men. *J. Geront.* 36:294–97, 1981.

61. Niinimaa, V., and Shephard, R. J. Training and oxygen conductance in the elderly: II The cardiovascular system. *J. Geront.* 33:362–67, 1978.

62. Norris, A. H., Shock, N. W., and Falzone, J. A. Relation of lung volumes and maximal breathing capacity to age and socio-economic status. In *Medical and Clinical Aspects of Aging,* ed. H.T. Blumenthal, pp. 163–71. New York: Columbia University Press, 1962.

63. Norris, A. H., Shock, N. W., Landowne, M., and Falzone, J. A. Pulmonary function studies: Age differences in lung volume and bellows function. *J. Geront.* 11:379–87, 1956.

64. Norris, A. H., Shock, N. W., and Yiengst, M. J. Age changes in heart rate and blood pressure responses to tilting and standardized exercise. *Circulation* 8:521–26, 1953.

65. Palmer, G. J., Ziegler, M. G., and Lake, C. R. Response of norepinephrine and blood pressure to stress increases with age. *J. Geront.* 33:482–87, 1978.

66. Pariskova, J., Eiselt, E., Sprynarova, S., and Wachtlova, M. Body composition, aerobic capacity and density of muscle capillaries in young and old men. *J. Appl. Physiol.* 31:323–25, 1971.

67. Pemberton, J., and Flanagan, E. G. Vital capacity and timed vital capacity in normal men over forty. *J. Appl. Physiol.* 9:291–96, 1956.

68. Perkins, L. C., and Kaiser, H. L. Results of short term isotonic and isometric exercise programs in persons over sixty. *Phys. Ther. Rev.* 41:633–35, 1962.

69. Petrofsky, J. S., and Lind, A. R. Aging, isometric strength and endurance, and cardiovascular responses to static effort. *J. Appl. Physiol.* 38:91–95, 1975.

70. Pollock, M. L., Carroll, J. F., Graves, J. E., Leggett, S. H., Braith, R. W., Limacher, M., and Hagberg, J. M. Injuries and adherence to walk-jog and resistance training programs in the elderly. *Med. Sci. Sports Exerc.* 23:1194–1200, 1991.

71. Retzlaff, E., and Fontaine, J. Functional and structural changes in motor neurons with age. In *Behavior Aging and the Nervous System,* eds. A. T. Welford and J. E. Birren. Springfield: Charles C. Thomas, 1965.

72. Rikli, R. E., and Edwards, D. J. Effects of a three-year exercise program on motor function and cognitive processing speed in older women. *Res. Q. Exerc. Sport* 62:61–67, 1991.

73. Rizzato, G., and Marazzini, L. Thoracoabdominal mechanics in elderly men. *J. Appl. Physiol.* 28:457–60, 1970.

74. Robinson, S. Experimental studies of physical fitness in relation to age. *Arbeitsphysiologie* 10:251–323, 1938.

75. Rockstein, M., Chesky, J. A., and Lopez, T. Effects of exercise on the biochemical aging of mammalian myocardium: I. Actomyosin ATPase. *J. Geront.* 36:294–97, 1981.

76. Saltin, B., Hartley, H., Kilbom, A., and Astrand, I. II. Physical training in sedentary middle-aged and older men. *Scand. J. Clin. Lab. Invest.* 24:323–34, 1969.

77. Sherwood, D. E., and Selder, D. J. Cardiorespiratory health, reaction time and aging. *Med. Sci. Sports* 11:186–89, 1979.

78. Shock, N. W. Current concepts of the aging process. *J.A.M.A.* 175:654–56, 1961.

79. Shock, N. W., Watkin, D. M., Yiengst, M. J., Norris, A. H., Gaffney, G. W., Gregerman, R. I., and Falzone, J. A. Age differences in the water content of the body as related to basal oxygen consumption in males. *J. Geront.* 18:1–8, 1963.

80. Sidney, K. H., and Shephard, R. J. Frequency and intensity of exercise training for elderly subjects. *Med. Sci. Sports* 10:125–31, 1978.

81. Simonson, E. Changes of physical fitness and cardiovascular functions with age. *Geriatrics* 12:28–39, 1957.

82. Smith, E. L., and Reddan, W. Physical activity—a modality for bone accretion in the aged. *Am. J. Roentgen.* 126:1297, 1977.

83. Spirduso, W. W. Exercise and the aging brain. *Res. Q. Exer. Sports* 54:208–18, 1983.

84. Spirduso, W. W., and Farrar, R. P. Effects of aerobic training on reactive capacity: An animal model. *J. Geront.* 36:654–62, 1981.

85. Starr, I. An essay on the strength of the heart and on the effect of aging upon it. *Am. J. Cardiol.* 14:771–83, 1964.

86. Suominen, H., Heikkinen, E., Liesen, H., Michel, D., and Hollmann, W. Effects of 8 weeks endurance training on skeletal muscle metabolism in 56–70-year-old sedentary men. *Eur. J. Appl. Physiol.* 37:173–80, 1977.

87. Suominen, H., and Rahkila, P. Bone mineral density of the calcaneus in 70–80-year-old male athletes and a population sample. *Med. Sci. Sports Exerc.* 23:1227–33, 1991.

88. Turner, J. M., Mead, J., and Wohl, M. E. Elasticity of human lungs in relation to age. *J. Appl. Physiol.* 25:664–71, 1968.

89. Tzankoff, S. P., and Norris, A. H. Effect of muscle mass decrease on age-related BMR changes. *J. Appl. Physiol.* 43:1001–6, 1977.

90. Vasiliyva, V. Y. The effect of physical exercise on the cardiovascular system of elderly persons. *Excerpta Medica Gerontology and Geriatrics* 5:5, no. 641. From papers presented at 2d conference on Gerontology and Geriatrics at Moscow, 1962.

91. Vogt, C., and Vogt, O. Aging of nerve cells. *Nature* 158:304, 1946.

92. Wahren, J., Saltin, B., Jorfeldt, L., and Pernow, B. Influence of age on the local circulatory adaptation to leg exercise. *Scand. J. Clin. Lab. Invest.* 33:79–86, 1974.

93. Wessel, J. A., and Van Huss, W. D. The influence of physical activity and age on exercise adaptation of women aged 20–69 years. *J. Sports Med. Phys. Fitness* 9:173–80, 1969.

94. Young, A. Exercise physiology in geriatric practice. *Acta Med. Scand. Suppl.* 711:227–32, 1987.

95. Young, J. C., Chen, M., and Holloszy, J. O. Maintenance of the adaptation of skeletal muscle mitochondria to exercise in old rats. *Med. Sci. Sports Exer.* 15:243–46, 1983.

Neuromuscular Fatigue

Historical Perspective

Importance of Neuromuscular Fatigue
Athletic Performance
Loss of Strength with Fatigue
Effect of Fatigue on Reflexes and Coordination
Effect of Fatigue on Industrial Workers

Physiology of Fatigue
Basic Nature of Fatigue

Central versus Peripheral Causes of Fatigue
Accumulation versus Depletion Hypotheses
Muscle Temperature Effect on Fatigue

Electromyographic Observations of Fatigue

Psychological Effects of Fatigue (Staleness)

The meaning of the word *fatigue* varies depending on the scientific discipline or clinical medical practice involved. In primary care, fatigue is the seventh most common symptom, accounting for more than 10 million office visits annually (11).

In the world of physical education and especially in the realm of athletic performance, we are constantly involved directly or indirectly with the concept of fatigue. In all events in which time or distance are criteria of success we are of necessity concerned with an endpoint largely determined by fatigue.

But what is fatigue? *Stedman's Medical Dictionary* defines it as "that state following a period of mental or bodily activity characterized by a lessened capacity for work and reduced efficiency of accomplishment, usually accompanied by a feeling of weariness, sleepiness or irritability; it may also supervene when from any cause energy expenditure outstrips restorative processes, e.g., lack of sleep or food" (47).

Simonson pointed out that fatigue is not an entity; there are various types of fatigue just as there are various types of work, involving different physiological functions to a different degree, different phenomena, different mechanisms, and different localizations (45).

However, for the purposes of exercise physiology, we will use the term fatigue to describe a transient decrease in working capacity that results from previous physical activity. We will further restrict our interest to dealing with neuromuscular fatigue, while fully recognizing the contributions of other systems such as the cardiovascular, pulmonary, and endocrine systems to the end result. Neuromuscular fatigue can be defined as a transient decrease in muscular performance usually seen as a failure to maintain or develop a certain expected force or power.

Historical Perspective

Early studies on muscle fatigue were carried out on animal preparations both on isolated muscle and *in situ*. Probably the first to study muscle fatigue in humans was Mosso, the Italian physiologist who in 1892 conceived the first ergograph that recorded excursions of the middle finger during fatiguing workbouts. A later version of the ergograph and the ergograms resulting from fatiguing workbouts as used by Hellebrandt and her coworkers (13) for evaluating wrist flexion fatigue are illustrated in chapter 22 (fig. 22.3). Mosso believed that muscle fatigue was basically of nervous origin. His opinion was based on the fact that mental (emotional) excitement had a salutary effect on the work done before fatigue intervened (1).

In the early years of the twentieth century many investigators examined the question of central versus peripheral location of fatigue. Central mechanisms were defined as proximal to the motor neurons (that is, mainly in the brain), while peripheral mechanisms were defined as residing within the motor units (that is, the motor neurons, the peripheral nerves, the motor endplates, and the muscle fibers themselves). The investigators used ergographs of various kinds patterned after that of Mosso. After thoroughly fatiguing the experimental muscle using various kinds of voluntary contraction (differing rates and both static and dynamic), and after demonstrating fatigue objectively on the ergograph, the investigators stimulated the muscle by electric shock to the motor nerve. Several investigators using this experimental paradigm found that after complete voluntary exhaustion, electrical stimulation at the motor nerve produced sizable contractions (for a review of this work see Simonson (45)). These findings constitute strong evidence for the central nervous system (CNS) as a primary site of fatigue but, of course, do not rule out peripheral sites such as the neuromuscular junction and the muscle fiber itself.

In 1954, Merton, using the adductor pollicis muscle, found that when fatigue had progressed to the point where even maximal electrical stimulation at the motor nerve could no longer produce evidence of a muscle twitch, the muscle action potentials were relatively unaffected (26, 27). He concluded that "fatigue is peripheral and is due to failure of muscle to contract when motor impulses reach it." He also concluded that the failure of muscle to respond is not due to blockage of impulses at the neuromuscular junction (NMJ) because there was no significant falling off in the voltage of the muscle action potentials (27).

To further confuse matters, Ikai and colleagues (17), using the same muscle preparation as Merton, demonstrated an enhancement of contractile force using electrical stimulation after voluntary contraction had produced a fatigue effect.

Bigland-Ritchie and coworkers (3) attempted to resolve the question, Does fatigue arise because the muscle machinery is failing or because the subject is not willing to go on driving it with the same motivation as at the start? Or more succinctly: central versus peripheral causation? They found that in sustained maximum voluntary contractions of the quadriceps, central fatigue may account for an appreciable proportion of the force loss, and they found no evidence that NMJ failure is a limiting factor. Five of their nine subjects consistently showed central fatigue while the rest did not. So we may conclude that both central and peripheral fatigue can be important factors although many individual differences are involved.

Importance of Neuromuscular Fatigue

Athletic Performance

Since World War II it has been commonly accepted in exercise physiology that oxygen delivery alone limits maximal exercise performance. Thus, performance limits, particularly during maximal but also during submaximal exercise have been explained largely in terms of O_2 transport and O_2 and fuel utilization. This tunnel vision has resulted in a failure to explore other factors determining muscle contractile function while we have concentrated on cardiovascular and respiratory limits to exercise performance.

Noakes (38), a renowned South African physiologist, has furnished a seminal review of the literature, which suggests that we should question whether O_2 limitation develops during maximal exercise. He suggests that if it does occur, it develops in only about 50% of test subjects. His views are based on considerable evidence that O_2 consumption has not plateaued in incremental work tests when in fact exhaustion has brought an end to exercise. His work and that reported by many other investigators suggest that the factors limiting maximal exercise performance might be better explained in terms of a failure of muscle contractility or *fatigue*.

Loss of Strength with Fatigue

The loss of strength with fatigue is, of course, the basis for the use of any of the ergographs that have been developed since Mosso's days. Using an ergograph the presence of fatigue is deduced from the loss in strength needed to lift a weight to full height seen at the beginning of exercise. Determining the fatigue factor during isometric contraction is also a matter of recording graphically the loss of maximal strength with the handgrip dynamometer when an effort is made to hold a maximal contraction (chap. 22, fig. 22.2).

Effect of Fatigue on Reflexes and Coordination

The effect of fatigue on reflex activity has been well known but somewhat neglected since the early work of Sherrington at the turn of the century. Sherrington demonstrated clearly the fading of a reflex with repeated stimulation, and the importance of his findings to our field can hardly be overemphasized (44). The phenomenon of mammalian reflex fatigue hinges on Sherrington's basic observation that conduction in the reflex arc is much more "fatigable" than is conduction in the nerve fiber itself. Where an axon may fail to respond to an artificial stimulus after say 100 trials, a reflex becomes inelicitable after far fewer trials, and the more interneurons or synapses are involved in the reflex arc, the more quickly it may become fatigued.

Since fatigue has rather dramatic effects on both strength and reflexes it is to be expected that it would also affect coordination in the complex movements involved in athletics. Anyone who has ever watched the degraded performance of marathon runners at the finish line needs no further evidence. However, this effect of fatigue has been quantitatively studied, and results from many early investigations suggest that the deterioration of motor performance with fatigue and its consequent increase in O_2 demand per unit work done is probably due to irradiation of motor impulses to neighboring motor nerve centers. These nerve centers cannot make any meaningful contribution to the job at hand and may indeed result in the incoordination that can be observed in extreme fatigue states (45).

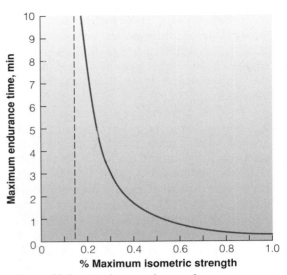

Figure 20.1   Maximum endurance time as a function of % force of maximal strength. (Source: Redrawn from W. Rohmert, "Ermittlung von Erholungspausen fur Statische Arbeit des Menschen" in *Int. Z. Angew. Physiol.* 18:123–164, 1960, Springer-Verlag, Heidelberg. Reprinted with permission.)

Effect of Fatigue on Industrial Workers

During World War II and for several decades after the war, German physiologists were actively researching pragmatic questions such as maximizing the output of industrial workers. The basic relationship of intensity to duration for static work is shown in figure 20.1. The essence of such a curve is its depiction of the fatigue phenomenon as it proceeds against varying forces. The more useful figure 20.2, from the work of Rohmert (42), shows the effect of both dynamic and static work in producing fatigue on the arm ergometer. The figure shows clearly that for any given length of work time (duration), static work is far more fatiguing than is dynamic work whether on an arm ergometer or in weight lifting. The difference is due to the fact that circulation is occluded with the static work, whereas dynamic work allows blood flow at least intermittently.

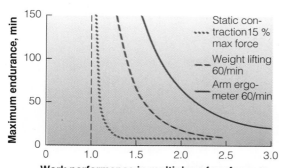

Figure 20.2 Effective work performance in multiples of performance at a level that can be sustained over several hours. (Source: Redrawn from W. Rohmert, *Zbl. Arb. Wiss.* 19:1–28, 1965, figure 5.)

It is obvious from the foregoing that the physical work rate that industrial workers can sustain for an eight-hour work shift must depend on the forces that the muscles are required to produce. Müller (35) showed that muscular fatigue could be observed quite reliably by calculating the mean heart rate increment (delta heart rate ΔHR) as a function of work time. When (ΔHR) was less than 0.1 bpm/min, work could be continued for an eight-hour workshift without undue muscle fatigue (41). Rohmert also developed equations from which the curves in figure 20.3 were drawn. From these curves we can see that static work at 25% of maximal voluntary contraction (MVC) can be maintained for an eight-hour shift if work intervals are interspersed with rest intervals twice as long, and work at 33% MVC can be maintained if the rest interval is three times as long. In applying these results to industrial work, the performance in grinding of cast iron, a static type of work, was improved and fatigue was reduced when the workers took appropriate pauses.

From the vantage point of metabolic factors, I. Astrand (2) found that work at 50% of $\dot{V}O_2$ max could be carried out for one hour

without fatigue at a steady state. Work prolonged to seven hours (seven times fifty minutes of work with ten-minute pauses and one hour for lunch) also could be carried out with a steady state of $\dot{V}O_2$, R.Q., lactate, and rectal temperature. However, the subjects became uncomfortable and showed increased HR by the end of the day. Michael, Hutton, and Horvath (29) concluded that when bicycling or walking for eight hours without interruption 35% of max $\dot{V}O_2$ is the limit that can be performed without undue fatigue.

Müller and Karrasch (36) compared the fatigue effect measured by HR increases brought about by 28,800 kgm of dynamic work over a one-hour period for various combinations of work intervals and rest intervals. For this level of work on the cycle ergometer (480 kgm/min if done without rest) the least fatigue was encountered when done without rest pauses. When the rest intervals were introduced, to maintain the hourly work rate of 28,800 kgm the minute work rates were necessarily increased, and fatigue became greater as the rest periods were lengthened because of the need for heavier loads during the work interval. Only when the rest intervals were kept short in a ratio of one:two (rest versus work) was fatigue avoided.

Physiology of Fatigue

Basic Nature of Fatigue

Notice in figure 20.2 that even though there are large differences in the curve parameters (that is, the large differences in rate of work that can be maintained for a given time) the curves all appear to have the same logarithmic mathematical relationship. The intensity-duration curve is even very similar if we plot velocity against time achieved for world records in running events. Simonson (45) explains this by suggesting that the relationship

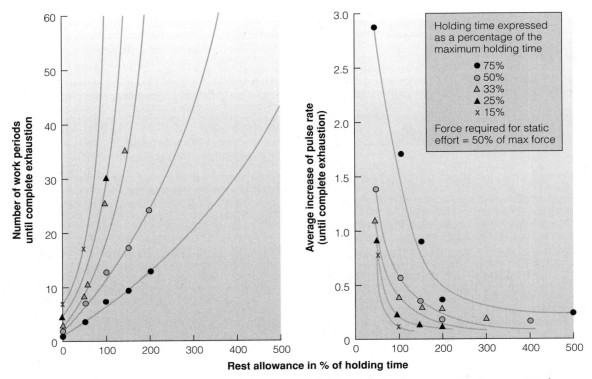

Figure 20.3   Influence of rest allowances for static work (holding a torsional moment of the lower arm). *Left:* number of work periods. *Right:* heart rate increment. (Source: Redrawn from W. Rohmert, ''Ermittlung von Erholungspausen fur Statische Arbeit des Menschen'' in *Int. Z. Angew. Physiol.* 18:123–164, 1960, Springer-Verlag, Heidelberg. Reprinted with permission.)

between intensity of work and endurance appears to be a fundamental characteristic of performance, largely independent of the type of work and determined by the speed of recovery during work. Thus, the time for recovery is zero during static work (above circulatory occlusion pressure) and varies in dynamic work according to the rest allowed between repetitive contractions during which blood can flow.

Central versus Peripheral Causes of Fatigue

The involvement of central or peripheral mechanisms in the development of fatigue is probably largely determined by the intensity of the workbout. EMG studies by Missiuro, Kirschner, and Kozlowski (31) on fifteen young men showed that a high-intensity workbout on an arm ergograph (approximately 50% MVC) that could be maintained for 1.5 to 3 minutes resulted in a *linear* increase of the integrated EMG (IEMG) of 2 1/2 to 3 times that recorded at the onset of the workbout. However, working at a low intensity (approximately 13% MVC) that could be maintained for 40 to 140 minutes, the resulting EMG response was much smaller and not linear and occurred in two or three rising waves and then diminished. The subject invariably stopped working at an EMG level 30% to 40% lower than the maximum reached at high intensity. We have found the same results in the authors' laboratories working with the quadriceps muscles on a bicycle ergometer. These findings strongly suggest that central factors are not involved to any great extent in high-intensity fatigue since the EMG voltage is still increasing at exhaustion. This result is consistent with fatigue of the contractile apparatus as found by Merton (26, 27). On the other hand, in fatigue brought about by low-intensity effort over a period of one to two hours at exhaustion, the EMG level is at submaximal value and diminishing, which suggests a failure in nervous system drive.

Although central factors are probably not of major importance in fatigue of short-term–high-intensity exercise, they may be operative even here as suggested by the "Setchenov phenomenon," which was first observed at the turn of the century, when it was found that more work could be produced after a pause with diverting activity than after a passive rest pause. Asmussen (1) explains this effect of diverting activity on the basis that during muscle fatigue, a feedback of nerve impulses from the fatigued muscles impinges on a part of the reticular formation in the brain and causes an inhibition of the voluntary effort. Diverting activity (either during the exercise or during the rest pause) on the other hand produced an increased inflow of impulses from nonfatigued parts of the body to the facilitatory part of the reticular formation, thus shifting the balance between inhibition and facilitation in a facilitatory direction.

Accumulation versus Depletion Hypotheses

With respect to what happens at the muscle site in fatigue, two of the original five hypotheses of Simonson (45) have remained tenable over the years. These two most attractive hypotheses regarding the cause of fatigue are: 1) the accumulation of metabolites, and 2) the depletion of energy-yielding substances.

Regarding the first hypothesis, the main metabolites of concern are lactate and its consequent increase in hydrogen ions, inorganic phosphate, and ammonia. Any one of these factors *could* be rationalized as limiting muscular performance as in fatigue, but unfortunately, the search for accumulation of substances with causal relationship to fatigue has limitations because concentrations in blood (which is all we can measure during exercise) may not reflect concentration in muscle or in other organs. It is quite possible that some substance accumulates in minute amounts in muscle and would escape blood analysis but could conceivably affect enzyme activity. At our present state of knowledge we can neither rule in nor rule out the accumulation hypothesis.

Regarding the second hypothesis, sometimes called the "depletion hypothesis," the depletion of energy sources such as glycogen, blood sugar, adenosine triphosphate (ATP), or creatine phosphate (CP) could also be seen as limiting muscular performance, and in certain limited experiments each can be shown to have an effect. Again, however, the evidence is unclear and in some cases contradictory. Also, there is no reason to believe that the accumulation and depletion theories are mutually exclusive. A large degree of interaction probably exists between these two fatigue mechanisms.

Possible Factors Operating in Accumulation Hypothesis

While the accumulation of lactate, hydrogen ions, inorganic phosphate, and ammonia could all contribute to fatigue, we will limit our discussion to the accumulation of lactate and its consequent increase in hydrogen ions (lowered pH) because this factor has not only theoretical implications but possible practical application in physical education and athletics as well.

It is well known that exercise of short duration and high intensity recruits fast glycolytic (FG) fibers and uses anaerobic glycolysis in the synthesis of ATP needed for muscle contraction. The result is accumulation of lactate in muscle and blood, with a concomitant increase in hydrogen ion concentration (lower pH). That this accumulation of H^+ ions results in failure of the muscle to maintain force has been demonstrated in the laboratory (24, 28, 30).

The possibility for improving the buffering of the lactic acid production and thereby improving human performance on the treadmill was recognized as long ago as 1937 by Dennig (6) in Germany. His experiments were well controlled and demonstrated that in ten subjects, use of alkaline salts improved treadmill performance by 10% to 30%. These results were corroborated by Jones and coworkers (18) in Canada some forty years later. Goldfinch, McNaughton, and Davies (12) found similar improvement in 400-meter racing times to result from alkalization. Interestingly, two later studies in Jones's laboratory failed to show benefits from alkalization, although acidification did decrease work output as would be predicted (20, 25).

The authors of this book and their colleagues (14) used an EMG approach to examine the effects of acid-base balance on the onset of fatigue (PWC_{FT}), a rather different approach, since the other investigators were evaluating *endurance* on short and long runs. The onset of fatigue was not affected by modifying acid-base balance in our laboratory. The best explanation for the divergent results is offered by McCartney and colleagues (25): ". . . the alterations in blood acid-base state had little influence on *muscle* pH. It is well known that the pH of resting muscle is unaltered by variations in plasma pH above pH 7.15. Thus the resting muscle pH just before the start of exercise may not have been altered." In the endurance study (18) the heavy exercise (90% $\dot{V}O_2$ max) was started after twenty minutes of lower intensity work. Thus, muscle pH was probably already reduced before the endurance exercise was begun and the buffering effect was therefore observable. The negative results from the authors' lab can

likely be explained on the same basis. Further research is needed and may provide us with an ergogenic aid that is both legal and effective (chap. 30).

Possible Factors Operating in Depletion Hypothesis

There is a large body of literature dealing with the depletion hypothesis, and it is both contradictory and confusing. Therefore, we will include here only the authors' interpretation of what is of greatest interest and importance to our field with no claims as to a comprehensive review.

For long-term athletic events such as the marathon running event and long-distance cycling events, there seems little doubt that muscle glycogen depletion must be a major (but not the only) determinant for the endpoint of the performance as discussed in chapter 3.

Hultman, Spriett, and Soderlund (16) have pointed out that the processes available for ATP resynthesis (the ultimate energy supply for muscle contraction) are creatine phosphate (CP) degradation, anaerobic glycolysis, and oxidative phosphorylation of carbohydrate (CHO) and fat. The maximal rates of ATP formation by these four processes are approximately 11, 5, 2, and 1 mmol ATP/sec, respectively. Hultman and colleagues point out further that at submaximal work intensity, glycogen utilization by oxidative phosphorylation dominates with increasing use of fat when the work load decreases. At no one work intensity, however, does the muscle utilize just one single fuel.

Callow, Morton, and Guppy (4) measured the utilization of CHO, lipid, protein, and also the plasma concentration of FFA, glucose, and lactate at intervals throughout fast marathon runs. They also concluded that CHO depletion is the cause of fatigue at this level of work.

For short duration muscle efforts at maximal or near maximal isometric contractions the story is quite different. In light of the data

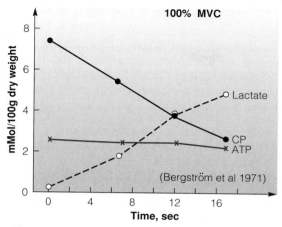

Figure 20.4   Changes in concentrations of ATP, CP, and lactate in vastus muscle during MVC until exhaustion.

from Hultman, Spriett, and Soderlund, which show the *rate* of energy supply (ATP formation) from anaerobic glycolysis to be less than half that of CP degradation, it is not surprising to find experimental evidence showing that under MVC the only substance undergoing a significant decrease is creatine phosphate (CP) (see fig. 20.4).

Muscle Temperature Effect on Fatigue

Clarke, Hellon, and Lind (5) varied bath temperature for the forearm over a range of 35° F to 108° F and measured endurance time at one-third MVC as a function of deep muscle temperature. They found the optimal deep muscle temperature for longest endurance time to be between 80° F and 86° F. At a muscle temperature of 103° F the endurance time fell 65%, while at a muscle temperature of 68° F, endurance fell by 80%. They postulate that the reduction of endurance at a temperature above 86° F is due to a more rapid accumulation of metabolites, while below 80° F they thought it to be due to an increasing number of muscle fibers becoming inoperative because of interference with neuromuscular transmission or

with some fundamental contractile properties of the muscle.

Electromyographic Observations of Fatigue

Many investigators have provided evidence that the electrical activity in muscle tissue increases as a function of time when the muscle works against a constant fatiguing force either isometrically (10, 19, 22, 39, 43) or isotonically (7, 31, 39, 43). DeVries (7) has shown that under certain experimental conditions the EMG voltage–time relation is linear for most subjects and that the slope of the line so determined has a close inverse relation to the endurance time versus a given load. Furthermore, the slope is directly proportional to the percentage of maximal voluntary contraction (MVC) represented by a given work load. More recently, Nagata (37) has shown that this increase in voltage–time ratio correlates well with the frequency shift in the EMG signal that occurs as a result of fatigue (21). It has also been shown that in pedaling a bicycle ergometer the integrated electromyogram (IEMG) from the quadriceps muscle can be used as a measure of the combined number of motor units involved and the nerve impulse frequency of the active muscles employed (3, 39).

Petrofsky (39), in agreement with earlier data by deVries (7), found that the amplitude of the IEMG taken over the quadriceps muscle during ergometer work rises in a relatively linear fashion with time if fatigue occurs. Figure 20.5 shows the results of a typical experiment in the authors' laboratory. It can be seen that for this subject riding the bicycle ergometer at work loads of 420 kgm/min and 840 kgm/min for two minutes induced no fatigue as deduced from the fact that the electrical output of the muscle did not increase over the work period. However, when the work load

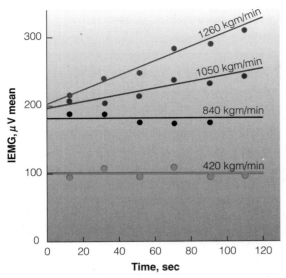

Figure 20.5   Effect of nonfatiguing work on the cycle ergometer (lower two curves) compared to fatiguing work (upper two curves).

was increased to 1,050 kgm/min a significant rate of rise in electrical output was seen, and work at 1,260 kgm/min necessitated even greater muscle activation (greater IEMG) to keep pedaling at this rate. The reason for this increased electrical activity in the muscle as fatigue progresses is thought to be a result of the combination of greater recruitment and higher innervation rate to make up for force losses as fatigued motor units drop out.

Using these principles the authors and their colleagues developed the PWC_{FT} test that was discussed in chapter 14 (9). This test was shown to be valid (9) and reproducible (8, 9) and feasible for fitness testing in older or unconditioned subjects (8). This method offers an entirely different endpoint to fatigue testing, that is, it measures the work capacity that can be maintained before the *onset of fatigue* in distinction to the duration a given workbout can be maintained, which involves subjective decisions on the part of subject and investigator.

The authors and their colleagues have begun a research program using this method to investigate the physiological bases of fatigue. At this point, neither manipulation of acid-base balance (14) nor energy stores (15) has proven to have a causal relation to the onset of fatigue (PWC_{FT}).

Psychological Effect of Fatigue (Staleness)

The phenomenon of "staleness" has long been known to result from overtraining, and its effect on performance is well recognized. In recent years, high school and college swimmers have been encouraged to use double and even triple workouts in their training regimens. It has been reported that the yearly incidence of staleness in college swimmers who train up to 14,000 meters per day is about 10% (32). Furthermore, the career prevalence of staleness in elite distance runners has been reported to be 60% (33). While it has long been known that overtraining is reflected in physiological changes in the cardiovascular, metabolic, and endocrine systems, such measurements are not readily available to coaches so they can take preventive measures. For this reason, the recent work of Morgan and co-workers (34) is very important to everyone involved with heavy distance training. They subjected twelve male college swimmers to an approximate doubling of daily training distance from 4,000 to 9,000 meters per day maintaining training intensity at 94% $\dot{V}O_2$ max for ten days. They found that monitoring mood states by psychometric methods (subjective report) accurately reflected the degree of physiological distress experienced by the swimmers. Thus, this simple method, feasible for coaches, can be of potential value in the prevention of staleness.

For the reader who desires greater breadth and depth on the subject of fatigue, several excellent reviews are available (1, 23, 45, 46).

Summary

1. The term "fatigue" is defined differently depending on the discipline. For physical education and athletics the term describes a transient decrease of working capacity resulting from previous physical activity.

2. Fatigue is not a single entity; there are various types of fatigue, as there are various types of work, involving different physiological functions to a different degree, different phenomena, different mechanisms, and different localizations.

3. Modern day investigation into the nature of fatigue in humans dates back to the Italian physiologist Mosso who developed the ergograph for objective measurement in 1892.

4. Whether fatigue originates at central or peripheral sites depends on the intensity and the nature of work (isometric versus dynamic), and there are probably individual differences as well.

5. Muscle contractility and susceptibility to fatigue are probably at least equally as important as O_2 transport in setting the limits in athletic performance.

6. The loss of strength with fatigue is the most readily observed physiological change and is the basis for ergographic measurements.

7. Fatigue causes slowing of conduction of nervous impulses through the reflex arc and this in concert with losses in strength causes dramatic losses in ability to coordinate physical actions at exhaustion.

8. A considerable body of knowledge exists regarding the effects of fatigue on work output of workers in industry. Proper use of rest pauses can optimize the output of heavy physical work in industry.

9. Regardless of the type of physical activity, muscles used, there appears to be a basic logarithmic relationship between intensity and duration of physical activity.

10. Available evidence suggests that in high-intensity activity lasting only for short duration (one to three minutes) fatigue probably originates in peripheral mechanisms, while in long term activity (thirty minutes or more) fatigue originates in central mechanisms. But there may be a strong interaction as well.

11. Two major hypotheses have been proposed for the causation of fatigue at the muscle level: 1) accumulation of metabolites and 2) depletion of energy substrate. There is evidence to support both hypotheses and neither has yet been ruled out.

12. Considerable evidence has been provided to support the importance of the accumulation of H^+ ions as a limiting factor in athletic performance, and therefore use of alkalinizers has been suggested as an ergogenic aid. However, there is still disagreement among investigators on this matter.

13. Carbohydrate depletion (in terms of muscle glycogen) is a major factor in the fatigue of long-term athletic events such as the marathon.

14. Depletion of high-energy phosphates such as creatine phosphate is probably a major factor in fatigue that is brought about very rapidly for near maximal intensity exercise.

15. The optimal deep muscle temperature for resistance to fatigue appears to lie between 80° F and 86° F. Fatigue occurs at a much greater rate at temperatures either above or below these values.

16. Electromyographic data can provide reasonably precise information regarding the onset of fatigue, and such data have the important advantage of objectivity in that they are free of any assumptions regarding the subject's level of cooperation.

17. The onset of fatigue as measured by EMG methods can be used as an endpoint for estimating PWC in subjects who are either incapable or unwilling to undergo the rigor of a maximal O_2 consumption test. Thus, the PWC_{FT} test has been developed for testing fitness in the elderly.

18. It has been shown that monitoring mood in athletes is a simple and feasible way to recognize the early manifestation of the physiological symptoms leading to the "staleness phenomenon."

References

1. Asmussen, E. Muscle fatigue. *Med. Sci. Sport.* 11:313–21, 1979.

2. Astrand, I. Aerobic work capacity in men and women with special reference to age. *Acta. Physiol. Scand.* 49:(Suppl 169), 1960.

3. Bigland-Ritchie, B., Jones, D. A., Hosking, G. P., and Edwards, R. H. T. Central and peripheral fatigue in sustained maximum contractions of human quadriceps muscle. *Clin. Mol. Med.* 54:609–14, 1978.

4. Callow, M., Morton, A., and Guppy, M. Marathon fatigue: The role of plasma fatty acids, muscle glycogen and blood glucose. *Eur. J. Appl. Physiol.* 55:654–61, 1986.

5. Clarke, R. S. J., Hellon, R. F., and Lind, A. R. The duration of sustained contractions of the human forearm at different muscle temperatures. *J. Physiol.* 143:454–73, 1958.

6. Dennig, H. Über Steigerung der körperlichen Leistungsfähigkeit durch eingriffe in den saurebasenhaushalt. *Deutsche Med. Wochenschrift.* 63:733–36, 1937.

7. deVries, H. A. Method for evaluation of muscle fatigue and endurance from electromyographic fatigue curves. *Am. J. Phys. Med.* 47:125–35, 1968.

8. deVries, H. A., Brodowicz, G. R., Robertson, L. D., Svoboda, M. D., Schendel, J. S., Tichy, A. M., and Tichy, M. W. Estimating physical working capacity and training changes in the elderly at the fatigue threshold (PWC_{FT}). *Ergonomics* 32:967–77, 1989.

9. deVries, H. A., Tichy, M. W., Housh, T. J., Smyth, K. D., Tichy, A. M., and Housh, D. J. A method for estimating physical working capacity at the fatigue threshold (PWC_{FT}). *Ergonomics* 30:1195–1204, 1987.

10. Edwards, R. G., and Lippold, O. C. J. The relation between the force and the integrated electrical activity in fatigued muscles. *J. Physiol.* 132:677–81, 1956.

11. Eichner, E. R. Chronic fatigue syndrome: Searching for the cause and treatment. *Physician and Sportsmed.* 17:142–52, 1989.

12. Goldfinch, J., McNaughton, L., and Davies, P. Induced metabolic alkalosis and its effects on 400-m racing time. *Eur. J. Appl. Physiol.* 57:45–48, 1988.

13. Hellebrandt, F. A., Skowlund, H. V., and Kelso, L. E. A. New devices for disability evaluation. *Arch. Phys. Med. Rehabil.* 29:21–28, 1948.

14. Housh, T. J., deVries, H. A., Johnson, G. O., Evans, S. A., and McDowell, S. The effect of ammonium chloride and sodium bicarbonate ingestion on the physical working capacity at the fatigue threshold. *Eur. J. Appl. Physiol.* 62:189–192, 1991.

15. Housh, T. J., deVries, H. A., Johnson, G. O., Evans, S. A., Tharp, G. D., Housh, D. J., and Hughes, R. J. The effect of glycogen depletion and supercompensation on the physical working capacity at the fatigue threshold. *Eur. J. Appl. Physiol.* 60:391–94, 1990.

16. Hultman, E., Spriett, L. L., and Soderlund, K. Biochemistry of muscle fatigue. *Biomed. Biochim. Acta.* 45:S97-S106, 1986.

17. Ikai, M., Yabe, K., Ishii, K. Muskelkraft und muskuläre ermüdung bei willkürlicher anspannung und elektricsher Reizung des Muskels. *Sportartz. un Sportmedizin.* 5:197–211, 1967.

18. Jones, N. L., Sutton, J. R., Taylor, R., and Toews, C. J. Effect of pH on cardiorespiratory and metabolic responses to exercise. *J. Appl. Physiol.* 43:959–64, 1977.

19. Knowlton, G. C., Bennett, R. L., and McClure, R. Electromyography of fatigue. *Arch. Phys. Med.* 32:648–52, 1951.

20. Kowalchuk, J. M., Heigenhauser, G. J. F., and Jones, N. L. Effect of pH on metabolic and cardiorespiratory responses during progressive exercise. *J. Appl. Physiol.* 57:1558–63, 1984.

21. Lindstrom, L., Magnussen, R., and Petersen, T. Muscular fatigue and action potential conduction velocity changes studied with frequency analysis of EMG signals. *Electromyography* 4:341–56, 1970.

22. Lippold, O. C. J., Redfearn, J. W. T., and Vuco, J. The electromyography of fatigue. *Ergonomics* 3:121–31, 1960.

23. MacLaren, D. P. M., Gibson, H., Parry-Billings, M., and Edwards, R. H. T. A review of metabolic and physiological factors in fatigue. *Exerc. Sport. Sci. Rev.* 17:29–68, 1989.

24. Mainwood, G. W., and Renaud, J. M. The effect of acid-base balance on fatigue of skeletal muscle. *Can. J. Physiol. Pharmacol.* 63:403–16, 1985.

25. McCartney, N., Heignehauser, G. J. F., and Jones, N. L. Effects of pH on maximal power output and fatigue during short-term dynamic exercise. *J. Appl. Physiol.* 55:225–29, 1983.

26. Merton, P. A. Voluntary strength and fatigue. *J. Physiol.* 123:553–64, 1954.

27. Merton, P. A. Problems of muscular fatigue. *Brit. Med. Bull.* 12:219–21, 1956.

28. Metzger, J. M., and Fitts, R. H. Role of intracellular pH in muscle fatigue. *J. Appl. Physiol.* 62:1392–97, 1987.

29. Michael, E. D., Hutton, K. E., and Horvath, S. M. Cardiorespiratory responses during prolonged exercise. *J. Appl. Physiol.* 16:987–1000, 1961.

30. Miller, R. G., Boska, M. D., Moussari, R. S., Carson, P. J., and Weiner, M. W. "P Nuclear Magnetic Resonance Studies of High Energy Phosphates and pH in Human Muscle Fatigue." *J. Clin. Invest.* 81:1190–96, 1988.

31. Missiuro, W., Kirschner, H., and Kozlowski, S. Electromyographic manifestations of fatigue during work of different intensity. *Acta Physiol. Polonica* 13:11–20, 1962.

32. Morgan, W. P., Brown, D. R., Raglin, J. S., O'Connor, P. J., and Ellickson, K. A. Psychological monitoring of overtraining and staleness. *Br. J. Sports Med.* 21:107–14, 1987.

33. Morgan, J. P., O'Connor, P. J., Sparling, P. E., and Pate, R. R. Psychological characterization of the elite female distance runner. *Int. J. Sports Med.* 8:124–31, 1987.

34. Morgan, W. P., Costill, D. L., Flynn, M. G., Raglin, J. S., and O'Connor, P. J. Mood disturbance following increased training in swimmers. *Med. Sci. Sport Exerc.* 20:408–14, 1988.

35. Müller, E. A. Ein Leistungs-pulsindex als Mass der Leistungsfähigkeit. *Arbeitsphysiologie* 14:271–84, 1950.

36. Müller, E. A., and Karrasch, K. Der Einfluss der Pausen-anordnung auf die Ermüdung bei Schwerarbeit. *Int. Z. Angew. Physiol.* 16:45–51, 1955.

37. Nagata, A. EMG power spectra during various levels of isometric contraction and fatigue. *Yokohama Medical Bulletin* 33:49–64, 1982.

38. Noakes, T. D. Implications of exercise testing for prediction of athletic performance: A contemporary perspective. *Med. Sci. Sport Exerc.* 20:319–30, 1988.

39. Petrofsky, J. S. Frequency and amplitude analysis of the EMG during exercise on the bicycle ergometer. *Eur. J. Appl. Physiol.* 41:1–15, 1979.

40. Rohmert, W. Ermittlung von Erholungspausen für statische Arbeit des Menschen. *Int. Z. Angew. Physiol.* 18:123–64, 1960.

41. Rohmert. W. Untersuchung statischer Haltearbeiten in achtstündigen Arbeitsversuchen. *Int. Z. Angew. Physiol.* 19:35–55, 1961.

42. Rohmert, W. Physiologische Grundlagen der Erhulungs-zeitbestimmung. *Zbl. Arbeit. Wiss.* 19:1–28, 1965.

43. Scherrer, J., and Bourguignon, A. Changes in the electromyogram produced by fatigue in man. *Am. J. Phys. Med.* 38:148–58, 1959.

44. Sherrington, C. S. *The Integrated Action of the Nervous System.* New Haven: Yale Univ. Press, 1947.

45. Simonson, E. *Physiology of Work Capacity and Fatigue.* Springfield, IL: Charles C. Thomas Publisher, 1971.

46. Simonson, E., and Weiser, P. C. *Psychological Aspects and Physiological Correlates of Work and Fatigue.* Springfield: Charles C. Thomas Publisher, 1976.

47. Stedman, T. L. *Stedman's Medical Dictionary.* Baltimore: The Williams and Wilkins Company, 1976.

PART **3**

Physiology of Training and Conditioning Athletes

21

Physiology of Muscle Strength

Physiology of Strength
    Hypertrophy versus Hyperplasia
    Morphological versus Neurological
        Factors in Strength Gain
    The Cross-Education Effect
    Disuse and Atrophy
    Bilateral Deficit in Strength
    Mechanical Factors in Strength
    The Necessary Stimulus for Strength
        Gain
    Joint Angle Specificity during
        Exercise
    Training Curves—The Time Course
        of Strength Development
Methods for Measurement and Training
    of Strength
    Isometric Training
    Advantages of Isometric Methods
    Methods in the Use of Isometric
        Contraction
    Cable Tension Strength Tests
    Isotonic Training

Training Methods Using Isotonic
    Contraction
Periodization
Measuring Strength by Isotonic
    Methods
Isokinetic Training
Plyometric Training
Concurrent Strength and Endurance
    Training
Variability in Strength/Individual
    Variability
Generality versus Specificity
Quantity and Quality of Muscle
    Tissue
Effect of Various Factors on Strength
    Age
    Gender
    Diurnal Variation
    Seasonal Effects
    Effects of Heat and Cold
    Psychological Factors
    Plasticity of the Human Body

The desirability of a *minimum quantity* of strength has long been recognized in athletics. However, the advantages of maximum levels of strength for all sports in which power is a factor were not recognized by physical educators, athletes, or coaches until quite recently. This strange neglect of the strength factor in athletes was the result of an unscientific acceptance by virtually everyone concerned that the development of large amounts of strength in the musculature (through activities such as weight training) inevitably resulted in a condition known as *muscle-bound.* Being muscle-bound was supposed to limit both range and speed of movement in those who participated in weight training. Therefore it was anathema to all but the most heretical coaches. This belief persisted until shortly after World War II.

At the end of World War II there was an acute need for rehabilitation procedures for restoring strength to various body segments of injured veterans. This need brought about a scientific evaluation of weight training procedures, and the pioneering work of De Lorme and Watkins (23) led to the acceptance of weight training for rehabilitation purposes. Acceptance of weight training by the medical profession apparently stimulated the research-oriented members of the physical education profession to put the muscle-bound hypothesis to the test by the scientific method. The results are now history, for many well-controlled investigations laid to rest the ghost of the muscle-bound myth. It is now generally accepted that properly conceived weight training programs not only do not slow or restrict joint motion but may even improve these factors while providing very substantial gains in strength.

The importance of strength in athletics is not always obvious. However, in an activity such as shot-putting, the need for maximum power is apparent. As discussed earlier, power is the rate of doing work (producing force). We may therefore think of power as the result of two factors: 1) strength to produce the force and 2) speed to increase the rate at which the force can be applied. In other words, we can improve an athlete's power in three different ways: 1) increase speed, strength remaining constant, 2) increase strength, speed remaining constant, and 3) improve speed and strength.

From practical experience in coaching, speed of movement improves rapidly in the training program to a plateau, from which it can be increased only with great difficulty. On the other hand, very few athletes have even begun to approach their maximum strength levels, and thus large gains in power are possible by improving strength while simply maintaining speed.

This chapter will discuss the physiological bases of strength and its improvement. It will culminate in a set of principles, based on our present knowledge, for the formulation of programs designed to improve the strength (and power) factor in athletes.

Physiology of Strength

Hypertrophy versus Hyperplasia

It is a well-known fact that when a muscle is trained with heavy resistance exercise, it grows larger in girth. This growth could be the result of either the enlargement of each muscle fiber (hypertrophy) or an increasing number of cells (hyperplasia). The latter was ruled out in the 1800s by Morpurgo. However, in recent years several investigators have reported fiber-splitting as the result of heavy resistance training, but no one has found evidence of true cell division (mitosis). For all practical purposes we can still accept hypertrophy as the basis for the growth of a muscle in response to heavy exercise.

It has been suggested (20) that eccentric contractions are necessary to simulate hypertrophy and, therefore, solely concentric training does not result in an increase in the size of the trained muscle. This hypothesis was supported by several studies (19, 27, 54, 65), which failed to demonstrate hypertrophy following concentric isokinetic training. Recently, however, Narici and colleagues (62) used magnetic resonance imaging to show significant increases (approximately 5% to 21%) in the cross-sectional area of the leg extensor muscles (quadriceps) following two months (four days per week) of concentric, isokinetic training. It is also interesting to note that each of the quadriceps muscles (vastus lateralis, vastus medialis, vastus intermedius, and rectus femoris) hypertrophied to a different degree. It is clear from these findings that hypertrophy does not require eccentric contractions.

We may, however, ask whether the hypertrophy is selective with respect to fiber type. The best evidence available suggests that heavy resistance exercise does result in a selective hypertrophy of the FT fibers (19, 76). Although there is no gain or loss of FT or ST fiber *numbers,* the selective hypertrophy of the FT fibers has been reported to bring about marginally significant changes in the cross-sectional *areas,* with the FT increasing by 5% to 12% as the ST decrease by roughly equivalent amounts (19). The increased area of FT fibers appears to be accounted for entirely by growth of the IIa (FOG) fibers, with no change in the IIb (FG) fibers.

Morphological versus Neurological Factors in Strength Gain

It has been shown that maximal electrical stimulation of human muscles can bring about approximately 30% greater expression of strength than can be elicited by maximal voluntary contraction (39). Therefore it is obvious that strength (or at least the *expression* of strength as we measure it) can also be improved by greater activation of the muscle tissue by central nervous system influences (29, 71). In young adults, neural factors account

for the greatest part of the early gain in strength (first three to four weeks), after which hypertrophy accounts for virtually all of the strength gain (35, 57, 59, 60). As pointed out in chapter 19, the elderly also have the capacity for significant hypertrophy as a result of strength training (11, 30).

The Cross-Education Effect

Before the turn of the century, psychologists demonstrated that training one limb resulted in significant improvements not only in the exercised limb but in the symmetrical, unexercised limb as well. This phenomenon, the cross-education effect or cross-training effect, was found to apply to both the learning of skills and the improvement of strength.

Cross-education has been thoroughly investigated for its usefulness in physical education and rehabilitation by Hellebrandt and her coworkers (36, 37, 38) and by Walters (83). Their work demonstrated the cross-education effect in relation to the gross motor activities of physical education. As a result of training one limb, they found that significant improvements in strength, endurance, and skill occurred not only in the trained limb but also in the contralateral (opposite), untrained limb. To produce a well-defined effect, it was necessary to go into an overload training condition. However, it seems that the nondominant arm could be trained as well by cross education with an overload condition as by direct practice with an underload. Furthermore, the nondominant arm sometimes gained as much in skill by cross-education as it did in direct practice, but this was not true for the dominant arm.

More recent studies (53, 74) have examined the effect of unilateral isokinetic strength training on the cross-education effect. Stevens and coworkers (74) found significant increases at contraction velocities of 0, 60, 120, 180, 240, and 300°/sec in the contralateral leg following unilateral leg extension and flexion training at 180°/sec. Krotkiewski and colleagues (53) reported increases at 0 and 120°/sec in the contralateral leg following unilateral leg extension training at 60°/sec. The cross-education effect on strength has been shown to result entirely from a greater ability to innervate previously inactive muscle fibers, with no evidence of muscle hypertrophy (59).

The rationale for this cross-education effect has not yet been clearly elucidated. However, from what we know of the motor pathways from the cortex, we can make logical deductions. As was pointed out in the description of the pyramidal system (chap. 5), 70% to 85% of the descending nerve fibers cross from one side to the other in their descent to synapse in the spinal cord. Some of the remainder seem to descend ipsilaterally, and it is known that ipsilateral effects are obtainable by stimulating the posterior premotor area of the cortex. Thus, it seems likely that the cross-education effect is brought about by an overflow of nervous activity from neurons in the motor cortex, which innervate the crossed pyramidal fibers, to a smaller number of neurons that supply the uncrossed fibers. Sufficient overflow apparently occurs only under the conditions of strong volition that are involved in overloading. It should also be pointed out that the untrained limb was frequently observed to produce isometric contractions during the training of its symmetrical partner. Technically, the untrained limb was not unexercised.

The implications of this work for the maintenance of muscle tone and prevention of atrophy in immobilized muscles is obvious. From the foregoing rationale, it will also be obvious that intact motor innervation is necessary for achieving the cross-education effect.

Disuse and Atrophy

Anyone who has had a limb in a cast can attest to the basic fact of muscular atrophy (shrinking of a muscle). Scientific evidence (28, 42) has shown that immobilization of a limb (whether mechanically, as by cast, or by denervation) results in decreased fiber size and (at least over a short period of time) in no loss in number of fibers. Thus we may say that all changes in muscle tissue brought about by training programs are impermanent, and that training must be carried on systematically throughout a lifetime. Otherwise, a degree of atrophy from disuse will set in.

There is growing evidence that stretch of muscle in vivo may not only retard atrophy of a denervated muscle but may even induce muscular hypertrophy (10, 33). Animal experiments provide a biochemical basis for this finding, in that amino acid transport into the stretched muscle is improved. Orthopedists now try to cast limbs in positions that allow the greatest resting muscle lengths.

Bilateral Deficit in Strength

The bilateral deficit refers to a decrease in the strength of a muscle group when the contralateral limb (same muscle group on the opposite side of the body) is concurrently performing a maximal contraction (29, 46). This can be demonstrated by determining the maximal strength for a specific movement in each limb (for example, a leg extension) unilaterally and then measuring the maximal strength in both limbs concurrently (bilaterally). The additive strength for the limbs measured individually is usually 5% to 25% greater than the strength when both limbs are measured concurrently (29). The bilateral deficit is more apparent in muscle groups that normally function in a reciprocal manner (contract in an alternating fashion such as the quadriceps during walking) than those which function concurrently (contract at the same time such as many functions of the arms) (29, 81).

It has been suggested that there is a neural basis for the bilateral deficit. When muscle groups on opposite sides of the body work concurrently to produce maximal force, the EMG from one of the muscle groups is less than if it were contracting maximally alone (46, 64, 80). The decrease in EMG is proportional to the bilateral deficit in force production. These findings suggest a neural inhibitory mechanism during maximal bilateral contractions.

It also appears that the bilateral deficit is modifiable with training if the training exercises utilize concurrent contractions of the same muscle groups on both sides of the body (29). Thus, familiarity with concurrent bilateral contractions affects the magnitude of the bilateral deficit. For example, Howard and Enoka (46) found a bilateral deficit in elite bicyclists (who normally train using reciprocal movements) and control subjects, but bilateral facilitation (increased bilateral strength compared to the sum of unilateral measurements) in weight lifters (who train using concurrent contractions).

Mechanical Factors in Strength

If strength development and muscle hypertrophy proceed together, we might expect to find no change in the ratio of strength per unit of cross section as training proceeds. Indeed, Hettinger and Mueller (40) found this to be true in their work with isometric training. Furthermore, it has been suggested that this ratio remains constant regardless of age or gender (68).

In any event, strength per unit of cross section is a theoretical concept, and it tells us little about the forces that can be produced at the ends of the bony lever systems. It will be recalled from earlier discussions that two factors interact to determine the force available at the end of a bony lever: 1) the length at which the muscle is working, and 2) the angle of pull. Figure 21.1 illustrates this in respect to the third-class lever that works at the elbow during elbow flexion. At full extension (180 degrees) where the muscle length is greatest, the angle of pull is poor. At full flexion (40 degrees), the muscle is at twice the disadvantage

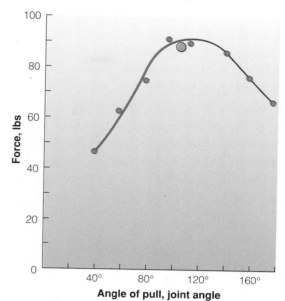

Figure 21.1 Relationship of force available in respect to joint angle for elbow flexion. (From Clarke, H. H. Relationship between Body Position and the Application of Muscle Power to Movement of the Joints, in *Archives of Physical Medicine and Rehabilitation* 31:81. © 1950 American Congress of Physical Medicine and Rehabilitation. Reprinted by permission.)

because it is both short and because it also works at a poor angle. The best combination of the two factors seems to be at approximately 115 degrees (16).

When a muscle works directly in pulling upon a bone (without going through a mechanical lever, as in pulling a rope over a pulley), the curve approximates a length-tension diagram in which the muscle length is the dominant factor in determining the force available. In figure 21.2 it is seen that the best force of contraction results when the hip is fully flexed at 50 degrees because this position has the hip extensors fully stretched. Thus it can be seen that the strength available for doing useful work varies from joint to joint and also with the angle of each joint. This is a very important point to bear in mind when one considers the effects of an exercise. It will be

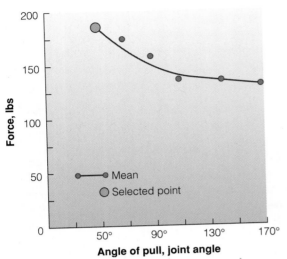

Figure 21.2   Relationship of force available in respect to joint angle for hip extension. (From Clarke, H. H. Relationship between Body Position and the Application of Muscle Power to Movement of the Joints, in *Archives of Physical Medicine and Rehabilitation* 31:81. © 1950 American Congress of Physical Medicine and Rehabilitation. Reprinted by permission.)

discussed in greater detail in a following section.

The Necessary Stimulus for Strength Gain

Our training procedures for the development of strength could undoubtedly be greatly improved if we knew precisely what quantity and quality of stimulus were required to bring about a training effect.

In a very general way, we know that we must bring about overload conditions to elicit the hypertrophic response (or strength gain). That is to say, we must load the muscle beyond its normal everyday use to bring about an adaptive response. The original work of Hettinger and Mueller (40) defined 20% maximal voluntary contraction (MVC) for 1 sec/day as the load required to prevent atrophy and 35% MVC as the threshold value at which a training response began to appear. However, holding muscle tensions between 35% and 100% MVC brings about many effects such as 1) increased tension in muscle and connective tissue, 2) gradual occlusion of blood flow, 3) increased local temperature, 4) hypoxia, and 5) increased levels of metabolic end products. The question is, Which of these factors provides the signal to elicit the hypertrophy response? Early thinking suggested hypoxia as the most likely signal, but that was ruled out by studies that showed no relationship between experimental occlusion and training effect when equal loads of tension were applied (39). At Harvard, Goldberg and associates (33) have done extensive work on this problem. After reviewing their own work and that of others, they point out that the factor that best explains all experimental observations with respect to muscle hypertrophy, including the fact that even passive stretching can improve protein turnover and amino acid transport and can stimulate muscle O_2 consumption, is that of tension development. However, the mechanisms by which tension development is coupled with the metabolic events remain to be discovered.

Joint Angle Specificity during Exercise

Considerable evidence is accumulating that suggests that strength gained is relatively specific to certain aspects of the training method.

Logan demonstrated that the strength training effect is specific to the angle at which the greatest resistance is applied (55). Of his three experimental groups (fifteen in each), one used weight resistance and one used spring resistance to strengthen the knee extensors, while the third group was a control. Using weight resistance, the greatest resistance was encountered from about 155 degrees to full extension, and with spring resistance (on this particular device) the greatest resistance was offered at 115 degrees. The weight training group made significantly greater gains than the spring resistance group when tested at 155 degrees, and the spring resistance group showed significantly greater gains when tested at 115 degrees.

It should be noted that these differences existed despite the fact that both groups exercised isotonically throughout the whole range of motion and that the only real difference in resistance at various angles was that of degree. These results implied that even greater differences in training due to joint angle specificity would be found as the result of isometric training, and this has indeed been the case. Two independent investigations (5, 31) have shown that strength tested at angles other than that at which isometric training took place may show gains less than 50% of that at the exercised angle. This difference in gains appeared when the test angle was as little as twenty degrees removed from the exercise angle. The lesser specificity for isotonic training has also been demonstrated (22).

It has also been shown that the rate of strength gain is greater when a muscle is trained isometrically at a short length compared with a long length. This was found to be true for all muscles tested: elbow flexor and extensor and wrist pronators and supinators (69).

Training Curves—The Time Course of Strength Development

The most definitive work in the area of the time course of strength development was done by Müller and Rohmert (61) at the Max Planck Institute in Dortmund, Germany. Unfortunately, their important work was published only in German and consequently has remained almost unknown in the United States. They showed that strength gain during isometric training approximates an exponential function with time: the rate of gain in strength at any given time is inversely proportional to the difference from the plateau value (*Endkraft*) to be achieved by that particular method of training. There is reason to believe this also applies to isotonic and isokinetic training. This

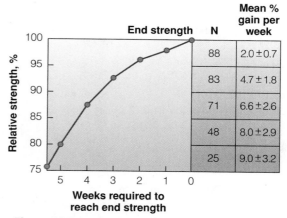

Figure 21.3   Gain in relative strength with isometric training of the trunk extensor muscles by one maximal contraction for one second daily. (Redrawn from the data of Mueller, E. A., and Rohmert, W. *Int. Z. Angew, Phsiol. einschl. Arbeitsphysiologie* 19:403, 1963. Reprinted by permission.)

means that the untrained individual gains at a much greater rate than the relatively trained one. Lack of appreciation of this fact has clouded most of the research directed to comparisons of different training methods.

The method used by Müller and Rohmert depends on the following relationships:

$$S_R = 100 \frac{S_B}{S_E} \text{ in percent}$$

where S_R = relative strength
S_B = strength at beginning of any training period of time
S_E = end strength, the plateau value achieved when strength gain over three to four weeks is less than standard error of measurement

Figure 21.3 illustrates this method. The important point is that beginning strength really has no physiological meaning. It depends to a very large extent on training status, which cannot be defined at the beginning of training. On the other hand, the end strength is a well-defined point, and if every subject is trained to

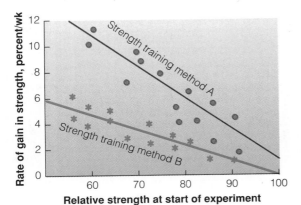

Figure 21.4   Conceptualization of the method of Müller and Rohmert for comparison of strength training methods.

this plateau value the weekly values of relative strength can be plotted as in figure 21.3.

To compare the effects of various training regimens, one then plots the mean weekly rate of strength gain as a function of relative strength at the start of training. This is shown in figure 21.4, where the mean total strength gain per week (V_{TOT}) is calculated as:

$$V_{TOT} = \frac{100 - S_R}{\text{weeks in training}}$$

Subjects who enter into training experiments have greatly varying levels of training status, and this method has the obvious advantage of controlling for these levels.

Methods for Measurement and Training of Strength

In general, there are in a physiological sense only five ways in which the contractile elements of muscle can produce force through the various bony levers available in the human body. They are 1) isometric contraction (a static contraction); 2) concentric isotonic contraction (shortening); 3) eccentric isotonic contraction (lengthening); 4) isokinetic contraction in which the angular velocity of the limb segment is constant; and 5) more or less normally accelerated movement against resistance, as applied in the use of the inertia wheel. Each of these types of muscle contraction can be used for both measurement and training purposes. Although many comparisons among methods have been attempted, none has yet been satisfactory from the standpoint of research design. For example, to achieve a meaningful comparison between isometric and isotonic methods of strength training one would need to equate 1) the training stimulus and 2) the trainability of the subjects, or at least assure randomization of trainability. To the authors' knowledge, no investigation has yet satisfied these requirements, although methods have been proposed for their accomplishment. The use of the force-time integral (72) would satisfy the first requirement, and the use of Müller and Rohmert's method would satisfy the second (61). Consequently we shall review various training methods without comment on their comparative effectiveness.

Isometric Training

Until quite recently, when individuals wanted to increase strength they usually used some form of weight lifting, applying the overload principle. In 1953, Hettinger and Müller published their work on isometric training (40). Their findings indicated that a maximum training effect could be obtained from one daily six-second isometric contraction against two-thirds of an individual's maximal contraction strength. Greater force, duration, or numbers of repetitions did not seem to increase the rate of strength gain, which they found averaged 5% per week when training was performed five times per week. Strength improved in various muscles from 33% to 181%.

Advantages of Isometric Methods

The chief advantages here are administrative in nature. If only one contraction is used per day as in the original work of Hettinger and Müller, great savings in time are possible. Furthermore, a little ingenuity can reduce the equipment needed to that already available in the gym or on the practice field. The elimination of the need for equipment such as barbells or dumbbells also makes it possible to work out larger groups in shorter periods of time.

However, work from the same German laboratory (61) has modified the original work of Hettinger and Müller, and it now appears that the rate of strength gain approximately doubles when maximal contraction strength is used instead of two-thirds maximum. Also, a higher end strength can be reached by increasing the number of six-second repetitions to between five and ten.

If these changes are made in the procedure, plus working each joint at three to four angles to eliminate the specificity problem, isometric results may well match isotonic results, but making these changes would nullify the advantage in time. It is also important to recall the discussion of chapter 7 in which the well-defined effect of isometric tension in raising the arterial blood pressure was pointed out. Isometric exercises must be considered potentially hazardous for people in cardiac rehabilitation or adult exercise programs because of the greater rise in blood pressure.

Methods in the Use of Isometric Contraction

The work of Müller and Rohmert (61) seems to be definitive, so there are few choices to be made as to frequency, intensity, and the like. Best results appear to be obtained by using maximal contraction strength, held for six seconds and repeated five to ten times daily. If a well-rounded workout is desired it is best to apply these contractions at varying points in the range of motion or, if the activity that is trained for demands strength or power, throughout the entire range of motion. In some cases, as in ballistic movements, analysis may indicate the need for maximal power at the beginning of the motion, and exercises should be designed accordingly.

Measurement of isometric tension is done easily, quickly, and is fairly precise, but does this measure the same capacity that is developed by isotonic exercise? A well-controlled study showed no significant correlation between isotonic and isometric measurements of strength gains (6). Even absolute strength, when measured by isotonic and isometric methods, yielded a correlation of only 0.622 to 0.800 (2, 6). The result of isotonic programs should therefore be measured isotonically and the results of isometric programs should be measured isometrically.

Cable Tension Strength Tests

Of all the methods for measuring isometric strength, probably the simplest and most widely used is the cable tension testing method of Clarke. Objectivity coefficients of 0.90 and above were obtained when the tests were administered by experienced testers. Thirty-eight such tests have been devised and validated for testing the various muscle groups of the body (15).

Isotonic Training

Probably the greatest advantage in isotonic methods is that strength gains are specific to the angle at which the resistance is encountered. Thus isotonic exercises can be designed to work the entire range of motion in one contraction, but several contractions would be needed at different angles to work the whole range of motion with isometric methods.

Another possible advantage of isotonic methods is that the individual sees work being done. This appears to be a psychological advantage for those who find a static contraction boring.

Training Methods Using Isotonic Contraction

Many combinations of resistance, repetitions, and number of sets are possible here, but let us first define our terms. *Repetitions* (although used incorrectly, the term is firmly entrenched in the literature) means the total number of executions. *Execution maximum* (EM) and *repetition maximum* (RM) can be used interchangeably and indicate the maximum weight that can be lifted for the indicated number of repetitions. That is, 10 EM (RM) is the greatest weight that can be lifted ten times. *One set* is the number of repetitions done consecutively, without resting.

The investigations performed in this area are not in close agreement, but a general picture seems to emerge. The classic work of De Lorme and Watkins (23) recommended the following program:

> 1 set of 10 repetitions with ½ 10 RM
> 1 set of 10 repetitions with ¾ 10 RM
> 1 set of 10 repetitions with full 10 RM

Other investigators have furnished support for the effectiveness of this method of weight training (3). However, systematic investigations of the value of varying numbers of repetitions seem to indicate that fewer repetitions may be even more effective: four, five, or six. Berger's data (7) in figure 21.5 provides rather good evidence that between four and eight repetitions provide maximal results in terms of strength gain. Another approach that has been validated under laboratory conditions as being very effective is that of doing ten repetitions in which each repetition is done against the maximum possible for that particular execution (8). Thus individuals start with their own 1 RM and use as large a weight as possible for each successive lift. In comparison with the use of one set of ten repetitions with

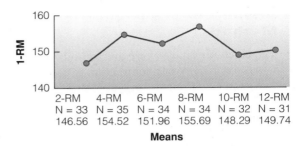

	2-RM	4-RM	6-RM	8-RM	10-RM	12-RM
	N = 33	N = 35	N = 34	N = 34	N = 32	N = 31
	146.56	154.52	151.96	155.69	148.29	149.74

Means

Figure 21.5   Mean strength resulting from weight training programs involving six different methods. (From Berger, R. A., in *Research Quarterly* 33:334. © 1962 American Alliance for Health, Physical Education and Recreation. Reprinted by permission.)

the full 10 RM, it was shown that significantly greater gain in strength was achieved, although the total work in foot-pounds was greater in the 10 RM groups. Muscle hypertrophy seems to be best brought about by the De Lorme and Watkins procedure (23). The optimal number of workouts per week is probably between three and five, depending on the amount of other vigorous activity a given individual may be indulging in (work or play) beyond the weight training program (32).

Recently, the American College of Sports Medicine (1) has recommended the following resistance training guidelines for the average healthy adult:

1. A minimum of eight to ten exercises involving the major muscle groups should be performed a minimum of two times per week.

2. A minimum of one set of eight to twelve repetitions to near fatigue should be completed.

These recommendations were based on time efficiency as well as the small additional benefit from a greater training volume.

Periodization

Periodizaton can be defined as systematic changes in the resistance, number of sets, and/

or number of repetitions performed during a chronic weight training program. It is generally accepted that varying the weight training protocol periodically is beneficial for optimal strength gains, in part by minimizing boredom and facilitating program adherence (52). Periodization has three major objectives (75):

1. Preparation of the athlete to achieve an optimal rate of improvement.
2. Preparation toward a definite goal.
3. Preparation for the main competitions associated with the ultimate goal.

The basic pattern of periodization involves starting with low-intensity (resistance) and high-volume (number of sets × repetitions × resistance) training during the preparation phase early in the season and shifting to high-intensity and low-volume training during the competition phase late in the season (52, 75). Although it has been suggested (75) that periodization is superior to conventional weight lifting protocols that do not vary the number of sets or repetitions, limited data are available to compare the efficacy of various periodization models (52).

Probably the simplest periodization model involves alternating intensity from one training session to the next using heavy (three to five RM), moderate (eight to ten RM) and light (twelve to fifteen RM) resistances (52). Other models involve changing the resistance every two to three weeks (52). The weight training variables (resistance, sets, repetitions, volume, and so on) can be manipulated in many different ways based on the individual goals of the athlete.

Measuring Strength by Isotonic Methods

Measuring isotonic strength involves a trial-and-error situation. For example, if we wish to determine the maximal weight that can be lifted by a muscle group, we may start with a weight that is estimated to be less than maximal and work up to the maximal in small increments. However, the number of trials needed to establish the maximum will vary from subject to subject (according to our "guessing" ability), and varying levels of fatigue will influence the maximum attained. This is hardly objective measurement, and consequently it is not often used for scientific purposes. Furthermore, isotonic testing determines the maximal amount of weight (1 RM) that can be lifted at the weakest point in the range of motion. For an isotonic attempt to be successful, it is necessary to move the resistance through the complete range of motion. The various points (joint angles) in the range of motion have different maximal force production capabilities. The point with the lowest force production capability is often called the "sticking point" (56). Isotonic testing determines the maximal amount of weight that can be lifted at the sticking point. Thus, the 1 RM value is a submaximal resistance at all joint angles other than the sticking point.

Isokinetic Training

In recent years, measurement of strength under conditions of constant angular velocity muscular contractions has become popular. This is called *isokinetic strength* measurement and probably got its impetus from the work of Asmussen and associates (2), who designed a device using strain gauges with which the force of contraction could be measured and recorded during movement, but also could be limited to constant angular velocity conditions. Figure 21.6 shows the results of their work in which it can be seen that, at all velocities, eccentric contraction can develop more force and concentric contraction less force than isometric contraction. They also showed that the correlation between maximum isometric and dynamic contraction was 0.80 at a velocity of 15% of arm length per second.

While this approach represents a distinct improvement over isometric tests and those using repeated measures of ability to lift weight, it still does not measure the quality of

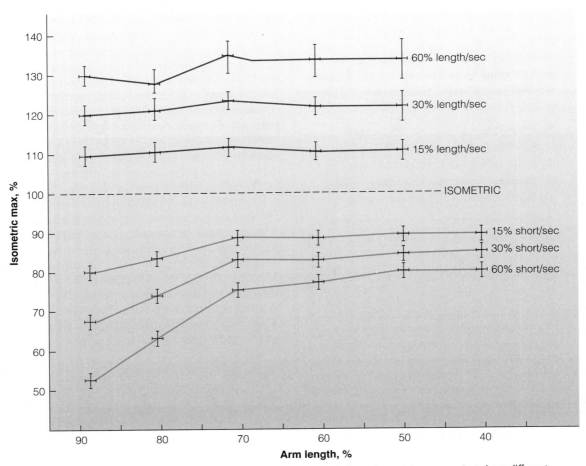

Figure 21.6   Concentric force (lower three curves) and eccentric force (upper three curves) at three different velocities of movement, expressed as percentages of isometric force in the different positions. Extended arm to the left. Horizontal and vertical bars denote ± 1 S.E.E. (From Asmussen, E., Hansen, O., and Lammert, O. *Communications from Testing and Observation Institute of the Danish National Association for Infantile Paralysis, 1965.*)

muscle that is really most important to athletic ability, the ability to produce force in accelerated movement that is typical of almost all skilled muscle action in sports. Interestingly, the basis for such measurement of force (strength) in accelerated movement against an inertia wheel was provided in the early 1920s by A. V. Hill (44). It hardly seems too early to rejuvenate the methods of Hill to study the production of force by muscles under game conditions, which are really not isometric or isokinetic but in fact necessitate the production of force in accelerating-decelerating movements.

Isokinetic testing and training are gaining popularity in clinical setting for rehabilitation following injury and/or surgery. Physical therapist and athletic trainers frequently utilize isokinetic testing for determining the readiness of athletes to return to practice and competition. Clinicians have begun to use isokinetic velocity spectrum training, which involves sets of maximal repetitions at many predetermined contraction velocities (66, 78). Theoretically, this type of training promotes increases in strength across the velocity spectrum.

Early isokinetic training studies indicated that increases in strength occurred only at contraction velocities that were equal to or less than the training velocity (54, 58). Furthermore, Ikai (48) found that training at 100% MVC improved force but not velocity; training at 30% to 60% MVC improved both force and velocity; training with no load and maximum velocity improved velocity but not force. This work was done with an inertia wheel and has great implications for the training of athletes. More recent isokinetic studies (13, 21, 53, 65, 77), however, have reported carryover in strength gains to contraction velocities that were substantially greater than as well as less than the training velocities. These studies indicate that the specificity of strength increases in response to constant velocity training is not as restrictive as was previously thought. Further research is necessary to compare the efficacy of velocity spectrum versus constant velocity training for promoting increases in strength at various speeds of muscular contraction.

Plyometric Training

Plyometric training is used by athletes to increase explosive muscular power. The origin of the term plyometric is unknown but may come from the Greek words pleythein, which means "to increase," or plio meaning "more" and metric meaning "to measure" (24). Plyometrics (also called the stretch-shortening cycle) involves stretching a muscle through an eccentric (lengthening) phase followed by a forceful concentric (shortening) contraction. This is accomplished through such exercises as depth jumps from an elevated stand,

bounding with loping strides, leaping over objects, and hopping on one or both feet (24). The eccentric phase of the exercise is a preparatory movement designed to increase the elastic energy stored in muscle and connective tissue (51). That is, when the athlete jumps from an elevated stand and lands on the floor, the quadricep muscles must absorb the weight of the body through an eccentric contraction that stretches the muscle. The subsequent concentric contraction of the quadriceps is then more forceful than it would be if it were not preceded by the eccentric phase of the movement.

Plyometric training studies have reported improved performance in anaerobic-type activities such as the high jump, long jump, triple jump, vertical jump, and 1 RM squat strength (9, 12, 17, 73). Therefore, plyometric training is particularly beneficial for athletes who compete in sports that require a high level of explosive power such as track and field, football, volleyball, basketball, and olympic-style weight lifting.

It is normally recommended that plyometrics be used as a supplement to other forms of training such as weight lifting and sprinting to enhance the functional capabilities of athletes (18, 24). As a supplement, it has been suggested that for advanced athletes, plyometric training be utilized no more than two times per week (24). Excessive use of plyometric training can result in overuse injuries such as tendinitis, particularly of the knee joint (24). Of the various plyometric techniques, the depth jump from an elevated stand is apparently most likely to cause injury (24).

Concurrent Strength and Endurance Training

Many athletes as well as nonathletes interested in health related fitness perform both strength and endurance training. In an attempt to enhance cardiorespiratory fitness as well as muscular strength, it is common for individuals to engage in aerobic activity several days per week and strength training on the same or alternate days. The revised guidelines from the American College of Sports Medicine (1) for developing and maintaining cardiorespiratory and muscular fitness in healthy adults have added a recommendation for moderate intensity strength training to the existing aerobic training protocol.

Several studies have examined the effects of concurrent strength and endurance training (4, 25, 43, 45, 47, 63, 70). In general, the results of these investigations indicated:

1. Concurrent strength and endurance training results in improvements in both muscular strength and aerobic capabilities.
2. The increases in muscular strength as a result of concurrent strength and endurance training tend to be less than those as a result of strength training alone.
3. There is no difference in the increase in aerobic power that results from concurrent strength and endurance training versus endurance training alone.

Clearly, concurrent strength and endurance training is beneficial for individuals interested in health related fitness. This may not be true, however, for strength and power athletes such as weight lifters, power lifters, and football players. Dudley and Fleck (26) have stated "It may be advised that athletes involved in pure strength/power type activities should not perform large volumes of endurance type training."

In addition, Chromiak and Mulvaney (14) have made the following recommendations:

1. The athlete and coach should be aware of the concept of training specificity, that is, training must emphasize the energy systems used in competition.
2. To increase muscular endurance, high volume weight training should be undertaken instead of moderate or long distance running or cycling.
3. Running should be limited to interval training of short distances and high intensity for athletes in sports that are primarily anaerobic.
4. Endurance athletes can benefit from strength training for injury prevention and enhanced performance.

Variability in Strength/Individual Variability

Strength can be expected to vary somewhat in an individual from day to day. The amount of this variability has been found to range from 1.5% to 11.6% for women and from 5.3% to 9.3% for men (calculated as the standard deviation from the mean) (82).

Generality versus Specificity

We often describe a person as strong or weak, implying that strength is a general quality and that all muscles are strong or weak to the same degree. Obviously the relationships of strength among the various muscles of any individual are not perfect, but there is a high degree of generality. When the strength of single muscle groups was correlated against the total of twenty-two representative muscle groups, all correlations were positive and were significant at better than 0.01 level of confidence. Muscle groups that correlated highest (most representative of general strength) were leg extensors, 0.89; hip flexors, 0.72; knee extensors, 0.70; handgrip, 0.69; and elbow flexors, 0.64 (79). Thus strength tests that use several of these muscle groups can estimate the general strength quite accurately.

Quantity and Quality of Muscle Tissue

It is apparent that *quantity* and *quality* enter into the determination of the ultimate strength of a muscle. When we relate the strength and size of the same muscle group in different subjects, we find substantial correlations. deVries has found this relationship to be between $r = 0.80$ to 0.90 for well-trained, nonobese young men in the elbow flexor group.

The quantity (or absolute muscle force) varies from muscle to muscle within an individual, however, and the quality of muscle tissue is best measured as strength per unit of physiological cross section. Physiological cross section is the same as anatomic cross section only when the muscle fibers are parallel to the tendon of the muscle. Otherwise it is obtained by dividing the volume of the muscle by the length (67). The mean strength per unit of cross section has been estimated for various muscle groups and varies from 4.36 kg/cm² for the rectus femoris (female) to 14.76 kg/cm² for the triceps muscle (male).

The available evidence indicates that in strength training programs the strength and size of muscles increase proportionately. Consequently it is the quantity (volume, not number of fibers) that increases, not the quality (40).

Effect of Various Factors on Strength

Age

As a child grows from infancy to adulthood, strength grows commensurately with the growth in the size of the muscles. Changes in the quality of muscle tissue seem to be small since almost all the gain in strength can be accounted for by the increased size (57). As discussed in chapter 18, children and adolescents respond favorably to strength training. Although experimental data are not available for the older segments of the population, it is quite probable that the decline in strength beyond age thirty can be attributed to decreased quantity of muscle tissue rather than to qualitative changes.

Gender

Most of the difference in strength between the genders can be accounted for by the difference in muscle size (68). It is possible that differences in motivation (culturally inspired) may be responsible for the observed qualitative differences and that in a histological sense no difference exists.

Diurnal Variation

A clear-cut picture of variation in grip strength with time of day has been presented. Figure 21.7 shows the diurnal variation in grip strength and its close relationship to the diurnal variation in oral body-temperature readings (84). The closeness of the relationship does not establish cause and effect, but other evidence (in relationship to athletic warm-up) tempts one to relate the two factors causally.

Another investigator, working with other muscles (including the elbow flexor and knee extensor groups), was unable to show a systematic variability in strength that was related to time of day in these muscles (79). It is possible there are differences from muscle to muscle.

Seasonal Effects

Experiments in Germany on twenty-one subjects who were observed for strength gains as a result of isometric training indicated seasonal variations. A minimum strength gain was found to occur in January and February, and a tenfold higher gain rate was observed in September and October. The investigators attributed this to changes in the diet: availability of fresh fruits and vegetables (41). This finding is interesting, but it requires verification by other investigators.

Effects of Heat and Cold

Immersion of the arm in hot water (120° F) for eight minutes resulted in small but significant gains in grip strength in eight of twelve

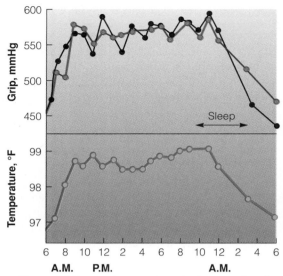

Figure 21.7 Diurnal variation of grip strength and body temperature. (From Wright, V., *Research Quarterly* 30:114. © 1959 American Alliance for Health, Physical Education and Recreation. Reprinted by permission.)

subjects. With the same subjects, immersion of the arm in cold water (50° F) resulted in a mean decrease in grip strength of 11%, which was highly significant (34). It would be of interest to extend these observations to varying temperatures and to other muscle groups.

Psychological Factors

It has long been known on empirical bases that strength, as expressed by voluntary maximal contractions, is limited by psychological factors before physiological limits are reached, and many examples illustrate this point. In one instance, a young man working under his car was pinned there when the jack failed. His mother, a woman of less-than-average size, lifted a corner of the car to release him. Unquestionably, her usual inhibitory processes were themselves inhibited, allowing her to exert her full physiological strength.

Some interesting experiments support this view. It was shown that forearm flexor strength can be significantly increased by the following factors:

1. A pistol shot from two to ten seconds before strength effort, +7.4%.

2. A subject shouting at application of force, +12.2%.

3. Hypnosis that suggests a greater strength, +26.5%. Hypnosis that suggested weakness brought about a significant decline in strength, 31.7% (49).

Plasticity of the Human Body

At the age of twenty-five one of the best U.S. weight lifters in the heavyweight class decided to discontinue his weight lifting career and to take up long-distance running. Three years later he ran the marathon distance in 3 hours, 3½ minutes. Figure 21.8 shows the changes in physique and performance that had taken place within the period under review. He lost 64 lb body weight; his strength (total snatch, and clean and jerk) declined by 196 lb; but per unit of body weight he was now slightly stronger (50).

Summary

Muscular Strength

1. Strength is a very important factor in any physical activity in which muscular forces move the body or move extraneous sports implements that have appreciable mass.

2. Athletic power is the rate of producing force. Power can usually be improved most by increasing the available force (strength).

3. Increased girth of muscle in response to training is the result of hypertrophy, largely of the fast twitch fibers.

4. Early responses to strength training are the result of better innervation, while

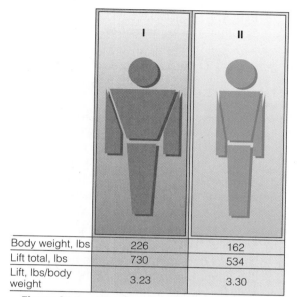

	I	II
Body weight, lbs	226	162
Lift total, lbs	730	534
Lift, lbs/body weight	3.23	3.30

Figure 21.8 Heavyweight weight lifting champion turned marathon runner. (Reprinted from the *American Corrective Therapy Journal* 33.2:61, 1979, with permission of the author and publisher.)

hypertrophy becomes the dominant factor after three to four weeks.

5. The overload principle means that gains in muscular strength and hypertrophy are brought about only when a muscle works against considerably greater resistance than that to which it is accustomed. For isometric training, a minimum resistance of one-third maximum contraction is required to furnish a training stimulus.

6. Strength gains are specific to the angle in the range of motion at which the resistance is met in training and also to the velocity of training.

7. The rate of strength gain is most rapid when a muscle has achieved only a small proportion of its possible maximal end strength. The rate of gain slows down as muscle strength approaches its maximal end strength.

8. The rate of strength loss after training ends is a very much slower process than strength gain. Retention of strength can probably be brought about by as little as one maximal contraction per week.

9. The strength of any muscle is the result of both the quantity and quality of the muscle tissue. Quality (strength per unit of cross-sectional area) varies considerably from muscle to muscle within an individual, but strength gains appear to be brought about largely by quantitative increases in fiber size.

10. To achieve maximal accuracy, strength testing should be applied under conditions that are constant in time of day, ambient temperature, and psychological factors.

Training Methodology and Isometric Training

1. Maximal contraction produces the fastest gains.

2. Duration of six seconds is optimal.

3. Higher end strength values can be attained by increasing repetitions from one to five to ten a day.

4. If a contraction strength less than the maximum is used, it should be based on a maximum that is measured weekly.

Training Methodology and Isotonic Training

1. All contractions should be made through the full range of motion.

2. For the development of *strength*, a program based on two or three sets of four to ten repetitions each, using maximum resistance for the number of repetitions, seems to rest on sound experimental bases.

3. For the development of *hypertrophy,* the De Lorme technique is probably most effective.

   1st set: 10 repetitions with ½ 10 RM
   2nd set: 10 repetitions with ¾ 10 RM
   3nd set: 10 repetitions with full 10 RM

4. Workouts should be scheduled no less than three and no more than five times weekly for optimal results.

5. The total exercise program should be scheduled so that no more than one workout per week approaches exhaustion.

References

1. American College of Sports Medicine. Position stand on: The recommended quantity and quality of exercise for developing and maintaining cardiorespiratory and muscular fitness in healthy adults. *Med. Sci. Sports Exerc.* 22:265–74, 1990.

2. Asmussen, E., Hansen, O., and Lammert, O. The relation between isometric and dynamic muscle strength in man. *Communications from the Testing and Observation Institute of the Danish National Association for Infantile Paralysis* 20:1–11, 1965.

3. Barney, V. S., and Bangerter, B. L. Comparison of three programs of progressive resistance exercise. *Res. Q.* 32:138–46, 1961.

4. Bell, G. J., Petersen, S. R., Wessel, J., Bagnall, K., and Quinney, H. A. Physiological adaptations to concurrent endurance training and low velocity resistance training. *Int. J. Sports Med.* 12:384–90, 1991.

5. Bender, J. A., and Kaplan, H. M. The multiple angle testing method for the evaluation of muscle strength. *J. Bone Joint Surg.* 45A:135–40, 1963.

6. Berger, R. A. Comparison of static and dynamic strength increases. *Res. Q.* 33:329–33, 1962a.

7. ———. Optimum repetitions for the development of strength. *Res. Q.* 33:334–38, 1962b.

8. Berger, R. A., and Hardage, B. Effect of maximum loads for each of ten repetitions on strength improvement. *Res. Q.* 38:715–18, 1967.

9. Blattner, S. E., and Noble, L. Relative effects of isokinetic and plyometric training on vertical jumping performance. *Res. Q.* 50:583–88, 1979.

10. Booth, F. W. Time course of muscular atrophy during immobilization of hindlimbs in rats. *J. Appl. Physiol.* 43:656–61, 1977.

11. Brown, A. B., McCartney, N., and Sale, D. G. Positive adaptations to weight-lifting training in the elderly. *J. Appl. Physiol.* 69:1725–33, 1990.

12. Brown, M. E., Mayhew J. L., and Boleach, L. W. Effect of plyometric training on vertical jump performance in high school basketball players. *J. Sports Med.* 26:1–4, 1986.

13. Caiozzo, V. J., Perrine, J. J. and Edgerton, V. R. Training-induced alterations of the in vivo force-velocity relationship of human muscle. *J. Appl. Physiol.* 51:750–54, 1981.

14. Chromiak, J. A., and Mulvaney, D. R. A review: The effects of combined strength and endurance training on strength development. *J. Appl. Sport Sci. Res.* 4:55–60, 1990.

15. Clarke, H. H., and Clarke, D. H. *Developmental and Adapted Physical Education.* Englewood Cliffs, N.J.: Prentice-Hall, 1963.

16. Clarke, H. H., Elkins, E. C., Martin, G. M., and Wakim, K. G. Relationship between body position and the application of muscle power to movements of the joints. *Arch. Phys. Med.* 31:81–89, 1950.

17. Clutch, D., Wilton, M., McGown, C., and Bryce, G. R. The effect of depth jumps and weight training on leg strength and vertical jump. *Res. Quart. Exer. Sport* 54:5–10, 1983.

18. Costello, F. *Bounding to the Top: The Complete Book of Plyometric Training.* West Bowie, MD: Athletic Training Consultants Inc., 1986.

19. Costill, D. L., Coyle, E. F., Fink, W. F., Lesmes, G. R., and Witzmann, F. A. Adaptations in skeletal muscle following strength training. *J. Appl. Physiol.* 46:96–99, 1979.

20. Cote, C., Simoneau, J., Lagasse, P., Boulay, M., Thibault, M., Marcotte, M., and Bouchard, C. Isokinetic strength training protocols: Do they induce skeletal muscle fiber hypertrophy? *Arch. Phys. Med. Rehabil.* 69:281–85, 1988.

21. Coyle, E. F., Feiring, D. C., Rotkis, T. C., Cote, W., Roby, F. B., Lee, W., and Wilmore, J. H. Specificity of power improvements through slow and fast isokinetic training. *J. Appl. Physiol.* 51:1437–42, 1981.

22. Darcus, H. D., and Salter, N. The effect of repeated muscular exertion on muscle strength. *J. Physiol.* 129:325–36, 1955.

23. De Lorme, T. L., and Watkins, A. L. *Progressive Resistance Exercise.* New York: Appleton-Century-Crofts, 1951.

24. Duda, M. Plyometrics: A legitimate form of power training? *Phys. Sportsmed.* 16:213–18, 1988.

25. Dudley, G. A., and Djamil, R. Incompatibility of endurance- and strength-training modes of exercise. *J. Appl. Physiol.* 59:1446–51, 1985.

26. Dudley, G. A., and Fleck, S. J. Strength and endurance training: Are they mutually exclusive? *Sports Med.* 4:79–85, 1987.

27. Duncan, P. W., Chandler, J. M., Cavanaugh, D. K., Johnson, K. R., and Buehler, A. G. Mode and speed specificity of eccentric and concentric exercise training. *J. Orthop. Sports Phys. Ther.* 11:70–75, 1989.

28. Eichelberger, L., Roma, M., and Moulder, P. V. Tissue studies during recovery from immobilization atrophy. *J. Appl. Physiol.* 18:623–28, 1963.

29. Enoka, R. M. Muscle strength and its development: New perspectives. *Sports Med.* 6:146–68, 1988.

30. Frontera, W. R., Meredith, C. N., O'Reilly, K. P., Knuttgen, H. G., and Evans, W. J. Strength conditioning in older men: Skeletal muscle hypertrophy and improved function. *J. Appl. Physiol.* 64:1038–44, 1988.

31. Gardner, G. W. Specificity of strength changes of the exercised and nonexercised limb following isometric training. *Res. Q.* 34:98–101, 1963.

32. Gillam, G. M. Effects of frequency of weight training on muscle strength enhancement. *J. Sports. Med. Phys. Fitness* 21:432–36, 1981.

33. Goldberg, A. L., Etlinger, J. D., Goldspink, D. F., and Jablecki, C. Mechanism of work-induced hypertrophy of skeletal muscle. *Med. Sci. Sports* 7:248–61, 1975.

34. Grose, J. E. Depression of muscle fatigue curves by heat and cold. *Res. Q.* 29:19–31, 1958.

35. Häkkinen, K., and Komi, P. V. Electromyographic changes during strength training and detraining. *Med. Sci. Sports Exer.* 15:455–60, 1983.

36. Hellebrandt, F. A. Cross education: Ipsilateral and contralateral effects of unimanual training. *J. Appl. Physiol.* 4:136–44, 1951.

37. Hellebrandt, F. A., Houtz, S. J., and Kirkorian, A. M. Influence of bimanual exercise on unilateral work capacity. *J. Appl. Physiol.* 2:446–52, 1950.

38. Hellebrandt, F. A., Parrish, A. M., and Houtz, S. J. Cross reduction: The influence of unilateral exercise on the contralateral limb. *Arch. Phys. Med.* 28:76–84, 1947.

39. Hettinger, T. Der Einfluss der Muskeldurchblutung beim muskeltraining auf den training-erfolg. *Arbeitsphysiologie* 16:95–98, 1955.

40. Hettinger, T., and Müller, E. A. Muskelleistung und Muskeltraining. *Arbeitsphysiologie* 15:111–26, 1953.

41. ———. Die Trainierbarkeit der Muskulatur. *Arbeitsphysiologie* 16:90–94, 1955.

42. Hettinger, T., and Müller-Wecker, H. Histologische und chemische Veränderungen der Skeletmuskulatur bei Atrophie. *Arbeitsphysiologie* 15:459–65, 1954.

43. Hickson, R. C. Interference of strength development by simultaneously training for strength and endurance. *Eur. J. Appl. Physiol.* 45:255–63, 1980.

44. Hill, A. V. The maximum work and mechanical efficiency of human muscles and their most economical speed. *J. Physiol.* 56:19–41, 1922.

45. Hortobagyi, T., Katch, F. I., and Lachance, P. F. Effects of simultaneous training for strength and endurance on upper and lower body strength and running performance. *J. Sports Med.* 31:20–30, 1991.

46. Howard, J. D., and Enoka, R. M. Maximum bilateral contractions are modified by neurally mediated interlimb effects. *J. Appl. Physiol.* 70:306–16, 1991.

47. Hunter, G., Demment, R., and Miller, D. Development of strength and maximum oxygen uptake during simultaneous training for strength and endurance. *J. Sports Med.* 27:269–75, 1987.

48. Ikai, M. Training of muscle strength and power in athletes. *Br. J. Sports Med.* 7:43–47, 1973.

49. Ikai, M., and Steinhaus, A. H. Some factors modifying the expression of human strength. *J. Appl. Physiol.* 16:157–63, 1961.

50. Jokl, P., and Jokl, E. Heavyweight weight lifting champion turned marathon runner. *Am. Corr. Ther. J.* 33:61, 1979.

51. Komi, P. V., and Bosco, C. Utilization of stored elastic energy in leg extensor muscles by men and women. *Med. Sci. Sports* 10:261–65, 1978.

52. Kraemer, W. J., and Fleck, S. J. Resistance training: Exercise prescription (part 4 of 4). *Phys. Sportsmed.* 16:69–81, 1988.

53. Krotkiewski, M., Aniansson, A., Grimby, G., Bjorntorp, P., and Sjostrom, L. The effect of unilateral isokinetic strength training on local adipose and muscle tissue morphology, thickness, and enzymes. *Eur. J. Appl. Physiol.* 42:271–81, 1979.

54. Lesmes, G. R., Costill, D. L., Coyle, E. F., and Fink, W. J. Muscle strength and power changes during maximal isokinetic training. *Med. Sci. Sports* 10:266–69, 1978.

55. Logan, G. A. Differential applications of resistance and resulting strength measured at varying degrees of knee flexion. Ph.D. diss., University of Southern Califoria, 1960.

56. Madsen, N., and McLaughlin, T. Kinematic factors influencing performance and injury risk in the bench press exercise. *Med. Sci. Sports Exerc.* 16:376–81, 1984.

57. McDonagh, M. J. N., Hayward, C. M., and Davies, C. T. M. Isometric training in human elbow flexor muscles. *J. Bone Joint Surg.* 65B:355–58, 1983.

58. Moffroid, M., and Whipple, R. Specificity of speed of exercise. *J. Amer. Phys. Ther. Assoc.* 50:1699, 1970.

59. Moritani, T., and deVries, H. A. The time course of strength gain: Neural factors versus muscular hypertrophy. *Am. J. Phys. Med.* 58:115–30, 1979.

60. ———. Neural factors versus hypertrophy in the time course of muscle strength gain in young and old men. *J. Geront.* 35:672–82, 1980.

61. Müller, E. A., and Rohmert, W. Die Geschwindigkeit der Muskelkraft Zunahme bei isometrischen Training. *Int. Z. Angew. Physiol.* 19:403–19, 1963.

62. Narici, M. V., Roi, G. S., Landoni, L., Minetti, A. E., and Cerretelli, P. Changes in force, cross-sectional area and neural activation during strength training and detraining of the human quadriceps. *Eur. J. Appl. Physiol.* 59:310–19, 1989.

63. Nelson, A. G., Arnall, D. A., Loy, S. F., Silvester, L. J., and Conlee, R. K. Consequences of combining strength and endurance training regimens. *Phys. Ther.* 70:287–94, 1990.

64. Ohtsuki, T. Decrease in grip strength induced by simultaneous bilateral exertion with reference to finger strength. *Ergonomics* 24:37–48, 1981.

65. Pearson, D. R. and Costill, D. L. The effects of constant external resistance exercise and isokinetic exercise training on work-induced hypertrophy. *J. Appl. Sport Sci. Res.* 2:39–41, 1988.

66. Quillen, W. F. Velocity spectrum rehabilitation with isokinetics: A protocol rationale for clinical knee rehabilitation. *Clin. Manag.* 2:9–10, 1982.

67. Ralston, H. J., Polissar, M. J., Inman, V. J., Close, J. R., and Feinstein, B. Dynamic features of human isolated voluntary muscle in isometric and free contractions. *J. Appl. Physiol.* 1:526–33, 1949.

68. Rodahl, K. Physical work capacity. *AMA Arch. Environ. Health* 2:499–510, 1961.

69. Rohmert, W., and Neuhaus, H. Der Einfluss verschiedener ruhelange des Muskels auf die Geschwindichkeit der Kraftzunahme durch isometrisches Training. *Int. Z. Angew. Physiol. einschl. Arbeitsphysiologie* 20:498–514, 1965.

70. Sale, D. G., Jacobs, I., MacDougall, J. D., and Garner, S. Comparison of two regimens of concurrent strength and endurance training. *Med. Sci. Sports Exerc.* 22:348–56, 1990.

71. Sale, D. G., McComas, A. J., MacDougall, J. D., and Upton, R. M. Neuromuscular adaptations in human thenar muscles following strength training and immobilization. *J. Appl. Physiol.* 53:419–24, 1982.

72. Starr, I. Units for the expression of both static and dynamic work in similar terms and their application to weight lifting experiments. *J. Appl. Physiol.* 4:21–29, 1951.

73. Steben, R. E., and Steben, A. H. The validity of the stretch shortening cycle in selected jumping events. *J. Sports Med.* 21:28–37, 1981.

74. Stevens, C. J., Costill, D. L., Benham, D., and Whitehead, T. Transfer of gains in muscle strength and endurance following unilateral isokinetic training. *Med. Sci. Sports Exerc.* 12:121, 1980.

75. Stone, M. H., O'Bryant, H., and Garhammer, J. A hypothetical model for strength training. *J. Sports Med.* 21:342–51, 1981.

76. Thorstensson, A. Observations on strength training and detraining. *Acta Physiol. Scand.* 100:491–93, 1977.

77. Timm, K. E. Investigation of the physiological overflow effect from speed-specific isokinetic activity. *J. Orthop. Sports Phys. Ther.* 9:106–10, 1987.

78. Timm, K. E., and Patch, D. G. Case study: Use of the Cybex II velocity in the rehabilitation of post surgical knees. *J. Orthop. Sports Phys. Ther.* 6:347–49, 1985.

79. Tornvall, G. Assessment of physical capabilities. *Acta Physiol. Scand.* 53, suppl. 210:1–102, 1963.

80. Vandervoot, A. A., Sale, D. G., and Moroz, J. R. Comparison of motor unit activation during unilateral and bilateral leg extension. *J. Appl. Physiol.* 56:46–51, 1984.

81. Vandervoot, A. A., Sale, D. G., and Moroz, J. R. Strength-velocity relationship and fatigability of unilateral versus bilateral arm extension. *Eur. J. Appl. Physiol.* 56:201–5, 1987.

82. Wakim, K. G., Gersten, J. W., Elkins, E. C., and Martin, G. M. Objective recording of muscle strength. *Arch. Phys. Med.* 31:90–100, 1950.

83. Walters, C. E. The effect of overload on bilateral transfer of motor skill. *Phys. Ther. Rev.* 35:567–69, 1955.

84. Wright, V. Factors influencing diurnal variation of strength of grip. *Res. Q.* 30:110–16, 1959.

22

Development of Muscular and Circulorespiratory Endurance

Endurance as a Factor in Human
   Performance
Local or Muscular Endurance
   Strength and Endurance
   *Measurement of Muscular
      Endurance*
   *Factors Affecting Muscular
      Endurance*
   Improvement of Muscular Endurance

General or Circulorespiratory Endurance
   Aerobic versus Anaerobic Work
   *Determinants of Circulorespiratory
      Endurance*
   *Physiological Changes Resulting
      from Training*
   *Training Methods for Distance
      Events*
   Marathon Running

The ability to persist in physical activity, to resist muscular fatigue, is referred to as endurance. If there is any one most important factor in human performance, it is endurance. It is probably the most important component of physical fitness in that it reflects the state of some of the physiological systems that are most important to the general health of an individual. In athletics, there are few sports in which endurance is not a factor, and in many sports all of the training and conditioning programs are directed toward this end.

In chapter 20, the physiological mechanisms thought to underlie fatigue were discussed. In a sense, endurance can be thought of as the ability to delay the onset of fatigue. The practical information presented in this chapter is based on our knowledge of the mechanisms of fatigue.

The concept of endurance is not altogether simple. Analyzing the parts involved in endurance is apt to mislead a student into thinking that the components are discrete elements, when in fact they are interwoven and interrelated and basically inseparable. Realizing that dividing the analysis of endurance into its several components is essentially artificial, we shall nevertheless make the analysis so that you can better understand the physiology involved.

Endurance as a Factor in Human Performance

A. Psychological elements
1. Motivation
2. Pain threshold
B. Physiological elements
1. Local endurance: involvement of only one, or several, localized muscle groups
   a. Strength of a particular muscle group

   b. Energy stores
   c. Peripheral circulatory factor
2. General endurance: whole body activity
   a. Strength of general musculature
   b. Energy stores
   c. Systemic circulatory factor
      (1) Aerobic activity: limited by maximal O_2 consumption
         (a) Respiratory function
         (b) Cardiac output
         (c) O_2 carrying capacity of blood
         (d) Vascularization of muscle tissues
         (e) Aerobic capacity of muscle tissue
      (2) Anaerobic activity
         (a) Muscle glycogen
         (b) ATP and CP stores
         (c) Alkaline reserve: blood buffers
   d. Efficiency of heat regulatory mechanisms
   e. Effectiveness of the nervous system in maintaining high levels of skill and coordination
3. Muscular efficiency: energy input required to bring about desired level of muscular performance

The psychological elements (although they are very important) are beyond the scope of this text, and muscular efficiency is discussed in detail in chapter 23. Thus the remainder of this chapter will be concerned with the physiology of endurance with respect to its two major components: 1) local or muscular endurance, and 2) general or systemic endurance.

Local or Muscular Endurance

Local muscular endurance, or the quality of maintaining a strenuous level of activity in a limited part of the body, is most important in such sports as gymnastics and wrestling. Holding a crucifix position on the rings or breaking a near pinning hold in wrestling exemplify this aspect of muscular performance.

Strength and Endurance

Let us consider for a moment the simplest possible illustration of muscular endurance. Let us concern ourselves with the maintenance of an isometric contraction of the elbow flexors against a load that is at least 60% of the *maximal* voluntary contraction (MVC). A load of this magnitude results in virtually complete occlusion of the blood vessels that supply the muscle tissue because the pressure of the contracted muscle exceeds systolic arterial pressure (47).

Under these conditions the duration of the isometric contraction may be limited by a finite energy supply or by the buildup of acid metabolic end products. Thus the contracting muscle group utilizes its only available sources of direct energy, the breakdown of ATP and creatine phosphate, and subsequently the energy available from the breakdown of glycogen. Neither of these energy sources can be replenished because circulation is occluded. Consequently the duration of this isometric contraction becomes a function of the amount of energy stored, the rate of energy depletion, and the concomitant drop in tissue pH that decreases the contractility of the muscle. The exact factor that actually sets the limit for duration of this isometric contraction is still in question. The work of Ahlborg and colleagues (1) suggests that depletion of muscle glycogen does not set the limit for isometric contraction. Depletion of high energy phosphates is possible, but at intermediate isometric tensions

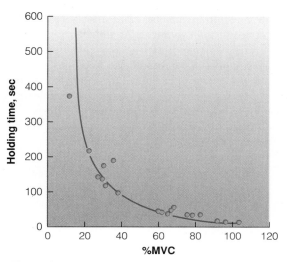

Figure 22.1   Relationship between observed holding times of contractions sustained to fatigue vs. percent MVC. (From Ahlborg, B., et al., in *Journal of Applied Physiology* 33:224. © 1972 American Physiological Society. Reprinted by permission.)

lactate buildup appears to be a likely cause (36). Decreases in pH *within the muscle cell* are a possible explanation for rapid fatigue from very heavy work (30). Such pH decreases in the muscle cell may reduce the binding capacity for calcium ion through an inactivation of the fibrillar protein, troponin (chap. 3).

Figure 22.1 illustrates the relationship of muscular endurance to the magnitude of the load imposed upon the muscle. Note that load is designated in terms of the percentage of MVC. This is necessary because strength is such a large factor in local muscular endurance. It is obvious that if a load of fifty pounds were used for subjects of widely varying strength, a weak subject would find that holding it required close to maximal contraction and the duration of the hold would be only a few seconds. For a very strong subject, the load would be light, and the duration might be several minutes (even longer if the contraction is below that which causes occlusion). Thus the test results would be more closely related to strength than to muscular endurance.

To further illustrate this fact, many investigators have found the relationship between strength and *absolute endurance* to be high, from $r = 0.75$ to $r = 0.97$, while the relationship between strength and *relative endurance* is practically nonexistent (6, 50) or even negative (31). Absolute endurance is measured by using the same load for everyone, whereas relative endurance is measured by using a given percentage of each individual's MVC (thus ruling out strength as a factor).

Measurement of Muscular Endurance

Maintenance of Isometric Tension

The simplest and most direct method has already been described, but another method that involves isometric tension is illustrated by figure 22.2. The subject holds a *maximal contraction,* and the effects of energy depletion on maximum strength are observed over time. It is also of interest to note that the effects of the circulatory factor do not become apparent (there are no differences between open circulation and circulation occluded by a pressure cuff) until the contraction strength falls below (approximately) 60% of MVC (this value is also supported by data for the arm musculature). However, the percentage of MVC at which occlusion occurs undoubtedly varies from muscle to muscle (it is probably very much lower in such muscles as the gastrocnemius, with bipennate fiber orientation). The plotting of these fatigue curves, however, is a laboratory procedure and does not lend itself readily to practical situations.

Recovery from Fatigue

It has been shown that recovery of maximal strength after isometrically induced fatigue is remarkably fast, being complete in about ten minutes. Interestingly, the recovery of endurance function is related to the tension of the

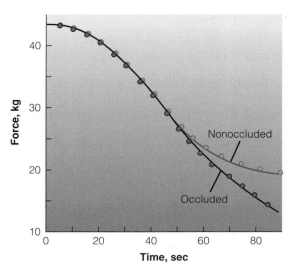

Figure 22.2   Isometric fatigue curves for forearm muscles. In subjects holding maximum voluntary contraction (MVC), the decrement in MVC is a function of fatigue. (From Royce, J., in *Research Quarterly* 29:204. © 1958 American Alliance for Health, Physical Education and Dance. Reprinted by permission.)

fatiguing contraction, whereas strength recovery is not (23).

Recently, Häkkinen and Myllyla (27) found that male endurance (cross-country skiers), power (judo and ski jumpers), strength (weight lifters), and control subjects recovered at different rates following fatigue induced by maintaining an isometric contraction at 60% of maximal capacity for as long as possible. Following three minutes of recovery, the groups had regained 93.4 (endurance), 84.5 (power), 80.5 (strength), and 89.0% (controls) of nonfatigued maximal isometric leg extension strength. The authors concluded that recovery from a fatiguing task is likely influenced by the specificity of previous training as well as the neuromuscular and metabolic characteristics of the individual.

Isotonic Testing by Ergographic Methods

F. A. Hellebrandt and her colleagues (29) have modified the classic Mosso ergograph into a very useful instrument for muscle endurance testing by isotonic methods (fig. 22.3). The main advantage in using this instrument is that the applied force is constant throughout the range of motion, and consequently the range of contraction decreases with increasing fatigue, resulting in fatigue curves or *ergograms* as in figure 22.4. It is possible to set up structured, progressive therapeutic exercise programs with this instrument, and so it has found use in physical medicine and rehabilitation work.

Strength–Decrement Index

H. H. Clarke (8) and his associates have demonstrated that as heavy work is performed over a sufficient period of time to bring about fatigue, decrements in the strength of the muscles involved can be observed with their cable-tension strength testing procedures. They have suggested the use of the percentage strength loss (of preexercise value) as a measure of the level of fatigue. Conversely, the *strength decrement index* (SDI) also provides information relative to muscular endurance.

Isokinetic Tests of Muscular Fatigue

The percent decline in peak torque as a result of repeated maximal isokinetic contractions has been used as a measure of muscular endurance (24, 40, 52). Normally, the test involves 40 to 60 maximal contractions with the percent decline calculated as the difference between the initial and final peak torque values divided by the initial peak torque times 100. A muscle group that fatigues quickly will exhibit a larger percent decline in peak torque than one which has a greater endurance capacity.

Thorstensson and Karlsson (52) reported a correlation of $r = 0.86$ between the percent decline in peak torque following fifty consecutive leg extension contractions at 180 degrees per second and the percent of fast twitch muscle fibers in the vastus lateralis. Thus, it is possible that isokinetic tests of muscular fatigue may be useful for noninvasive estimates

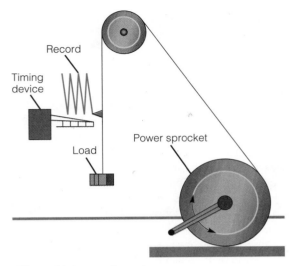

Figure 22.3   A schematic representation of Kelso-Hellebrandt ergograph. (From Hellebrandt, F. A., Skowlund, H. V., and Kelso, L. E. A. "New Devices for Disability Evaluation" in *Archives of Physical Medicine and Rehabilitation* 29:21. © 1948 American Congress of Physical Medicine and Rehabilitation. Reprinted by permission.)

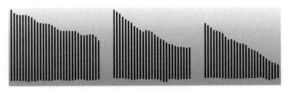

Wrist flexion

Figure 22.4   Ergograms from three workouts of wrist flexion showing increasing levels of fatigue from left to right. (From Hellebrandt, F. A., Skowlund, H. V., and Kelso, L. E. A. "New Devices for Disability Evaluation" in *Archives of Physical Medicine and Rehabilitation* 29:21. © 1948 American Congress of Physical Medicine and Rehabilitation. Reproduced with permission of the Archives of Physical Medicine and Rehabilitation.)

of fiber type characteristics as well as for monitoring changes in endurance capacity as a result of training.

Electromyographic Evaluation of Fatigue

It has been shown that as normal human muscles maintain a constant isometric tension, the electrical activity in the muscle increases as the muscle fatigues (17). The most obvious explanation for this phenomenon is that as the contraction continues and fatigue occurs, each motor unit is able to contribute less force to the contraction. Consequently more and more motor units must be recruited to maintain the same level of tension. deVries has found that the rate of increase in electrical activity with time is highly correlated with isometric endurance measured on a hydraulic dynamometer. This relationship may have practical value for estimating muscular endurance in subjects who are unable or unwilling to cooperate fully in testing.

Factors Affecting Muscular Endurance

1. *Age.* Relatively little information is available concerning the effect of age on muscular endurance. Rich has shown that there seems to be no greater fatigability in young children than in older (high school age) children (44). Evans (19) has shown that older men fatigue more rapidly than young, although the loss of endurance is smaller than expected.

2. *Gender.* Most available data seem to agree that there is no significant difference in muscular endurance due to gender, if the strength factor is ruled out. Indeed, recent data suggest that relative endurance may be superior in the female because of a higher critical occluding tension (32). However, it is also possible that MVC of the female does not come as close to true

physiological maximum as does that of the male, due to cultural differences and/or less experience in exerting MVC. Thus any percent MVC would represent a lower true fraction of capacity and thus account for the greater endurance time.

3. *Temperature.* It appears that rate of fatigue and total amount of work done (handgrip dynamometer) are adversely affected by immersion of the arm for eight minutes in a water bath at 120° F (26). The effects of cold were shown to be advantageous, until a muscle temperature of 80° F was reached. This appears to be an optimal temperature, since temperatures below this produce poorer performance (9).

4. *Cross-education effect.* It has been demonstrated that training one limb brings about changes in its untrained partner (33). When the endurance of the trained limb was increased 966%, the untrained contralateral limb improved by 275%. A recent study by Kannus and coworkers (34) examined the effect of seven weeks of unilateral isokinetic leg flexion and extension training on muscular endurance (defined as the work performed during the last five contractions in a twenty-five repetition test) of both the trained and contralateral limbs. The results indicated that 15% to 17% increases in endurance for the trained limb were associated with 5% to 7% increases in the contralateral limb. It is clear that there is a cross-education effect for muscular endurance, but the increases in the contralateral limbs are substantially less than those of the trained limb.

5. *Circulation.* Twenty-nine weeks of isometric training has been shown to bring about a decrease in the ratio of blood flow debt per unit of exercise

effort (54). This is in agreement with
the work of Rohter, Rochelle, and
Hyman (45), who have shown
significant improvement in muscle blood
flow as the result of the training regimen
of college swimmers. It seems highly
probable that improved peripheral
circulation, by virtue of improved
vascularization of active muscle tissue, is
one of the important mechanisms in the
development of improved muscular
endurance levels.

Improvement of Muscular Endurance

In a classic piece of work with which every
student of physical performance should
become familiar, Hellebrandt and Houtz (28)
provided definitive answers to some of the basic
questions that must be answered to place
exercise programs upon a scientific, system-
atized basis. Using ergographic procedures,
they performed 620 experiments that tested
different training procedures on wrist flexion
and extension. They used thirty-second workbouts alternated with thirty-second rest periods, each bout consisting of twenty-five
isotonic contractions.

When experimentation with successively
heavier loads is conducted, *work curves* can be
plotted in which the work done (kilogram-
meters) is seen to rise to an *optimum load,* then
fall again. Thus in figure 22.5 it can be seen
that at the initial test, 2.0 kg allowed the best
combination of $F \times D$ (force times distance,
distance being the result of the number of repetitions and the height lifted for each repetition as recorded on the ergogram). As more
weight was loaded in subsequent tests, the distance suffered by more than was gained in
weight moved, and therefore the product of
$F \times D$ decreased. Resistances less than the
value that brings about the optimal load constitute an *underload,* and a greater-than-
optimal load constitutes an *overload.* The

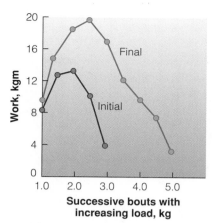

Figure 22.5   Work curve showing the total work
done in successive workbouts as a function of load.
(From Hellebrandt, F. A., and Houtz, S. J., "Mechanisms
of Muscle Training in Man" in the *Physical Therapy
Review* 36:371. © 1956 American Physical Therapy
Association. Reprinted by permission of the publisher
and authors.)

initial and *final curves* of figure 22.5 show
the improvement in one of their subjects in
six practice periods. It can be seen that
strength, power, and endurance improve
simultaneously.

Figure 22.6 demonstrates the need for
overload conditions in developing muscular
endurance. The two groups performed the
same number of contractions per day (250),
three times a week for eight weeks, the only
difference being that one group trained with
an underload and one with an overload.

Comparison was also made of two groups
that worked with underload and overload conditions when the total work done per day was
held constant. In other words, the group that
trained with an overload (twenty-five repetitions with the twenty-five repetition maximum
[RM]) did fewer total bouts than the group
that trained with an underload, so that work
in terms of $F \times D$ was equal for all subjects.
Again, figure 22.7 demonstrates the need for
overload conditions.

It would be very desirable to pursue such
avenues of investigation for other muscle

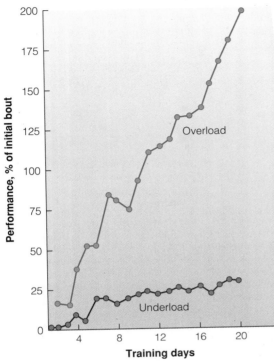

Figure 22.6   Effects of underload and overload in improving muscular endurance. (From Hellebrandt, F. A., and Houtz, S. J., "Mechanisms of Muscle Training in Man" in the *Physical Therapy Review* 36:371. © 1956 American Physical Therapy Association. Reprinted by permission of the publisher and authors.)

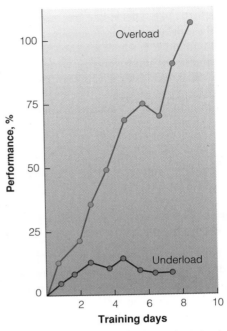

Figure 22.7   Effects of underload and overload of force overcome at each contraction when the total work done is held constant. Lower curve represents underload; upper curve represents overload. (From Hellebrandt, F. A., and Houtz, S. J., "Mechanisms of Muscle Training in Man" in the *Physical Therapy Review* 36:371. © 1956 American Physical Therapy Association. Reprinted by permission of the publisher and authors.)

groups and indeed for overall body activity. Only with such systematic investigations can the training and conditioning of athletes become a science.

The results of work on the training effects of strength versus endurance workouts is of interest. Clarke and Stull (7, 51) conducted two series of training experiments, one of which used low resistance and high repetitions, a combination that is ordinarily considered to be *endurance-type training*. In the other experiment they used the De Lorme technique of heavy resistance and low repetitions (*strength-type training*). Surprisingly, the gains in strength were as great from endurance training as from strength training, and the gains in absolute endurance were also similar in the two training experiments, although relative endurance did not change. Two other investigations support their findings (16, 49), which leads to the conclusion that the first order of business in improving athletes' muscular endurance is to optimize their strength. Since heavy resistance training such as weight training is more time efficient, this would seem to be the method to choose.

General or Circulorespiratory Endurance

When we change our frame of reference from a localized movement, such as elbow flexion or leg extension, to an activity that involves gross body movement, such as running or swimming, we change from local involvement of a small percentage of the body's musculature to a movement that involves a large percentage of body musculature with many muscle groups working simultaneously. In local situations, muscle endurance is limited by a combination of energy supply and peripheral vascularization. The central systems of supply are never extended to a large degree. In gross body activity, it is the central systems of respiration, circulation, and heat dissipation and the nervous system and the homeostatic mechanisms, in addition to peripheral muscle function, that are likely to establish the limits of performance.

Aerobic versus Anaerobic Work

When work begins, anaerobic energy sources are used during the transition to *steady state,* as was described in chapter 12. If the work load is greater than maximal aerobic power, anaerobic mechanisms continue to contribute until maximum O_2 debt is achieved, at which point the exercise must end or slow down. The percentage contribution of aerobic and anaerobic energy depends on the nature of the exercise, as shown in figure 22.8.

Activities of an explosive nature that last only a few seconds at most (such as the shot put) depend mainly on the immediate energy sources (ATP and CP). If the activity is maximal and must be continued for a period of up to one minute duration, such as the 100-meter

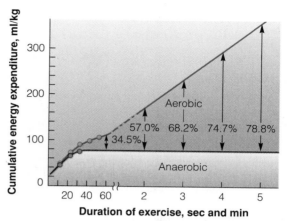

Figure 22.8   The relative importance of oxygen debt and steady oxygen intake during maximum exercise of varying duration. (From Shephard, R. J., in *Journal of Sports Medicine and Physical Fitness* 10:73. © 1970 International Federation of Sportive Medicine. Reprinted by permission.)

freestyle swim or running events from 100 to 400 meters, then the energy source is largely from glycolysis. Maximal performance in events lasting longer than one minute is increasingly dependent on aerobic metabolism. Consequently, $\dot{V}O_2$ max and the lactate threshold become ever more important in determining performance (chap. 12).

In reality, most athletic events involve both aerobic and anaerobic energy sources, the proportions depending on the speed and duration of the event. It can be estimated, for example, that sprints are about 90% anaerobic and distance runs are about 90% aerobic. Other athletic events fall in between (fig. 22.8).

The importance of all this in our discussion of endurance is that, again, different factors are involved (even for a gross body activity) that depend on the speed and duration of an athletic event. The remainder of this chapter, then, is directed toward athletic events in which the energy supply is largely aerobic (events of several minutes' duration or longer).

Determinants of Circulorespiratory Endurance

Energy Substrate

As was discussed in chapter 3, exhaustion in lengthy, severe bicycle ergometer rides seems to occur when muscle biopsy techniques show muscle glycogen to be depleted. Thus, there seems little doubt that muscle glycogen depletion is one factor that *can* set the limits of endurance. However, it must be recognized that bicycle exercise places most of the load on relatively few muscles. Costill and coworkers (12, 13) have raised the interesting question of whether glycogen depletion is also a factor under conditions of endurance-type *running events,* where the load is distributed over a greater muscle mass. Since substantial amounts of muscle glycogen were found after both prolonged (ten miles) and short (maximal O_2 consumption test) exhaustive runs on the treadmill, glycogen depletion is an unlikely explanation for the fatigue at exhaustion in such efforts. Furthermore, in a subsequent study involving three consecutive days of such efforts, they found that subjects were able to initiate the ten-mile run on the third day with leg muscle glycogen concentrations lower than those measured after termination of running on the first day.

Pernow and Saltin (41) have shown the importance of *free fatty acids* (FFA) as an energy substrate. When subjects performed bicycle ergometer work to exhaustion (1 to 1.5 hours duration), it was shown that when the glycogen stores are reduced, prolonged work can still be performed by the same muscles, but only if the intensity of the work is less than 60% to 70% maximum $\dot{V}O_2$ and the supply of FFA is adequate. Elimination of both muscle glycogen and FFA seriously impairs the ability for prolonged work.

Maximum O_2 Consumption (Max Aerobic Power or $\dot{V}O_2$ max)

Except in a marathon run lasting several hours, or in athletic events that overload limited muscle masses (as the bicycle ergometer), the limiting factor in endurance is probably O_2 supply or tissue O_2 utilization rather than oxidizable substrate. We may think of the possible limiting factors for O_2 supply as 1) external respiration and 2) gas transport. The available evidence suggests that the limiting factor for high level athletic performance is some combination of gas transport and tissue O_2 utilization.

Gas transport can be limited by 1) cardiac output, 2) vascular dynamics, and 3) O_2-carrying capacity of the blood (hemoglobin concentration and number of erythrocytes per unit of blood). All of these factors, operating in concert, can be evaluated by the maximal O_2 consumption test described earlier in this book (chap. 14). This test, along with anaerobic threshold or lactate threshold, are the best predictive measures of success in endurance-type athletic events. High correlations have been demonstrated between aerobic power and time on a 4.7-mile run ($r = 0.83$) (10) and endurance time on a bicycle test ($r = 0.78$) (56). Even higher correlations ($r = 0.94$) have been reported in predicting marathon times from anaerobic threshold measurements (43).

Genetic Factor

As was discussed in chapter 12, training can bring about substantial improvement in aerobic capacity and thus markedly improve performance, but genetic factors ultimately set the ceiling. Record-breaking performance is not to be expected unless the genetic endowment for O_2 transport is considerably better than average to begin with. In fact, it has been shown that not only is the ultimate capacity for athletic performance genetically determined but that the rate of response to training also depends largely on genetic factors (5, 42).

Bouchard and colleagues (4) are examining the genetic influences in exercise performance and trainability by considering the following:

1. Genetic variations in gene products (enzymes, antigenic specificities, carrier proteins, and so on).

2. Fragment length polymorphism generated by restriction enzymes in nuclear DNA.

3. Fragment length polymorphism in mitochondrial DNA.

The results of these lines of research will provide valuable information regarding the genetic component of physical performance.

Motivation

In an interesting experiment on the influence of motivation on physiological parameters limiting work capacity, Wilmore (55) tested the PWC of twenty-two college-age males on a bicycle ergometer on three occasions, two control and one experimental. On the experimental test the subjects were motivated by competition. As might be expected, the performances were significantly better in the competitive situation, but there were *no significant differences* in the maximum *physiological responses* such as heart rate, maximum ventilation, or O_2 consumption. It can be concluded that the maximal values for the physiological variables are essentially fixed for a given individual at a given time at a given training level and that the supramaximal performances elicited by motivation were the result of increased anaerobic rather than aerobic power, which may be the result of reduced psychological inhibitions allowing greater tolerance to anaerobic metabolites.

Physiological Changes Resulting from Training

Continual, methodical stressing of the human organism by subjecting it to progressively increasing work loads results in responses that are seemingly directed toward making its reaction to the challenges of increased metabolic rates ever more successful. The physiological changes brought about by training can be summarized as follows:

1. Lower resting heart rate.

2. Lower heart rate for any submaximal work load.

3. Greater maximal cardiac output.

4. Greater maximal stroke volume.

5. Lower ventilation equivalent (less ventilation required per unit O_2 utilized).

6. Greater maximal O_2 consumption.

7. Less utilization of anaerobic energy sources for a given work load.

8. Capacity for greater O_2 debt (probably due to a combination of improved alkaline reserve and greater willingness to bear pain).

9. Less displacement of physiological function by any given level of work load and faster recovery to baseline values after completion of exercise.

Training Methods for Distance Events

Table 22.1 provides information concerning several methods of training for distance running. It is important to recognize that during a year of training, a distance runner will probably use many, if not all, of the methodologies listed in the table. The relative emphasis on one type of training versus another is dependent on the goals of the athlete and the timing of major competitions.

Daniels (15) has identified three key points regarding the training of distance runners:

1. There are many types of training for distance running, each one varying in intensity and duration. The coach and athlete first must set goals and then determine the best training regimen to reach those goals.

Table 22.1   The Types of Training Listed Below are Arranged by Intensity, from Easiest to Hardest (Slowest to Fastest).

	Easy (E)	Long (L)	Tempo (T)	Cruise (C)	Interval (I)	Reps (R)
Purpose	• Warmup • Recovery • Cooldown • Early season build-up	• Skeletal and cardiac muscle adaptation	• Improve endurance by raising lactate threshold		• Improve $\dot{V}O_2$ max	• Improve speed and running economy
Intensity	• Conversational, 70% of $\dot{V}O_2$ max		• Comfortably hard • 86% of $\dot{V}O_2$ max • 15 seconds *per mile* slower than 10 K race pace		• 5 K race pace or slightly slower • 95%–100% of $\dot{V}O_2$ max	• 5 seconds *per* 400 m faster than interval pace or race pace, whichever is fastest
Duration of Each Work Bout	• 20–60 minutes	• 60–120 minutes	• 20 minutes	• 3–10 minutes	• 1/2–5 minutes	• 30–90 seconds
Recovery Time Between Work Bouts	• Not applicable	• Not applicable	• Not applicable	• 1 minute	• 1 to 1 work:rest ratio	• 1 to 5 work:rest ratio
Number of Work Bouts in One Session	• Not applicable	• Not applicable	• Not applicable	• Repeat work bouts until quality work totals 8% of 1 weekly mileage; not over 6 miles/session		• 5% of weekly mileage; not over 5 miles/session

From Daniels, J. *Training Distance Runners—A Primer*. Gatorade Sports Science Exchange. 1(11), 1989.

2. Each runner's strengths and weaknesses must be considered in the development of a training program. Place early season emphasis on weaknesses and late season emphasis on strengths.

3. An effective training program results from efficient long-range planning, the judicious use of rest and recovery days, and gradual increases in training intensity and duration.

Long Slow Distance (LSD) Training

The purpose of LSD training is to develop the cardiorespiratory system and cirulatory blood supply to the active muscles as well as enhance the muscles' metabolic characteristics. Normally, LSD training is performed for one to two hours at an intensity equal to approximately 65% to 70% of $\dot{V}O_2$ max. In terms of running velocity, this intensity usually corresponds to one to two minutes slower than the athletes 10 kilometer race pace (15).

Use of Lactate Threshold in Training Programs

It has been suggested by German investigators that the aerobic–anaerobic transition is bounded by the *aerobic threshold* at the point where blood lactate reaches 2.0 mM/l and by the *anaerobic threshold* at the point of reaching 4.0 mM/l. As pointed out in chapter 12, there are semantic problems with these terms but their concepts are of interest. They suggest that, theoretically, the optimum load intensity for endurance training should be in the neighborhood of loads that result in 4 mM/l of lactate (the so-called anaerobic threshold), because under these conditions there is strong stimulation of oxidative metabolism in skeletal muscle cells with minimal stress. They conclude that endurance training at the aerobic threshold (2 mM/l) will only maintain the state of physical condition, while training at the anaerobic threshold (4 mM/l) is required for improvement (38). Evidence for these conclusions is unclear, but German swimmers training according to these concepts have been very successful. Australian swimmers appear to be using a similar but more complex approach in developing their training regimens (53).

With respect to distance running, training at the lactate threshold is also called tempo-pace or cruise interval training (15). Tempo-pace training refers to continuous workbouts of approximately twenty minutes duration while cruise intervals are discontinuous and usually last three to ten minutes with one minute rest periods (total distance for a cruise interval session should not exceed six miles; table 22.1.) The typical intensity for trained runners at the lactate threshold (used for both tempo-pace and cruise intervals) is approximately 85% of $\dot{V}O_2$ max or a running velocity of fifteen to twenty seconds per mile slower than the 10 kilometer race pace (15).

Interval Training

Interval training consists of short periods of work alternating with short rest intervals, as opposed to workbouts that are continuous. Thus an individual training for a 1,500-meter swim, instead of swimming long distances continuously, might be trained largely on 100-meter swims that are swum faster. The endurance (or training) factor would be gained through manipulation of 1) the speed at which the 100s are negotiated and 2) the total number of 100s accomplished, plus 3) the duration of the rest interval.

From the standpoint of the exercise physiologist, interval training makes very good sense indeed. Obviously, one of the primary goals of a conditioning program is to achieve the greatest possible work load with the smallest physiological strain (fatigue), and that this can best be achieved through the methods of interval training is supported on physiological bases. Astrand and coworkers (2) found that a work load (2,160 kgm/min) that could be tolerated for an hour when done intermittently resulted in exhaustion in nine minutes when done continuously. Thus the total work done continuously was 19,400 kgm, while the work done intermittently was 64,800 kgm.

The level of physiological stress can be evaluated best by the heart rate and blood lactate levels achieved. In the continuous work the heart rate reached 204 bpm and blood lactate rose to 150 mg percent. In the intermittent work, in which more than three times as much work was done, heart rate did not exceed 150 bpm and blood lactate was 20 mg percent, which indicates that very little of the work was done anaerobically.

More recent work has confirmed these theoretical advantages for interval training (22), and it has also been shown that by shortening the pause (rest) interval to thirty to forty-five seconds, the training stimulus to both cardiopulmonary and muscle glycolytic systems can be greatly increased (37). Thus one of the advantages of interval training lies in the *simultaneous* development of both aerobic and anaerobic power. Both are essential to many sports.

In spite of these obvious theoretical advantages for interval training over continuous training, when the methods are compared under careful experimental conditions for practical training effect, no clear advantage has been found (25, 39, 46, 48) in favor of interval training. However, interval training methods are advantageous in that interval training is usually conducted at a higher pace and therefore favors the use of the same recruitment patterns and muscle fiber types as does the actual event. In addition, both aerobic and anaerobic functions can be trained simultaneously.

The work of the Astrands and their colleagues (2) also sheds light on what constitute desirable intervals. The same work load when done in alternating three-minute intervals of work and rest required heart rates of 188 bpm and blood lactate of 120 mg percent, but alternating intervals of thirty seconds raised these values to only 150 and 20, respectively. The value of the thirty-second work interval, which is often recommended, is thus borne out on experimental bases.

As an extension of this work, the effect of changing the length of the rest interval was also investigated (3). It was shown that the physiological stressfulness of the training is not highly related to the duration of the rest interval. Only small increases in blood lactate were observed when the rest interval was decreased from four minutes to thirty seconds, although the total work done increased fourfold.

Although maximal training effect on the circulatory system probably demands maximal loading of the O_2 transport system, this does not necessarily mean that the athlete's performance must be maximal in terms of *speed* of running or swimming. Karlsson, Astrand, and Ekblom (35) have shown that as an athlete approaches maximum performance (speeds), there is a considerable range, possibly from 80% to 100%, of maximum performance capability (speed of running, and so on)

at which O_2 consumption is at its maximum, although the production of lactic acid rises rapidly over this same range. Since they also found a declining O_2 pulse at the highest levels of work, the data suggest that training the O_2 transport system is best carried out at a work rate that is short of maximal performance but will still fully load the O_2 transport system. Such a small reduction in speed implies less fatigue (lower levels of lactate) and thus permits an increase in training volume.

To summarize, interval training for events that are largely *aerobic* can be developed around work intervals ranging from thirty seconds to five minutes with alternating rest intervals of approximately the same duration. It must be realized that the shorter the interval the greater the training effect on anaerobic capacity, and the longer the interval the more effective for aerobic capacity, so the selection of interval depends to a large extent on the exact nature of the event trained for. It must also be remembered that the shorter intervals allow very large total work loads to be handled. It is deVries's experience with swimmers that such workouts should be reserved for bringing athletes to peak performance. Using intervals of thirty to sixty second swims can bring high school and college swimmers to a peak in four to six weeks. If such workouts are used too early in the season or over too long a period, they may result in staleness.

Repetition (REP) Training

Repetition (REP) training is intended to improve speed and running economy (15). Generally, REP training involves an intensity that is greater than that used for interval training with individual workouts lasting 30 to 90 seconds. Daniels (15) has recommended that REP training be performed at an intensity equal to three to five seconds per 400 meters faster than interval training pace, particularly when training for races longer than 5,000 meters *or* up to five seconds per 400 meters faster than current race pace (using the race of primary importance as the standard). The ratio of work to recovery intervals should be 1:5. As indicated in table 22.1, the total distance performed during a REP training session should be less than or equal to five miles.

Fartlek Training

Fartlek training has also been called "speed play" because the athlete varies the speed of running frequently during a session (15). The foundation of Fartlek training is an easy continuous running pace interspersed with short, high-intensity bursts. Frequently, this form of training is performed over a varied terrain where the pace is, in part, determined by running up or down hills (15). Fartlek training is, generally, not highly structured; the athlete decides when, how much, and for how long to alter the running speed.

"Hypoxic Training" for Swimmers

For many years swimming coaches have used changes in the frequency of breathing as a training mechanism. Breathing once every stroke cycle in the crawl stroke means breathing every second arm stroke and consequently breathing on the same side. Most coaches realized long ago that turning the head from the midline to breathe resulted in slower times. Therefore they experimented with controlled frequency breathing (CFB) in which the swimmer breathed every fourth or sixth stroke and even less frequently in high school 50-yard sprints. Others also used breathing every third stroke to combine CFB with achieving a more symmetrical swim style. However, in recent years it was proposed that this less frequent breathing constituted what was called "hypoxic training" in the belief that the reduction in inspired air resulted in a decreased O_2 delivery to the musculature.

Controlled experiments, however, have shown that as ventilatory volume decreases in CFB, O_2 extraction and tidal volume increase to maintain a constant $\dot{V}O_2$ for a given speed of swimming. Estimated alveolar partial pressure of O_2 decreased while CO_2 increased.

Thus the training could be called "hypercapnic training" but not "hypoxic training" (18). If there are any performance advantages to such training they would be associated with an improved tolerance to high alveolar levels of CO_2 rather than to hypoxia as had been suggested.

Determinants of Success in Distance Events

It has been shown that distance running performance is strongly related to $\dot{V}O_2$ max ($r = -.84, -.87, -.88$ for 1-, 2-, 6-mile runs, respectively). The percentage of slow twitch (ST) muscle fibers contributes less strongly ($r = -.52, -.54, -.55$ for 1-, 2-, 6-mile runs). Muscle enzyme patterns correlate poorly but may be more important as far as intraindividual changes in training state (21). At a given constant speed of running, the percentage of $\dot{V}O_2$ max required is highly related to performance ($r = -0.94$) (14, 43). Well-trained distance runners can also maintain a high percentage of $\dot{V}O_2$ max without substantial increases in plasma lactate (20).

Analysis of Pace as an Indicator of Training Needs

In middle-distance and distance athletic events, where pace is established on a voluntary basis, considerable insight can be gained into training needs by comparing *split times* with those of championship performances in the same event. If an athlete's split times, for example, are in the same proportion as those of championship performance but slower for each split, further improvement probably depends on increased power or better technique. In this case, off-season weight training and interval training, with rate as the variable for progression, should be utilized.

On the other hand, if an athlete meets the championship pace on the first splits but fades badly late in the race, the fault probably stems from circulorespiratory factors, and endurance work is needed (such as increasing the number of repeats of an interval training workout).

Marathon Running

Running in a marathon (42 km or 26.2 miles) has become the ultimate achievement for many newly converted runners. Therefore, physical educators should become familiar with some of the physiology involved in this activity. Costill has furnished an excellent review on this topic (11).

1. *Desirable physical characteristics.* The ideal marathoner should be small in stature with a small bony frame and minimal fat. Both fat and bony structure constitute dead weight to be moved at a cost in energy.

2. *Desirable physiological characteristics.* As has been discussed for distance events in general, a large $\dot{V}O_2$ max is essential. In addition, a large fraction of ST fibers in the leg muscles and the ability to utilize a large fraction of the $\dot{V}O_2$ max are important.

3. *Running efficiency.* Since oxygen (and, to a lesser extent, energy substrate) must be transported by the circulatory system, higher maximal limits can be set by the more efficient neuromuscular mechanisms, other things being equal. Differences in the mechanical efficiency of running, even among skilled distance runners, may be as large as 50% (chap. 23).

4. *Physiological responses.* The marathon run is an extremely costly event in terms of energy consumption, with an average cost of about 2,400 kcal for the 26.2 miles. Energy consumption increases if the wind is blowing or if the terrain is hilly. One might think that the loss going uphill is regained on the downhill stint, but this is not the case because the gain is not so large as the loss.

Circulatory response requires near-maximal levels of heart rate, stroke volume, and cardiac output even under normal weather conditions. Adverse weather conditions such as high heat and humidity therefore necessitate slowing the pace so that the circulatory system can meet the demand for the additional circulation required for thermoregulation. Even under normal conditions, rectal temperature rises to about 104° F and may go as high as 106° F.

Naturally, under such conditions fluid losses are extremely high, averaging about one liter per square meter body surface per hour. Despite these high fluid losses, which may range from eight to twelve pounds weight loss, even ad lib fluid ingestion cannot keep up with the loss rate because of a limited rate of gastric emptying. Even the partial fluid replacement that is possible is extremely important in stabilizing rectal temperature (11).

Prediction of Marathon Time from Anaerobic Threshold

Rhodes and McKenzie (43) have shown that marathon times can be rather accurately predicted from anaerobic threshold (AT) measurements. Eighteen marathoners ranging from moderately trained to highly trained were tested on a treadmill to determine their AT. The average predicted time was 2:53:49, while the average actual time was 2:52:06. The correlation between predicted and measured times was $r = 0.94$.

Summary

Muscular Endurance

1. An optimal level of strength should be developed in the endurance training program. This allows a muscle group to work at lower percentages of its all-out capacity and thus significantly increases endurance (*absolute endurance*).

2. The *overload principle* applies to muscular endurance as well as to strength. Repetitions with easy work loads do not bring about optimal improvement in muscular endurance.

3. In general, suitable overload training brings about improvement in strength and muscular endurance simultaneously.

4. If either the duration of work load or the *total work* is held constant, overload training brings about far greater improvement than underload training, in strength and in endurance.

5. Overload training should not reach the point where the range of motion is curtailed.

6. The *power* (work per unit time) of muscular contraction seems to be more important than the total amount of work in bringing about a training effect.

Circulorespiratory Endurance

1. The limits of human circulorespiratory endurance are set by such psychological factors as motivation and willingness to take pain and by many physiological factors. The most important physiological factors are oxygen transport and the metabolic capacity of the involved muscle tissue.

2. At the beginning of an endurance workout, anaerobic energy sources are used until the transition to steady state is accomplished, at which point the energy is supplied almost entirely aerobically.

3. Immediate energy sources (particularly CP) can be depleted during very high intensity exercise in less than twenty seconds.

4. Events of several minutes' duration or longer are almost entirely aerobic.

5. The limiting factors in circulorespiratory endurance are primarily O_2 transport and O_2 utilization in the skeletal muscles. Energy substrate depletion can be a limiting factor if small muscle masses are used over very long periods (several hours).

6. Interval training concepts rest on sound theoretical bases. More work can be done per workout for any given physiological stressfulness if it is done intermittently rather than continuously.

7. Thirty-second workbouts are most advantageous, and the rest interval is probably best set by physiological stress as measured by heart rate. The rest interval has been adequate when the resting heart rate has returned to 120 bpm.

8. Experimental evidence is still inconclusive with respect to the practical advantages of interval training over continuous training in terms of increased PWC or $\dot{V}O_2$ max.

9. Success in distance running is strongly related to a) $\dot{V}O_2$ max, b) percentage of ST muscle fibers, and c) percentage of $\dot{V}O_2$ max required at a given speed of running.

10. Training progress can be hampered by exercising to complete exhaustion. Workouts should not exceed intensity and duration levels that allow recovery from fatigue in several hours.

11. Athletes should not be brought along too fast early in the season for fear of hitting peak performances before championship events. In general, the early season workout progressions should gradually increase the number of repetitions. Late in the season the rate for each repetition is the important variable.

12. If split times are proportional to record performances, further improvement probably depends on improvement of strength (power) or technique. If split times fade badly in comparison with record performances, circulorespiratory endurance needs improvement.

13. The physiology of marathon running is discussed with emphasis upon the limitations of the human organism in such activity under adverse conditions.

References

1. Ahlborg, B., Ekelund, L. G., Guarnieri, G., Harris, R. C., Hultman, E., and Nordesjo, L-O. Muscle metabolism during isometric exercise performed at constant force. *J. Appl. Physiol.* 33:224–28, 1972.
2. Astrand, I., Astrand, P-O., Christensen, E. H., and Hedman, R. Intermittent muscular work. *Acta Physiol. Scand.* 48:448–53, 1960.
3. ———. Myohemoglobin as an oxygen store in man. *Acta Physiol. Scand.* 48:454–60, 1960.
4. Bouchard, C., Chagnon, M., Thibault, M. C., Boulay, M. R., Marcotte, M., Cote, C., and Simoneau, J. A. Muscle genetic variants and relationship with performance and trainability. *Med. Sci. Sports Exerc.* 21:71–77, 1989.
5. Bouchard, C., and Lortie, G. Heredity and endurance performance. *Sports Med.* 1:38–64, 1984.
6. Caldwell, L. S. Relative muscle loading and endurance. *J. Engineering Psychol.* 2:155–61, 1963.
7. Clarke, D. H., and Stull, G. A. Endurance training as a determinant of strength and fatigability. *Res. Q.* 41:19–26, 1970.
8. Clarke, H. H., Shay, C. T., and Mathews, D. K. Strength decrement index: A new test of muscle fatigue. *Arch. Phys. Med. Rehabil.* 36:376–78, 1955.
9. Clarke, R. S. J., Hellon, R. F., and Lind, A. R. The duration of sustained contractions of the human forearm at different muscle temperatures. *J. Physiol.* 143:454–73, 1958.
10. Costill, D. L. The relationship between selected physiological variables and distance running performance. *J. Sports Med.* 7:61–66, 1967.
11. Costill, D. L. Physiology of marathon running. *J.A.M.A.* 221:1024–29, 1972.
12. Costill, D. L., Bowers, R., Branam, G., and Sparks, K. Muscle glycogen utilization during prolonged exercise on successive days. *J. Appl. Physiol.* 31:353–56, 1971.
13. Costill, D. L., Sparks, K., Gregor, R., and Turner, C. Muscle glycogen utilization during exhaustive running. *J. Appl. Physiol.* 31:353–56, 1971.
14. Costill, D. L., Thomason, H., and Roberts, E. Fractional utilization of the aerobic capacity during distance running. *Med. Sci. Sports* 5:248–52, 1973.
15. Daniels, J. Training distance runners— A primer. *Gatorade Sports Sci. Exch.* 1(11), 1989.
16. De Lateur, B. J., Lehman, J. F., and Fordyce, W. E. A test of the De Lorme axiom. *Arch. Phys. Med. Rehabil.* 49:245–48, 1968.
17. deVries, H. A. Method for evaluation of muscle fatigue and endurance from electromyographic fatigue curves. *Am. J. Phys. Med.* 47:125–35, 1968.
18. Dicker, S. G., Lofthus, G. K., Thornton, N. W., and Brooks, G. A. Respiratory and heart rate responses to tethered controlled frequency breathing swimming. *Med. Sci. Sports Exer.* 12:20–23, 1980.

19. Evans, S. J. An electromyographic analysis of skeletal neuromuscular fatigue with special reference to age. Ph.D. diss., Physical Education, University of Southern California, 1971.

20. Farrell, P. A., Wilmore, J. H., Coyle, E. F., Billing, J. E., and Costill, D. L. Plasma lactate accumulation and distance running performance. *Med. Sci. Sports* 11:338–44, 1979.

21. Foster, C., Costill, D.L., Daniels, J. T., and Fink, W. J. Skeletal muscle enzyme activity, fiber composition and $\dot{V}O_2$ max in relation to distance running performance. *Eur. J. Appl. Physiol.* 39:73–80, 1978.

22. Fox, E. L., Robinson, S., and Wiegman, D. L. Metabolic energy sources during continuous and interval running. *J. Appl. Physiol.* 27:174–78, 1969.

23. Funderburk, C. F., Hipskind, S. G., Welton, R. C., and Lind, A. R. Development of and recovery from fatigue induced by static effort at various tensions. *J. Appl. Physiol.* 37:392–96, 1974.

24. Gray, M. C., and Chandler, J. M. Percent decline in peak torque production during repeated concentric and eccentric contractions of the quadriceps femoris muscle. *J. Orthop. Sports Phys. Ther.* 10:315–23, 1989.

25. Gregory, L. W. The development of aerobic capacity: A comparison of continuous and interval training. *Res. Q.* 50:199–206, 1979.

26. Grose, J. E. Depression of muscle fatigue curves by heat and cold. *Res. Q.* 29:19–31, 1958.

27. Häkkinen, K., and Myllyla, E. Acute effects of muscle fatigue and recovery on force production and relaxation in endurance, power and strength athletes. *J. Sports Med.* 30:5–12, 1990.

28. Hellebrandt, F. A., and Houtz, S. J. Mechanisms of muscle training in man. *Phys. Ther. Rev.* 36:371–83, 1956.

29. Hellebrandt, F. A., Skowlund, H. V., and Kelso, L. E. A. New devices for disability evaluation. *Arch. Phys. Med. Rehabil.* 29:21–28, 1948.

30. Hermansen, L., and Osnes, J. B. Blood and muscle pH after maximal exercise in man. *J. Appl. Physiol.* 32:304–8, 1972.

31. Heyward, V. Influence of static strength and intramuscular occlusion on submaximal static muscle endurance. *Res. Q.* 46:393–402, 1975.

32. Heyward, V., and McCreary, L. Comparison of the relative endurance and critical occluding tension levels of men and women. *Res. Q.* 49:301–7, 1978.

33. Hodgkins, J. Influence of unilateral endurance training on contralateral limb. *J. Appl. Physiol.* 16:991–93, 1961.

34. Kannus, P., Alosa, D., Cook, L., Johnson, R. J., Renstrom, P., Pope, M., Beynnon, B., Yasuda, K., Nichols, C., and Kaplan, M. Effect of one-legged exercise on the strength, power and endurance of the contralateral leg. *Eur. J. Appl. Physiol.* 64:117–26, 1992.

35. Karlsson, J., Astrand, P-O., and Ekblom, B. Training of the oxygen transport system in man. *J. Appl. Physiol.* 22:1061–65, 1967.

36. Karlsson, J., Funderburk, C. F., Essen, B., and Lind, A. R. Constituents of human muscle in isometric fatigue. *J. Appl. Physiol.* 38:208–11, 1975.

37. Keul, J. The relationship between circulation and metabolism during exercise. *Med. Sci. Sports* 5:209–19, 1973.

38. Kindermann, W., Simon, G., and Keul, J. The significance of the aerobic-anaerobic transition for the determination of work load intensities during endurance training. *Eur. J. Appl. Physiol.* 42:25–34, 1979.

39. Knuttgen, H. G., Nordesjo, L-O., Ollander, B., and Saltin, B. Physical conditioning through interval training with young male adults. *Med. Sci. Sports* 5:220–26, 1973.

40. Montgomery, L. C., Douglass, L. W., and Deuster, P. A. Reliability of an isokinetic test of muscle strength and endurance. *J. Orthop. Sports Phys. Ther.* 10:315–22, 1989.

41. Pernow, B., and Saltin, B. Availability of substrates and capacity for prolonged heavy exercise in man. *J. Appl. Physiol.* 31:416–22, 1971.

42. Prud'homme, D., Bouchard, C., Leblanc, C., Landry, F., and Fontaine, E. Sensitivity of maximal aerobic power to training is genotype dependant. *Med. Sci. Sports Exer.* 16:489–93, 1984.

43. Rhodes, E. C., and McKenzie, D. C. Predicting marathon time from anaerobic threshold measurements. *Physician and Sportsmed.* 12 (Jan.):95–98, 1984.

44. Rich, G. Q. Muscular fatigue curves in boys and girls. *Res. Q.* 31:485–98, 1960.

45. Rohter, F. D., Rochelle, R. H., and Hyman, C. Exercise blood flow changes in the human forearm during physical training. *J. Appl. Physiol.* 18:789–93, 1963.

46. Roskamm, H. Optimum patterns of exercise for healthy adults. *Can. Med. Assoc. J.* 96:895–900, 1967.

47. Royce, J. Isometric fatigue curves in human muscle with normal and occluded circulation. *Res. Q.* 29:204–12, 1958.

48. Saltin, B. Intermittent exercise: Its physiology and practical application. John R. Emens Lecture, Ball State University, Muncie, Indiana, Feb. 20, 1975.

49. Shaver, L. G. Effects of training on relative muscular endurance in ipsilateral and contralateral arms. *Med. Sci. Sports* 2:165–71, 1970.

50. Start, K. B., and Graham, J. S. Relationship between the relative and absolute isometric endurance of an isolated muscle group. *Res. Q.* 35:193–204, 1964.

51. Stull, G. A., and Clarke, D. H. High resistance, low repetition training as a determiner of strength and fatigability. *Res. Q.* 41:189–93, 1970.

52. Thorstensson, A., and Karlsson, J. Fatiguability and fibre composition of human skeletal muscle. *Acta. Physiol. Scand.* 98:318–22, 1976.

53. Treffene, R. J., Dickson, R., Craven, C., Osborne, C., Woodhead, K., and Hobbs, K. Lactic acid accumulation during constant speed swimming at controlled relative intensities. *J. Sports Med. and Phys. Fitness* 20:244–54, 1980.

54. Vanderhoof, E. R., Imig, C. J., and Hines, H. M. Effect of muscle strength and endurance development on blood flow. *J. Appl. Physiol.* 16:873–77, 1961.

55. Wilmore, J. H. Influence of motivation on physical work capacity and performance. *J. Appl. Physiol.* 24:459–63, 1968.

56. ———. Maximal oxygen intake and its relationship to endurance capacity on a bicycle ergometer. *Res. Q.* 40:203–10, 1969.

23

Efficiency of Muscular Activity

Aerobic versus Anaerobic Efficiency

Running Economy
  Age
  Fiber Type
  Altitude
  Gender
  Psychological State
  Body Mass
  Trainability of Running Economy

Effect of Speed on Efficiency
  Simple Movements
  Running
  Walking
  Cycling
  Storage of Elastic Energy

Effect of Work Rate on Efficiency

Effect of Fatigue on Efficiency

Diet and Efficiency

Effects of Environmental Temperature

Effect of Wind on Running Efficiency

Effect of Obesity on Efficiency

The Looseness Factor

Acceleration-Deceleration versus Smooth
  Movement

Pace and Efficiency

Efficiency of Positive and Negative Work

For the engineer and the physicist, definition of the efficiency of a machine is quite simple.

$$\text{Efficiency} = \frac{\text{Output}}{\text{Input}}$$
$$= \frac{\text{Work done by machine}}{\text{Work done on the machine}}$$

The physiologist usually uses the same concept in the following terms.

$$\text{Efficiency} = \frac{\text{Work output}}{\text{Energy expended}}$$

In practice, energy expended is measured indirectly by oxygen consumption, which is converted into heat units (calories), and work output, which is measured in foot-pounds (ft-lb) or kilogram-meters (kgm) and can also be converted into heat units (3,087 ft-lb or 427 kgm = 1 kcal) so one may work with similar units. This is a simple procedure for activities in which the work output is easily measured as force times distance, such as riding a bicycle ergometer or lifting the body weight in bench-stepping.

Problems arise, however, in defining the baseline from which to measure the energy input (the denominator of our efficiency equation). Should we use the gross $\dot{V}O_2$ during the exercise in question, or should we subtract the resting value of $\dot{V}O_2$, in which case we would have "net efficiency"? Gross efficiency and net efficiency have been the classic methods employed, but each results in artifactual errors of computation—gross efficiency because it includes resting $\dot{V}O_2$, which is not really attributable to the exercise, and net efficiency because the appropriate resting value is impossible to measure precisely, as will be shown below. Gaesser and Brooks (33) have shown clearly that erroneous conclusions may be derived from the classic approach. At the present time there is ongoing dialogue concerning the best approach for the measurement of efficiency. Two new methods have been proposed, and we can define the differences in methods as follows:

1. Gross efficiency $= \dfrac{\text{Work output}}{\text{Energy expended}}$
   $$= \frac{W}{E} \times 100$$

2. Net efficiency $= \dfrac{\text{Work output}}{\substack{\text{Energy expended above} \\ \text{that at rest}}}$
   $$= \frac{W}{E - e} \times 100$$

3. Work efficiency $= \dfrac{\text{Work output}}{\substack{\text{Energy expended above} \\ \text{that in unloaded cycling}}}$
   $$= \frac{W}{E_L - E_U} \times 100$$

4. Delta efficiency $= \dfrac{\Delta \text{Work output}}{\Delta \text{Energy expended}}$
   $$= \frac{\Delta W}{\Delta E} \times 100$$

Where W = caloric equivalent of external work done
E = gross caloric expenditure including resting expenditure
e = resting caloric expenditure
E_L = caloric expenditure under load
E_U = caloric expenditure in unloaded pedaling
ΔW = caloric equivalent of increment in work output above previous work rate
ΔE = increment in caloric expenditure above that at previous work rate

These different methods result in quite different values of efficiency under the same experimental conditions on a bicycle ergometer, with gross efficiency showing a range of 7.5% to 20.4%, net efficiency 9.8% to 24.1%, and delta efficiency 24.4% to 34.0%. Work efficiency proved difficult to apply because of the difficulty in obtaining a true zero work pedaling condition (33).

13 hp Total oxygen consumption
- 7.8 hp Waste in recovery
  - Developing tension
  - Maintaining tension
- 5.2 hp Initial energy
  - Shortening energy
  - Waste

Useful work 2.95 hp
- Gravity .... 0.1 hp
- Velocity changes 0.5
- Acceleration of limbs 1.68
- Deceleration of limbs 0.67

Friction loss
Waste
Fixation

Since caloric expenditure goes up at least in proportion to (linearly with) and probably more rapidly than does work rate (33, 40), efficiency must either remain constant or decrease with increasing work rate. Gaesser and Brooks (33) showed that delta efficiency produced this result, while the use of gross or net values showed increasing values of efficiency with increasing work rate due to the artifacts of calculation. Thus delta efficiency seems to be the best method. Work efficiency would be equally satisfactory if a true zero work unloaded pedaling device were available. Unfortunately, all presently available ergometers in deVries's experience provide anywhere from 20 to 35 watts of resistance due to such factors as friction and inertia when set at zero load.

If efficiency values are needed for application in nutritional studies where gross energy expenditure is the matter of concern, then gross efficiency is the measure to be used.

The problem becomes more complex when activities such as walking and running are considered because large proportions of the working forces are dissipated in reciprocal movements of the arms and legs.

Fenn (32) has demonstrated that even the more difficult problems are capable of solution by applying motion picture recording and subsequent analysis of the forces involved in accelerating and decelerating the various body segments. His analysis (shown above) of the forces and energy involved in running is of interest.

This classic work of Fenn has been improved upon by Winter (66), who has further refined the calculation of the numerator of the efficiency equation by accounting for the internal work done by the limbs themselves.

The efficiency of machines varies between 10% and 20% in steam engines, 20% and 30% in gasoline engines, and 80% and 90% in electric motors. The mechanical efficiency of humans varies from less than 10% to 30% or even 40% or more, depending on the activity and method of calculation.

It would be well at this point to consider in which athletic activities efficiency plays an important role. Obviously, any event that involves endurance will be very much influenced by the factor of muscle efficiency. Thus we are talking largely about running events greater than a quarter mile and swimming events beyond 100 yards.

In the events where a single explosive effort is required, such as the shot put, power rather than efficiency is the critical factor. In sprint events efficiency of movement is of some importance but is probably secondary to the need for power.

An analogy from the automotive world seems appropriate. In a drag race (an acceleration contest), one does not care how many miles per gallon of gas (efficiency) the machine achieves; *power* is all-important. For an economy run, however, power is unimportant; miles per gallon determines the winner.

Thus this chapter can be considered a continuation of the last chapter in that it also is mainly concerned with endurance. The maximum speed at which humans can run distance events depends largely on the rate at which they can supply energy (limited by maximal O_2 consumption) and on their efficiency in using this energy.

Aerobic versus Anaerobic Efficiency

The efficiency of work done anaerobically has been reported to be only about half that of work done aerobically (5, 18, 19). However, the work of Gladden and Welch (34) suggests that anaerobic metabolism is no less efficient than aerobic metabolism. In any event, efficiency does in fact decrease as the power output (work rate) increases (31, 33, 40). This may be the result of a true decrease in muscular efficiency, or an increased metabolic overhead (cost of heart and lung function and the like, which are not measured as work output), or both.

Running Economy

There are large differences in running economy from individual to individual. Figure 23.1 shows the differences in O_2 consumption for runners of varying skill as studied by Dill, Talbot, and Edwards in 1930. The famous marathoner of that time, Clarence DeMar, had the lowest O_2 consumption at 26 ml/kg·min^{-1}, while the less skilled runners went 54% higher, requiring as much as 40 ml/kg·min^{-1} for the same run.

Running economy (efficiency) has been defined as "the aerobic demand ($\dot{V}O_2$) of submaximal running" (54). In recent years, there has been an increased interest in running economy because of its relationship with distance running performance (54). In particular, running economy has been shown to be a good predictor of endurance performance in highly trained runners who have comparable $\dot{V}O_2$ max values. For example, Conley and Krahenbuhl (20) found that for highly trained, national level runners, 65% of the variance in 10-kilometer race performance was accounted for by differences in running economy, while $\dot{V}O_2$ max was a much weaker determinant of success.

Many factors may influence running economy including age, fiber type, altitude, gender, psychological state, and body mass.

Age

Children are less economical runners than adults but improve steadily throughout childhood and adolescence (48). Krahenbuhl and Williams (48) have suggested that children and adults differ in running economy for three primary reasons:

1. Children have higher resting metabolic rates.
2. Children have greater ventilatory equivalents for oxygen.
3. Children have disadvantageous stride rates and stride lengths.

Fiber Type

It is unclear if there is an association between fiber type and running economy (54). Williams and Cavanagh (64) found no difference in fiber type characteristics in male runners who exhibited varying levels of running economy. Bosco, Montanari, and Ribacchi (7), however, reported a significant relationship ($r = 0.60$) between percent fast twitch fibers and the oxygen cost of running in athletes. That is, at the same running velocity, athletes with a high percentage of fast twitch fibers required more oxygen than those with a high percentage of slow twitch fibers.

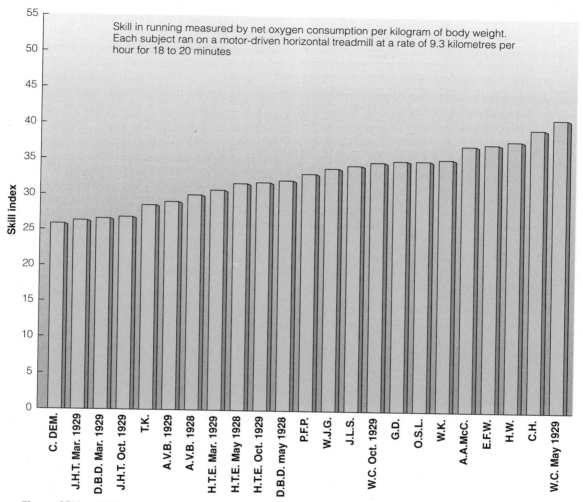

Figure 23.1 Skill in running. Each man ran at the same rate on the horizontal treadmill. In contrast with the relatively uniform cost of walking at 90 m/min the cost varied widely. The most efficient was Clarence DeMar, the famous marathoner of that time, 1929. (From Dill, D. B., Talbot, and Edwards., in *Journal of Physiology* 69:267. © 1930 Cambridge University Press. England. Reprinted by permission.)

Altitude

Apparently the oxygen cost of submaximal exercise is lower at altitude than sea level (24, 38, 54). Morgan and Craib (54) have suggested that this may be due to "lowered overall work of breathing due to the reduced air density at altitude and environmental differences in anaerobic energy contribution." Economy during track running is also better at altitude than sea level, possibly due to a decreased energy cost associated with the less dense air.

Gender

Daniels and Daniels (23) reviewed the available evidence concerning gender differences in running economy. With respect to elite male and female runners, they concluded that:

1. Males are more economical than females at common velocities of running.
2. No difference exists in running economy between males and females at typical, relative (% $\dot{V}O_2$ max) race intensities.
3. Among males and females of equal $\dot{V}O_2$ max, males are more economical, both at common velocities and at common relative intensities of running.
4. Among males and females of equal running economy, males have a greater $\dot{V}O_2$ max and a greater running velocity at $\dot{V}O_2$ max.

Psychological State

Psychological state may influence running economy but the presently available evidence is not conclusive (22). If there is an effect, it appears that reduced tension is associated with improved running economy (65, 69).

Body Mass

Martin and Morgan (51) reviewed the literature regarding the association between body mass and running economy. The authors concluded that "larger individuals are more economical per unit of body mass than smaller individuals."

Trainability of Running Economy

In their recent review, Morgan and Craib (54) indicated that there is conflicting evidence regarding the trainability of running economy from both cross-sectional studies of trained versus untrained subjects or elite versus non-elite athletes as well as longitudinally as a result of exercise training and/or instruction related to proper running technique. The authors stated that "It is possible that training exerts a minor influence on economy and that

economical runners are endowed with an anatomical or genetic makeup that produces an economical running style and favors success in longer running events."

With respect to children, Krahenbuhl and Williams (48) stated that "Running economy in later childhood fails to respond to either short-term instruction on the techniques of running or short-term participation in running training. Long-term participation in running training may augment improvements in running economy that occur naturally with age."

Effect of Speed on Efficiency

Simple Movements

In a classic 1922 experiment of muscle physiology, A. V. Hill (41) provided evidence of an optimum speed of movement below which efficiency falls slowly and above which it falls rapidly. It must be cautioned, however, that this work was done on a simple contraction of isolated muscle groups.

Running

In another important experiment in 1926, Sargent (59) determined the oxygen consumption of a subject who ran 120 yards at varying rates of speed, up to an all-out sprint. His results indicated that O_2 consumption increased as the 3.8th power of speed. This would mean that O_2 consumption increases almost sixteen times when speed is doubled. This would also mean a tremendous loss of efficiency as running speed increases. Many theories of pace and so on have been built on this concept.

Sargent's subject, however, ran anaerobically, and his O_2 consumption was calculated as O_2 debt based on the O_2 consumption after the race. From this was subtracted the resting rate measured *before* the run. It has, however, been demonstrated that resting consumption after exercise remains considerably higher for six to eight hours after exercise, and this higher metabolism is not related to the O_2 debt incurred during the run. Consequently, Sargent's calculations resulted in erroneously high O_2 consumptions because he had subtracted too low a baseline value from the recovery O_2 consumption rates.

More recent work (29, 30, 36, 50) shows that the rate of increase in energy demand is only *proportional* to increases in speed. Thus efficiency remains constant in spite of changes in speed for all distance events (45). The linear relationship between $\dot{V}O_2$ and running velocity has been used to examine gender and event differences in running economy as well as predict distance running performance (23, 53).

Stride length and the amount of vertical movement appear to be important determinants of running efficiency. In a comparison of good and poor runners in Japan, it was found that the better performers 1) used a longer stride, 2) had a faster stride, and 3) had a greater forward lean. Most important, they found that in the 5,000-meter event the poor performers did 17,968 kgm of vertical work (wasted energy) while the better performers did only 9,407 kgm of vertical work (52).

Two groups of investigators working with untrained subjects found that each individual has an optimal stride length and that the tendency is toward overstriding (inefficient) rather than understriding (10, 17).

Cavanagh and Williams (16) concluded that *well-trained* runners are very likely to run with a combination of stride length and stride frequency that is extremely close to their optimal condition. Therefore, in most cases a coach would be wise not to dictate a particular stride profile for an athlete—although Cavanagh and Williams did find that in *isolated cases* adjustment of stride patterns could result in reductions in $\dot{V}O_2$ and thus improved performance.

Trained male runners appear to be more efficient than trained females, although the differences found were not large—10% or less (9, 43).

Walking

The most economical rate of walking has been found to be 4 km/hr (2.4 mph) (11), at which the energy consumption is about one-half kilocalorie per kilometer walked per kilogram of body weight. The energy consumption for aerobic running is about twice that value, regardless of speed.

Walking more slowly than 4 km/hr apparently causes energy to be wasted in static components of muscle activity because weight is supported too long in respect to the useful work. Walking faster causes energy consumption to increase faster than the useful work done and efficiency again falls off, presumably because of a disproportionate increase of energy wasted in accelerating and decelerating body parts.

As a result of the increasing inefficiency at increasing rates, energy consumption of walking at about 8 km/hr (4.8 mph) becomes greater than that required for running, so that running is more efficient than walking above 8 km/hr.

Cycling

Using total work loads on bicycle ergometers that were equated for energy cost, Henry (39) found that 69 rpm resulted in work output of 620 kgm/min, while 116 rpm produced only 95 kgm/min. The difference in efficiency is obvious. Earlier workers had reported that 70 rpm is the most efficient pedaling rate. However, more recent work shows that the most efficient pedaling rate increases with increases in power output (work rate) from 42 rpm at a light load of 40.8 watts to 62 rpm at a heavy load of 327 watts (60). These differences among investigators are probably due to the different flywheel masses involved on the different ergometers. A small flywheel mass would require higher peak force output by the leg muscles.

Interestingly, Hagberg and coworkers (37) found the average preferred pedaling rate for *experienced racing cyclists* to be 91 rpm, which is considerably above all of the preceding data. This can be explained by the fact that previous studies had either used subjects who were non-cyclists, or they used cyclists who were studied on cycle ergometers, not on their regular racing bicycle. Hagberg, on the other hand, found 91 rpm to be the most efficient rate for trained cyclists riding their own racing equipment on a treadmill.

Storage of Elastic Energy

An explanation seems called for to rationalize the fact that many forms of physical activity have an optimum rate above which increased speed demands disproportionately greater energy expenditure. The efficiency of running, on the other hand, seems to be unaffected by speed.

Early workers, such as Fenn (32) and Hubbard (44), discussed the possibility of the storage of mechanical energy in the muscles and tendons. The extension of a muscle and tendon that are antagonistic in one phase of reciprocating movement might store the kinetic energy of the protagonist as potential energy, which is released when the antagonist contracts.

It has been demonstrated in a laboratory preparation that such a storage of energy can and does occur (13). When a contracted muscle was forcibly stretched, a substantial amount of the work done in stretching the muscle appeared to be available in the work done in the subsequent contraction. Further-more, the sooner the contraction followed the forced stretch the greater was the increase in work performed. It must be realized that this phenomenon could bring about considerable economy in quickly reciprocating movements, as in running, but the economy would be less as the rate slows because of the greater length

of time during which the contracted muscle exerts tension (uses energy) against the stretching. It has been calculated by the same investigators that this elastic work may contribute as much as half of the total mechanical work performed in running (12). More recent work from the same laboratory has corroborated this concept and extended it into the realm of human arm and leg movement (14, 63). Using an electronic force platform, Thys, Faraggiana, and Margaria (63) studied subjects in deep-knee-bending exercise under two conditions 1) rebounding, where they bounced back up immediately after assuming the full squat position, thus using the elastic energy stored in stretching the leg extensors in the subsequent contraction, and 2) nonrebounding exercise, identical except that the exercise stopped for a fraction of a second in the full squat position, thus allowing the elastic energy to be dissipated as heat. They found the rebounding movement to have faster maximum speed of movement (20%), more power (29%), and better efficiency (37%). This appears to be an important factor to apply in athletics wherever pertinent. These facts seem to offer the best explanation for why the efficiency of running does not decrease with increasing speed (15).

It has also been suggested that there are gender differences in the storage of elastic energy. Although the leg extensors of the male can sustain much higher stretch loads, the female may be able to utilize a greater portion of the stored elastic energy in jumping (47).

Effect of Work Rate on Efficiency

It appears from available data that if speed is held constant, the work rate (or power output) probably affects work efficiency or delta efficiency very little, at least at the light and moderate loads that have been used in investigations (33, 40).

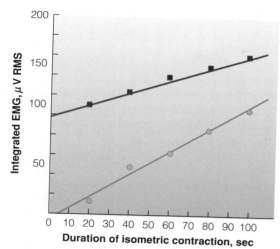

Figure 23.2 Illustration of increased electrical activity as a function of time when 40% of maximal voluntary contraction strength is maintained isometrically in the elbow flexors. Open circles represent data for a subject whose maximal duration was 127 seconds; squares represent subject with maximal duration of 338 seconds.

Effect of Fatigue on Efficiency

It has been pointed out that the electrical activity of a muscle increases with time even though it maintains constant tension. Figure 23.2 illustrates this fact. The best explanation for this is that, as fatigue occurs, more and more motor units are required to do the same piece of work. It is obvious that the recruitment of more units should result in greater energy consumption. Since the force *output* remains constant, the increased energy *input* must result in lowered efficiency. This will be important to our discussion of pace and efficiency.

A recent investigation by Morgan and co-workers (55) examined the effect of a 30-minute treadmill run at 89% of $\dot{V}O_2$ max on running economy in male distance runners. The results indicated that a prolonged (30

minutes) maximal run had no effect on running economy or related biomechanical factors. Further research is necessary, however, to determine the effect of repeated exhaustive exercise bouts on the oxygen cost of submaximal running (54).

Diet and Efficiency

There appears to be agreement among various investigators that the efficiency of muscular work is greatest when carbohydrate supplies the energy for muscular contraction. However, the differences due to this factor are small, probably not more than 5%.

Effects of Environmental Temperature

It has been shown that moderate work performed at 100° F ambient temperature requires an average 13.3% higher metabolic rate than work performed at 85° F. When work was heavy, the increase was 11.7% (21). The difference between work loads is probably not significant.

This decreased efficiency is undoubtedly the result of the increased load on the circulatory system for meeting the demand for increased peripheral circulation to transport heat from the core to the skin (increased heart rate, and so on).

Effect of Wind on Running Efficiency

The energy cost of overcoming air resistance even on a calm day outdoors was calculated to require additional energy to the extent of 7.8% for sprinting (10 m/sec), 4% for middle distances (6 m/sec), and 2% for the marathon (5 m/sec) (25). One might think that the wind effect would help as much on the downwind part of the course as it hurts on the headwind side of the track, but this is not the case. Mathematics shows that the help received is not nearly so great as the losses. It has been estimated that for a wind speed equal to running velocity, the overall cost is a loss of about four seconds per lap (25).

Of potential interest to runners is the concept of drafting. Drafting involves running directly behind another runner (usually 1 to 2 meters) so that the wind and air resistance is reduced and energy expenditure is conserved. The limited available evidence indicates that drafting may reduce the energy cost of running by three to six percent (49, 56). This level of energy savings may be beneficial, particularly at the end of a distance event. Drafting is even more important where velocity is greater as in ice skating and bicycling competition.

Effect of Obesity on Efficiency

Dempsey and coworkers (26) compared the exercise responses of fourteen normal young men with fourteen obese young men. It was shown that the obese required 2.01 liters/min of O_2 at a work load of 650 kgm/min, while the normals used only 1.54 liters/min for a slightly higher work load. Thus the obese required 30% more energy to do the job. For the moderately obese, the difference is probably not significant (67).

The Looseness Factor

Athletes and coaches frequently speak of being *loose* or *tight* in such activities as sprint running and swimming. It has been suggested that a tight runner can be thought of as one whose movements are impeded by the resistance of antagonistic muscles and their connective tissues due to a lack of flexibility. deVries has

investigated this possibility by controlled experiments in which four subjects ran ten 100-yard sprints. Five of the sprints were run under normal conditions of flexibility, and five were run after flexibility of trunk flexion, ankle flexion, and ankle extension had been significantly improved by static stretching. No significant differences in speed or oxygen consumption were found (28).

Interestingly, Gleim, Stachenfeld, and Nicholas (35) found that an index associated with flexibility of the trunk and lower extremities was negatively related ($r = -0.43$) to aerobic energy costs during walking and running. These findings indicated that "tightness" (lack of flexibility) resulted in improved economy. The authors suggested that lower levels of flexibility may reduce unproductive movements and thereby decrease the aerobic demands of the activity. Clearly, much additional research is necessary to clarify the relationship between flexibility and the oxygen cost of submaximal exercise.

Acceleration-Deceleration versus Smooth Movement

In some activities (such as swimming) the smoothness of movement is important to efficiency. In swimming the butterfly stroke, for example, if constant velocity could be maintained throughout the various events of the single-stroke cycle (the pull, the arm recovery, and the leg drive), maximum efficiency would be achieved. This is so because at a constant speed, a constant amount of energy is required to overcome the resistance of the body's movement through the water. This resistance is called *drag*. If the stroke is coordinated so that the leg drive sustains the velocity achieved by the arm pull during the recovery phase of the arms, only the force of drag must be overcome. If the coordination is such that the swimmer comes to a virtual standstill during arm recovery, then, in addition, the body must

Table 23.1 Comparison of Energy Requirements for One Stroke (in Arbitrary Units) (V = Velocity in ft/sec; V^2 is an Estimate of Energy Consumption)

Consecutive 1/10-second Periods	Ideal Swimmer		National Record Holder		Inexperienced Swimmer	
	V	V^2	V	V^2	V	V^2
0–0.1	6.07	36.54	8.00	64.00	11.10	123.21
0.1–0.2	6.07	36.54	6.72	45.13	8.63	74.48
0.2–0.3	6.07	36.54	6.63	43.96	6.12	37.45
0.3–0.4	6.07	36.54	4.92	24.21	3.08	9.49
0.4–0.5	6.07	36.54	4.42	19.54	1.00	1.00
0.5–0.6	6.07	36.54	6.22	38.69	5.76	33.18
0.6–0.7	6.07	36.54	5.33	28.41	4.35	18.92
0.7–0.8	6.07	36.54	4.92	24.21	3.21	10.30
0.8–0.9	6.07	36.54	4.84	23.43	2.42	5.86
0.9–1.0	6.07	36.54	6.22	38.69	6.55	42.90
1.0–1.1	6.07	36.54	8.52	72.59	14.52	210.83
Mean	6.07		6.07		6.07	
Total energy units used for one stroke		405.24		422.86		567.62

be *accelerated* by each arm pull. The energy required for acceleration is very costly because it varies as the square of the velocity. To double the velocity, then, requires four times the energy output.

To illustrate this concept, table 23.1 was prepared from an experiment in which de Vries measured the velocity of outstanding butterfly swimmers for each 0.10 second in their stroke cycles (27). For the sake of comparison, arbitrary energy units were calculated for 1) an ideal swimmer, swimming so smoothly that no acceleration-deceleration occurs, 2) a national record holder, whose highest velocity was 1.94 times his slowest velocity, and 3) an inexperienced swimmer, whose highest velocity was 14.52 times his slowest velocity (not unusual).

Although all three swimmers achieved an *average* velocity of 6.07 feet per second for the stroke that was analyzed, even the champion used 4% more energy than was necessary, and the inexperienced swimmer used 40% more. Furthermore, it has been shown that drag increases disproportionately above 5 or 6 feet per second, so that the actual differences in efficiency would be even greater than those predicted (4).

Pace and Efficiency

The question of how best to pace an endurance event cannot be answered simply. First, we have seen that efficiency for most activities (but apparently not running) falls off beyond some optimum rate of speed. Second, the fatigue level must be considered, inasmuch as efficiency falls off rapidly as fatigue brings about greater recruitment of muscle fibers to do the same job and possibly interferes with neuromuscular coordination.

In events that are largely aerobic (two-mile or more run), a constant rate is probably the most efficient. This is true even in running in which efficiency does not seem to vary with speed (aerobic condition). Even though the varying rates may be equally efficient, the *changes in rate* cost additional energy.

Constant rate does not necessarily mean running or swimming equal split times. For example, it is typical in distance swimming that the number of strokes per minute remains constant throughout the 1,500-meter swim, but each successive 100 meters shows a small decrement in speed—two or three seconds, or more, depending on the swimmer. This is the result of the fatigue process. Even though cadence remains the same, the force developed—and consequently the *distance per stroke*—decreases.

For middle-distance running events, some very interesting evidence *against* the constant rate has been presented by Robinson and colleagues (58), who ran two men on three different pace plans. Each man ran one trial at constant speed, one trial with a fast first minute and slower remainder, and one trial with a slow first minute and faster remainder. In both men, it was found that the slow start and faster finish resulted in slightly less O_2 consumption than the constant rate and in considerably less than the fast start and slower remainder. The overall time for the three pace plans was kept constant on the treadmill.

They also showed in another experiment that when three men ran to exhaustion in from 2.58 to 3.37 minutes, each man's O_2 consumption increased from 60% to 143% during the last half minute, as the lactic acid rose to high levels.

Thus the explanation for the results in the pace experiment seems to be that starting out fast results in an earlier accumulation of lactic acid, and thus more of the race is run inefficiently (68). On this basis, it would seem wise to run middle-distance races in which high O_2 debts are encountered on a pace plan that postpones the O_2 debt until late in the race. However, more recent studies that measured O_2 consumption to compare similar pace plans did not entirely support Robinson's data. Adams and Bernauer (3) found the steady pace to be significantly less demanding. Kollias and coworkers (46) found no difference between steady state and slow-fast pace, but a fast-slow pace required significantly greater O_2 consumption than either of the other two conditions. Summarizing the evidence from these three metabolic studies with two radiotelemetry studies on the cardiac cost of similar pace plans (8, 61) leaves us with complete agreement only on the fact that the fast-slow pacing creates greater physiological demands for middle-distance runs. Whether the slow-fast pace is better than the steady pace will be finally resolved only by further investigation.

Efficiency of Positive and Negative Work

Positive work is done when muscle contraction provides force that works through a distance, and this is associated with the concentric contraction of muscle. Negative work results when an extrinsic force overcomes the force developed by muscle contraction, and thus the muscle lengthens during contraction (eccentric contraction). By definition, positive work lifts a weight; negative work lowers a weight to its resting place. These definitions are not altogether satisfactory, however, for if we continue increasing the velocity with which we lower the weight until we accelerate its lowering to 32 ft/sec^2, all of the work would be done by gravitational force. A very slow lowering, on the other hand, could require a large degree of effort in a physiological sense. Undoubtedly, efforts by biophysicists will improve our definitions of these terms. In the meantime, some very interesting findings revolve about these definitions.

Negative work requires 10% to 30% less energy than positive work (62). Electromyographic evidence suggests that reduced muscle fiber activation during eccentric contractions compared to concentric contractions may contribute to the lower energy cost (2, 62). Interestingly, however, negative work requires less energy than positive work even during maximal activation of isolated muscle where the number of muscle fibers involved is the same (57). Based on these findings, Stauber (62) has suggested that two factors contribute to the reduced energy cost of negative work:

1. Altered recruitment of motor units (reduced EMG).

2. Decreased energy use of the active muscles that develop tension while being stretched.

A. V. Hill and his coworkers discovered the surprising fact that application of external mechanical work to a living muscle cell can reverse the normal biochemical processes (1, 42). Their experiments suggest that an absorption of energy by muscle tissue occurs during the forced extension of the contractile component when the muscle is in isometric contraction. Experiments on intact human muscles have supported these findings.

Asmussen (6) studied a man's energy expenditure in riding a bicycle uphill and downhill on a treadmill. He found it required from three to nine times as much energy to pedal uphill (positive work) as it did to resist the force of gravity in backpedaling downhill (negative work).

Abbott, Bigland, and Ritchie (2) found similar results. They used a pair of subjects on two bicycle ergometers, coupled in opposition (back to back) so that all of the positive work of one subject was dissipated as negative work in the other. Although the subjects used the same leg muscles in similar movements at identical speeds, at 35 rpm the O_2 consumption for positive work was 3.7 times that of negative work. This ratio increased with the speed of pedaling.

Summary of Principles for Coaching

1. Improve the skills involved first.

   A. Eliminate *unnecessary movements.*

   B. Eliminate *unnecessary muscle activity*—within even the necessary movement.

      1. Maintain relaxation in antagonistic muscles.

      2. Relax even the prime movers when possible. For example, convert tension movements into ballistic movements wherever possible. Thus even the prime movers can relax during a large portion of the movement.

   C. Make all movements in the *correct directions.* For example, an arm pull that moves laterally from the body in swimming the crawl wastes a considerable part of its total force.

   D. Apply only the *necessary amount of power;* too forceful an effort is usually wasteful.

   E. Use *muscles that are best suited to the activity.* For example, use the larger leg muscles in lifting heavy weights rather than the weaker back muscles.

   F. Use the *optimum speed* if time is not a factor.

2. Improve physical condition so that a given level of work results in less fatigue. Better condition delays fatigue; fatigue increases energy cost.

3. Avoid costly acceleration. Maintain a constant cadence if possible, even though fatigue may result in progressively slower split times.

4. Use a high carbohydrate, low fat, normal protein diet.

5. Pace (for a distance event) should adhere to principle three. For middle-distance events that incur large oxygen debts, a gradually accelerating pace may have advantages.

References

1. Abbott, B. C., Aubert, V. M., and Hill, A. V. Absorption of work by muscle stretched during single twitch or short tetanus. *Proc. R. Soc. Lond.* 139: 86–104, 1951.

2. Abbott, B. C., Bigland, B., and Ritchie, J. M. Physiological cost of negative work. *J. Physiol.* 117:380–90, 1952.

3. Adams, W. C., and Bernauer, E. M. The effect of selected pace variations on the oxygen requirement of running a 4:37 mile. *Res. Q.* 39:837–46, 1968.

4. Alley, L. E. An analysis of water resistance and propulsion in swimming the crawl stroke. *Res. Q.* 23:253–70, 1952.

5. Asmussen, E. Aerobic recovery after anaerobiosis in rest and work. *Acta Physiol. Scand.* 11:197–210, 1946.

6. ———. Experiments on positive and negative work. In *Fatigue,* eds. W. F. Floyd and A. T. Welford. London: H. K. Lewis and Co., 1953.

7. Bosco, C., Montanari, G., and Ribacchi, R. Relationship between the efficiency of muscular work during jumping and the energetics of running. *Eur. J. Appl. Physiol.* 56:138–43, 1987.

8. Bowles, C. J., and Sigerseth, P. O. Telemetered heart rate responses to pace patterns in the one-mile run. *Res. Q.* 39:36–46, 1968.

9. Bransford, D. R., and Howley, E. T. Oxygen cost of running in trained and untrained men and women. *Med. Sci. Sports* 9:41–44, 1977.

10. Burke, E. J., and Berger, R. A. Energy cost of running at three different stride lengths. *N. Z. J. HPER* 9:96–99, 1976.

11. Cavagna, G. A., Saibene, F. P., and Margaria, R. External work in walking. *J. Appl. Physiol.* 18:1–9, 1963.

12. ———. Mechanical work in running. *J. Appl. Physiol.* 19:249–56, 1964.

13. ———. Effect of negative work on the amount of positive work performed by an isolated muscle. *J. Appl. Physiol.* 20:157–58, 1956.

14. Cavagna, G. A., Dusman, B., and Margaria, R. Positive work done by a previously stretched muscle. *J. Appl. Physiol.* 24:21–32, 1968.

15. Cavagna, G. A., and Kaneko, M. Mechanical work and efficiency in level walking and running. *J. Physiol.* 268:467–81, 1977.

16. Cavanagh, P. R., and Williams, K. R. The effect of stride length variation on oxygen uptake during distance running. *Med. Sci. Sports Exer.* 14:30–35, 1982.

17. Cavanagh, P. R., Williams, K. R., and Hodgson, J. L. The effect of stride length variation on O_2 uptake during distance running. *Med. Sci. Sports* 10:63, 1978.

18. Christensen, E. H., and Hogberg, P. The efficiency of anaerobical work. *Arbeitsphysiologie* 14:249–50, 1950.

19. ————. Steady state, O_2 deficit and O_2 debt at severe work. *Arbeitsphysiologie* 14:251–54, 1950.

20. Conley, D. L., and Krahenbuhl, G. S. Running economy and distance running performance of highly trained athletes. *Med. Sci. Sports Exer.* 12:357–60, 1980.

21. Consolazio, C. F., Matoush, L. D., Nelson, R. A., Torres, J. B., and Isaac, G. J. Environmental temperature and energy expenditure. *J. Appl. Physiol.* 18:65–68, 1963.

22. Crews, D.J. Psychological state and running economy. *Med. Sci. Sports Exerc.* 24:475–82, 1992.

23. Daniels, J., and Daniels, N. Running economy of elite male and elite female runners. *Med. Sci. Sports Exerc.* 24:483–89, 1992.

24. Daniels, J., Foster, C., Daniels, S., and Krahenbuhl, G. Altitude and human performance with special consideration of the aerobic demands of running. Proceedings of the NCPEAM/ NAPECW National Conference, pp. 61–67, 1977.

25. Davies, C. T. M. Effects of wind assistance and resistance on the forward motion of a runner. *J. Appl. Physiol.* 48:702–9, 1980.

26. Dempsey, J. A., Reddan, W., Balke, B., and Rankin, J. Work capacity determinants and physiologic cost of weight supported work in obesity. *J. Appl. Physiol.* 21:1815–20, 1966.

27. deVries, H. A. A cinematographical analysis of the dolphin swimming stroke. *Res. Q.* 30:413–22, 1959.

28. ————. The "looseness" factor in speed and O_2 consumption of an anaerobic 100-yard dash. *Res. Q.* 34:305–13, 1963.

29. Dill, D. B. Comparative physiology of oxygen transport. *J. Sports Med. Phys. Fitness* 3:191–200, 1963.

30. ————. Oxygen used in horizontal and grade walking and running on the treadmill. *J. Appl. Physiol.* 20:19–22, 1965.

31. Donovan, C. M., and Brooks, G. A. Muscular efficiency during steady-state exercise; II. Effects of walking speed and work rate. *J. Appl. Physiol.* 43:431–39, 1977.

32. Fenn, W. O. Frictional and kinetic factors in the work of sprint runners. *Am. J. Physiol.* 92:583–610, 1930.

33. Gaesser, G. A., and Brooks, G. A. Muscular efficiency during steady-rate exercise: Effects of speed and work-rate. *J. Appl. Physiol.* 38:1132–39, 1975.

34. Gladden, L. B., and Welch, H. G. Efficiency of anaerobic work. *J. Appl. Physiol.* 44:564–70, 1978.

35. Gleim, G. W., Stachenfeld, N. S., and Nicholas, J. A. The influence of flexibility on the economy of walking and jogging. *J. Orthop. Res.* 8:814–23, 1990.

36. Hagan, R. D., Strathman, T., Strathman, L., and Gettman, L. R. Oxygen uptake and energy expenditure during horizontal treadmill running. *J. Appl. Physiol.* 49:571–75, 1980.

37. Hagberg, J. M., Mullin, J. P., Grese, M. D., and Spitznagel, E. Effect of pedaling rate on submaximal exercise responses of competitive cyclists. *J. Appl. Physiol.* 51:447–51, 1981.

38. Hagerman, F., Addington, W., and Gaensler, E. Severe steady state exercise at sea level and altitude in Olympic oarsman. *Med. Sci. Sports* 7:275–79, 1975.

39. Henry, F. M. Individual differences in O$_2$ metabolism of work at two speeds of movement. *Res. Q.* 22:324–33, 1951.

40. Hesser, C. M., Linnarsson, D., and Bjurstedt, H. Cardiorespiratory and metabolic responses to positive and negative and minimum load dynamic leg exercise. *Resp. Physiol.* 30:51–67, 1977.

41. Hill, A. V. The maximum work and mechanical efficiency of human muscles and their most economical speed. *J. Physiol.* 56:19–41, 1922.

42. ———. Production and absorption of work by muscle. *Science* 131:897–903, 1960.

43. Howley, E. T., and Glover, M. E. The caloric costs of running and walking one mile for men and women. *Med. Sci. Sports* 6:235–37, 1974.

44. Hubbard, A. W. An experimental analysis of running and a certain fundamental difference between trained and untrained runners. *Res. Q.* 10:28–38, 1939.

45. Ito, A., Komi, P. V., Sjodin, B., Bosco, C., and Karlsson, J. Mechanical efficiency of positive work in running at different speeds. *Med. Sci. Sports Exer.* 15:299–308, 1983.

46. Kollias, J., Nicholas, W. C., Buskirk, E. R., and Mendez, J. Oxygen requirements for running at moderate altitude. *J. Sports Med.* 10:27–35, 1970.

47. Komi, P. V., and Bosco, C. Utilization of stored elastic energy in leg extensor muscles by men and women. *Med. Sci. Sports* 10:261–65, 1978.

48. Krahenbuhl, G. S., and Williams, T. J. Running economy: Changes with age during childhood and adolescence. *Med. Sci. Sports Exerc.* 24:462–66, 1992.

49. Kyle, C. Reduction of wind resistance and power output of racing cyclists and runners travelling in groups. *Ergonomics* 22:387–97, 1979.

50. Margaria, R., Cerretelli, P., Aghemo, P., and Sassi, G. Energy cost of running. *J. Appl. Physiol.* 18:367–70, 1963.

51. Martin, P. E., and Morgan, D. W. Biomechanical considerations for economical walking and running. *Med. Sci. Sports Exerc.* 24:467–74, 1992.

52. Miyashita, M., Miura, M., Murase, Y., and Yamaji, K. Running performance from the viewpoint of aerobic power. Paper to International Symposium on Environmental Stress, Santa Barbara, CA, September 1, 1977.

53. Morgan, D. W., Baldini, F. D., Martin, P. E., and Kohrt, W. M. Ten kilometer performance and predicted velocity at $\dot{V}O_2$ max among well-trained male runners. *Med. Sci. Sports Exerc.* 21:78–83, 1989.

54. Morgan, D. W., and Craib, M. Physiological aspects of running economy. *Med. Sci. Sports Exerc.* 24:456–61, 1992.

55. Morgan, D. W., Martin, P. E., Baldini, F. D., and Krahenbuhl, G. S. Effects of a prolonged maximal run on running economy and running mechanics. *Med. Sci. Sports Exerc.* 22:834–40, 1990.

56. Pugh, L. The influence of wind resistance in running and walking and the mechanical efficiency of work against horizontal and vertical forces. *J. Physiol.* (Lond.) 213:255–76, 1971.

57. Rall, J. A. Energetic aspects of skeletal muscle contraction: Implications of fiber types. In *Exercise and Sport Sciences Reviews,* ed. R. L. Terjung. New York: MacMillan, pp. 33–74, 1985.

58. Robinson, S., Robinson, D. L., Mountjoy, R. J., and Bullard, R. W. Fatigue and efficiency of men during exhausting runs. *J. Appl. Physiol.* 12:197–202, 1958.

59. Sargent, R. M. The relation between O_2 requirement and speed in running. *Proc. R. Soc. Lond.* 100:10–22, 1926.

60. Seabury, J. J., Adams, W. C., and Ramey, M. R. Influence of pedalling rate and power output on energy expenditure during bicycle ergometry. *Ergonomics* 20:491–98, 1977.

61. Sorani, R. P. The effect of three different pace plans on the cardiac cost of 1320-yard runs. Ph.D. diss., Physical Education, University of Southern California, 1967.

62. Stauber, W. T. Eccentric action of muscles: Physiology, injury, and adaptation. In *Exercise and Sport Sciences Reviews,* ed. K. B. Pandolf. Baltimore: Williams and Wilkins, pp. 157–85, 1989.

63. Thys, H., Faraggiana, T., and Margaria, R. Utilization of muscle elasticity in exercise. *J. Appl. Physiol.* 32:491–94, 1972.

64. Williams, K., and Cavanagh, P. Relationship between distance running mechanics, running economy, and performance. *J. Appl. Physiol.* 63:1236–45, 1987.

65. Williams, T. J., Krahenbuhl, G. S., and Morgan, D. W. Mood state and running economy in moderately trained male runners. *Med. Sci. Sports Exerc.* 23:727–31, 1991.

66. Winter, D. A new definition of mechanical work done in human movement. *J. Appl. Physiol.* 46:79–83, 1979.

67. Wolfe, L. A., Hodgson, J. L., Barlett, H. L., Nicholas, W. C., and Buskirk, E. R. Pulmonary function at rest and during exercise in uncomplicated obesity. *Res. Q.* 47:829–38, 1976.

68. Yates, J. W., Gladden, L. B., and Cresanta, M. K. Effects of prior dynamic leg exercise on static effort of the elbow flexors. *J. Appl. Physiol.* 55:891–96, 1983.

69. Ziegler, S. G., Klinzing, J., and Williamson, K. The effects of two stress management training programs on cardiorespiratory efficiency. *J. Sport Psychol.* 4:280–89, 1982.

24

Speed

Intrinsic Speed of Muscle Contraction

Force–Velocity Relationship

Specificity of Speed

Strength and Speed

Flexibility and Speed

Body Mechanics and Speed in Running

Body Mechanics and Speed in Swimming

Physiological Considerations in the
      Design of Running Tracks

Gender Differences in Speed of
    Movement

Variation of Speed with Distance in
    Running and Swimming

Limiting Factors in Speed
    Speed of Single Muscle Contraction
    Speed of Gross Motor Movements

Methods for Improving Sprint Speed

Speed of movement is very important in athletics. It is worthy of careful analysis so that we can better understand this aspect of human performance and thus be in a better position to improve this function in athletes.

First, we must realize that, basically, speed is the result of applying force to a mass. Second, speed usually implies movement at a *constant* rate. The movement of a body (human or otherwise) at a constant rate requires sufficient driving force to balance the forces that resist movement. An airplane must have just enough force to overcome the friction of air drag to maintain a constant speed. If more than this balancing amount of force is applied, acceleration occurs (speed increases with time); if less, the aircraft decelerates.

In the human body the resisting force has several components. We can think of a balance of positive and negative forces in respect to propulsion of the body or any of its parts (the same physical laws apply). The positive force that propels the body is provided by muscular contractions, aided in some cases by the storage of elastic energy (see chap. 23). The negative forces depend on the nature of the activity.

In running, for example, it was shown in chapter 23 that the 2.95 hp of useful work (positive force) developed by the muscles were used to balance the negative forces as follows: 1) gravity, 0.1 hp; 2) velocity changes, 0.5 hp; 3) acceleration of limbs, 1.68 hp; and 4) deceleration of limbs, 0.67 hp. Had this run been performed on the track instead of on a treadmill, another negative force, air resistance—possibly as much as 0.5 hp—would have had to be overcome, and the positive or propelling force needed for maintaining a constant rate of speed would have been 3.45 hp.

From the above considerations we might hypothesize that speed can be improved by either increasing the positive or by decreasing the negative factors. In a practical sense, this suggests that improving strength would be the most important positive factor. The negative factors might be reduced through improved neuromuscular coordination (skill) and flexibility, which might conceivably decrease the values of the factors listed above. We shall examine these possibilities in this chapter.

Intrinsic Speed of Muscle Contraction

As has been pointed out, muscles differ in their ability to produce fast movement. This, of course, reflects the differences in their makeup with respect to proportions of fast twitch (FT) and slow twitch (ST) fibers as discussed in chapters 2, 3, and 4. Thus there are considerable intrinsic differences between the postural extensor muscles and the faster flexor muscles within a given individual. There are also interindividual differences in speed of movement for the same muscle group or type of movement, and speed of contraction also varies greatly from one animal species to another, approximately in inverse ratio to size. This variability in speed persists even in animals deprived of innervation, so that at least in simple movements, the differences in speed of contraction must be intrinsic to the muscle tissue itself. But is this intrinsic difference the result of different lengths of sarcomeres or differences in the velocity of actin filaments sliding past myosin filaments? It seems clear that sarcomere length is relatively constant, not only among human individuals but also among vertebrates in general (18). The sliding velocity of the filaments may vary about threefold, and this seems to account for differences in speed of contraction (4).

Several factors influence the speed of contraction of a muscle fiber. Of these, the primary factors that are believed to differentiate ST and FT fibers in terms of speed of contraction include the following (43):

1. The level of actomyosin ATPase activity. Inherently, FT fibers have greater activity of this enzyme and therefore

liberate the stored energy from ATP more effectively.

2. ST fibers have poorly developed sarcoplasmic reticulum that may interfere with the rate of calcium release and muscle contraction.

3. There may be slight differences in the myosin molecule in FT and ST fibers.

4. There may be differences in the ability of calcium to bind with troponin between FT and ST fibers.

Comparing the intrinsic speeds of different muscles requires that we equate them by fiber length. Obviously, a muscle fiber that is ten times longer than another fiber can shorten at one end ten times as fast, although intrinsic properties are the same.

Although evidence is lacking, it seems very likely that ultimate maximal speed capacity is limited by the intrinsic speed of an individual's muscle tissue and by the efficacy of that person's neuromuscular coordination patterns. Neither factor is amenable to changes as large as those that affect strength and endurance.

Force–Velocity Relationship

It has been shown with experimental muscle preparations that the force available from a muscle's shortening decreases as the rate of shortening increases. Figure 24.1 illustrates this relationship, which has important implications for athletics.

The shape of the curve in figure 24.1 also leads us to conclude that there must be an *optimum speed* at which a muscle can produce its greatest *power* and greatest *efficiency*. It has been found that this optimum speed is approximately one-third of the maximum speed at which it can shorten under zero load (16). Kaneko (20) has shown that maximum power is developed when force and velocity are both about 35% of their maximum values. Data

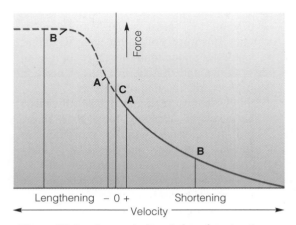

Figure 24.1 Force-velocity relation of contracting muscle: to the right, shortening; to the left, lengthening. C, at zero speed, represents an isometric contraction. A and A' are at the same velocity of shortening and lengthening. So are B and B'. (From Hill, A. V., "The Mechanics of Voluntary Muscle," in *Lancet* 261:947. © 1951 Lancet Ltd., England. Reprinted by permission of the publisher and author.)

from deVries's laboratory shown in figure 24.2 are in essential agreement.

Another important implication pertains to the vulnerability to athletic injury. Hill (15) has pointed out that if a rapid flexor movement is made and the object is suddenly wrenched in the opposite direction, the muscle or its attachments may be torn. This can happen because the forces of the muscle in the lengthening movement could be increased several times beyond what they were in shortening before a reflex inhibition (from the inverse myotatic reflex) could take place. This sudden increase in the forces, which is predicted from figure 24.1, could well exceed the elastic limits of the tissues. Figure 24.1 shows clearly that a virtually instantaneous change from a shortening contraction at point *B* to a lengthening contraction at point *B'* results in a severalfold increase in forces within the muscle involved. This is the basis for many athletic injuries.

From the standpoint of human performance in the intact individual, there are two

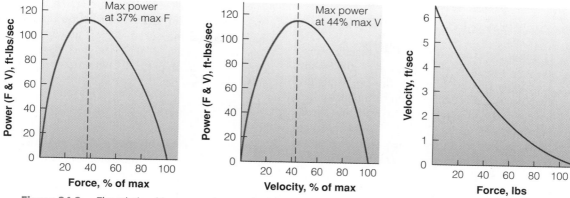

Figure 24.2   The relationships among force, velocity, and power produced in healthy young men in elbow flexion.

aspects of speed. The first (really acceleration) is related to how fast an athlete can accelerate from a standstill (for example, a football lineman's charge or the start of a sprint event). This factor is an important determinant of speed for the first five or ten yards. It is probably determined by the shape of an individual's force-velocity curve. A recent investigation by Mero (29) emphasized the importance of muscular strength to the sprint start. On the other hand, for distances more than twenty yards, the most important determinant is the maximal movement rate, which is in turn limited by intrinsic speed and neuromuscular coordination. Therefore, an individual could conceivably be a slow starter with a good 100-yard speed, or a fast starter with a poor 100-yard time, or indeed be proficient in football, tennis, and other sports, where quick-starting movements are important, but be a poor 100-yard sprinter.

In experienced sprint athletes, however, there is a close relationship ($r = -0.68$ to -0.81) between starting velocity and 100-meter running time. Thus, in competitive sprinters, muscular strength contributes to a successful start and the start is closely related to overall running performance (29).

Specificity of Speed

It is commonplace in physical education and athletics to speak of an individual as fast or slow, but evidence is accumulating that speed has very little generality. Indeed, an individual with a fast arm movement may well have slow leg movement. In fact, this specificity extends even to the type of task and the direction of movement (3, 13, 37).

It has been shown, for example, that speed is 87% or 88% specific to the limb (37). Even within a limb, speed is 88% to 90% specific to the direction of movement. This means there is practically no correlation between the speeds with which one can perform an arm movement and a leg movement and only a small relationship between speed of movement in a forward arm swing and a backward arm swing. This might lead us to describe an individual as fast in a backward swing of the right leg! Obviously this makes no sense, but neither does it make sense to speak of a fast or slow individual. We can speak of a fast runner, but we are not justified in assuming the same individual can throw a fast ball in baseball.

Strength and Speed

It might be expected from the preceding discussions that strength and speed of movement are highly related; however, the experimental evidence is controversial. Four different studies have agreed in findings that strength and speed are unrelated (2, 13, 14, 39). However, all of these studies were concerned with the same movement pattern, the horizontal adductive arm swing. Farrar and Thorland (11) also found no significant relationships for flexion and extension of the thigh or leg versus 40- and 100-yard sprint times in college-age males. Nelson and Fahrney (31), however, have shown rather strong significant and consistent correlations in three experimental subject groups of $r = 0.74$, 0.79, and 0.75 between strength and speed of elbow flexion. In addition, Kenney (24) found that isokinetic arm extension (at the shoulder joint) strength was significantly correlated ($r = -0.47$) with 50-yard sprint swimming (front crawl stroke) performance in male collegiate swimmers. Thus a final decision on strength–speed relationships must await further research.

Interestingly, if movements are resisted by substantial loads on a tested limb, sizable relationships between strength and speed (up to 0.76) can be demonstrated (44). This leads us to think of speed in terms of the neuromotor specificity that has been demonstrated in so many other aspects of human performance. What we are saying, in effect, is that various speeds of movement against varying loads require different neuromotor coordination patterns. Thus, if we measure strength statically, we might expect higher correlations between strength and speed as we slow the speed (or increase the load) to more closely approximate static contraction. And this, we find, is what happens.

Carrying our discussion further requires that we visualize two strength factors: one a *static strength,* as we usually measure it by

dynamometer or cable tensiometer, and the other a dynamic or *strength in action* factor, which must be measured during movement. Each may involve a separate and distinct neural coordination pattern. Dynamic strength can be described as:

$$F = \frac{2md}{t^2}$$

where F is the force of contraction, m is the mass moved, d is the distance, and t is the time. This approach has been widely used by F. M. Henry and his collaborators at the University of California at Berkeley (13, 14). In this approach the mass is measured and the distance moved is timed electrically so that F, the force of contraction (or strength, if a maximal effort is made), can be calculated. Although the relationship between dynamic strength and speed is very close, it is hard to define. In calculating a correlation, the results are spurious because distance is usually a constant and mass varies very little. In effect, one would be correlating speed against itself.

Now for the most practical question: Can we improve speed of movement by improving strength? Even though there is no relationship between the static strength level of achievement and speed at any given time, considerable evidence (9, 16, 40) indicates a strong relationship between gain in strength and gain in speed. It has been shown that gains in strength, whether brought about by isometric or isotonic training, are associated with significant gains in speed of movement. The gain in speed has also been demonstrated to result from both strength training that used the same movement as was tested and from training that merely improved the strength of the involved muscles but avoided training in the same movement.

Interestingly, Francis and Tipton (12) found that the knee-jerk reflex time is improved by physical conditioning of the involved muscles. A significant 5% improvement in reflex time was shown after six weeks of weight training, although there appeared to be no correlation between strength and reflex time or between improvement in strength and reflex time. Thus, while the mechanism remains obscure, there seems to be good reason to include strength training in a training regimen for speed. Furthermore, it must be realized that in most speed events there is a period of acceleration to attain maximum velocity, as in running the 100-yard sprint. Since acceleration of the body's mass is by definition dependent on strength (acceleration = force/mass), there can be no question of the importance of optimizing strength (force) in the practical coaching situation (assuming strength increases to a proportionally greater degree than mass).

Flexibility and Speed

As we have pointed out, logic tells us that improving flexibility should decrease the negative forces (resistance) involved in running and thus improve the speed. However, experiments by deVries—in which speed and oxygen consumption during a 100-yard dash were measured—failed to confirm this hypothesis (8). Even though range of motion was significantly improved, the short-term effect on speed was not significant.

In another experiment, in which the long-term effects of supplementing sprint training with flexibility work and weight training were investigated, it was found that neither weight training nor flexibility added to the gains in speed of the sprint training program. When both were used, however, the gains in speed were significantly better than those by sprint training alone (9).

It must be realized that stopwatch errors in timing a 100-yard dash can be 1% to 2%, and the changes brought about by an improved range of motion are not likely to be much larger than this. So the question cannot be considered closed.

Body Mechanics and Speed in Running

The area of body mechanics and speed in running has not yet been exhaustively investigated, but some experiments have been performed and their results are interesting.

Bringing about many accelerations and decelerations of the limbs at exactly the right time, at exactly the right rate, and with precisely the appropriate amount of force to run well obviously requires exquisite neuromuscular coordination patterns. One of the basic questions about running—Is the maximum speed limited by the maximum rate of leg alternation?—was answered by a simple but clever experiment by Slater-Hammel (38), who demonstrated that the rates of leg alternation in sprinting were 3.10 to 4.85/sec. Because considerably higher rates are possible in cycling (5.5 to 7.1), he concluded that speed in running is not limited in this way.

In another interesting kinesiological analysis of running, Hubbard (17) demonstrated that improvement results from increasing the length of stride rather than the rate of movement. Applying the formula for dynamic strength, $F = 2md/t^2$, we see that this requires more dynamic strength because d increases while t and m remain the same. Thus F, the force required (strength), must be greater. Again, we see that strength is a factor in speed.

Photographic analyses have shown that efficient running is also characterized by a high knee lift, a long running stride, and placement of the feet beneath the runner's center of gravity (7).

Use of the electrogoniometer (37), which provides electrical recording of joint angle changes, has shown that experienced distance runners increase both stride length and frequency when increasing velocity from running a 440 in 2:12 to running a 440 in 60.9 seconds. Stride length is more important at the lower speeds, while frequency becomes more important at the higher speeds. The only joint function that may become limiting appears to be that of hip flexion since it is the only joint angle that increases markedly at the higher speeds. Thus the track coach would be well advised to include flexibility work in the regimen for distance runners, such as the static stretching techniques described in the following chapter (chap. 25).

Body Mechanics and Speed in Swimming

Craig and Pendergast (5) performed a very interesting series of studies relating 1) stroke rate, 2) distance per stroke, and 3) velocity achieved by the swimmer. They found that in all four competitive stroke specialities, increased speed of swimming was achieved by a combination of increasing stroke rate and decreasing distance per stroke. This seems to imply that simply stroking faster and disregarding efficiency of stroking is the way to go, but this is not the case. The decreasing distance per stroke found is not a *cause* for going faster but rather the *result* of stroking faster. This is borne out by their finding that the individual who had the longest distance per stroke in slow swims had the greatest maximum all-out swim speed—and vice versa: poor distance per stroke results in poor maximum speed. These results support the idea (which every swim coach probably knows) that improving performance involves considerable practice swimming with slow stroke rates in order to develop greater distance per stroke. In support of this concept, a recent study by Toussaint (42) concluded that "on average the better swimmer distinguishes himself from the poorer one by a greater distance per stroke rather than a higher stroke frequency." Improving the distance per stroke should probably be accomplished early in the season, while establishing power and efficiency at race speeds should be emphasized in the late season.

Physiological Considerations in the Design of Running Tracks

McMahon (27) at Harvard University studied the physiological bases of running speed from the engineering viewpoint. When the university decided to build a new indoor track (completed in 1977), the Harvard track coach and the planning office sought his advice. The most important question was how much compliance to build into the track surface. On a springy track the time spent rebounding from the surface is increased so that the runner is slowed down. One might therefore suppose that the hardest surface is the fastest, but that did not turn out to be the case. They found in some interesting experiments that if they "tuned" the resiliency (compliance) of the track surface to the elastic and mechanical properties of the human runner, running speed could be increased.

How much compliance should be built into the track? They found that the most useful way to measure running speed (from the engineering viewpoint) was the ratio of step length (distance the body moves forward while one foot is on the ground) to ground contact time. On a tuned track, the ground contact time should be minimized and the step length maximized. At a track stiffness of approximately twice that of the runner's legs, the two factors determining running speed come together in optimal fashion. Theory dictated enhanced performances of 2% to 3%. In actuality, the runner's speed advantage on the new track averaged 2.91% (28).

Gender Differences in Speed of Movement

In sports such as running and swimming, records show women's speed to be 85% to 90%

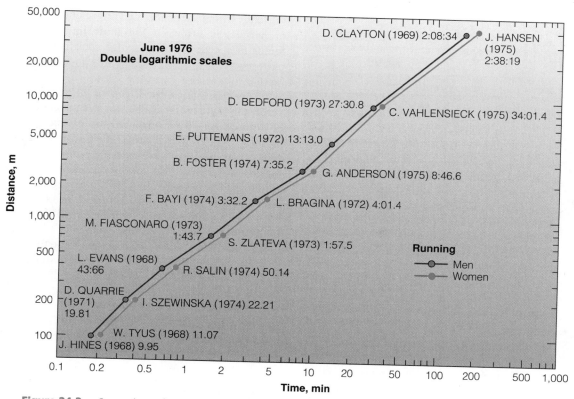

Figure 24.3 Comparison of men's and women's world records in running (100 m-42,200 m). (From Jokl, P., and Jokl, E., in *Journal of Sports Medicine and Physical Fitness* 17:213. © 1977 Federation Internationale de Medicine Sportive. Reprinted by permission.)

that of men, but that this reflects true differences in speed of movement per se is questionable. First, it has been shown that speed depends to a large extent on strength, so that the difference in speed may merely reflect the gender differences in strength. Second, the selection of women for sports represents a much smaller population of athletes, and it is possible that the fastest women athletes have not been found.

Jokl and Jokl (19) have plotted the times for running as they relate to the distance of the event for men and women, using world record times up to 1976. The relationship is simplified by using a double logarithmic plot. Figure

24.3 shows that there is an 11% difference for the 100-meter run, with gradually increasing differences up to 23% slower performance for women on the marathon. It is reasonable to assume that the women athletes are selected from a smaller fraction of their total population, so that no physiological conclusions can be drawn.

In controlled experiments, arm speed was found to be 17% slower in women than in men. But when the length of the arm was removed as a factor, the gender difference was only 5%. This is probably a good evaluation of true gender differences in speed of movement.

Variation of Speed with Distance in Running and Swimming

Jokl and Jokl (19) have analyzed and compared world records through 1976 in swimming and running. It is interesting to note that their data (fig. 24.4) show that the decline in speed with distance is greater in running than in swimming. In terms of duration, the 1,500-meter running event and the 400-meter freestyle swimming event are comparable. But the swim velocity has fallen about 10% from maximal velocity, whereas run time has fallen by 30%. The differences in rates of decline of velocity become greater with increasing distances, and on the whole, runners seem to lose speed at rates almost three times greater than swimmers.

Jokl and Jokl explain this difference on the basis of three advantages enjoyed by the heart in swimming over running exercise: 1) weightlessness, 2) horizontal body position, and 3) cooling effect of the water.

At first one would think that the first two items are really the same in that the horizontal body position and weightlessness both should act to increase venous return. But evidence is presented to show that body immersion creates a separate and additive effect on heart size, over and above that of the horizontal position. In addition to these two factors, the cooling effect of the water should hold the vasodilatation of the skin to a minimum and thus further improve the venous return.

Limiting Factors in Speed

Speed of Single Muscle Contraction

As described earlier in this chapter, in a simple contraction of a muscle, intrinsic speed of the muscle, which depends on physiochemical properties, is probably the most important factor in speed. Neuromuscular coordination patterns are a smaller, though still important, factor.

Sprint activities are of course largely anaerobic by nature (fig. 22.8) and as such could be limited by either mechanisms of energy production or by the accumulation of the end products of the anaerobic activity. Among the factors that might limit energy production are 1) energy substrate levels, 2) glycolytic enzyme activity, or 3) muscle fiber-type composition. Parkhouse and McKenzie, after a thorough review of available evidence (34), concluded that alterations in any of these factors by training are of insufficient magnitude to account for the enhanced performance of sprint-trained athletes. Therefore, they suggest that sprint training improves anaerobic performance capacity by increasing buffering capacity, which would counteract the deleterious effects on performance of decreasing muscle pH resulting from anaerobic activity. In line with this thinking, improving buffering by chemical intervention has been shown to improve performance (chap. 30).

Given the potential influence of anaerobic metabolic factors in sprint running performance, Tharp and coworkers (41) examined the relationships between 50-yard dash times and anaerobic power and capacity as measured by the Wingate Anaerobic Test in 10- to 15-year old males (see chapter 14 for a discussion of the Wingate Anaerobic Test). The results indicated that 50-yard dash times were only moderately correlated ($r = -0.53$ for both anaerobic power and capacity) with these indirect measures of anaerobic metabolic capabilities. When body weight was considered, however, the correlations were increased ($r = -0.66$ for anaerobic power and $r = -0.68$ for anaerobic capacity). It is also likely that the magnitude of the relationships between 50-yard dash times and anaerobic power

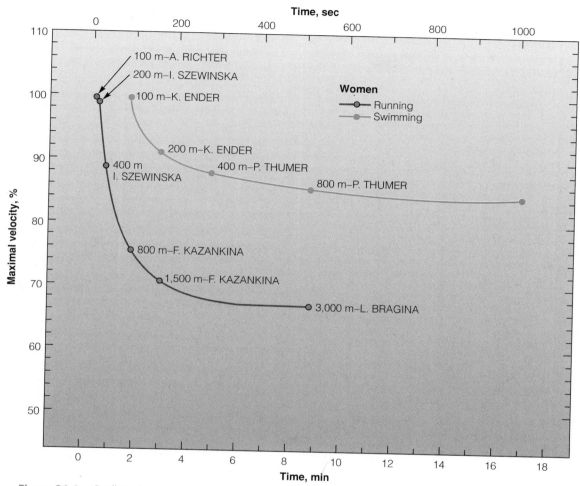

Figure 24.4 Decline of running and swimming speed with distance (women) based on world records in swimming (100 m–1,500 m) and running (100 m–3,000 m), expressed as percentage values of maximal velocity per unit of time (as of August 1976). 100 m world record = 100% maximal velocity. (From Jokl, P., and Jokl, E., in *Journal of Sports Medicine and Physical Fitness* 17:213. © 1977 Federation Internationale de Medicine Sportive. Reprinted by permission.)

and capacity reflected the fact that a cycle ergometer test (Wingate) was used to predict running performance.

A.V. Hill (16) has pointed out the importance of muscle temperature. An animal's muscle contraction can be quickened about 20% by raising its body temperature 2° C. He suggests that such an increase might be brought about in a sprinter by diathermy, and he raises the interesting question whether an athlete might not then do 100 yards in 8.0 seconds.

Speed of Gross Motor Movements

Many important factors act and interact in determining gross motor movements. In lightly loaded and simple movements, the limitations are probably similar to those of a single muscle contraction. In lightly loaded movements of greater complexity, it is likely that ability to coordinate neuromotor patterns would set the upper limits.

In heavily loaded but simple movements, the strength factor is probably dominant. In heavily loaded and complex movements, the limits are undoubtedly set by an interaction of strength and neuromotor coordination.

Methods for Improving Sprint Speed

There has been considerably less research re lated to methods for improving sprinting performance than endurance capabilities. Given the relative lack of scientifically derived data it is not surprising that much of the currently available information with regard to improving sprinting performance is based on conventional wisdom. For example, there are many descriptions of methods that have been used to train athletes for the improvement of speed (1, 6, 25, 26, 30, 32, 33, 35, 36). Some of these techniques are based on the recommendations of successful athletes (32) and coaches (6, 25, 26, 36), while others use novel approaches based on a logical relationship with sprinting performance (1, 30, 33, 35). Much additional research is necessary to fully evaluate the effectiveness of various training techniques for improving sprint speed.

Two of the most commonly used methods for improving sprinting speed include: 1) *sprint-resisted training,* in which sprint running is simulated with added resistance, the aim being to improve the dynamic strength factor, and 2) *sprint-assisted training,* where the effort is directed toward improving the rate of leg alternation. The first method uses devices such as uphill running and weighted clothing. The second method uses downhill running, towing behind an auto at velocities above maximum unassisted, and treadmill

running at supramaximal rates (possible because of decreased air resistance). Dintiman (10) has provided an excellent review of the literature in this area for the interested reader.

Recent investigations by Karvonen and colleagues (21, 22, 23) found that two to three weeks of training at a moderate altitude (1,850 to 1,900 meters above sea level) significantly improved 300-meter sprint running performance. These preliminary data suggest an advantage to sprint training at high altitudes, and this concept deserves further study.

Summary of Principles for Coaching

1. The strength of the prime and assistant movers used in an activity should be developed to an optimum level, preferably by dynamic movements that are closely related to the skill.

2. If speed is desired, the skill should be practiced at rates at least as fast as those to be used in competition. Faster-than-competition rates can be practiced by several different methods. For sprinters, it can be accomplished by downhill running, auto towing, or treadmill running.

3. Flexibility should be improved until range of motion is such as to ensure that no resistance to movement can occur in the skill under consideration.

4. Warming-up should be long and vigorous enough to bring about increased deep-muscle temperature. Ordinarily this will require sweating.

5. A skill should be analyzed on the basis of kinesiological principles, and all improper applications of positive forces should be corrected. Any unnecessary accelerations and decelerations or movements in the vertical dimension should be eliminated.

6. If the speed of movement is greater than that of middle-distance running, air resistance can become an important negative factor and should be held to a minimum whenever possible. For example, use the crouch position in ice skating and bicycle racing.

References

1. Chu, D. A., and Panariello, R. A. Jumping into plyometrics. *NSCA Journal* 10:73, 1988.

2. Clarke, D. H. Correlation between strength/mass ratio and the speed of an arm movement. *Res. Q.* 31:470–74, 1960.

3. Clarke, D. H., and Henry, F. M. Neuromotor specificity and increased speed from strength development. *Res. Q.* 32:315–25, 1961.

4. Close, R. I. Dynamic properties of mammalian skeletal muscles. *Physiol. Rev.* 52:129–97, 1972.

5. Craig, A. B., and Pendergast, D. R. Relationship of stroke rate, distance per stroke, and velocity in competitive swimming. *Med. Sci. Sports* 11:278–83, 1979.

6. Cross, T. Technique drills for speed development. *NSCA Journal* 13:35–39, 1991.

7. Deshon, D. E., and Nelson, R. C. A cinematographical analysis of sprint running. *Res. Q.* 35:451–55, 1964.

8. deVries, H. A. The "looseness" factor in speed and O_2 consumption of an anaerobic 100-yard dash. *Res. Q.* 34:305–13, 1963.

9. Dintiman, G. B. Effects of various training programs on running speed. *Res. Q.* 35:456–63, 1964.

10. ———. Techniques and methods of developing speed in athletic performance. In *Proceedings of the International Symposium on the Art and Science of Coaching,* eds. L. Percival and J. W. Taylor, vol. 1, pp. 97–139. Willowdale, Canada: F.I. Productions, 1971.

11. Farrar, M., and Thorland, W. G. Relationship between isokinetic strength and sprint times in college-age men. *J. Sports Med. Phys. Fitness* 27:368–72, 1987.

12. Francis, P. R., and Tipton, C. M. Influence of a weight training program on quadriceps reflex time. *Med. Sci. Sports* 1:91–94, 1969.

13. Henry, F. M. Factorial structure of speed and static strength in a lateral arm movement. *Res. Q.* 31:440–47, 1960.

14. Henry, F. M., and Whitley, J. D. Relationships between individual differences in strength, speed and mass in an arm movement. *Res. Q.* 31:24–33, 1960.

15. Hill, A. V. The mechanics of voluntary muscle. *Lancet* 261:947–51, 1951.

16. ———. The design of muscles. *Br. Med. Bull.* 12:165–66, 1956.

17. Hubbard, A. W. An experimental analysis of running and a certain fundamental difference between trained and untrained runners. *Res. Q.* 10:28–38, 1939.

18. Huxley, H. E. Factors limiting the maximum tensions and maximal speed of shortening of muscles. Chap. 7 in *Structure and Function of Muscle,* ed. G.H. Bourne. New York: Academic Press, 1972.

19. Jokl, P., and Jokl, E. Running and swimming world records. *J. Sports Med. Phys. Fitness* 17:213–29, 1977.

20. Kaneko, M. The relation between force, velocity and mechanical power in human muscle. *Res. J. Phys. Educ.* (Japan) 14:141–45, 1970.

21. Karvonen, J., Peltola, E., Naveri, H., and Harkonen, M. Lactate and phosphagen levels in muscle immediately after a maximum 300 m run at sea level. *Res. Quart. Exerc. Sport* 61:108–10, 1990.

22. Karvonen, J., Peltola, E., and Saarela, J. The effect of sprint training performed in a hypoxic environment on specific performance capacity. *J. Sports Med. Phys. Fitness* 26:219–29, 1986.

23. Karvonen, J., Peltola, E., Saarela, J., and Nieminen, M. Changes in running speed, blood lactic acid concentration and hormone balance during sprint training performed at an altitude of 1860 metres. *J. Sports Med. Phys. Fitness* 30:122–26, 1990.

24. Kenney, K. B. The relationship between selected physiological variables and sprint swimming performance. Unpublished masters thesis, University of Nebraska–Lincoln, 1988.

25. Korchemny, R. Training with the objective to improve stride length. *NSCA Journal* 10:21–25, 1988.

26. Korchemny, R. Training with the objective to improve stride length, Part II. *NSCA Journal* 10:61–64, 1988.

27. McMahon, T. A. Using body size to understand the structural design of animals: Quadripedal locomotion. *J. Appl. Physiol.* 39:619–27, 1975.

28. McMahon, T. A., and Greene, P. R. Fast running tracks. *Sci. Am.* 239:148–63, 1978.

29. Mero, A. Force-time characteristics and running velocity of male sprinters during the acceleration phase of sprinting. *Res. Quart. Exerc. Sport* 59:94–98, 1988.

30. Morrow, L. J. Single leg strength: Its relationship to speed enhancement. *NSCA Journal* 8:64–65, 1986.

31. Nelson, R. C., and Fahrney, R. A. Relationship between strength and speed of elbow flexion. *Res. Q.* 36:455–63, 1965.

32. Olinekova, G. Improving running speed: From the sprints to the marathon. *NSCA Journal* 4:6–9, 1982.

33. Oviatt, R., and Hemba, G. Oregon State: Sandblasting through the PAC. *NSCA Journal* 13:40–46, 1991.

34. Parkhouse, W. S., and McKenzie, D. C. Possible contribution of skeletal muscle buffers to enhanced anaerobic performance: A brief review. *Med. Sci. Sports Exer.* 16:328–38, 1984.

35. Pauletto, B. The speed chute. *NSCA Journal* 13:47–48, 1991.

36. Ruisz, E. Soviet sprint training. *NSCA Journal* 9:34–35, 1987.

37. Sinning, W. E., and Forsyth, H. L. Lower limb actions while running at different velocities. *Med. Sci. Sports* 2:28–34, 1970.

38. Slater-Hammel, A. Possible neuromuscular mechanisms as limiting factors for leg movement in sprinting. *Res. Q.* 12:745–57, 1941.

39. Smith, L. E. Individual differences in strength, reaction latency, mass and length of limbs and their relation to maximal speed of movement. *Res. Q.* 32:208–20, 1961.

40. ———. Influence of strength training on pre-tensed and free arm speed. *Res. Q.* 35:554–61, 1964.

41. Tharp, G. D., Newhouse, R. K., Uffelman, L., Thorland, W. G., and Johnson, G. O. Comparison of sprint and run times with performance on the Wingate anaerobic test. *Res. Quart. Exerc. Sport* 56:73–76, 1985.

42. Toussaint, H. M. Differences in propelling efficiency between competitive and triathlon swimmers. *Med. Sci. Sports Exerc.* 22:409–15, 1990.

43. Vrbova, G. Influence of activity on some characteristic properties of slow and fast mammalian muscles. *Exercise and Sports Sciences Reviews* 7:181–213, 1979.

44. Whitley, J. D., and Smith, L. E. Velocity curves and static strength-action strength correlations in relation to the mass moved by the arm. *Res. Q.* 34:379–95, 1963.

25

Flexibility

Physiology of Flexibility
  What Sets the Limits of Flexibility?
  Physical Properties of Connective
    Tissue
  Static versus Dynamic Flexibility
    (Stiffness)
  Stretch Reflexes and Flexibility
Measuring Flexibility
  Static Flexibility
  Dynamic Flexibility
  Effects of Anthropometric
    Measurements on Measurement of
    Flexibility

Methods for Improving Range of Motion
  Static Stretching Method versus
    Ballistic Method
  Proprioceptive Neuromuscular
    Facilitation (PNF)
Weight Training and Flexibility
Factors Affecting Flexibility
  Activity
  Gender
  Age
  Temperature
  Ischemia

Flexibility can be most simply defined as the range of possible movement in a joint (as in the hip joint) or series of joints (as when the spinal column is involved). The need for flexibility varies with the athletic endeavor, but in some activities it is all-important. A hurdler must have the best possible hip flexion–hip extension flexibility. In competitive swimming, shoulder and ankle flexibility can be decisive factors. And a diver who cannot execute a deep pike position will never achieve outstanding success.

Even for the armchair athlete, flexibility is important because graceful movement in walking and running are unlikely without it. More importantly, considerable evidence indicates that maintenance of good joint mobility prevents or to a large extent relieves the aches and pains that grow more common with increasing age.

It should be recognized from the outset that flexibility is specific to a given joint or combination of joints. As with speed of movement, an individual is a composite of many joints, some of which may be unusually flexible, some inflexible, and some average. Accordingly, it would be incorrect to speak of a flexible individual (14).

Physiology of Flexibility

What Sets the Limits of Flexibility?

For some joints the bony structure sets a very definite limit on range of motion. For example, extension of the elbow joint and the knee joint are limited in this fashion. Also, in a very heavily muscled person it is likely that flexion of the elbow and knee joints is limited by the bulk of the intervening muscle. These are mechanical factors that cannot be greatly modified, and therefore they are of only academic interest.

In such joints as the ankle joint or hip joint, however, the limitation of range of motion is imposed by the soft tissues: 1) muscle and its fascial sheaths; 2) connective tissue, with tendons, ligaments, and joint capsules; and 3) the skin. This, then, is where our interest lies, for these factors can be modified by physical methods, and they are important factors in human performance.

Physical Properties of Connective Tissue

If a resting excised muscle is stretched passively (no contraction), the greater the length the greater the force required to hold the stretch. It has been shown that this resistance does not lie in the contractile elements of the muscle but is due almost entirely to the fascial sheath that covers the muscle and the sarcolemma of the muscle fiber (1, 29). Thus it is the fascial investments of muscle tissue with which we are concerned in the pursuit of flexibility.

What are the relative contributions of the various soft tissues (listed above) in limiting our movement? An ingenious experiment by Johns and Wright (17) was directed toward the problem of joint stiffness. deVries has recalculated their data to estimate the percentage contributions of the various tissues in resisting wrist flexion and extension in the cat (they showed that these functions in a cat are very similar to those of humans). Table 25.1 shows the results of these calculations. It can be seen that the most important factors limiting free movement are 1) muscles (and their fascial sheaths), 2) the joint capsule, and 3) the tendons. It must be remembered that this data applies directly only to the wrist joint, but in other joints where ligaments play a more prominent role, as in the ankle joint, these structures are no doubt equally important.

Table 25.1	Estimated Contribution of Various Tissues in Resisting Wrist Flexion and Extension in the Cat			
Tissue	**Extension—48°** **Torque Required**		**Flexion + 48°** **Torque Required**	
	gram cm	% total	gram cm	% total
1. Skin	−70	11.2	−45*	−8.7
2. Extensor muscles	−35	42.4	0	36.9
3. Flexor muscles	−230		190	
4. Tendon	−70	11.2	170	33.0
5. Joint capsule	−220	35.2	200	38.8
Total	−625	100	515	100

*Skin aided in flexing the joint.
Calculated from the data of R. J. Johns, and V. Wright. Relative importance of various tissues in joint stiffness. *Journal of Applied Physiology* 17:824–28, 1962.

Physical Properties Important to Stretching Theory

Animal studies have shed considerable light on the responses of connective tissue to stretching procedures. Experiments on rat tail tendon, for example, have provided data that can probably be cautiously extrapolated to human connective tissues. It was found that the time required to stretch such tissue a given amount varies inversely with the forces applied. That is, a low-force stretching method requires more time to produce a given elongation than does a higher force method. However, it was also shown that the proportion of elongation that remains after stretching is greater for the low-force, long-duration stretch (33, 34). The epitome of low-force, long-duration stretching is, of course, static stretching, as has been advocated in this textbook since its inception. On the other hand, ballistic stretching, as shown in figure 25.3, represents a relatively high-force method. Warren and coworkers (33, 34) have also shown that for the same amount of tissue elongation accomplished, the high-force methods produce more structural weakening than the slow, low-force methods.

In agreement with much human experience, the laboratory studies also showed that within the range of normal human deep-muscle temperatures, the amount of structural weakening produced by a given amount of tissue elongation varies inversely with the temperature. This emphasizes the importance of using warm-up procedures before stretching (chap. 27). Unfortunately, many coaches and athletes have been misled into using static stretching as a warm-up. Athletes and others should be advised to "break a sweat" by slow jogging, brisk walking, or other mild exercise before attempting *any* stretching procedures, otherwise the very procedure designed to *prevent* muscular problems may itself become a *source* of problems.

Static versus Dynamic Flexibility (Stiffness)

It is obvious that the ability to flex and extend a joint through a wide range of motion (which is measured virtually in a static position) is not necessarily a good criterion of the stiffness or looseness of that same joint as this applies to the ability to move the joint quickly with little resistance to the movement. Range of motion is one factor—the only one that has been widely investigated at this point. How easily the joint can be moved in the middle of the range of motion, where the speed is necessarily greatest, is quite another factor.

We should therefore consider two separate components of flexibility: 1) *static flexibility,* which is what we ordinarily measure as range of motion, and 2) *dynamic flexibility,* which has been investigated in respect to stiffness in joint disease (37) but has been neglected in physical education. It may be hypothesized that the flexibility of motion may be of much greater importance to physical performance than the ability to achieve an extreme degree of flexion or extension of a joint! Hardy and Jones (10) have suggested that dynamic flexibility may be particularly important for speed events.

The method for such investigations was developed by Wright and Johns (37) for laboratory work. With their methods, the physical factors that contribute to joint stiffness and therefore limit dynamic flexibility have been identified and their relative contributions measured (in finger and wrist joints only). They investigated the effects of *elasticity, viscosity, inertia, plasticity,* and *friction* in normal and in diseased joints. It was found that inertia and friction were negligible; viscosity accounted for only one-tenth the torque used in moving the joint passively; and elasticity and plasticity were the major factors. These forces are wasted on the stretching of connective tissues.

Stretch Reflexes and Flexibility

The stretch reflexes as they apply to the stretching of body components for improving static flexibility were discussed at length in chapter 5, but we remind the reader that a muscle that is stretched with a jerky motion responds with a contraction whose amount and rate vary directly with the amount and rate of the movement that causes the stretch. This is the result of the myotatic reflex that originates in the muscle spindle.

On the other hand, a firm, steady, static stretch invokes the inverse myotatic reflex, which brings about inhibition not only of the muscle whose tendon organ was stretched but also of the entire functional group of muscles involved. It has been shown, for example, that the amount of *tension increase* for a given amount of stretch is more than doubled by a quick stretch, as compared to slow stretch (32), when the degree of stretching is the same.

Some therapists have suggested the use of tension in the agonist either before or when stretching the antagonist to take advantage of the inhibition brought about by *reciprocal inhibition,* the neuromuscular function that serves to turn off one of a pair of muscles when its opponent is activated in reciprocating type movements. However, a study using EMG techniques recently reported by Moore and Hutton (26) showed that for most subjects the lowest levels of innervation during passive stretching were attained by the static stretching technique. Attempts at implementing the reciprocal inhibition principle were not so effective in reducing activation as was the static method. This work seems to support the use of static stretching.

Measuring Flexibility

Static Flexibility

In general, static flexibility can be measured in two ways: 1) by *goniometry,* the *direct measurement* of the angle of the joint in its extremes of movement, and 2) by *indirect measurement* of joint angles through measurement of how closely one body part can be brought into opposition with another body part or some other reference point.

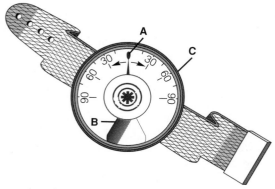

Figure 25.1 Drawing illustrating the principle of Leighton's flexometer. *A* indicates needle; *B* indicates weight that keeps needle vertical; *C* indicates housing that rotates in respect to needle with movement of body part. (From Leighton, J. R., "An Instrument and Technique for Measurement of Range of Joint Motion," in *Archives of Physical Medicine and Rehabilitation* 36:571. © 1955 American Congress of Physical Medicine and Rehabilitation. Reprinted by permission.)

Goniometry, in its classic form, uses a protractorlike device to measure the angle of the joint at both ends of its movement range, but it suffers from the serious disadvantage that body parts are not regular geometric forms, and a good deal of subjectivity is introduced during measurements in deciding where the axis of a bony lever may be. A simple but ingenious device, Leighton's *flexometer,* overcomes this disadvantage to a large extent (fig. 25.1). It is a small instrument that is strapped onto a body part and records range of motion in respect to a perpendicular established by gravity. Reliability coefficients well above 0.90 have been reported (20, 21).

The sit and reach test of Wells and Dillon (36) has been widely used as a test of back and leg flexibility. In the long sitting position, subjects slide their hands forward on a table that is approximately of shoulder height to the limit of their reach. The distance reached by the fingertips is the score on this test. A reliability of 0.98 has been reported for young adults and 0.83 for middle-age and older adults (30).

Dynamic Flexibility

Wright and Johns (37) developed a method to measure the stiffness of normal and diseased joints that uses laboratory devices to measure the forces (torque) needed to move a joint through various ranges of motion at varying speeds. Although this method has not yet been applied to research in physical performance, it seems to have distinct possibilities for such use. It seems highly probable that this measurement can tell us more about potential performance in speed events than can static flexibility.

Effects of Anthropometric Measurements on Measurement of Flexibility

One of the criticisms leveled at tests that use the indirect principle for measurement of static flexibility is that the measurement depends too heavily on anthropometric measurements. For example, it can be argued that an individual with a long upper body and arms and with short legs might have little trouble with such trunk flexion tests as touching the floor with the fingertips.

Several investigators have attacked this problem with respect to young men (35) and women (2, 12, 23), elementary school boys (24), as well as middle-age and older adults (30) but have found no meaningful relationships between static flexibility and various measurements and ratios of body parts. It appears that static flexibility can be measured indirectly, with no significant interference from varying anthropometric measurements.

With respect to flexibility of the lower back and posterior thighs measured by the sit and reach test, Smith and Miller (31) found that a "head-up" position produced significantly greater flexibility scores than a "head-down" position. The authors concluded, however, that the "difference was quite small and would preclude any recommendation that one head position be specified over another."

Methods for Improving Range of Motion

Static Stretching Method versus Ballistic Method

The question of which methods are most advantageous for improving range of motion has received very little attention. The conventional calisthenic exercises used for this purpose have usually involved bobbing, bouncing, or jerky movements in which one body segment is put in movement by active contraction of a muscle group and the momentum then arrested by the antagonists at the end of the range of motion. Thus the antagonists are stretched by the dynamic movements of the agonists. Because momentum is involved, this may be called the *ballistic method*.

On the other hand, the methods of yoga suggested to deVries the possibility of better application of the available knowledge regarding the stretch reflexes (chap. 5). Although the static stretch methods developed by deVries (5) are in many cases derived from Hatha Yoga, and both depend on the same physiological principles (though unknown to yoga), there are also enough differences so that the term *static stretch* was coined to separate the methods. The most important differences are: 1) static stretching should be considered a generic term for the use of held stretches that apply neurophysiological principles to strictly physical and physiological uses, whereas yoga is a system of abstract meditation and mental concentration pursued for spiritual as well as physiological purposes; 2) static stretching is based on neurophysiological principles with better health and performance as the goals, whereas yoga is based on spiritual principles and pursued not only to achieve better health and performance but also to attain union with the supreme spirit of the universe; and 3) yogic stretching has been directed largely to the joints and musculature of the trunk, whereas static stretching is equally concerned with the limb muscles (6).

The static stretching method involves holding a static position for thirty to sixty seconds during which specified joints are locked into a position that places the muscles and connective tissues passively at their greatest possible length. Since the neurophysiology of the stretch reflexes suggests advantages in static stretching procedures, a study was undertaken in deVries's laboratory to compare the ballistic and static methods (5). The difference in the two stretching methods is illustrated by figures 25.2 and 25.3. The ballistic exercises were taken—to a large extent—from Kiphuth's (18) exercises for stretching swimmers. The static exercises were developed to best utilize the inverse myotatic reflex and were designed to parallel the ballistic exercises in the affected muscles and joints.

It was found that both methods resulted in significant gains in static flexibility (in seven thirty-minute training periods) in trunk flexion, trunk extension, and shoulder elevation. There was no significant difference between methods. We may therefore conclude that static stretching is just as effective as the conventional ballistic methods, but the former offers three distinct advantages: 1) there is less danger of exceeding the extensibility limits of the tissues involved; 2) energy requirements are lower; 3) although ballistic stretching is apt to cause muscular soreness, static stretching after exercise will not; in fact, the latter relieves soreness (chap. 26). It is important to note, however, that static stretching before exercise does not prevent muscular soreness (13).

It is also of interest that the changes brought about by stretching exercises persist for a considerable period of time (eight weeks or more) after stretching is discontinued (25). Furthermore, Chapman has shown that dynamic as well as static flexibility can be significantly improved by exercise in the old as well as in the young (4). This finding would

1. Upper trunk stretcher

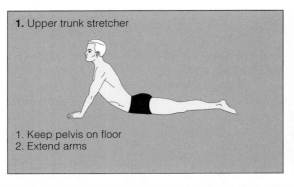

1. Keep pelvis on floor
2. Extend arms

2. Lower trunk stretcher

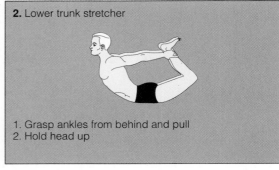

1. Grasp ankles from behind and pull
2. Hold head up

3. Lower back stretcher

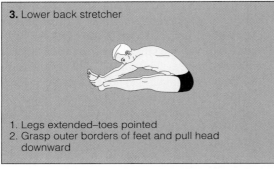

1. Legs extended–toes pointed
2. Grasp outer borders of feet and pull head downward

4. Upper back stretcher

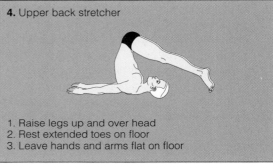

1. Raise legs up and over head
2. Rest extended toes on floor
3. Leave hands and arms flat on floor

5. Trunk twister

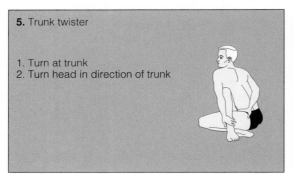

1. Turn at trunk
2. Turn head in direction of trunk

6. Gastrocnemius stretcher

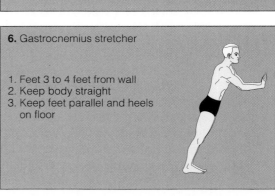

1. Feet 3 to 4 feet from wall
2. Keep body straight
3. Keep feet parallel and heels on floor

7. Toe pointer

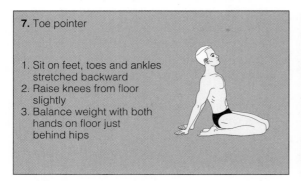

1. Sit on feet, toes and ankles stretched backward
2. Raise knees from floor slightly
3. Balance weight with both hands on floor just behind hips

8. Shoulder stretcher

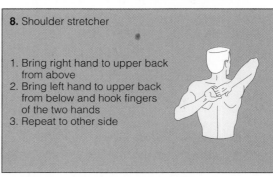

1. Bring right hand to upper back from above
2. Bring left hand to upper back from below and hook fingers of the two hands
3. Repeat to other side

Figure 25.2   Illustration of the static stretching methods used in deVries's laboratory.

1. Trunk lifter

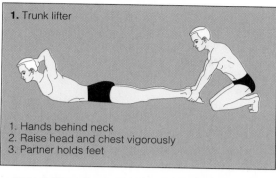

1. Hands behind neck
2. Raise head and chest vigorously
3. Partner holds feet

2. Leg lifter

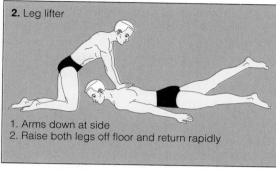

1. Arms down at side
2. Raise both legs off floor and return rapidly

3. Trunk bender

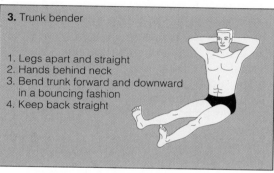

1. Legs apart and straight
2. Hands behind neck
3. Bend trunk forward and downward in a bouncing fashion
4. Keep back straight

4. Upper back stretcher

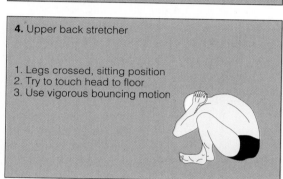

1. Legs crossed, sitting position
2. Try to touch head to floor
3. Use vigorous bouncing motion

5. Trunk rotator

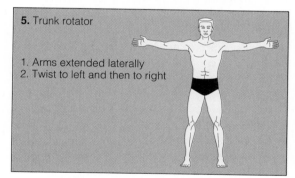

1. Arms extended laterally
2. Twist to left and then to right

6. Gastocnemius stretcher

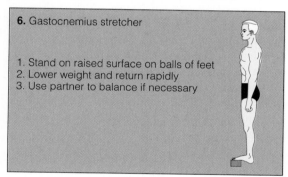

1. Stand on raised surface on balls of feet
2. Lower weight and return rapidly
3. Use partner to balance if necessary

7. Single leg raiser

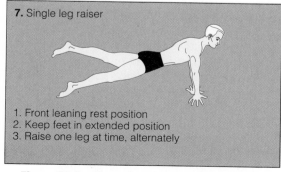

1. Front leaning rest position
2. Keep feet in extended position
3. Raise one leg at time, alternately

8. Arm and leg lifter

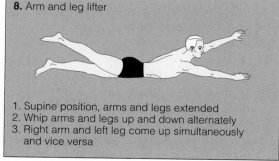

1. Supine position, arms and legs extended
2. Whip arms and legs up and down alternately
3. Right arm and left leg come up simultaneously and vice versa

Figure 25.3   Illustration of the ballistic stretching exercises against which the static stretching method was compared experimentally.

appear to have some importance in gerontology, since declining joint mobility creates
many problems for the elderly.

Proprioceptive Neuromuscular Facilitation (PNF)

Proprioceptive neuromuscular facilitation
(PNF) is a rationale for improving muscle
compliance during stretching exercises by
stretching a muscle immediately after a maximal contraction. There are several variations
of PNF techniques used by athletes and nonathletes for maintaining and/or increasing
flexibility as well as in clinical settings for restoring the range of motion following injury.
Probably the most common PNF procedures
involve contract-relax (CR) and contract-relax
with agonist-contraction (CRAC) stretching
techniques (8, 9). Etnyre and Lee (8) have described the CR technique as "isometrically
contracting the lengthened muscle then relaxing and further passively lengthening the
muscle" and the CRAC technique as "identical to CR except that during the final
stretching phase the muscle opposite the one
stretched is concentrically contracted."

Theoretically, contractions of the stretched
(antagonist) or opposite (agonist) muscles
should serve to facilitate autogenic and reciprocal inhibition, respectively. Thus, it should
be possible to increase the length of the
stretched muscle because of the inhibition to
contraction.

Etnyre and Lee (8) have suggested that
there should be an additive effect of the inhibitory influences as utilized in the CRAC technique. Hutton (16), however, has pointed out
that maximum or near maximum contraction
prior to the onset of muscle stretch should exacerbate muscle stiffness rather than increase
compliance. This is so because following a tetanic contraction, both monosynaptic reflexes
and muscle unit responses are potentiated (15),
a phenomenon referred to as "post-tetanic
twitch potentiation" or PTP. Furthermore,

recent surface electromyographic studies
(26, 27) have reported that contraction of the
agonist muscles resulted in an increase in the
electrical activity of the stretched muscle
group.

Paradoxically, however, the CRAC technique produced greater flexibility than static
or CR stretching even though there was apparently no reciprocal inhibition (26, 27).
Etnyre and Abraham (7) addressed this paradox using both surface and implanted wire
electrodes in the soleus and tibialis anterior
muscles. It was found that during dorsiflexion,
no activity from the wire electrode was observed in the soleus muscle but there was delayed activity measured by the surface
electrode. The authors concluded that "in this
study the tracings from the surface electrodes,
which gave the appearance of co-contraction
between antagonist muscles, were actually
cross-talk between the electrodes." Therefore,
although inferences regarding the presence of
cross-talk in previous studies that have used
surface EMG procedures and demonstrated a
lack of reciprocal inhibition (26, 27) should be
made with caution, the findings of Etnyre and
Abraham suggest that methodological considerations may have accounted for the seemingly paradoxical increase in flexibility as a
result of CRAC stretching techniques without
reciprocal inhibition.

There are conflicting results regarding the
effectiveness of PNF techniques compared to
static or ballistic stretching. Hutton (15) and
Hartley-O'Brien (11) found no advantage to
PNF compared with other conventional
stretching methods. Furthermore, Hardy and
Jones (10) found that "in terms of short term
improvements of dynamic range of motion,
appropriately chosen ballistic stretching techniques can be just as effective as PNF-based
techniques."

Etnyre and Lee (9), however, reported that
PNF techniques, including both CR and
CRAC, were more effective than static
stretching for increasing flexibility for hip
flexion and shoulder extension in both males

and females. Furthermore, in a recent review, Etnyre and Lee (8) stated "Based upon applications and experimental procedures among the various comparative investigations, PNF methods are more efficient than static or ballistic stretching techniques." This conclusion was based largely on their findings that "Of the 10 comparative studies which equated the amount of time stretching, nine found the PNF methods produced a greater range of motion than static or ballistic stretching methods, which suggests that the PNF methods should be considered generally more effective and more efficient." Etnyre and Lee went on to say, however, that "the problem of which stretching method is most effective is still not clearly resolved. Also, the effectiveness of each method on muscle groups other than the hamstring and lower back muscles has not been adequately addressed."

Although recent evidence supports the effectiveness of PNF techniques, further research is necessary before a definitive recommendation can be made regarding the use of static stretching or PNF.

Weight Training and Flexibility

Many investigators have shown that weight training has no harmful effects on either speed or range of movement when properly pursued, but an interesting study by Massey and Chaudet (22), which supports these findings, indicates the need for capable guidance. In an experiment designed to evaluate the effects of weight training on range of movement, they found no appreciable effects in general, but they did find a significant decrease in ability to hyperextend the arms at the shoulder joint, a movement for which no exercise had been included. It is very probable that inclusion of an exercise for hyperextension would have prevented this decrease in mobility.

Very heavy resistance exercise can, under certain circumstances, result in a restriction of range of motion. This factor, however, is not inherent in weight training, and it can be prevented by inclusion of the proper exercises and performance throughout the full range of motion. As Massey and Chaudet pointed out, it appears that weight lifting increases range of movement in the joints that are exercised, but may restrict range of movement in the areas not exercised. Therefore, a well-rounded workout is necessary when heavy resistance methods are used.

Factors Affecting Flexibility

Activity

It has been found that active individuals tend to be more flexible than inactive individuals (25). This is in accord with the well-known fact that connective tissues tend to shorten when they are maintained in a shortened position (as when a broken limb is placed in a plaster cast).

Gender

The results of two investigations agree that among elementary school age children, girls are superior to boys in flexibility (19, 28). It is likely that this difference exists at all ages and throughout adult life.

Age

The results of many tests indicate that elementary school age children become less flexible as they grow older, reaching a low point in flexibility between ten and twelve years of age (3, 19, 28). From this age upward, flexibility seems to improve toward young adulthood, but it never again achieves the levels of early childhood. Dynamic flexibility apparently grows steadily poorer, from childhood on, with increasing age (37). There are also age-related decreases in static flexibility of the head, shoulder, ankle, and hip joints in males and females between the ages of forty-five and seventy-five years (30).

Temperature

Dynamic flexibility is improved 20% by local warming of a joint to 113° F, and it is decreased 10% to 20% by cooling to 65° F (26). Experience indicates that static flexibility is probably similarly affected by temperature changes.

Ischemia

Dynamic flexibility is markedly reduced by arterial occlusion for twenty-five minutes (37). The physiology underlying this phenomenon has not been elucidated, but it appears to have important implications for the study of joint disease.

Summary

1. Two types of flexibility should be recognized: 1) *static flexibility,* a measure of range of motion, and 2) *dynamic flexibility,* a measure of the resistance to motion offered by a joint. (The following principles apply to static flexibility only because dynamic flexibility has not yet received the attention of physical educators.)
2. Flexibility can be limited by bone structure or by the soft tissues. When it is limited by soft tissues, great improvements can be brought about by the proper stretching methods.
3. After improvements have been brought about, cessation of the exercise program is not immediately accompanied by regression of flexibility. The effects of a stretching program are relatively long lasting (at least eight weeks).

4. Stretching by jerking, bobbing, or bouncing methods invokes the stretch reflexes, which actually oppose the desired stretching.
5. Stretching by static methods invokes the inverse myotatic reflex, which helps relax the muscles to be stretched.
6. Static stretching methods have been shown to be just as effective as the ballistic methods.
7. Static stretching is safer than ballistic methods because it does not impose sudden strains upon the tissues involved.
8. Ballistic stretching methods frequently cause severe soreness in muscles. Static stretching does not usually cause soreness; it may, indeed, relieve soreness when it has occurred.
9. Static stretch positions should be held for thirty to sixty seconds for best results.
10. All stretching procedures should be preceded by warm-up exercise such as easy jogging or brisk walking to assure a rise in deep muscle temperature, indicated by the onset of sweating.
11. In light of item 10, stretching is best done at the end of the workout if the objective is physical fitness. To optimize athletic performance stretching should be done both before and after the workout (but not before warming up).

References

1. Banus, M. G., and Zetlin, A. M. The relation of isometric tension to length in skeletal muscle. *J. Cell. Comp. Physiol.* 12:403–20, 1938.
2. Broer, M. R., and Galles, N. R. G. Importance of relationship between various body measurements in

performance of toe-touch test. *Res. Q.* 29:253–63, 1958.

3. Buxton, D. Extension of the Kraus-Weber test. *Res. Q.* 28:210–17, 1957.

4. Chapman, E. A., deVries, H. A., and Swezey, R. Joint stiffness: Effects of exercise on young and old men. *J. Geront.* 27:218–21, 1972.

5. deVries, H. A. Evaluation of static stretching procedures for improvement of flexibility. *Res. Q.* 33:222–29, 1962.

6. ———. *Health Science: A Positive Approach.* Glenview, IL: Scott, Foresman & Co., 1979.

7. Etnyre, B. R., and Abraham, L. D. Antagonist muscle activity during stretching: A paradox re-assessed. *Med. Sci. Sports Exerc.* 20:285–89, 1988.

8. Etnyre, B. R., and Lee, E. J. Comments on proprioceptive neuromuscular facilitation stretching techniques. *Res. Quart. Exerc. Sport* 58:184–88, 1987.

9. Etnyre, B. R., and Lee, E. J. Chronic and acute flexibility of men and women using three different stretching techniques. *Res. Quart. Exerc. Sport* 59:222–28, 1988.

10. Hardy, L., and Jones, D. Dynamic flexibility and proprioceptive neuromuscular facilitation. *Res. Quart. Exerc. Sport* 57:150–53, 1986.

11. Hartley-O'Brien, S. J. Six mobilization exercises for active range of hip flexion. *Res. Q.* 51:625–35, 1980.

12. Harvey, V. P., and Scott, G. D. Reliability of a measure of forward flexibility and its relationship to physical dimensions of college women. *Res. Q.* 38:28–33, 1967.

13. High, D. M., Howley, E. T., and Franks, B. D. The effects of static stretching and warm-up on prevention of delayed-onset muscle soreness. *Res. Quart. Exerc. Sport* 60:357–61, 1989.

14. Hupperich, F. L., and Sigerseth, P. O. The specificity of flexibility in girls. *Res. Q.* 21:25, 1950.

15. Hutton, R. S. Acute plasticity in spinal segmental pathways with use: Implications for training. Paper presented to Kyoto Satellite Symposium, July 26, 1981.

16. ———. Neuromuscular physiology. In *Current Therapy in Sports Medicine,* eds. R. P. Welch and R. J. Shephard, Toronto: B. C. Decker, Inc., pp. 1–4, 1985.

17. Johns, R. J., and Wright, V. Relative importance of various tissues in joint stiffness. *J. Appl. Physiol.* 17:824–28, 1962.

18. Kiphuth, R. J. H. *Swimming.* New York: A. G. Barnes & Co., 1942.

19. Kirchner, G., and Glines, D. Comparative analysis of Eugene, Oregon, elementary school children using the Kraus-Weber test of minimum muscular fitness. *Res. Q.* 28:16–25, 1957.

20. Leighton, J. R. A simple objective and reliable measure of flexibility. *Res. Q.* 13:205–16, 1942.

21. ———. An instrument and technic for the measurement of range of joint motion. *Arch. Phys. Med. Rehabil.* 36:571, 1955.

22. Massey, B. H., and Chaudet, N. L. Effects of systematic heavy resistance exercise on range of joint movement in young male adults. *Res. Q.* 27:41–51, 1956.

23. Mathews, D. K., Shaw, V., and Bohnen, M. Hip flexibility of college women as related to length of body segments. *Res. Q.* 28:352–56, 1957.

24. Mathews, D. K., Shaw, V., and Woods, J. B. Hip flexibility of elementary school boys as related to body segments. *Res. Q.* 30:297–302, 1959.

25. McCue, B. F. Flexibility of college women. *Res. Q.* 24:316, 1953.

26. Moore, M. A., and Hutton, R. S. Electromyographic evaluation of muscle stretching techniques. *Med. Sci. Sports* 12:322–29, 1980.

27. Osternig, L. R., Robertson, R. N., Troxel, R. K., and Hansen, P. Differential responses to proprioceptive neuromuscular facilitation (PNF) stretch technique. *Med. Sci. Sports Exerc.* 22:106–11, 1990.

28. Phillips, M. Analysis of results from the Kraus-Weber test of minimum muscular fitness in children. *Res. Q.* 26:314–23, 1955.

29. Ramsey, R. W., and Street, S. The isometric length tension diagram of isolated skeletal muscle fibers of the frog. *J. Cell. Comp. Physiol.* 15:11, 1940.

30. Shephard, R. J., Berridge, M. On the generality of the "sit and reach" test: An analysis of flexibility data for an aging population. *Res. Quart. Exerc. Sport* 61:326–30, 1990.

31. Smith, J. E., and Miller, C. V. The effect of head position on sit and reach performance. *Res. Quart. Exerc. Sport* 56:84–5, 1985.

32. Walker, S. M. Delay of twitch relaxation induced by stress and stress relaxation. *J. Appl. Physiol.* 16:801–6, 1961.

33. Warren, C. G., Lehmann, J. F., and Koblanski, J. N. Elongation of rat tail tendon: Effect of load and temperature. *Arch. Phys. Med. Rehabil.* 52:465–74, 1971.

34. ———. Heat and stretch procedures: An evaluation using rat tail tendon. *Arch. Phys. Med. Rehabil.* 57:122–26, 1976.

35. Wear, C. L. Relationships of flexibility measurements to length of body segments. *Res. Q.* 34:234–38, 1963.

36. Wells, K. F., and Dillon, E. K. Sit and reach, a test of back and leg flexibility. *Res. Q.* 23:115–18, 1952.

37. Wright, V., and Johns, R. J. Physical factors concerned with the stiffness of normal and diseased joints. *Bull. Johns Hopkins Hosp.* 106:215–31, 1960.

26

Physiology of Muscle Soreness— Cause and Relief

Immediate versus Delayed Muscle Pain

Theoretical Basis for Delayed Onset
    Muscle Soreness (DOMS)
    Mechanical Trauma Theory
    Acute Inflammation Theory
    Local Ischemia Theory
    Spasm Theory

Attempt at Unification and
    Simplification: Practical Aspects
    for Coach and Athlete

Physiology Underlying Static Stretching

Prevention of Muscular Soreness
    Warm-Up
    Progression in Training Programs
    Chronic Exercise Training
    Types of Activity
    Static Stretching

Relief of Muscular Soreness
    Static Stretching
    Acute Exercise
    Anti-Inflammatory Drugs

Severe Muscle Problems

Immediate versus Delayed Muscle Pain

It is common experience that physical over-exertion results in pain. In general, two types of pain are associated with severe muscular efforts: 1) pain during and immediately after exercise, which may persist for several hours, and 2) a localized soreness, which usually does not appear until twenty-four to forty-eight hours later.

The first type of pain is probably due to the diffusible end products of metabolism acting upon pain receptors, but this is not a very serious problem because it is of short duration and is relieved by cessation of exercise or by short periods of rest.

The second type of pain called delayed onset muscle soreness (DOMS) can become chronic under certain conditions and is at least annoying enough to constitute a deterrent to further exercise. This localized and delayed muscle soreness, or *lameness,* sometimes called a *myositis,* is usually not serious enough to require medical attention. However, when the overexertion is great enough and involves muscles that are confined within relatively tight fascial structures, the problem may become severe enough to require medical attention and often surgical procedure to relieve the pain and to prevent even more serious results (5, 22, 51, 56, 66). Indeed one physician alone has reported on a series of sixty-one patients suffering from chronic muscle problems resulting from overuse of such muscles (51). Thus the DOMS problem is very important to coaches and physical educators.

Theoretical Basis for Delayed Onset Muscle Soreness (DOMS)

At this time, neither the causative factor nor the cellular mechanisms are firmly established, but the past twenty years have provided a great deal of information related to the problem of DOMS. In recent years, widespread use of electron microscopy and more sophisticated histochemistry methods has generated a huge amount of information to provide a better description of the cellular results of muscular overexertion.

In the past editions of this text, deVries discussed the theoretical bases for the onset of the events leading to DOMS in terms of a controversy between muscle spasm versus structural damage. There is now a voluminous body of literature based on very good experimental evidence that DOMS is indeed accompanied by structural damage whose extent is closely related to the level of pain experienced (21, 24, 25, 26, 29, 37, 42, 57, 65, 67). Fortunately, an excellent review of this abundant literature has been provided by Armstrong (4), who has also proposed the model for a *mechanical trauma* theory of causation based on work in his laboratory along with work reported from many other laboratories throughout the world. At present this theory seems to be the most widely accepted, but there appears to be equally good evidence to support a theory of causation based on *local ischemia* as the etiological agent.

Mechanical Trauma Theory

The mechanical trauma theory as proposed by Armstrong (4) suggests the following sequence of events in the production of DOMS:

1. High mechanical forces produced during muscular exercise, particularly in

eccentric exercise when forces are distributed over relatively small cross-sectional areas of the muscles, cause disruption of structural proteins in muscle fibers and connective tissue in series between the active cross-bridges and the bony attachments.

2. Structural damage to the sarcolemma or alterations in the permeability of the cell membrane, resulting from the high mechanical forces, is accompanied by net influx of Ca^{++} from the interstitium. This abnormal influx of Ca^{++} has several deleterious effects on the muscle fiber (13, 63, 68). When abnormally high Ca^{++} levels exist in the cell, the mitochondria accumulate the ion, which inhibits cellular respiration (68).

   This initiates a cycle of events in which reduced ability to produce ATP compromises the cell's ability to actively extrude Ca^{++}. Thus, this destructive cycle results in impairment of oxidative phosphorylation and abnormally high Ca^{++} concentrations in the cell. High Ca^{++} concentrations in the muscle cells have been shown to activate a calcium-dependent proteolytic enzyme that preferentially degrades Z-discs (13) and troponin and tropomyosin (14).

3. The progressive deterioration of the sarcolemma in the post-exercise period would be accompanied by diffusion of intracellular components into the interstitium and plasma. These substances, as well as the products of collagen breakdown (50), would serve to attract monocytes (4) that convert to macrophages and to activate mast cells and histocytes in the injured areas. Accompanying these processes would be activation of endogenous lysosomal proteases (55) that degrade other specific muscle proteins (59).

4. The accumulation of histamine, kinins, and potassium in the interstitium in the regions of group IV free nerve endings, resulting from the active phagocytosis and cellular necrosis as well as elevated pressure from tissue edema and increased local temperature, could then activate the nociceptors (pain receptors) and result in the sensation of DOMS.

Acute Inflammation Theory

In a recent review, Smith (62) examined the possibility that acute inflammation is the underlying mechanism of DOMS. The author listed seven similarities between acute inflammation and DOMS:

1. Three of the cardinal signs of acute inflammation—pain, swelling, and loss of function—are observed during DOMS.

2. Similar cellular infiltrates have been noted. In particular, the macrophage, an essential component of the inflammatory process, predominates at the site of injury. In both instances this occurs at twenty-four and forty-eight hours after the initiation of tissue disruption.

3. Fibroblasts have been seen in association with both events.

4. Increased lysosomal activity occurs during both events.

5. The progression in the size of the lesion occurs in both instances for about forty-eight hours.

6. Increased levels of interleukin-1 and acute phase proteins occur after both events.

7. Signs of healing are observed at approximately seventy-two hours.

Based on these similarities, Smith proposed the following sequence of events with respect to DOMS:

1. Connective and/or contractile tissue disruption occurs during exercise that involves unaccustomed eccentric muscle action.

2. Within a few hours, there is a significant elevation in circulating neutrophils.

3. Neutrophils migrate to the site of injury and predominate for several hours (not clearly established in the exercise literature).

4. The next wave of white blood cells, the monocytes, emigrates to the injured area between six and twelve hours after exercise (not established in the exercise literature). They are present in large numbers at twenty-four hours, peak in number at forty-eight hours, and are generally no longer seen at seventy-two hours.

5. On exposure to the inflammatory environment, macrophages begin synthesizing large quantities of prostaglandin E_2 (PGE_2) (not established in the exercise literature), which results in significant increases in serum PGE_2.

6. PGE_2 sensitizes type III and IV "pain" afferents (not established in the exercise literature).

7. In an attempt to explain why DOMS is not experienced during rest but rather in response to movement or palpation, Smith proposes the following scenario. Edema associated with DOMS does not produce a significant increase in intramuscular pressure at rest in a compliant compartment. However, movement or palpation may exacerbate even small increases in pressure and thus provides a mechanical stimulus for "pain" receptors already sensitized by PGE_2. Thus, the combination of increased pressure and hypersensitization produces the sensation of DOMS. Figure 26.1 describes the time course of events in DOMS based on the acute inflammatory response.

Local Ischemia Theory

First it must be realized that the degeneration/regeneration of muscle fibers observed and reported after two to three hours of experimental ischemia is entirely similar to that resulting from overexertion during exercise (2, 34, 40, 41, 56, 60, 61, 64). Second, it is well known that DOMS can occur after overexertion involving long duration with only moderate intensity of contraction, which would not seem likely to bring about tissue destruction because of too high a tension production. Clinical investigators have found that chronic DOMS can result from such atraumatic activities as *ordinary walking* (51) and rowing (27). On the other hand, it has been known at least since 1939 (7) that even moderate muscle contractions can result in sufficient tissue pressure to bring about significant decreases in muscle blood flow. More recent experiments have shown the importance of tissue pressure increases in bringing about levels of ischemia that, when occurring in muscles with restricting fascia, can become serious enough to necessitate fasciotomy (surgical procedure to relieve the pressure) (5, 51, 66). Such increased tissue pressure, if not relieved, can result in permanent muscle and nerve damage.

It appears that any trauma capable of inducing initial swelling of muscle tissue is capable through cyclic reinforcement of producing widespread arterial shutdown (22). The cyclic reinforcement is thought to be a vicious cycle, resulting from increased tissue pressure that causes edema that causes further increase in tissue pressure and so on (22, 51, 66). It has long been known that even under normal conditions the volume of skeletal muscle increases during exercise due to

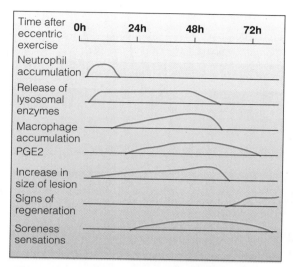

Time after eccentric exercise	0h	24h	48h	72h

Neutrophil accumulation

Release of lysosomal enzymes

Macrophage accumulation

PGE2

Increase in size of lesion

Signs of regeneration

Soreness sensations

Figure 26.1 Proposed sequence of events in DOMS based on the acute inflammatory response. (From L. L. Smith, "Acute Inflammation: The Underlying Mechanisms in Delayed Onset Muscle Soreness?", *Medicine and Science in Sports and Exercise*, vol. 23, issue 5, pp. 542–551, 1991, © by The American College of Sports Medicine.)

both localized swelling of muscle cells (36) and the increased fluid volumes (51).

The evidence against the local ischemia theory rests largely on findings that the muscle contractions that cause the greatest degree of soreness, that is, eccentric contractions, require a relatively low expenditure of energy (3, 6, 57, 58). Schwane and coworkers had subjects run down an inclined treadmill and on a level treadmill at the same speed and for the same duration on two different occasions. Downhill running required significantly lower $\dot{V}O_2$ and produced less lactic acid but resulted in greater DOMS (57, 58). These findings seem to argue against the ischemia hypothesis if we consider the muscle as a whole. But DOMS does not affect all of a muscle. Only very localized parts of the muscle become painful and under these conditions small areas of muscle could well be ischemic without measurable increases in the total muscle's $\dot{V}O_2$ or

lactic acid production. Indeed, the total muscle's $\dot{V}O_2$ and lactic acid production could well decrease as reported in the presence of localized ischemia because eccentric contractions use far fewer motor units (8).

In light of the above discussion, the case for mechanical trauma being the initial causal agent for DOMS seems less attractive than the case for localized ischemia. The remaining steps postulated by the Armstrong model could just as well follow localized ischemia as mechanical trauma, though (as recognized by Armstrong) they remain to be proven. Furthermore, there is other experimental evidence concerning DOMS that was presented by deVries some years ago as the "spasm theory," which can be rationalized with the localized ischemia theory but whose supporting data are at odds with the concept of mechanical disruption of tissue as the first step in the DOMS syndrome.

Spasm Theory

deVries proposed the spasm theory after observing typical muscle fatigue curves in excised muscles (fig. 4.4). It is readily seen that, in addition to the decrement in amplitude of contraction with increasing fatigue, an increasing inability to achieve complete relaxation is typical. Significantly, this may end in contracture. Evidence has shown that the same phenomenon occurs in the intact human muscle. Petajan and Eagan (49) interpreted their findings as showing the tendency of the untrained muscle after intense exercise to remain in the contracted condition, since the increased intramuscular pressure of exercise limits the availability of factors important to the recovery process. For these reasons, deVries proposed the spasm theory: the delayed localized soreness that occurs after unaccustomed exercise is caused by tonic, localized spasm of motor units. A rationale based on considerable physiological evidence was constructed to support this hypothesis. First, it had been shown that exercise above a minimal level caused a degree of ischemia in the active muscles (20, 54). Second, ischemia can cause muscle pain, probably by transfer of *P substance* (52, 53) across the muscle cell membrane into the tissue fluid where it gains access to free nerve endings. Third, the pain brings about a reflex tonic muscle contraction, which prolongs the ischemia, and a vicious cycle is born. Evidence has been presented (48) that supports the concept of spasm caused by painful stimuli. This hypothesis agrees with the thinking of medical clinicians, who have suggested that many of the aches and pains of organic disease and anxiety states result from muscle spasm.

From the standpoint of the physical educator and athletic coach, the spasm theory was attractive in that the aforementioned vicious cycle had a vulnerable aspect that allowed one to apply simple corrective measures for relief. Competitive swimmers and swimming coaches know that swimmer's cramp (gastrocnemius) is promptly relieved by gently forcing the cramped muscle into its longest possible state and holding it there for a moment. This relief of cramp by stretching has also been demonstrated experimentally (48). It is very likely that the inverse myotatic reflex (chap. 5), which originates in the Golgi tendon organs, is the basis for this relief.

The first experimental study to test the spasm theory (15) was done on seventeen college-age subjects, who did a four-minute standard exercise (designed to produce soreness) that consisted of wrist hyperextension against a resistance of 9½ pounds. Both arms were exercised simultaneously. Immediately after exercise, and at intervals thereafter, the wrist flexors and extensors of the nondominant arm were stretched by static methods. The dominant arm, which was not stretched, developed significantly greater levels of soreness for the group. The greatest soreness levels were found twenty-four and forty-eight hours after

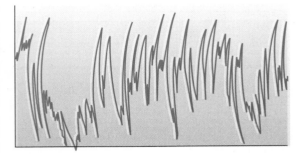

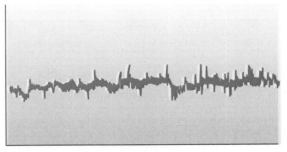

Figure 26.2   Effects of static stretching on muscle soreness of the shin-splint type. *Upper trace:* electrical activity before stretching. *Lower trace:* electrical activity after stretching. Symptomatic relief accompanied the decrease in electrical activity.

the exercise. The difference in soreness between stretched and unstretched arms was significant for both of these observations.

During the same period electromyographic equipment was designed to achieve very high sensitivity so that small differences in resting muscle tissue activity could be observed. Use of this instrumentation showed that static stretching markedly reduced resting EMG activity in six of seven subjects who had chronic muscular problems of the shin-splint type (fig. 26.2). Symptomatic relief seemed to parallel lowered EMG values (16). The subject who was atypical showed a marked rise in electrical activity and increased levels of pain. It was hypothesized that in this case structural damage had indeed occurred—a truly ruptured muscle.

This introduced the interesting possibility that ruptured muscles could be differentiated from those that are merely in spasm by applying static stretch and observing the EMG changes. To test this hypothesis, eighteen subjects—three of whom had medically verified ruptured muscles—were tested by the same technique. Of the fifteen subjects who showed no evidence of a torn muscle, thirteen had lowered levels of electrical activity after static stretching, while the three subjects with torn muscles showed higher levels (17).

In the last experiment (with more sophisticated EMG equipment, described in chap. 4), it was possible to bring about muscular soreness experimentally and to relieve it by static stretching, with the entire series of physiological changes in electrical state of the muscle under EMG observation (18). Figure 26.3 illustrates the course of events in fifteen subjects (eleven males, four females) who did arm curls (ten sets, with ten repetition maximum) with the right arm. The left arm was unexercised and thus furnished a control for comparison.

The relationship between the soreness that was present after forty-eight hours and the increased electrical activity (evidence of increased muscular activity or local spasm) is clearly shown in figure 26.3. When soreness appeared, activity increased 98% over the biceps and 62% over the brachialis (this included some biceps activity). The relief of soreness by static stretching is also shown. Immediately after the forty-eight-hour EMG observation both arms were stretched, and EMG recordings were again taken immediately after the stretching. Again, large decreases in electrical activity paralleled the symptomatic relief.

The rise in resting electrical activity in the exercised muscle and the relatively unchanged activity in the paired, unexercised muscle is difficult to explain on any other basis than a tonic local muscle spasm.

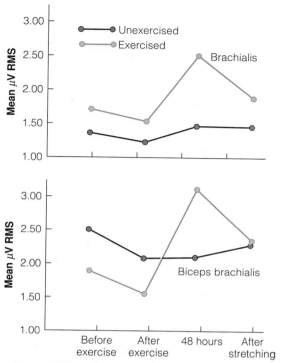

Figure 26.3   Effects of static stretching on experimentally induced soreness. Note that the electrical activity is virtually brought back to presoreness values by the static stretching. Symptomatic relief usually parallels the decreased electrical activity.

EMG data were also examined over a four year period in thirty-one athletes who were referred by coaches, trainers, and physicians because of muscle injuries (18). These data were also quite conclusive in showing a very well-defined rise in EMG during the soreness phenomenon, and a return to more normal resting values after treatment as a spasm.

Thus the evidence for increased EMG activity during the delayed muscle soreness phenomenon is strong. In addition, it has been shown that when muscle pain is brought about by saline injection, EMG changes reflect this pain quite faithfully (12).

Unfortunately, subsequent investigators who attempted to replicate the EMG data of deVries did not achieve the level of sensitivity required to observe the small changes deVries reported. Figure 26.3 shows that the changes deVries observed were in the range of 1 to 3 microvolts. Such electrophysiological changes can be measured only with unipolar electrode leads and a very high level of amplifier sensitivity, which in turn requires working in a well-constructed Faraday cage. The frequency band pass of the amplifier must be focused on the part of the spectrum of interest, for example, 10 to 250 Hz. No subsequent investigator has met these requirements, and therefore it is not surprising that later investigators have not achieved similar findings (1, 44, 47).

Attempt at Unification and Simplification: Practical Aspects for Coach and Athlete

The "law of parsimony" suggests that when looking at potential solutions to a problem, one should first look to the simplest rather than the more complex solution. In this light we can postulate a relatively simple model for the development of DOMS that would be consistent with all the well-established experimental findings, although this does not imply complete understanding of the underlying mechanism for each step. Basically the model to be proposed here accepts the fact of structural damage that is now well established but sees it as a *result* of ischemia rather than a *causal factor* in itself. That blood flow to a muscle during vigorous exercise can be reduced at least to the point of relative ischemia (if not complete ischemia in some parts of a muscle) seems to be well established, as discussed earlier.

Thus in deVries's opinion the following model best fits the available data in the most parsimonious manner:

1. Vigorous overload exercise (with respect to *either intensity or duration*) results in a swelling of the muscle both at the cell level and the gross muscle level. Every weight trainer has observed the "pumping up" of the exercised muscle.

2. This swelling of muscle tissue increases tissue pressure.

3. Increasing tissue pressure creates pressure against the arteries, arterioles, and the microcirculation, which results in at least a degree of ischemia throughout the whole muscle and quite possibly total ischemia in the more poorly supplied fasciculi of the muscle.

4. Ischemic areas eventually result in cell necrosis, with release of cellular components into the tissue fluids and concomitant increases in osmotic pressure.

5. The increased osmotic pressure would of course result in a further increase in tissue pressure. Thus a vicious cycle is born that conceivably has a time course that fits the observed twenty-four to forty-eight-hour delay found in DOMS.

6. As in the Armstrong model, the pain is explained to be a result of the tissue edema and inflammatory processes.

Actually this model can be easily rationalized with the Armstrong (4) model and disagrees with it only with respect to the original causation. This localized ischemia model avoids the difficulty of explaining how seemingly nontraumatic exercise can bring about severe DOMS. Furthermore, this model is also consistent with the increased electrical activity found in deVries's laboratory. Cobb and coworkers (12) demonstrated the close parallels between pain and electrical activity. The increased electrical activity that represents incompletely relaxed muscle during DOMS, as reported from deVries's laboratory, may thus represent a result of the DOMS instead of the cause as we originally postulated before muscular structural damage had been verified. In any event, the increased resting muscle activity could only act to exacerbate the vicious cycle that is hypothesized here. This ischemia model is also consistent with the findings of relief of DOMS from static stretching, as discussed in the following paragraphs. The mechanical trauma model, on the other hand, is totally inconsistent with such findings. That static stretching is effective has now been corroborated by research in China. Using the electron microscope, Changping (11) reported that "static stretch could inhibit the ultrastructural alteration or accelerate the ultrastructural recovery in muscles after unaccustomed exercise."

The fact that static stretching can often provide relief from both traumatic and delayed soreness is also consistent with such a theoretical position. This latter fact is probably most important for physical educators, coaches, and athletes because the static stretching relief of muscle pain rests on a great deal of human experience plus experimental research findings (15, 16, 17, 18, 48). Absence of effect from static stretching has also been reported by Buroker and Schwane (9). The difference in findings is difficult to explain although the research paradigms were dissimiliar.

Physiology Underlying Static Stretching

To test the spasm theory, several different lines of investigation were pursued in deVries's laboratory. First, it was hypothesized that, if the spasm theory had merit, the simple stretching technique that relieves a swimmer's cramp in the calf muscle should also be effective in providing prevention and relief for any sore muscle that can be put on stretch. Therefore a stretching technique was designed to take best possible advantage of the following neurophysiological concepts (chap. 5).

1. There are two components to the spindle reflex: phasic and static (35, 45).

2. The amount and rate of the phasic response in the spindle reflex are proportional to the amount and rate of stretching (45).

3. The Golgi tendon receptor organs have a relatively high threshold, but when innervated bring about inhibition of not only the muscle in which the receptors are situated but also the entire functional muscle group (43).

4. Steady stretch depresses the monosynaptic response, even when the tendon organs are not active (30).

5. The amplitude of EMG in large human muscles characteristically diminishes when they are stretched (31).

6. Reduced amplitude of EMG in large muscles upon stretching is related to tendon organ activity in human muscle (39).

deVries's system of *static stretching* was developed around the six concepts outlined above: a body position is held that locks the joints around the sore muscle in a position of greatest possible muscle length and with as little concomitant muscle activity as possible (many Yoga exercises have been found useful since they use the same principle). This procedure results in the least possible reflex stimulation to the involved muscle. A *bouncing stretch,* on the other hand, invokes stretch reflexes whose end result (contraction of the sore, stretched muscle) is undesirable. The duration used in most cases has been two sets at two minutes each with a one-minute rest intervening. Figure 26.4 illustrates the stretching principle for the gastrocnemius muscle.

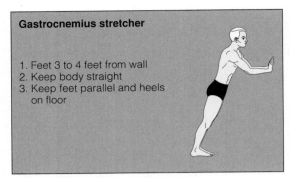

Gastrocnemius stretcher

1. Feet 3 to 4 feet from wall
2. Keep body straight
3. Keep feet parallel and heels on floor

Figure 26.4   Illustration of the static stretching method as applied in deVries's laboratory for relief of experimentally caused soreness (and also used for accidental soreness).

Prevention of Muscular Soreness

The aforementioned theoretical considerations allow us to bring theory and practice to bear on the problem of preventing muscle pain.

Warm-Up

It has long been the popular opinion of coaches and athletes that *warm-up processes* serve to prevent muscle soreness. This was supported in an experiment in which deVries investigated the effects of flexibility upon O_2 consumption during 100-yard sprints. The subjects ran under conditions of no warm-up, as a control situation, compared with a static stretching flexibility warm-up. In this experiment, two of the four subjects developed very sore muscles as the result of running without warm-up. This would seem to support the necessity for warm-up.

A recent study by High, Howley, and Franks (28), however, found that warm-up had no effect on DOMS. In this study, a group of subjects who performed warm-up exercises and static stretching prior to a step test reported nearly identical soreness ratings as subjects who performed only the test (no stretching or warm-up). Based on these findings, the authors stated "This study failed to show that static stretching and/or warm-up before exercise has a significant effect on the perception of DOMS following the exercise."

Progression in Training Programs

In the many experiments and pilot studies conducted in deVries's laboratory, one factor especially stands out in regard to muscle soreness: soreness seems to occur only when large overloads of intensity or endurance are imposed upon an individual muscle. In fact, one of the difficult problems to overcome in setting up systematic experimentation was development of standard exercises that would result in high levels of soreness in large percentages of the subjects. Thus if sore muscles are to be avoided, a *gradual increase* of work load should be planned, so that no one workout represents too great an overload for the physical condition of the musculature.

Chronic Exercise Training

Chronic training reduces the DOMS response to a given exercise (4). Apparently, repeated bouts of exercise result in a training effect that dramatically reduces the symptoms associated with DOMS. Newham, Jones, and Clarkson (46) had subjects perform eighty maximal eccentric contractions of the elbow flexors (one every fifteen seconds for twenty minutes) on three occasions each separated by two weeks. The authors reported that "muscle tenderness was greatest after the first bout and thereafter progressively decreased." In addition, plasma levels of creatine kinase (a muscle fiber enzyme that, when found in the plasma, reflects tissue damage) were elevated after the first exercise bout but remained unchanged following the second and third workbouts. Findings consistent with these have also been reported by Jones and Newham (33) for forearm flexion exercises and Byrnes and coworkers (10) following repeated bouts of downhill running.

Presently, however, the physiological mechanism by which exercise training reduces the DOMS response is unknown.

Types of Activity

Some types of muscular activity are more likely to result in sore muscles than others. The following activities are most likely to result in soreness:

1. Eccentric muscle contractions, as in downhill running (10, 58, 59).

2. Vigorous muscle contractions while a muscle is in a shortened condition. This often results in muscle cramp (48).

3. Muscle contractions that involve jerky movements. In this case, a muscle is temporarily overloaded when a full load is placed on it before enough motor units have been recruited (fig. 24.1).

4. Muscle contractions that involve repetitions of the same movement over a long period of time (endurance imposed on a limited number of muscle fibers). This repetitious movement causes even more soreness if a slight rest interval is allowed between repetitions because the bout can be disproportionately increased in length and a greater total work load is demanded.

5. Bouncing-type stretching movements. At the end of a ballistic motion, the movement is stopped by the muscle and connective tissues, which brings about reflex contraction at the time the muscle is being forcefully elongated.

Static Stretching

On many occasions it is impossible to avoid some of the conditions that predispose toward sore muscles, but in such situations a brief (ten-minute) period of static stretching after the workout can bring about a significant degree of prevention. deVries has described a well-rounded static stretching program for this purpose elsewhere (19). In any event, application of the principles of kinesiology will enable a professionally trained coach or physical educator to design the exercise for a specific situation.

For example, in a running situation where shin splints may be expected, the muscles involved are the flexors of the ankle joint. Consequently, the athletes are put into a kneeling position, with the ankles extended (plantar flexed). Then the full weight of the body is brought to bear—gently—on the muscle by rocking back onto the ankles. This position is held a minimum of one minute, with *no bouncing*.

Relief of Muscular Soreness

Static Stretching

When a muscle becomes painful twenty-four to forty-eight hours (or more) after unaccustomed exercise, relief can usually be provided by the following procedure.

1. Determine (by palpation) which muscle or muscles are involved.

2. Determine the nature of the activity that brought about the situation.

3. Determine the muscular attachments of the involved muscle or muscles by consulting a textbook of anatomy or kinesiology.

4. Devise a simple position in which the attachments are held as far apart as possible with the least possible effort.

5. Have the subject hold this position for two-minute periods, with a one-minute rest period intervening. If the pain is severe, this should be repeated two or three times daily.

This procedure has proven effective even in chronic muscular problems (15, 18).

Acute Exercise

Acute exercise temporarily reduces the symptoms of DOMS (4). The mechanism associated with the reduced pain during exercise is unknown, but some researchers' hypotheses are listed below (4):

1. Adhesions resulting from injury in the sore muscles are broken, thereby reducing the sensation of pain.
2. Acute exercise causes increased blood flow and/or temperature in the muscle.
3. Endogenous opioids released during exercise have an analgesic effect.
4. Increased afferent input from large, low-threshold sensory units in the muscle may interfere with pain sensations.
5. Exercise directs attention to the activity and away from the pain.

Anti-Inflammatory Drugs

Inflammation normally accompanies DOMS. The model of DOMS proposed by Smith (62) suggests that upon exposure to the inflammatory environment, macrophages synthesize prostaglandins which add to the sensation of pain. Recent investigations (23, 32, 38) have examined the effect of anti-inflammatory drugs (flurbiprofen and aspirin) on the muscle soreness associated with DOMS. These drugs act to suppress prostaglandin synthesis and activity. The somewhat conflicting results of these studies have shown that flurbiprofen has no effect on DOMS and aspirin reduces soreness at forty-eight hours but not at twenty-four hours after exercise. Additional research is necessary before the effectiveness of anti-inflammatory drugs on DOMS will be known.

Severe Muscle Problems

None of the foregoing discussion should be construed as suggesting that all painful muscles are due to ischemia. Nor is it suggested that muscles cannot, under certain conditions, be torn (ruptured). It is obvious that a muscle can be put under such great, sudden strain that some of the tissue exceeds its elastic limits and ruptures, but this probably occurs much less often than athletes and coaches seem to think.

In any event, muscular pain that is severe or that persists longer than a few days should be diagnosed by a physician, as should any muscle injury in which deformation or severe swelling and/or inflammation occurs.

Summary

1. Two types of muscle pain result from overexertion: (a) pain during and immediately after exercise, which is probably due to diffusion of metabolites into the tissue spaces, and (b) a localized, delayed soreness that appears in twenty-four to forty-eight hours.

2. Overwhelming evidence for structural damage is now available from investigators showing biochemical, histological, and ultrastructural changes in muscle tissue to accompany DOMS.

3. The *mechanical trauma* theory for DOMS proposes a model in which the original causal factor is the disruption of muscle tissue due to high mechanical forces required during muscle contraction. The structural damage results in a net calcium influx into the muscle cell that ultimately activates a calcium-dependent proteolytic enzyme that degrades Z discs and troponin and tropomyosin. Deterioration of the sarcolemma results in diffusion of intracellular components into the tissue fluids and plasma and consequently an inflammatory process that brings about the pain experienced in DOMS.

4. The acute inflammation theory is based on the similarities between DOMS and inflammation.

5. The *local ischemia* theory for DOMS proposes a model in which (a) muscle overuse (of either intensity or duration) causes increased tissue pressure; (b) increased tissue pressure results in localized ischemia; and (c) localized ischemia causes the observed structural damage. Structural damage results in the inflammatory processes that cause further increases in tissue pressure, creating a vicious cycle whose end result is DOMS when the tissue pressure (and possible tissue irritants) are sufficient to excite the type IV nerve endings.

6. The local ischemia theory is consistent with earlier findings of increased electrical activity in sore muscles (spasm theory), postulated earlier as being causal. It is also consistent with the findings of prevention or relief (or both) of DOMS by static stretching. The mechanical trauma theory is difficult to rationalize with these findings.

7. Several factors are important in the prevention of sore muscles: (a) proper *warm-up* may reduce soreness; (b) workouts should be designed with *progressive* increases in work load; (c) activity that involves vigorous muscle contraction with the muscle in a shortened condition, jerky movements, long-term repetition of a movement, or bouncing-type stretching is most likely to produce muscular soreness.

8. *Static stretching* has been found to be effective in providing relief of muscular soreness.

References

1. Abraham, W. M. Factors in delayed muscle soreness. *Med. Sci. Sports* 9:11–20, 1977.

2. Arcangeli, P., Digliesi, V., Masala, B., Serra, M. V., and Congilu, A. Metabolism of skeletal muscle following incomplete ischemia. *Angiology* 24:114–22, 1973.

3. Armstrong, R. B., Ogilvie, R. W., and Schwane, J. A. Eccentric exercise-induced injury to rat skeletal muscle. *J. Appl. Physiol.* 54:80–93, 1983.

4. Armstrong, R. B. Mechanisms of exercise-induced delayed onset muscular soreness: A brief review. *Med. Sci. Sports Exer.* 16:529–38, 1984.

5. Ashton, H. The effect of increased tissue pressure on blood flow. *Clin. Orthop. Relat. Res.* 113:15–26, 1975.

6. Asmussen, E. Observations on experimental muscular soreness. *Acta Rheumatol. Scand.* 2:109–16, 1956.

7. Barcroft, H., and Millen, J. L. E. The blood flow through muscle during sustained contraction. *J. Physiol.* 97:17–31, 1939–40.

8. Bigland-Ritchie, B., and Woods, J. J. Integrated electromyogram and oxygen uptake during positive and negative work. *J. Physiol.* 260:267–77, 1976.

9. Buroker, K. C., and Schwane, J. A. Does post exercise static stretching alleviate delayed muscle soreness? *Phys. Sportsmed.* 17:65–83, 1989.

10. Byrnes, W. C., Clarkson, P. M., White, J. S., Hsieh, S. S., Frykman, P. N., and Maughan, R. J. Delayed onset muscle soreness following repeated bouts of downhill running. *J. Appl. Physiol.* 59:710–15, 1985.

11. Changping, D. Effects of acupuncture and static stretch on ultrastructural alterations in skeletal muscle during delayed muscle soreness. Paper to 1984 Olympic Scientific Congress, Eugene, Oregon, July 26, 1984.

12. Cobb, C. R., deVries, H. A., Urban, R. T., Leukens, C. A., and Bagg, R. J. Electrical activity in muscle pain. *Am. J. Phys. Med.* 54:80–87, 1975.

13. Cullen, M. J., and Fulthorpe, J. J. Phagocytosis of the A band following Z line and I band loss. *Pathology* 138:129–43, 1982.

14. Dayton, W. R., Reville, W. J., Goll, D. E., and Stromer, M. H. A Ca^{++} activated protease possibly involved in myofibrillar protein turnover. *Biochemistry* 15:2159–67, 1976.

15. deVries, H. A. Electromyographic observations of the effects of static stretching upon muscular distress. *Res. Q.* 32:468–79, 1961a.

16. ———. Prevention of muscular distress after exercise. *Res. Q.* 32:177–85, 1961b.

17. ———. Treatment of muscular distress in athletes. *Proceedings of the 65th Annual College Physical Education Association Meeting.* Kansas City, December, 1961c.

18. ———. Quantitative electromyographic investigation of the spasm theory of muscle pain. *Am. J. Phys. Med.* 45:119–34, 1966.

19. ———. *Health Science: A Positive Approach.* Glenview, IL: Scott, Foresman & Co., 1979.

20. Dorpat, T. L., and Holmes, T. H. Mechanisms of skeletal muscle pain and fatigue. *Arch. Neurol. Psychiatry* 74:628–40, 1955.

21. Dressendorfer, R. H., and Wade, C. E. The muscular overuse syndrome in long-distance runners. *Physician and Sportsmed.* 11 (Nov.):116–30, 1983.

22. Eaton, R. G., and Green, W. T. Volkmanns ischemia: A volar compartment syndrome of the forearm. *Clin. Orthop. Relat. Res.* 113:58–64, 1975.

23. Francis, K. T., and Hoobler, T. Effects of aspirin on delayed muscle soreness. *J. Sports Med.* 27:333–37, 1987.

24. Friden, J., Sjostrom, M., and Ekblom, B. A morphological study of delayed muscle soreness. *Experientia* 37:506–7, 1981.

25. ———. Myofibrillar damage following intense eccentric exercise in man. *Int. J. Sports Med.* 4:170–76, 1983.

26. Hagerman, F. C., Hikida, R. S., Staron, R. S., Sherman, W. M., and Costill, D. L. Muscle damage in marathon runners. *Physician and Sportsmed.* 12 (Nov.):39–48, 1984.

27. Hansen, K., Bjerre-Knudsen, J., Brodthagen, U., Jordal, R., and Pauley, P-E. Muscle cell leakage due to long distance training. *Europ. J. Appl. Physiol.* 48:177–88, 1982.

28. High, D. M., Howley, E. T., and Franks, B. D. The effects of static stretching and warm-up on prevention of delayed-onset muscle soreness. *Res. Quart. Exerc. Sport* 60:357–61, 1989.

29. Hikida, R. S., Staron, R. S., Hagerman, F. C., Sherman, W. M., and Costill, D. L. Muscle fiber necrosis associated with human marathon runners. *J. Neurol. Sci.* 59:185–203, 1983.

30. Hunt, C. C. The effect of stretch receptors from muscle on the discharge of motoneurons. *J. Physiol.* 117:359–79, 1952.

31. Inman, B. T., Ralston, H. J., Saunders, J. B., Feinstein, B., and Wright, E. W. Relation of human electromyogram to muscular tension. *Electroencephalogr. Clin. Neurophysiol.* 4:187–94, 1952.

32. Janssen, E., Kuipers, H., Verstappen, F., and Costill, D. Influence of an anti-inflammatory drug on muscle soreness. *Med. Sci. Sports Exerc.* 15:165, 1983.

33. Jones, D. A., and Newham, D. J. The effect of training on human muscle pain and damage. *J. Physiol.* 365:76P, 1985.

34. Karpati, G., Carpenter, S., Melmed, C., and Eisen, A. A. Experimental ischemic myopathy. *J. Neurol. Sci.* 23:129–61, 1974.

35. Katz, B. Depolarization of sensory terminals and the initiation of impulses in the muscle spindle. *J. Physiol.* 111:261–82, 1950.

36. Kilburn, K.H. Muscular origin of elevated plasma potassium during exercise. *J. Appl. Physiol.* 21:675–78, 1966.

37. Knochel, J. P. Rhabdomyolysis and myoglobinuria. *Ann. Rev. Med.* 33:435–43, 1982.

38. Kuipers, H., Keizer, H. A., Verstappen, F. T. J., and Costill, D. L. Influence of a prostaglandin-inhibiting drug on muscle soreness after eccentric work. *Int. J. Sports Med.* 6:336–39, 1985.

39. Libet, B., Feinstein, B., and Wright, E. W. Tendon afferents in autogenic inhibition. *Fed. Proc.* 14:92, 1955.

40. Mäkitie, J., and Teravainen, H. Histochemical studies of striated muscle after temporary ischemia in the rat. *Acta Neuropath.* 37:101–9, 1977a.

41. ———. Ultrastructure of striated muscle of the rat after temporary ischemia. *Acta Neuropath.* 37:237–45, 1977b.

42. Matin, P., Lang, G., Caretta, R., and Simon, G. Scintographic evaluation of muscle damage following extreme exercise: Concise communication. *J. Nucl. Med.* 24:308–11, 1983.

43. McCouch, G. P., Deering, I. D., and Stewart, W. B. Inhibition of knee jerk from tendon spindles of crureus. *J. Neurophysiol.* 13:343–50, 1950.

44. McGlynn, G. H., Laughlin, N. T., and Filios, S. P. The effect of electromyographic feedback on EMG activity and pain in the quadriceps muscle group. *J. Sports Med.* 19:237–44, 1979.

45. Mountcastle, V. B. Reflex activity of the spinal cord. In *Medical Physiology,* ed. P. Bard, chap. 60. St. Louis: C. V. Mosby, 1961.

46. Newham, D. J., Jones, D. A., and Clarkson, P. M. Repeated high-force eccentric exercise: Effects on muscle pain and damage. *J. Appl. Physiol.* 63:1381–86, 1987.

47. Newham, D. J., Mills, K. R., Quigley, B. M., and Edwards, R. H. T. Pain and fatigue after concentric and eccentric muscle contractions. *Clin. Sci.* 64:55–62, 1983.

48. Norris, F. H., Jr., Gasteiger, E. L., and Chatfield, P. O. An electromyographic study of induced and spontaneous muscle cramps. *Electroencephalogr. Clin. Neurophysiol.* 9:139–47, 1957.

49. Petajan, J. H., and Eagan, C. J. Effect of temperature and physical fitness on the triceps surae reflex. *J. Appl. Physiol.* 25:16–20, 1968.

50. Postlewaite, A. E., and Kang, A. H. Collagen and collagen peptide induced chemotaxis of human blood monocytes. *J. Exp. Med.* 143:1299–1307, 1976.

51. Reneman, R. S. The anterior and the lateral compartmental syndrome of the leg due to intensive use of the muscles. *Clin. Orthop. Relat. Res.* 113:69–80, 1975.

52. Rodbard, S. Pain associated with muscular activity. *Am. Heart J.* 90:84–92, 1975.

53. Rodbard, S., and Farbstein, M. Improved exercise tolerance during venous congestion. *J. Appl. Physiol.* 33:704–10, 1972.

54. Rohter, F. D., and Hyman, C. Blood flow in arm and finger during muscle contraction and joint position changes. *J. Appl. Physiol.* 17:819–23, 1962.

55. Salminen, A., and Vihko, V. Effects of age and prolonged running on proteolytic capacity in mouse cardiac and skeletal muscles. *Acta Physiol. Scand.* 112:89–95, 1981.

56. Sanderson, R. A., Foley, R. K., McIvor, W. D., and Kirkaldy-Willis, W. H. Histological response on skeletal muscle ischemia. *Clin. Orthop. Relat. Res.* 113:27–35, 1975.

57. Schwane, J. A., Johnson, S. R., Vandenakker, C. B., and Armstrong, R. B. Delayed-onset muscular soreness and plasma CPK and LDH activities after downhill running. *Med. Sci. Sports Exer.* 15:51–56, 1983.

58. Schwane, J. A., Watrous, B. G., Johnson, S. R., and Armstrong, R. B. Is lactic acid related to delayed-onset muscle soreness? *Physician and Sportsmed.* 11:124–31, 1983.

59. Schwartz, W. N., and Bird, J. W. C. Degradation of myofibrillar proteins by cathepsins B and D. *Biochem. J.* 167:811–20, 1977.

60. Shannon, A. D., Adams, E. P., and Courtice, F. C. The lysosomal enzymes acid phosphatase and B glucuronidase in muscle following a period of ischemia. *Aust. J. Exp. Biol. Med. Sci.* 52:157–71, 1974.

61. Sheridan, G. W., and Matsen, F. A. An animal model of the compartmental syndrome. *Clin. Orthop. Relat. Res.* 113:36–42, 1975.

62. Smith, L. L. Acute inflammation: The underlying mechanism in delayed onset muscle soreness? *Med. Sci. Sports Exerc.* 23:542–51, 1991.

63. Soybel, D., Morgan, J., and Cohen, L. Calcium augmentation of enzyme leakage from mouse skeletal muscle and its possible site of action. *Res. Commun. Chem. Path. Pharmacol.* 20:317–29, 1978.

64. Stenger, R. J., Spiro, D., Scully, R. E., and Shannon, J. M. Ultrastructural and physiologic alterations in ischemic skeletal muscle. *Am. J. Pathol.* 40:1–20, 1962.

65. Vihko, V., Salminen, A., and Rantamaki, J. Exhaustive exercises, endurance training and acid hydrolase activity in skeletal muscle. *J. Appl. Physiol.* 47:43–50, 1979.

66. Whiteside, T. E., Haney, T. C., Morimoto, K., and Harada, H. Tissue pressure measurements as a determinant for the need of fasciotomy. *Clin. Orthop. Relat. Res.* 113:43–51, 1975.

67. Williams, M. H., and Ward, A. J. Hematological changes elicited by prolonged intermittent aerobic exercise. *Res. Q.* 48:606–16, 1977.

68. Wrogeman, K., and Pena, S. D. J. Mitochondrial calcium overload: A general mechanism for cell necrosis in muscle diseases. *Lancet* 27:672–73, 1976.

27

Warming Up

Practice Effect versus Physiological
   Warm-Up

Physiology of Warming Up
   General versus Local Heating
   Rectal versus Muscle Temperature
   O_2 Consumption and Warm-Up
   Blood Flow through the Lungs

Types of Warm-Up
   Passive versus Active
   Related and Unrelated Warm-Up
     Methods
   Intensity and Duration of Warm-Up
   Overload Warm-Up

Effect of Warm-Up on Various Athletic
   Activities
   Speed
   Strength
   Muscular Endurance
   Circulorespiratory Endurance
   Power
   Throwing
   Swimming

Duration of the Warm-Up Effect

Recovery between Events

Warm-Up and Prevention of Muscle
   Injury

Warm-Up and Heart Function

Until relatively recently, the value of warming up had not been challenged. On the basis of theoretical concepts, warming up was accepted by virtually all coaches and athletes. However, much scientific interest has lately been directed toward 1) its value in athletics, 2) elucidation of its physiological nature, and 3) comparisons of the effectiveness of various warm-up procedures.

Unfortunately, the various investigators have used different methods, so that the type, intensity, and duration of the warm-ups have varied, as has the physical activity in which the level of performance was to be affected. Consequently the work of the investigators can seldom be compared, and confusion has resulted. Some investigations have been equivocal, some poorly controlled, and still others have used so little warm-up activity (in terms of intensity and duration) that no conceivable physiological changes could have been brought about. On the other hand, because some of the experiments have been properly conducted and are quite definitive in certain respects, we will try to derive some principles by which physical educators and coaches can guide their professional activities.

Practice Effect versus Physiological Warm-Up

A great source of confusion is the fact that the effects of practice in improving a skill are frequently confused with the actual warming up in which physiological changes are brought about. Unquestionably, if skill and accuracy are important factors in a physical activity, practice can bring about improvement in performance. The question considered in this chapter has to do with the physiological aspects of warming up.

Physiology of Warming Up

On theoretical grounds it might be expected that a warming-up that results in increased blood and muscle temperatures should improve performance through the following mechanisms: 1) muscles relax and contract faster, 2) lower viscous resistance in the muscles increases efficiency, 3) hemoglobin gives up more oxygen at higher temperatures and also dissociates much more rapidly, 4) myoglobin shows temperature effects similar to those of hemoglobin, 5) metabolic process rates increase with increasing temperature, and 6) resistance of the vascular bed decreases with increasing temperature.

Gutin and his coworkers have suggested another rationale for the use of warm-up, based on a mobilization hypothesis (1, 2, 23, 24). They view prior exercise (PE) as a mobilizing stimulus for the systems involved in O_2 transport, thereby allowing the subject to reach a high level of aerobic metabolism more quickly during the subsequent athletic task. This reduces the initial O_2 deficit (chap. 12, fig. 12.5), thus leaving more of the anaerobic capacity for later use. The hypothesis was supported by a recent investigation by Roberts and colleagues (43), which reported lower muscle and blood lactate accumulation as a result of a two minute cycle ergometer sprint ride at 120% of $\dot{V}O_2$ max following a ten minute warm-up than without the warm-up period. Furthermore, Hetzler and coworkers (25) found that a twenty minute walking warm-up prior to forty minutes of treadmill running at 65% of $\dot{V}O_2$ max, resulted in a greater percentage of energy production from fat metabolism than without the warm-up. The increased contribution from fat metabolism resulted in a sparing of carbohydrates during the exercise. These findings (25) may have implications for athletes involved in long duration moderate intensity activities as well as individuals involved in weight loss programs.

General versus Local Heating

Three well-controlled investigations found substantial and significant improvements in performance (1% to 8%) when the entire body was heated so that rectal and muscle temperatures were increased (3, 14, 36). This heating can be accomplished actively by vigorous exercise of various kinds, or passively by hot baths, showers, Turkish baths, or diathermy. However, local heating of only the involved limb has been shown to result in earlier fatigue and lessened work output in that limb (15, 22). It has also been shown that in local heating, the factor of major importance is probably the distribution of blood between the skin and the underlying muscles, if both are served by the same large artery (37, 38).

It seems likely, then, that the explanation for the different effects of local and general heating lies in the fact that in local heating a large vasodilation effect is possible in the skin to the detriment of circulation through the underlying muscle. This could well result in the amount of decreased performance actually observed. On the other hand, heating of the entire body must exert some, or all, of the beneficial effects stated previously, while the vasodilatation effect on the skin cannot be nearly so large and may not occur to any great extent when a large proportion of the musculature is active.

On the basis of all the available evidence, there seems little doubt that general heating of the body that results in increased core (rectal) and muscle temperatures improves performance.

Theoretical evidence has shown that the effect of temperature on the force-velocity curve (chap. 4, fig. 4.9) is such that a rise in muscle temperature of 5° C should increase velocity and maximum power by about 10%

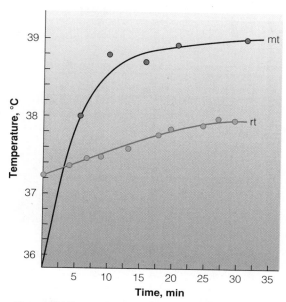

Figure 27.1   Temperature measured in lateral vastus muscle (mt) and in rectum (rt) during a work of 660 kgm/min. (From Asmussen, E., and Boje, O., in *Acta Physiologica Scandinavica* 10:1. © 1945 Scandinavian Physiological Society, Stockholm. Reprinted by permission.)

(9). This is in agreement with the empirical evidence from the earlier studies.

Rectal versus Muscle Temperature

Figure 27.1 illustrates the changes in muscle and rectal temperature that occur as the result of warming up by riding the cycle ergometer at a moderate load. It can be seen that the greatest part of the increase in muscle temperature occurs in the first five minutes, with rectal temperature increasing more gradually and steadily for thirty minutes.

Figure 27.2 shows the same temperature data and relates the two temperatures to performance time for a sprint on the cycle ergometer. Because performance has shown its greatest improvement during the time that muscle temperature has increased markedly and rectal temperature has increased very

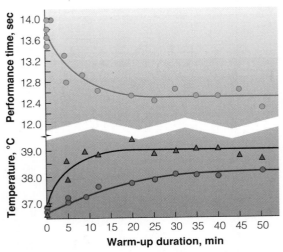

Figure 27.2   Effect of *duration* of warm-up on performance time; ●———● is performance time for sprint; ▲———▲ is muscle temperature; ○———○ is rectal temperature. (From Asmussen, E., and Boje, O., in *Acta Physiologica Scandinavica* 10:1. © 1945 Scandinavian Physiological Society, Stockholm. Reprinted by permission.)

little, Asmussen and Boje (3) consider muscle temperature to be the more important factor. This contention has been supported by Carlile (14), who found no positive relationships between rectal temperature and swimming times.

More recent work has further corroborated this early work (29, 31), and we may therefore conclude that any procedure that significantly raises deep muscle temperature will improve performance.

On the other hand, it has been shown that if a subject is warmed up in such a fashion as to raise rectal temperature, and muscle temperature is allowed to return to normal while rectal temperature is still elevated (rectal temperature returns to normal much more slowly), performance is still somewhat improved over control conditions (36). Thus we must say that both muscle and blood temperatures are important, but muscle temperature probably has the greater effect.

O_2 Consumption and Warm-Up

It has been shown that maximal oxygen uptake is slightly higher after warming up, compared with cold conditions, but that the O_2 necessary for a given amount of work is reduced (3, 48). This seems to indicate that efficiency is improved as a result of warming up. Presently, however, there is no conclusive data available regarding the effect of warm-up or increases in core and muscle temperature on the oxygen cost of running (running economy) (35).

deVries has attempted to separate the effects of temperature from those of increased mobility (flexibility) in warming up for 100-yard dashes. When flexibility was improved by static stretching so as to eliminate the temperature and circulatory factors, no improvement in efficiency could be demonstrated (19). Thus it seems that the improvement in efficiency is probably temperature-related.

The mobilization hypothesis of Gutin, Andzel, and coworkers has been tested in a number of investigations (1, 2, 23, 24). On the basis of all available data it would appear that the hypothesis is tenable but only with respect to athletic tasks in which the initial work loads are maximal or supramaximal. It is of questionable value in endurance tasks where aerobic power is important (23). Prior exercise (PE), the term used by these investigators to distinguish it from true temperature warm-up effects, appears to be effective only under very specific conditions: 1) the PE must be approached in very gradual fashion; 2) the PE must be at an intensity below anaerobic threshold (heart rate = 140 has proven successful); and 3) most important, the beneficial effect is available for only thirty to sixty seconds after the PE. The objective of the PE is to mobilize the O_2 transport function without depleting phosphagen energy and/or stored O_2 supplies (chap. 12). Their data suggest that a thirty- to sixty-second rest between PE and the athletic task is sufficient to replenish the O_2 stores and phosphagen energy while still retaining a partial mobilization effect. Rest intervals longer than sixty seconds are ineffective and may decrease subsequent performance.

Blood Flow through the Lungs

An investigation of the effects of exercise on pulmonary blood flow showed that a period of moderate exercise, such as might be used for warming up, results in a decrease of total pulmonary resistance of about 13% (54). This decrease was highly significant. The reduced resistance to blood flow and its concomitant improvement of lung circulation could make an important contribution to the warm-up phenomenon.

Types of Warm-Up

Passive versus Active

In regard to whole-body warm-up and large-muscle activity, there seems little doubt that any procedure that increases rectal and muscle temperatures will improve subsequent athletic performance. This warm-up effect has been demonstrated for active warm-up brought about by such diverse activities as running, bicycle riding, bench-stepping, or calisthenics. Passive heating by hot baths, hot showers, Turkish baths, or diathermy has also been found effective.

Related and Unrelated Warm-Up Methods

Related warm-up is any procedure that involves the athletic activity itself, or something close to it. *Unrelated warm-up* is any procedure designed to bring about the desired physiological changes without involving the actual movement itself. Investigations in this area are somewhat inconclusive, but it can be assumed on the basis of common sense that if the desired physiological changes can be achieved by use of related warm-up procedures, these are preferable to unrelated procedures in that a practice effect would also be gained. In many athletic events, however, the activity is not well suited for warming up (jumping), or it is too fatiguing.

Intensity and Duration of Warm-Up

Burke (13) has demonstrated that optimal combinations of intensity and duration are needed to bring about the desired warm-up effect. Too little work does not achieve optimal levels of temperature, and too much warm-up can result in impaired performance due to fatigue. More recent work has shown that warm-up intensity of 75% $\dot{V}O_2$ max or more can impair performance instead of enhance it (17). The interaction of the effects of warm-up and fatigue in untrained young girls is shown clearly in the work of Richards (fig. 27.3). The girls warmed up with varying durations (one to six minutes) of bench-stepping prior to a vertical jump test. It can be seen that the warm-up effect is greater than the fatigue effect when the warm-up is carried out for one to three minutes. Longer warm-up results in more loss to fatigue than is gained in warm-up benefit (42). However, figure 27.4 shows that in a *well-conditioned* athlete, a very heavy load can be used for as long as thirty minutes, with ever-increasing muscle temperature and constantly improving performance. It should be pointed out that for the average child or poorly conditioned athlete a thirty-minute warm-up at an intensity of 1,600 kgm/min (fig. 27.4) would result in complete exhaustion. Recent evidence, indeed, shows that warm-up for sixty minutes at intensity below anaerobic threshold (AT) is ineffective, while an intensity above AT impairs subsequent performance (20).

Bonner (12) has shown that the two-factors theory of Richards (warm-up versus fatigue effects) also holds for increasing levels

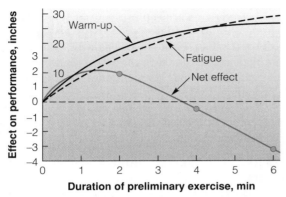

Figure 27.3   Effect of *length* of preliminary exercise on jumping performance. The inner numbers refer to the magnitude of the exponential factors. (From Richards, D. K., in *Research Quarterly* 39:668. © 1968 American Alliance for Health, Physical Education and Recreation. Reprinted by permission.)

of intensity as well as increasing durations of warm-up. For a given athletic task there is a specific combination of intensity and duration that results in best performance.

Obviously, the intensity and duration of warm-up also must be adjusted to the individual athlete. As a rule of thumb, one can look for signs of development of heat from within, which in a normal environment is indicated by perspiration. For those who wish to be more scientific, an increase in rectal temperature of 1° or 2° F appears desirable.

Overload Warm-Up

A common practice in baseball is to swing two or three bats in preparation for a turn at bat. Although this is more a practice effect than a true warm-up, it has interesting implications in both a practical and a scientific sense. It has been shown that throwing an 11-ounce baseball for a warm-up results in significantly improved velocity in subsequent tests with a ball of regulation weight (52). The neurophysiology of this phenomenon has not yet been elucidated. It is also possible that psychological effects are important.

Effect of Warm-Up on Various Athletic Activities

Speed

A number of investigators have shown various types of warm-up effective in improving the speed of running (10, 48), cycling (3), and arm speed (41). Other investigators, however, have found no improvement from various warm-up procedures in these activities (13, 27, 30, 32). This conflicting evidence leaves the picture rather unclear. Unfortunately, none of the investigators who found no improvement had measured muscle or rectal temperature, so we cannot be sure that a true physiological warm-up had occurred.

On the other hand, the only study that attempted psychological control over the subjects found no improvement, and it is possible that the improvements the other investigators found were caused by psychological factors. Conclusions must await further research.

Strength

An interesting picture emerges in respect to strength. The two investigators who used whole-body warm-up found significant increases in strength after warm-up (3, 13), while the three investigators who applied only local heat found no improvement after warm-up (15, 22, 47). It is therefore tempting to hypothesize that strength changes depend on central nervous system changes that are brought about by temperature change, circulatory change, or both.

On the basis of this evidence, plus evidence related to jumping and swimming, it seems that strength can be improved by a general body warm-up. But again the explanation of the underlying physiology awaits further investigation.

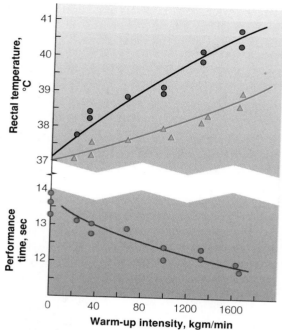

Figure 27.4   Effect of *intensity* of thirty-minute warm-up on performance time; ●——● is sprint performance time; ▲——▲ is rectal temperature; ○——○ is muscle temperature. (From Asmussen, E., and Boje, O., in *Acta Physiologica Scandinavica* 10:1. © 1945 Scandinavian Physiological Society, Stockholm. Reprinted by permission.)

Muscular Endurance

Asmussen and Boje (3), using whole-body heating, found that increased muscle temperature brought about improvement in times for riding a stationary bicycle. The work load of 9,860 kgm would take about five minutes, and it must therefore be considered to have an element of muscular endurance.

All other investigators have used only local-muscle warm-up. Their results agree that increasing the local-muscle temperature by warming up, either actively or passively, results in no improvement (46, 47) or in a decrement in endurance (15, 22, 37, 38).

There is also agreement on the finding that local cooling that reduces skin temperature results in better endurance for the underlying

muscle groups (15, 22, 37, 38). The rationale for this improvement was discussed earlier in this chapter.

Circulorespiratory Endurance

Grodjinovsky and Magel (21) found that only a vigorous warm-up consisting of five minutes of jogging, eight calisthenic exercises, plus a sprint of one-tenth mile improved time in the one-mile run. Warm-up without the sprint had no significant effect.

Power

One of the best measures of human power is the vertical jump, and complete agreement exists among four investigations on warming up for jumping (33, 39, 40, 42). Significant improvements, ranging from 2.6% to 20.0%, were found to result from the following warm-ups: massage, running in place, isometric stretching, deep knee bends, and stool-stepping. These findings, moreover, could be predicted on the basis of the strength findings, for power is really the expression of strength (force) per unit of time.

In addition, Inbar and Bar-Or (28) reported that a fifteen-minute intermittent warm-up on a treadmill (thirty seconds on, thirty seconds off) resulted in a 7% increase in mean power as measured by the Wingate Anaerobic Test (see chapter 14 for a description of the Wingate Anaerobic Test). Interestingly, the intermittent warm-up was more effective than a fifteen-minute equicaloric continuous warm-up (7).

Throwing

Because throwing has a strength factor (dynamic strength), this activity would also be expected to show improvement as the result of warm-up, and three investigations in this area support this contention. Improvement was shown to result from overload warm-up (52), related warm-up (34, 44), and unrelated warm-up (34).

Swimming

All investigations in this area show that swimming times can be improved by warming up. Hot showers of eight minutes' duration resulted in about 1.0% improvement in 40-yard times and 1.5% improvement in 220-yard times (14). Hot baths of from fifteen to eighteen minutes improved performance in the 400-meter freestyle and the 200-meter breaststroke by 2.1% to 3.9%, and in the 50-meter freestyle by as much as 2.0% (36).

Jogging and cycle ergometer work improved subsequent swim times by 0.6% to 2.2% (36). Short-wave diathermy improved swimming times by 1.3% to 1.9%, and cold baths decreased performances by 3.6% to 6.3% (36). One investigator found improvement from a related warm-up (swimming) but not from an unrelated warm-up (51).

deVries attempted to compare the values of commonly used warm-up procedures for highly skilled varsity swimmers for 100-yard times in their specialty strokes. It was found that a 500-yard swim was the only warm-up that brought about significant improvement for the group as a whole (1.0%). It was also found that calisthenic warm-ups produced the best improvement (2.0%) for the butterfly and breaststroke men and that it impaired the performance of the freestylers and backstrokers (18). This phenomenon points up the need for *individualizing* warm-up procedures.

Duration of the Warm-Up Effect

In some athletic events it is not possible to warm up after the program has begun—for example, swimming meets in which there is only one pool. A very practical question, then, is how long a warm-up effect persists. This question cannot be answered for the practice effect, but for temperature changes in muscle tissue it has been shown that this effect persists for forty-five to eighty minutes (36, 37).

Recent evidence is in disagreement and suggests that a rest interval between warm-up and the athletic event eliminates the warm-up effect (16).

Recovery between Events

In many athletic competitions such as swimming and track and field an athlete competes in more than one event, and the events may be separated by various periods of time. How does the athlete best recover between events to achieve optimal performance in each event?

Physiologically the problem is that the intense muscular activity of the first event results in the production of lactic acid (LA), which inhibits the mobilization of free fatty acids and retards the rate of glycolysis by inhibiting the activity of such enzymes as lactic dehydrogenase and phosphofructokinase. Therefore the removal of LA between events becomes critical.

The breathing of 100% O_2 to enhance lactate removal has been attempted, but two groups of investigators have shown this to be ineffective (49, 53).

In recent years, it has been found that not only is LA taken up by the heart, liver, brain, and kidney, but most important it is taken up by exercising muscle. Therefore one might hypothesize that the LA level could be reduced fastest by exercising the involved muscles during recovery at a rate that would optimize LA uptake by the muscles without causing any LA production (that is, exercising below anaerobic threshold). Recent evidence from five different investigations shows that this is indeed the case (8, 11, 49, 50, 53). Thus exercising during recovery the same muscles used in the preceding event at a rate of 30% to 50% of $\dot{V}O_2$ max permits the highest possible skeletal muscle blood flow without producing additional LA. It has been shown that the fastest rate of reduction of LA occurs when exercise is at about 32% of $\dot{V}O_2$ max, but even self-selected rates of exercise (about 50% $\dot{V}O_2$ max) were almost as effective (8). Thus easy jogging after a running event or easy swimming between swimming events for a period of ten to fifteen minutes should bring about optimal recovery between events.

Warm-Up and Prevention of Muscle Injury

Although there is still some uncertainty about the value of warm-up in improving performance, warming up has been retained as standard practice on the grounds that it might prevent injury to muscles. However, there is no direct evidence to support this contention, although considerable data exists showing that deep muscle temperature and compliance should be very important factors in the incidence of athletic injuries (45). The lack of evidence is understandable: no investigator would intentionally subject his or her subjects to experiments designed to bring about injury.

Quite unintentionally, objective evidence has become available in deVries's laboratory. In an unrelated study, four college-age male subjects ran 100-yard dashes (against time) to measure metabolic efficiency (19). When the subjects ran without warming up (control procedure), two of them developed muscular soreness that might have become severe in the absence of appropriate preventive measures. Thus it seems that muscle injury is indeed a real possibility when vigorous exercise is not preceded by proper warming up to bring about increased body temperatures. A recent study by High, Howley, and Franks (26), however, found that static stretching and/or warm-up prior to an exhaustive step test had no effect on the subjects' perception of delay-onset muscle soreness (DOMS) twenty-four hours following the exercise bout. The authors concluded that prior "static stretching and/or warm-up does not prevent DOMS resulting from exhaustive exercise." This is not to be confused with the effect of static stretching after the exercise, which has been found to be beneficial (chap. 26).

Warm-Up and Heart Function

The potential for injury to skeletal muscles by vigorous exercise without warm-up has been well recognized. Until recently, however, no one has questioned the effect of strenuous exercise without warm-up on the heart—the most important muscle of all. Barnard and his colleagues at UCLA (4, 5, 6) have conducted two important studies in this regard. In the first study (5) they ran forty-four healthy, asymptomatic individuals, ages twenty-one to fifty-two on a severe ten-second treadmill test without prior warm-up. Immediately after the run, 68% of the men had abnormal ECG changes. When two minutes of easy jogging preceded the sudden strenuous exercise, the abnormal ECG changes were eliminated or reduced in severity in almost all cases.

In a second study (6) they showed that the ECG abnormalities were the result of abnormally large increases in blood pressure that greatly increased the work of the heart (chap. 6). When their subjects were given a fifteen- to twenty-minute warm-up prior to the sudden exercise, the ECG abnormalities were again eliminated or reduced in almost all cases. They concluded that the adaptation of coronary blood flow to a rapid increase in the work of the heart is not instantaneous and that periods of myocardial ischemia may occur even in normal hearts. These findings alone underscore the need for adequate warm-up before sudden strenuous exercise.

Summary

Although all the results are not yet in for the warming-up phenomenon, intelligent coaches and athletes use the best available evidence to govern their activities, and the best available evidence justifies the following principles for warming up.

1. Whole-body warm-up of appropriate intensity and duration that raises muscle and blood (rectal) temperatures can significantly improve athletic performance.

2. Whenever possible, a *related warm-up* that raises muscle and blood temperatures is preferred over an unrelated warm-up so that a practice effect can be achieved simultaneously.

3. Warming up is important for preventing muscle soreness or injury.

4. Warming up is most important to protect the heart from ischemic changes that otherwise occur with sudden strenuous exercise.

5. Warming-up procedures must be suited to the individual.

6. Warming-up procedures must be suited to the athletic event.

7. A combination of intensity and duration of warm-up must be achieved that produces temperature increases in the deep tissues without undue fatigue. Sweating is an indication of increased internal temperature. For high-level competitive performances, the additional effort of taking the rectal temperature appears worthwhile. An increase of 1° or 2° F is desirable.

8. If active, related warm-up is impossible, passive heating can be used effectively.

9. Warming-up appears to be most important (makes the greatest contribution) in activities that directly involve strength and is less important in events that have a large element of power or acceleration of body weight.

10. Overload warm-up may be valuable for events in which neuromuscular coordination patterns are of major importance.

11. Tissue temperature changes brought about by warming up probably persist for forty-five to eighty minutes.

References

1. Andzel, W. D. The effects of moderate prior exercise and varied rest intervals upon cardiorespiratory endurance performance. *J. Sports Med. Phys. Fitness* 18:245–52, 1978.

2. Andzel, W. D., and Gutin, B. Prior exercise and endurance performance: A test of the mobilization hypothesis. *Res. Q.* 47:269–76, 1976.

3. Asmussen, E., and Boje, O. Body temperature and capacity for work. *Acta Physiol. Scand.* 10:1–22, 1945.

4. Barnard, R. J. Warm-up is important for the heart. *Sports Med. Bull.* (ACSM), January 1975.

5. Barnard, R. J., Gardner, G. W., Diaco, N. V., MacAlpin, R. N., and Kattus, A. A. Cardiovascular responses to sudden strenuous exercise—heart rate, blood pressure and ECG. *J. Appl. Physiol.* 34:833–37, 1973.

6. Barnard, R. J., MacAlpin, R., Kattus, A. A., and Buckberg, G. D. Ischemic response to sudden strenuous exercise in healthy men. *Circulation* 48:936–42, 1973.

7. Bar-Or, O. The Wingate anaerobic test: An update on methodology, reliability and validity. *Sports Med.* 4:381–94, 1987.

8. Belcastro, A. N., and Bonen, A. Lactic acid removal rates during controlled and uncontrolled recovery exercise. *J. Appl. Physiol.* 39:932–36, 1975.

9. Binkhorst, R. A., Hoofd, L., and Vissers, C. A. Temperature and force-velocity relationship of human muscles. *J. Appl. Physiol.* 42:471–75, 1977.

10. Blank, L. B. Effects of warm-up on speed. *Athletic J.* 10:45–46, 1955.

11. Bonen, A., and Belcastro, A. N. Comparison of self-selected recovery methods on lactic acid removal rates. *Med. Sci. Sports.* 8:176–78, 1976.

12. Bonner, H. Preliminary exercise: A two-factor theory. *Res. Q.* 45:138–47, 1974.

13. Burke, R. K. Relationships between physical performance and warm-up procedures of varying intensity and duration. Ph.D. diss., University of Southern California, 1957.

14. Carlile, F. Effect of preliminary passive warming-up on swimming performance. *Res. Q.* 27:143–51, 1956.

15. Clarke, R. S. J., Hellon, R. F., and Lind, A. R. The duration of sustained contractions of the human forearm at different muscle temperatures. *J. Physiol.* 143:454–73, 1958.

16. DeBruyn-Prevost, P. The effects of various warming-up intensities and durations upon some physiological variables during an exercise corresponding to WC$_{170}$. *Eur. J. Appl. Physiol. Occup. Physiol.* 43:93–100, 1980.

17. DeBruyn-Prevost, P., and Lefebvre, F. The effects of various warming-up intensities and durations during short maximal anaerobic exercise. *Eur. J. Appl. Physiol. Occup. Physiol.* 43:101–7, 1980.

18. deVries, H. A. Effects of various warm-up procedures on 100-yard times of competitive swimmers. *Res. Q.* 30:11–20, 1959.

19. ———. The looseness factor in speed and O$_2$ consumption of an anaerobic 100-yard dash. *Res. Q.* 34:305–13, 1963.

20. Genovely, H., and Stamford, B. A. Effects of prolonged warm-up exercise above and below anaerobic threshold on maximal performance. *Eur. J. Physiol. Occup. Physiol.* 48:323–30, 1982.

21. Grodjinovsky, A., and Magel, J. R. Effect of warm-up on running performance. *Res. Q.* 41:116–19, 1970.

22. Grose, J. E. Depression of muscle fatigue curves by heat and cold. *Res. Q.* 29:19–31, 1958.

23. Gutin, B., Horvath, S. M., and Rochelle, R. D. Physiological response to endurance work as a function of prior exercise. Abstracted in *Med. Sci. Sports* 10:50, 1978.

24. Gutin, B., Stewart, K., Lewis, S., and Kruper, J. Oxygen consumption in the first stages of strenuous work as a function of prior exercise. *J. Sports Med. Phys. Fitness* 16:60–65, 1976.

25. Hetzler, R. K., Knowlton, R. G., Kaminsky, L. A., and Kamimori, G.H. Effect of warm-up on plasma free fatty acid responses and substrate utilization during submaximal exercise. *Res. Q. Exerc. Sport* 57:223–28, 1986.

26. High, D. M., Howley, E. T., and Franks, B. D. The effects of static stretching and warm-up on prevention of delayed-onset muscle soreness. *Res. Q. Exerc. Sport.* 60:357–61, 1989.

27. Hipple, J. Warm-up and fatigue in junior high school sprints. *Res. Q.* 26:246–47, 1955.

28. Inbar, O., and Bar-Or, O. The effects of intermittent warm-up on 7–9 year-old boys. *Eur. J. Appl. Physiol.* 34:81–89, 1975.

29. Kaijser, L. Oxygen supply as a limiting factor in physical performance. In *Limiting Factors of Human Performance,* ed. J. Keul. Stuttgart: G. Thieme, 1973.

30. Lotter, W. S. Effects of fatigue and warm-up on speed of arm movements. *Res. Q.* 30:57–65, 1959.

31. Martin, B. J., Robinson, S., Wiegman, D. L., and Aulick, L. H. Effect of warm-up on metabolic responses to strenuous exercise. *Med. Sci. Sports* 7:146–49, 1975.

32. Massey, B., Johnson, W. R., and Kramer, G. F. Effect of warm-up exercise upon muscular performance using hypnosis to control the psychological variable. *Res. Q.* 32:63–71, 1961.

33. Merlino, L. Influence of massage on jumping performance. *Res. Q.* 30:66–74, 1959.

34. Michael, E., Skubic, V., and Rochelle, R. Effect of warm-up on softball throw for distance. *Res. Q.* 28:357–63, 1957.

35. Morgan, D. W., and Craib, M. Physiological aspects of running economy. *Med. Sci. Sports Exerc.* 24:456–61, 1992.

36. Muido, L. The influence of body temperature on performances in swimming. *Acta Physiol. Scand.* 12:102–9, 1946.

37. Nukada, A. Hauttemperatur und Leistungsfähigkeit in Extremitaten bei statischer Haltearbeit. *Arbeitsphysiologie* 16:74–80, 1955.

38. Nukada, A., and Müller, E. A. Hauttemperatur und Leistungsfahigkeit in Extremitaten bei dynamischer Arbeit. *Arbeitsphysiologie* 16:61–73, 1955.

39. Pacheco, B. A. Improvement in jumping performance due to preliminary exercise. *Res. Q.* 28:55–63, 1957.

40. ———. Effectiveness of warm-up on exercise in junior high school girls. *Res. Q.* 30:202–13, 1959.

41. Phillips, W. H. Influence of fatiguing warm-up exercises on speed of movement and reaction latency. *Res. Q.* 34:370–78, 1963.

42. Richards, D. K. A two-factor theory of the warm-up effect in jumping performance. *Res. Q.* 39:668–73, 1968.

43. Robergs, R. A., Pascoe, D. D., Costill, D. L., Fink, W. J., Chwalbinska-Moneta, J., Davis, J. A., and Hickner, R. Effects of warm-up on muscle glycogenolysis during intense exercise. *Med. Sci. Sports Exerc.* 23:37–43, 1991.

44. Rochelle, R. H., Skubic, V., and Michael, E. Performance as affected by incentive and preliminary warm-up. *Res. Q.* 31:499–504, 1960.

45. Sapega, A. A., Quedenfeld, T. C., Moyer, R. A., and Butler, R. A. Biophysical factors in range of motion exercise. *Physician and Sportsmed.* 9 (Dec.):57–65, 1981.

46. Sedgewick, A. W. Effect of actively increased muscle temperature on local muscular endurance. *Res. Q.* 35:532–38, 1964.

47. Sedgewick, A. W., and Whalen, H. R. Effect of passive warm-up on muscular strength and endurance. *Res. Q.* 35:45–59, 1964.

48. Simonson, E., Teslenko, N., and Gorkin, M. Einfluss von Vorübungen auf die Leistung beim 100 m. lauf. *Arbeitsphysiologie* 9:152–65, 1936.

49. Stamford, B. A., Moffatt, R. J., Weltman, A., Maldonado, C., and Curtis, M. Blood lactate disappearance after supramaximal one-legged exercise. *J. Appl. Physiol.* 45:244–48, 1978.

50. Stamford, B. A., Weltman, A., Moffatt, R., and Sady, S. Exercise recovery above and below anaerobic threshold following maximal work. *J. Appl. Physiol.* 51:840–44, 1981.

51. Thompson, H. Effect of warm-up upon physical performance in selected activities. *Res. Q.* 29:231–46, 1958.

52. Van Huss, W. D., Albrecht, L., Nelson, R., and Hagerman, R. Effect of overload warm-up on the velocity and accuracy of throwing. *Res. Q.* 33:472–75, 1962.

53. Weltman, A., Stamford, B. A., Moffatt, R. J., and Katch, V. L. Exercise recovery, lactate removal and subsequent high intensity exercise performance. *Res. Q.* 48:786–96, 1977.

54. Widimsky, J., Berglund, E., and Malmberg, R. Effect of repeated exercise on the lesser circulation. *J. Appl. Physiol.* 18:983–86, 1963.

28

Environment and Exercise

Physiology of Adaptation to Heat and
    Cold
Exercise in the Cold
    Cold Acclimatization
    Human Limitations in Cold
        Environments
    Effect of Cold on Performance
Exercise in the Heat
    Hot, Dry Environment
    Hot, Humid Environment

Human Limitations in the Heat
    Effects of Age, Gender, and Obesity
Acclimatization to Hot Environments
Fluid and Electrolyte Replacement
Exercise at High Altitudes
    Limitations in Performance at High
        Altitudes
    Acclimatization
    Administration of Oxygen to
        Improve Performance

The efficiency of the human organism in various forms of work or exercise may vary between 15% and 40%. This means that, of the energy consumed, only 15% to 40% is converted into useful work, while the remaining energy (60% to 85%) is wasted as heat energy. This wasted heat energy must be dissipated; otherwise the body temperature will rise unduly. Furthermore, in a hot climate the body also absorbs heat from its environment. These two factors tend to increase the body heat stores and thus increase body temperature.

Physiology of Adaptation to Heat and Cold

There are four means by which the body can maintain thermal balance by losing heat to the environment.

1. **Conduction.** Heat exchange by conduction is accomplished through contact between one substance and another substance. The rate of exchange is determined by the temperature difference between the two substances and by their thermal conductivities. For example, the body loses heat in this manner when submerged in cold water.

2. **Convection.** In convection, heat is transferred by a moving fluid (liquid or gas). Thus in the example of a man submerged in cold water, the heat that is transferred from the body to the water by conduction is carried away from the body by convection (the water that has been warmed rises, making way for new molecules to be heated by conduction, and so on).

3. **Radiation.** The process of heat transfer by means of electromagnetic waves is radiation. These waves can pass through air without imparting much heat to it; however, when they strike a body, their energy is largely transformed into heat. This is the means by which the sun heats the earth, which also explains why one can be perfectly comfortable in air that is below the freezing point if one receives enough solar radiation. (Skiing in high mountains in subtropical latitudes is an example. The air may be cold due to the altitude, yet the sun's declination is such that it transfers considerable radiant heat.)

4. **Evaporation.** Changing a liquid into a gas is called evaporation, or vaporization, and requires large amounts of heat energy. Thus while one kilocalorie can raise the temperature of one liter of water one degree centigrade, it takes 580 kilocalories to evaporate one liter of water at body temperature. These 580 kilocalories are taken from the surroundings. This of course is the principle that underlies the operation of a kitchen refrigerator. Human beings function much as refrigerators when they leave a swimming pool and the atmosphere absorbs the water on their skin.

Thus it seems that people's problems in adjusting to their thermal environment are twofold: 1) heat dissipation in hot climates and 2) heat conservation in cold climates. We can gain heat from two sources: environment and metabolism. We can lose heat from one, two, or more of the following factors: conduction, convection, radiation, and evaporation.

Under normal indoor atmospheric conditions, resting individuals maintain body temperature equilibrium within narrow limits. In this situation heat gain is entirely due to metabolism, and heat loss is estimated to occur approximately 40% by convection, 40% by radiation, and 20% by evaporation (insensible perspiration). Conduction is usually negligible. Input is balanced by output, and body temperature remains constant—at, or close to, 98.6° F. In fact, within the range of about 30°

F to 170° F environmental temperature, the body temperature of a nude human is maintained at a constant temperature within about 1° F of normal resting temperature. This very precise regulatory function is brought about by nervous feedback mechanisms operating through the temperature regulatory center *(thermostat)* in the hypothalamus. The temperature receptors that feed into this thermostat sense the body temperature 1) at the preoptic area of the anterior hypothalamus, 2) in the skin, and 3) probably in some of the internal organs.

When the body temperature is too high, the thermostat in the hypothalamus, having received the error signals from the temperature sensors, increases the rate of heat loss from the body in two principal ways: 1) by stimulating the sweat glands to secrete, which results in evaporative heat losses from the body, and 2) by inhibiting the sympathetic centers in the posterior hypothalamus, thus reducing the vasoconstrictor tone of the arterioles and microcirculation in the skin. This allows vasodilatation of the skin vessels and thus better transport of metabolic heat to the periphery for cooling.

When the body temperature is too low, mechanisms are brought into play to 1) produce more metabolic heat and 2) conserve the heat produced within the body. Heat production is increased by hypothalamic stimulation of 1) shivering, which can increase metabolic rate by two to fourfold, 2) catecholamine release, which increases the rate of cellular oxidation, and 3) the thyroid gland, which increases metabolic rates considerably. Heat conservation is brought about by vasoconstriction of the skin vessels and abolition of the sweating response.

Exercise in the Cold

Excellent reviews of the physiological factors associated with exercise in the cold have been provided by Pate (38), Sutton (48), and Young (52).

Some sports and athletic activities are of necessity carried on in cold environments. Skiing and ice skating depend on snow and ice, and many other sports, such as football and soccer, are occasionally played in very cold weather. A cold environment ordinarily poses few problems for athletes because increased metabolic heat produced by the activity soon warms them to a normal *operating temperature*. Heat dissipation to the atmosphere occurs easily by radiation, convection, and when sweating starts, by evaporation.

The chief problem in this situation is to prevent sudden changes in temperature (chilling). Athletic dress is extremely important, especially when there are intermittent periods of activity and rest (as in football). Athletes must be dressed in attire that 1) keeps them comfortably warm while they are waiting to perform and warming up, and 2) can be removed (in part) after warm-up has been accomplished.

It is possible for metabolic rates to increase by as much as twenty-five to thirty times basal values in very vigorous activity. This means that even in the coldest weather (no wind) an athlete has large heat loads to dissipate if a sport is extremely vigorous. Many athletes sweat profusely even in cold environments, so the clothing worn during actual participation (and after warm-up) should be as light as possible in weight and provide as little barrier to passage of water vapor (sweat) as possible. Otherwise, sweat will accumulate on the skin or in soaked jerseys, thus leading to chilling in the time between the end of exercise and showering.

In winter sports that are less physically active such as hiking, snowmobiling, ice fishing, and so on, metabolic heat contributes less to the body heat and clothing becomes even more important. For short exposure it has been shown that heavily insulating the hands and feet prevents cold discomfort, while overinsulating the hands and feet in comparison with the torso for longer exposures may result in decreasing core temperature and shivering (27). More thermal insulation over the torso than the hands and feet complements the normal physiological heat conservation mechanisms and maintains core temperature. The popular down-filled vest is excellent for this purpose. It has also been found that superficial warming of the hand will stimulate blood flow to it, but blood flow will not return to the foot unless the whole body is sufficiently warm. Therefore, we see again how important torso protection is even for protection of the feet from cold damage (28).

Cold Acclimatization

It is well known that continued exposure to cold environments results in greater ability to withstand cold. However, the physiological adjustments are not yet well defined. The most important factor is the maintenance of *core temperature* (rectal temperature, which reflects the temperature of the central nervous system and deep viscera). Core temperature is maintained at a fairly constant 99° F even though skin temperature may fall from its normal average temperature of 92° F to as low as 60° F.

On the basis of the earlier discussion, it is seen that the body can react to cold 1) by reduction of heat loss and 2) by increased metabolism. When a resting and naked human is cooled from a comfortable environment of 85° F to approximately 72° F, no increase in metabolism occurs, and heat is conserved by vasoconstriction of cutaneous blood vessels that prevents loss of the heat carried by the blood from the core. Below 72° F, increased metabolism results from shivering. The involuntary contraction of the muscles in shivering may raise the metabolic rate from two to four times the resting rate.

For these reasons investigators have looked for changes in basal metabolic rates, peripheral circulation, and skin temperature as indicators of acclimatization. The results are controversial. An increased basal metabolic rate (BMR) of 35% in Korean women who dive for commercial purposes in winter water (temperature 50° F) has been observed (26), and Eskimos have been found to have a higher BMR than Caucasians: 46 kcal/m²·hr⁻¹ compared with 37 kcal/m²·hr⁻¹ (32). However, experiments on personnel during expeditions into antarctic regions have failed to find significant BMR changes.

Local adaptation to cold has been shown in the fishermen of Gaspé Bay, Canada, who gave lower pressor responses to immersion of hands and feet in ice water than did controls (31). It is interesting to note that hypnosis suppressed shivering, lowered the heart rate, and improved vigilance-task performance significantly over the controls during cold exposure at 40° F (29).

It seems likely that adaptation to cold is composed of physiological and psychological factors, and it may well be that the interaction between the two—as well as the type of physiological changes—varies from individual to individual.

Human Limitations in Cold Environments

Ability to withstand cold environments varies widely with individuals. Truly remarkable resistance to cold has been claimed by some of the adherents of religions that practice religious pilgrimages, such as Yoga. In one such pilgrimage, which was observed under scientific conditions (39), a Nepali pilgrim was uninjured by four days of exposure at 15,000 to 17,000 feet, where temperatures ranged between 5° F and 9° F at night, although he wore only light clothing and no shoes or gloves. It was found that his resistance to cold depended upon elevated metabolism.

Table 28.1	The Combined Effect of Wind and Temperature (Wind Chill Factor). Data Supplied by National Safety Council.

Wind Speed MPH	When the Thermometer Reads (degrees Fahrenheit)											
	50	40	30	20	10	0	−10	−20	−30	−40	−50	−60
	the Temperature Equals This in Its Effect on Exposed Flesh											
Calm	50	40	30	20	10	0	−10	−20	−30	−40	−50	−60
5	48	37	27	16	6	−5	−15	−26	−36	−47	−57	−68
10	40	28	16	4	−9	−21	−33	−46	−58	−70	−83	−95
15	36	22	9	−5	−18	−36	−45	−58	−72	−85	−99	−112
20	32	18	4	−10	−25	−39	−53	−67	−82	−96	−110	−121
30	28	13	−2	−18	−33	−48	−63	−79	−94	−109	−125	−140
40	26	10	−6	−21	−37	−53	−69	−85	−100	−116	−132	−148

Little danger if properly clothed	Danger of freezing exposed flesh	Great danger of freezing exposed flesh

From L. A. Brouha, "Effect of Work on the Heart," chapter 21 in *Work and the Heart*, edited by F. F. Rosenbaum and E. L. Belknap, 1959. Reprinted with permission of J. B. Lippincott Company.

Table 28.1 shows the combined effect of wind and temperature, the windchill factor as it is usually called. It can be seen that a temperature of −20° F with no wind is not likely to cause tissue damage (frostbite) for a properly clothed individual. But there is danger of freezing exposed flesh at the same temperature if the wind is blowing 5 to 20 mph and even greater danger with higher winds. Vigorous exercise moderates the windchill factor by virtue of the metabolic heat produced, but it requires a tenfold increase (10 METS) over resting metabolism to maintain thermal balance if the temperature is −20° C with a wind of 9 mph (23).

Body build and tissue proportions are important factors in determining an individual's ability to withstand cold. Other things being equal, the more rotund *(endomorphic)* a person, the less surface area he or she has in relation to volume (mass of tissues). Consequently, heat loss occurs at a slower rate than in a person of angular *(ectomorphic)* build. Furthermore, fat tissue is an excellent insulator against heat loss. These two factors make the round, fat person better able to withstand cold; conversely, the tall, thin person is better able to dissipate heat (and remain cool) in a hot climate.

Effect of Cold on Performance

During maximal exercise if core and muscle temperatures fall below normal, endurance, $\dot{V}O_2$ max, and HR all decrease linearly with decreasing body temperature. In well-trained male subjects, it was shown that $\dot{V}O_2$ max declined by 5% to 6% per degree centigrade decline in core temperature. Time to exhaustion on a cycle ergometer declined by 20% per degree centigrade, and HR declined 8 bpm per degree centigrade (7).

Exercise in the Heat

Exercise in hot climates is a more serious problem than exercise in the cold. In a cold climate the increased metabolic heat production combats the increased heat loss to the environment, but in a hot climate metabolism and environment combine to increase heat gain in body tissues. The problem is further complicated by the fact that when environmental temperature approaches skin temperature (approximately 92° F), heat loss through convection and radiation gradually comes to an end, so that at temperatures above skin temperature the *only* means for heat loss is *evaporation of sweat*. Radiation and convection reverse their direction and add heat to the body.

Sweating, then, is the only avenue for heat loss at temperatures above skin temperature, and it is the most important avenue at temperatures that approach skin temperature. At this point it is most important to understand that the mere process of sweating is not in itself effective in dissipating heat; *liquid sweat must be converted to a gas by evaporation before any heat loss occurs*. Sweat that merely rolls off is virtually ineffective, but large heat losses can result when the weather is so dry that the liquid evaporates from the skin rapidly. Under such conditions sweating is imperceptible. For these reasons, exercise in the heat will be discussed as two separate and distinct environmental problems: hot and dry environment, and hot and humid environment. Recent reviews by Sawka and Young (43), Sutton (48), and Young (52) have provided information concerning the thermoregulatory, cardiovascular, and metabolic factors associated with exercise in hot environments.

Hot, Dry Environment

When a person works or plays in a hot and dry environment, cooling of the skin is brought about by evaporation of sweat. There is no problem because dry air can absorb considerable moisture before becoming saturated. Cooling the skin is not the desired end result, however; it is the *internal environment* that must be cooled at all costs. To retain a normal core temperature, heat must be transported from the core to the skin, and this requires adjustments from the normal, resting circulatory state. As we discussed earlier (chap. 7), the arteriovenous anastomoses of the microcirculation open up, along with precapillary sphincters, to increase flow through the skin and subcutaneous tissues. This results in greater volumes of slow-moving blood in and close to the skin for better transfer of heat to the evaporative surfaces, and thus in better cooling.

Along with the improved cooling, however, the volume of the circulatory system has increased by a considerable amount. Under these conditions, venous return to the heart is somewhat impaired, and this results in a decreased stroke volume (in accord with Starling's law). To maintain a constant cardiac output for the demands of both exercising muscles and skin circulation, the heart rate must increase (42, 50). Because increases in rate depress cardiac efficiency, exercise at temperatures close to or above skin temperature can impose very severe loads on the cardiovascular system, even when the air is relatively dry.

Since the entire process of heat dissipation now depends on elimination of water in perspiration, it is obvious that dehydration is a distinct possibility. How important this factor can be has been pointed out by Adolph (2) and his associates, who note that a man walking in the desert (temperature 100° F) will lose approximately one quart of water per hour. Furthermore, their extensive desert experimentation indicates that voluntary thirst results in adequate water replacement during rest but *not* during work or exercise.

Hot, Humid Environment

When the air surrounding an individual is not only hot but is also loaded with moisture, evaporative cooling is impaired because evaporation cannot take place unless volumes of air are available to take up the water vapor given off. To illustrate this, let us take the extreme example where the air is completely saturated

(100% relative humidity) and the air temperature is higher than the skin temperature. Under these conditions no heat dissipation can occur. Consequently, the metabolic heat accumulates and raises body temperature, until death ensues (108° F to 110° F).

One may therefore conclude that the problems in a hot, dry atmosphere are related to increased cardiovascular loads and dehydration if water intake is insufficient. In a hot, humid climate the same problems exist and are aggravated by a lessened ability to unload water vapor into an already loaded ambient atmosphere. These facts are illustrated in figure 28.1, where the hot, wet environment is 90° F and 85% relative humidity and the hot, dry environment is 100° F and 25% relative humidity—compared with the normal or control environment (room temperature) of 72° F and 42% relative humidity. It is clear that although the temperature is lower in the hot, wet situation, it is considerably more stressful in terms of heart rate response than the hot, dry climate.

Human Limitations in the Heat

Listed below are some problems that can be caused by exercising in the heat with which coaches, trainers, and athletes should be familiar (36).

Heat Stress
The sum of the metabolic and environmental heat loads. The total thermal load is related to the exercise intensity (metabolic load), the environmental temperature, and the evaporative potential of the environment (itself related to the ambient water vapor pressure, or humidity).

Heat Strain
The bodily effect of heat stress, that is, the relative elevation of body core temperature, average skin temperature, and heart rate over that occurring in a cool environment.

Heat Exhaustion
The fatigue that develops during exercise in the heat. This fatigue may be caused by excess body heat, which occurs when the rate of heat loss from the body is not sufficient to balance the body's rate of heat production and/or gain from the environment. Heat exhaustion may also be caused by dehydration, which can lead to an inability to maintain adequate blood flow to the contracting skeletal muscles.

Heat Stroke
A potentially fatal disorder that occasionally follows heat exhaustion. It is characterized by a lack of consciousness (coma) following exertion and by clinical symptoms of damage to the central nervous system, liver, and kidneys.

The combination of hot weather and strenuous physical activity resulted in almost 200 deaths from heat stroke in recruits at training centers in the United States during World War II. In just one summer (1952) there were approximately 600 heat casualties at one Marine Corps recruit training center (33). From August 1959 to October 1962, twelve heat stroke deaths were reported in football players, seven in high school and five in college (18). These statistics do not appear to be improving and show the need for physical educators and coaches to be more familiar with the physiological effects of combinations of heat stress and physical activity.

First, we need to define the problem. Unfortunately, we cannot evaluate the heat stress of any given situation by simply reading the thermometer because, as was pointed out earlier, the transfer of heat into or out of the body depends on the balance of heat gain from metabolism and environment against heat loss to the environment. Thus we need information regarding not only temperature but also humidity, air movement, and heat gain from solar radiation. What is really needed is one index that is sensitive to all of the above factors, giving us an *effective temperature* that tells the whole story of heat stress. Such an index was developed by Yaglou (51) in 1927 and has

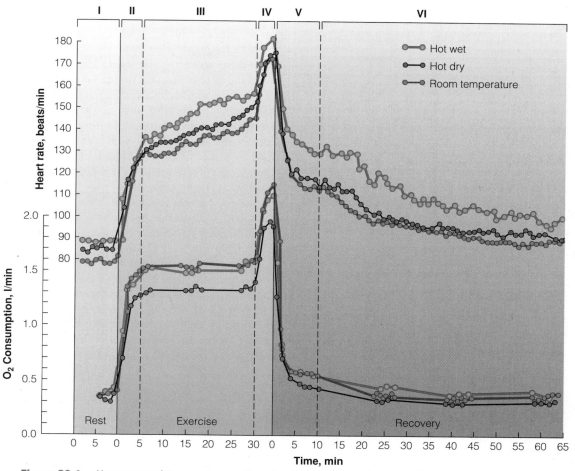

Figure 28.1 Heart rate and oxygen consumption of male subjects pedaling a bicycle ergometer at 540 kgm/min during phases II and III, and at 720 kgm/min during phase IV, in the different environments. (From L. A. Brouha, "Effect of Work on the Heart," chap. 21 in *Work and the Heart,* edited by F. F. Rosenbaum, and E. L. Belknap, Copyright © 1959 Harper & Row Publishers, Inc.)

gained wide usage in industry and in the military. His effective temperature, or ET, was defined as that temperature with 100% relative humidity and still air that brings about an equivalent physiological response to the environment under observation. It was later corrected for radiation effect and was then called *corrected effective temperature,* or CET. Estimation of CET requires the reading of three instruments, *dry bulb, wet bulb,* and *globe* thermometers, plus the necessary calculations. Botsford (8) developed the *wet globe thermometer* (WGT), which exchanges heat with the surroundings by conduction, convection, evaporation, and radiation essentially the same way a perspiring human does (fig. 28.2). So one reading of the temperature of the globe without further calculation (WGT) provides a

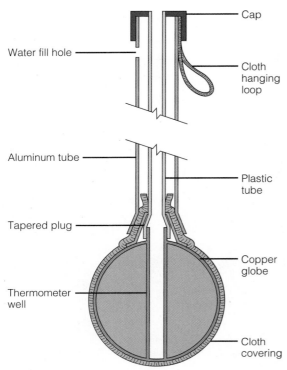

Water fill hole

Cap

Cloth hanging loop

Aluminum tube

Plastic tube

Tapered plug

Copper globe

Thermometer well

Cloth covering

Figure 28.2   Sectional sketch showing construction of the wet globe thermometer (not to scale). (From Botsford, J. H., in *American Industrial Hygiene Association Journal* 32:1. © 1971 American Industrial Hygiene Association. Reprinted by permission.)

comprehensive measure of the cooling capacity of the work environment.* This instrument provides a simple readout and consequently should be placed in every institution where heat stress can conceivably become a problem in conducting physical education or athletics. Figure 28.3 shows Botsford's compilation of data for maximal allowable WGT at various metabolic rates with deVries's extrapolations to caloric value of various athletic activities.

Recently a similar instrument has come on the market that makes the same measurements and in addition provides an electrical output for recording purposes (25).†

One note of caution should be added. All of the data on which figure 28.3 is based were taken on subjects who wore no artificial barriers to vapor loss during sweating. The uniform worn by football players creates a great load by virtue of its weight and, more important, it cuts off about 50% of the player's evaporative surface area. This was shown to increase the sweat loss by 78%. Thus the uniform both adds to the metabolic heat load and simultaneously prevents transfer of the heat away from the body (18).

To emphasize this point, deVries has used the temperature and humidity data relating to the football heat stroke deaths reported by Fox and coworkers (18) to estimate the WGT at the time of each football fatality. Since only temperature and humidity were available, the estimates were based on an 8-mph breeze and no radiant effect.

Figure 28.3 suggests a maximal WGT of about 64° F for a metabolic rate of 2,000 Btu/hr, which probably is a good approximation of the metabolic rate during football. But table 28.2 shows that only two of the nine fatalities occurred above that level of heat stress. This suggests 1) that the heat stress was considerably greater for uniformed football players than for equivalent metabolic levels of lightly clothed individuals, from whom the data were taken, and 2) that the data of figure 28.3 must be used very conservatively with respect to football players.

The feasibility of reducing heat stress casualties through enlightened control of activity when heat loads are hazardous has been shown in the Marine Corps recruit training program

---

*This instrument is now commercially available from Howard Engineering Co., P.O. Box 3164, Bethlehem, PA 18017

---

†This instrument is called the Reuter-Stokes RSS-211D heat stress monitor and is available from Reuter-Stokes, Cambridge, Ontario, Canada.

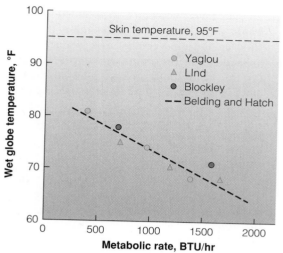

Figure 28.3   Maximum wet globe temperatures for continuous work according to various authorities. Approximate metabolic rates would be about 500 Btu or 125 kcal/hr for standing at ease, 1,000 Btu or 250 kcal for light calisthenics, 1,500 Btu or 375 kcal for playing singles tennis, and 2,000 Btu or 500 kcal for heavy activity in football, basketball, or handball. (From Botsford, J. H., in *American Industrial Hygiene Association Journal* 32:1. © 1971 American Industrial Hygiene Association. Reprinted by permission.)

(33). They reduced the weekly heat casualty rate from 12.4 to 4.7 per 10,000 recruits by instituting a program involving the following precautions:

1. Curtailed activity when heat loads are high.
2. A gradual breaking-in period for the first week or two.
3. Increased emphasis on physical fitness.
4. Allowing water ad libitum.
5. Replacement of salt.
6. Loosening of uniform regulations to allow T-shirts and so on.

Listed below are some practical considerations for reducing the likelihood of heat-related illnesses (36).

Education

It is important to understand that the heat produced during exercise cannot be readily dissipated from the body in a hot and/or humid environment. Exercise intensity should be moderated in the heat.

Table 28.2	Estimations of the ET and WGT at the Time of Each Football Fatality				
Football Fatality	**Dry Bulb Temp °F**	**Wet Bulb Temp °F**	**Relative Humidity**	**Effective Temp (ET)**	**Wet Globe Temp (WGT)**
1	64	64	100%	52	52
2	90	75	50	77	67
3	85	76	62	74	64
4	75	67	75	63	59
5	82	73	68	71	62
6	85	71	50	72	63
7	83	72	60	71	62
8	93	76	45	79	68
9	81	75	78	71	62

From E. L. Fox et al. *Research Quarterly* 37:333, 1966.

Clothing

Clothing adds insulation to the body and reduces the effective surface area for heat transfer. It is important to minimize clothing to provide an optimal skin surface area from which evaporation can occur.

Hydration

Progressive dehydration reduces sweating and blood flow to the skin and leads to excessive body heating. It is essential to keep well hydrated before, during, and following exercise in the heat.

Fitness

Physical training and heat accumulation can expand blood volume and provide a more sensitive heat dissipation response to an increase in body core temperature. The majority of heat illness victims are novice runners, the elderly, and those with circulatory or respiratory disorders. These are people who have become unfit by choice or due to an inability to remain active. People at risk should avoid extremes of heat or activity.

This area of concern is so important that the American College of Sports Medicine has seen fit to issue a position statement regarding distance running in the heat (table 28.3).

Effects of Age, Gender, and Obesity

Age

It has been shown that prepubertal girls (17, 21) and prepubertal boys (6, 24) have less tolerance for exercise in the heat than do adults. This appears to be true even when subjects are matched for aerobic power and working at the same proportion of their maximal capacity (17). There is also evidence that elderly people do not respond as well to heat exposure as do young people (16, 46). Although there seems little doubt that children and older adults are more susceptible to heat stress, the physiological mechanisms responsible for their lower

tolerance are not fully understood. Drinkwater and Horvath (16) suggest that for children the greater heat risk is due to the instability of an immature cardiovascular system, while for the elderly the problem is more likely related to their decreased aerobic capacity.

Gender

Earlier work suggested that at all ages females are less heat tolerant than are males (24, 46). However, recent studies have shown that there are few differences in male and female responses to heat stress when they are matched for $\dot{V}O_2$ max. Therefore it seems that the earlier work largely reflected lower fitness levels in the women (4, 24, 45). However, there are gender differences in that females tolerate hot-wet climates better than males, while males tolerate hot-dry conditions better than females (45). This finding is largely explained by the fact that, on the average, females have a higher ratio of body surface area to weight. This is an advantage in hot-wet climates but a disadvantage under hot-dry conditions. This is so because heat production is mainly weight dependent, whereas heat dissipation is related to the skin surface area. Since evaporation is not a factor in a hot-wet environment, the more surface area available for radiation and convection losses in relation to heat production, the better the adjustment. In hot-dry conditions, a high ratio of surface area to weight is disadvantageous because it allows more heat gain by convection and radiation. During distance road races the incidence of heat illness is about the same in men and women (24).

Obesity

As might be expected, exercise in the heat is more stressful for the obese than the lean individual (22, 24). This can be explained on a simple dimensional basis. Heat production is related to the *volume* of metabolizing tissue, which is a cubic function. The ability to dispose of the heat is related to the skin surface *area,* which is only a square function. Therefore the rounder (the more endomorphic) an individual becomes, the greater the difference in growth of volume in proportion to skin area and the poorer the capacity for heat dissipation.

Acclimatization to Hot Environments

In these days of rapid transportation, individual athletes and whole teams frequently travel far enough for their competitions to encounter a severe climatic change. Going from a cold to a hot climate will bring about a considerable decrement in performance if the event involves heavy demands on the cardiovascular system.

For these reasons, coaches and exercise physiologists have explored the possibility of bringing about improved heat tolerance by physical conditioning in a normally cool environment. Considerable controversy has arisen concerning the possible magnitude of such an acclimatization procedure, but there is little doubt that heat tolerance can be improved to some extent by conditioning alone. Thus appropriate conditioning can improve the function of the sweating mechanism and expand the plasma volume (44). Also the sensitivity of the sweating response is increased, so the sweating occurs at lower skin and core temperatures. Thus the trained individual stores less heat in the transient phase of starting to exercise in the heat, arrives at a thermal steady state sooner, and maintains a lower internal temperature at equilibrium (34). In the long term then, the results of physical conditioning for heat acclimatization per se are cooler skin and core temperatures, which in turn reduce the level of skin blood flow needed for regulation of body temperature (41). This results in a greater portion of the cardiac output being available to muscle blood flow, which is what improves performance in the heat.

The controversy concerning the magnitude of the acclimatization effect through training in a cool environment has probably resulted from three factors: 1) inadequate controls of the physical characteristics of subjects by some investigators, 2) differences in the heat tolerance tests used, and 3) differences in the intensity and duration of training used (20).

When these problems are resolved, there appears to be reasonable agreement that the best improvement in heat tolerance results from intensive interval or continuous training at intensities greater than 50% $\dot{V}O_2$ max for eight to twelve weeks (20, 37). Utilization of such procedures appears to produce about 50% of the total adjustment resulting from actual heat acclimatization (37). This is true for women as well as men (9).

Thus the evidence seems clear. When competition is scheduled for a different, hot climate, artificial acclimatization is a must for preventing serious decrements in performance. This can be accomplished by progressively increasing workouts in an artificial hot room over four or five days.

Even after full acclimatization has been brought about, two other precautions should be followed for maintaining optimum health and performance in hot climates. First, and most important, athletes must maintain adequate intakes of water. The simplest way to check this is by recording weight records under consistent conditions. Dehydration shows up quickly as a loss in weight, and any weight loss of more than two or three pounds should be corrected by encouraging fluid consumption. Second, athletes should be encouraged to decrease the protein in their diet because the specific dynamic action of protein digestion causes more heat formation than the other foodstuffs. Inclusion of more foods with high water and mineral content, such as fruits and salads, is also advisable. Evidence (30) also suggests that ingestion of 250 to 500 mg of vitamin C daily increases heat tolerance.

Table 28.3	The American College of Sports Medicine Position Stand on Prevention of Heat Injuries During Distance Running

Position Stand

It is the position of the American College of Sports Medicine that the following RECOMMENDATIONS be employed by directors of distance runs or community fun runs.

1. **Medical Director**

   A medical director knowledgeable in exercise physiology and sports medicine should coordinate the preventive and therapeutic aspects of the running event and work closely with the race director.

2. **Race Organization**

   a. Races should be organized to avoid the hottest summer months and the hottest part of the day. As there are great regional variations in environmental conditions, the local weather history will be most helpful in scheduling an event to avoid times when an unacceptable level of heat stress is likely to prevail. Organizers should be cautious of unseasonably hot days in the early spring, as entrants will almost certainly not be heat acclimatized.

   b. The environmental heat stress prediction for the day should be obtained from the meteorological service. It can be measured as wet bulb globe temperature (WBGT), which is a temperature/humidity/radiation index. If WBGT is above 28° C (82° F), consideration should be given to rescheduling or delaying the race until safer conditions prevail. If below 28° C, participants may be alerted to the degree of heat stress by using color-coded flags at the start of the race and at key positions along the course.

   c. All summer events should be scheduled for the early morning, ideally before 8:00 A.M., or in the evening after 6:00 P.M., to minimize solar radiation.

   d. An adequate supply of water should be available before the race and every 2 to 3 km during the race. Runners should be encouraged to consume 100 to 200 ml at each station.

   e. Race officials should be educated as to the warning signs of an impending collapse. Each official should wear an identifiable arm band or badge and should warn runners to stop if they appear to be in difficulty.

   f. Adequate traffic and crowd control must be maintained at all times.

   g. There should be a ready source of radio communications from various points on the course to a central organizing point to coordinate responses to emergencies.

3. **Medical Support**

   a. **Medical Organization**

   The Medical Director should alert local hospitals and ambulance services to the event and should make prior arrangements with medical personnel for the care of casualties, especially those suffering from heat injury. The mere fact that an entrant signs a waiver in no way absolves the organizers of moral and/or legal responsibility. Medical personnel supervising races should have the authority to evaluate, examine, and/or stop a runner who displays the symptoms and signs of impending heat injury, or who appears to be mentally and/or physically out of control for any other reason.

b. Medical Facilities

    i. Medical support staff and facilities should be available at the race site.

    ii. The facilities should be staffed with personnel capable of instituting immediate and appropriate resuscitation measures. Apart from the routine resuscitation equipment, ice packs and fans for cooling are required.

    iii. Persons trained in first aid, appropriately identified with an arm band, badge, etc., should be stationed along the course to warn runners to stop if they exhibit signs of impending heat injury.

    iv. Ambulances or vans with accompanying medical personnel should be available along the course.

    v. Although the emphasis in this stand has been on the management of hyperthermia, on cold, wet, and windy days athletes may be chilled and require "space blankets," blankets, and warm drinks at the finish to prevent or treat hypothermia.

4. Competitor Education

The education of fun runners has increased greatly in recent years, but race organizers must not assume that all participants are well informed or prepared. Distributing guidelines at the preregistration, publicity in the press, and holding clinics/seminars before runs are valuable.

The following persons are particularly prone to heat illness: the obese, unfit, dehydrated, those unacclimatized to the heat, those with a previous history of heat stroke, and anyone who runs while ill. Children perspire less than adults and have a lower heat tolerance. Based on the above information, all participants should be advised of the following.

a. Adequate training and fitness are important for full enjoyment of the run and also to prevent heat-related injuries.

b. Prior training in the heat will promote heat acclimatization and thereby reduce the risk of heat injury. It is wise to do as much training as possible at the time of day at which the race will be held.

c. Fluid consumption before and during the race will reduce the risk of heat injury, particularly in longer runs such as the marathon.

d. Illness prior to or at the time of the event should preclude competition.

e. Participants should be advised of the early symptoms of heat injury. These include clumsiness, stumbling, excessive sweating (and also cessation of sweating), headache, nausea, dizziness, apathy, and any gradual impairment of consciousness.

f. Participants should be advised to choose a comfortable speed and not to run faster than conditions warrant.

g. Participants are advised to run with a partner, each being responsible for the other's well-being.

Fluid and Electrolyte Replacement

We are indebted to Costill and his coworkers at Ball State University for considerably improving our understanding of the needs for fluid and electrolyte replacement in athletes who must train or compete in the heat.

Until very recently, it had been believed that the loss of electrolytes such as sodium, potassium, and chloride in heavy sweating had to be replaced by taking salt pills or using various "athletic drinks" that included these electrolytes in their makeup. However, Costill and colleagues (11) have shown that such practice is of minimal value for athletes who are losing water at a rate of 3% of body weight daily or less, if they are permitted to eat and drink ad libitum. Work by Dressendorfer and coworkers supports these findings (15). However, in some occupational and athletic situations, it is possible to lose more than 8% of body weight by heavy sweating, and it seems unlikely that such losses could be replaced without electrolyte supplementation. Losses of fluids and electrolytes up to 3% body weight are made up by normal mineral ingestion in food, together with a greatly reduced rate of excretion by the kidneys and the formation of a hypotonic sweat (much lower salt concentration).

Another important fact is that little exchange of water occurs in the stomach, and therefore the rate of movement of fluids from the stomach to the intestine is very important in fluid replacement. Many factors can affect the rate of gastric emptying, the more important being the volume, temperature, and sugar content of the drink. Costill and Saltin (12) showed that a drink volume of about 400 to 600 ml leaves the stomach more rapidly than smaller volumes and that a cold drink (5° C) leaves more rapidly than a warm one (35° C).

Most important, they found that heavily sugared drinks in combination with high-intensity exercise (over 70% $\dot{V}O_2$ max) may combine to block gastric emptying. It should be realized, however, that relative needs for fluids and carbohydrates vary greatly with the athletic event and climatic conditions. In mild exercise in severe heat, fluid replacement is the major concern, and therefore the sugar should be minimized to assure good gastric emptying. But in very heavy exercise over long durations in a cool environment (for example, distance running), maintaining the energy stores may become more important than gastric emptying rate if dehydration is no longer a problem.

These findings seem to cast considerable doubt on the value of the commercially available athletic drinks. A direct comparison of three of the more popular drink brands against plain water showed that none was as effective in gastric emptying as water and one that was heavily sugared significantly slowed gastric emptying (13). Recently, however, Nadel (35) has stated "Rehydration will occur more rapidly when beverages containing sodium—the major electrolyte lost in sweat—are consumed. Ingesting a beverage containing sodium allows the plasma sodium to remain elevated during the rehydration period and helps maintain thirst while delaying stimulation of urine production. The rehydration beverage should also contain glucose or sucrose because these carbohydrates provide a source of energy for working muscles, stimulate fluid absorption in the gut, and improve beverage taste." Furthermore, Gisolfi (19), has stated "the presence of glucose in a sport drink significantly enhances fluid absorption from the lumen of the small intestine; however, sodium must be present in the intestinal lumen for glucose transport to occur."

Costill suggests the following guidelines for hot weather competition and training (10):

1. *Hot-weather competition*—Use cold, palatable drinks in volumes of 3 to 10

ounces that are low in sugar concentration (less than 2.5 gm/100 ml of water).

2. *Precompetition*—Drink 13.5 to 20 ounces (two to three glasses) of the above drink thirty minutes before the competition starts.

3. *During competition*—Drink 3 to 6 ounces at ten- to fifteen-minute intervals.

4. *Postcompetition*—Salt foods moderately and use fruit juices such as orange juice and tomato juice to replace electrolytes lost in sweat.

More recent recommendations by Nadel (35) are generally consistent with those of Costill and provide additional guidelines to help athletes maintain proper hydration during practice and competition in hot weather.

1. Weigh in without clothes before and after exercise, especially during hot weather. For each pound of body weight lost during exercise, drink 2 cups of fluid.

2. Drink a rehydration beverage containing sodium to quickly replenish lost body fluids. The beverage should also contain 6% to 8% glucose or sucrose.

3. Drink 2.5 cups of fluid two hours before practice or competition.

4. Drink 1.5 cups of fluid fifteen minutes before the event.

5. Drink at least 1 cup of fluid every fifteen to twenty minutes during training and competition.

6. Do not restrict fluids before or during an event.

7. Avoid beverages containing caffeine and alcohol because they increase urine production and add to dehydration.

Use of the above guidelines should protect the athlete who must train or compete in the heat.

Exercise at High Altitudes

Our travels to find athletic competition often involve not only changes in temperature and humidity but large changes in altitude as well. It has been known since the turn of the century and the advent of aviation that whenever humans ascend to higher altitudes they encounter lower atmospheric pressures. Because oxygen maintains a constant 20.93% of decreasing total pressure regardless of altitude, a gradually decreasing partial pressure drives oxygen into the blood. This decreasing availability of oxygen to the tissues would be expected to hamper physical performance, and indeed it does.

The O_2 saturation of arterial blood at sea level approaches 100%, even under conditions of exercise. But at 19,000 feet saturation is only 67% at rest, and exercise at this altitude may drop the value below 50% (49). We do not have to go to this extreme altitude, however, to find changes that may be of great importance in athletic competition. At 3,000 feet even acclimatized subjects have lost 5% of their aerobic power, and at 6,500 feet 15% (3). More recent data by Squires and Buskirk are in close agreement (47).

This decreased aerobic power (maximum O_2 consumption) is brought about by a combination of factors, probably the most important of which are reduction in O_2 saturation of arterial blood, decreased cardiac output, and the higher cost of increased lung ventilation. The impaired lung diffusion is the result of the lowered O_2 pressure gradient. The decreased cardiac output is undoubtedly due to the hypoxic myocardium. The lung ventilation is increased progressively with altitude. All this results from the necessity of breathing more air to attempt to get the same number of molecules of O_2. The increased effort of the respiratory muscles increases their O_2 consumption and lowers their efficiency. Recent reviews (40, 43, 48, 52) have described various aspects of exercise at altitude.

Limitations in Performance at High Altitudes

Not all athletic performances suffer because of the hypoxia of higher altitudes. Obviously, athletes participating in *one maximal effort* activities, such as the shot put, long jump, and high jump, do not suffer because they do not depend on O_2 transport. Furthermore, events of less than one minute's duration, such as the 100- and 220-yard dashes, are also performed very largely anaerobically. Consequently performances are unimpaired, but recovery times are longer.

In any event that lasts one minute or more aerobic power is more important, and this importance increases as duration increases (fig. 22.8). Considerable losses in performance may be expected in such events unless athletes have had adequate time for acclimatization.

Acclimatization

The need for artificially increasing the available oxygen at higher altitudes has been recognized by the Federal Aviation Authority. In aircraft that are not pressurized, regulations require breathing *aviator's oxygen* at altitudes above 12,500 feet. Experiments in low-pressure chambers (to simulate high altitude) have shown that without additional oxygen the average individual may remain conscious *at rest* (with varying degrees of impairment) for about thirty minutes at 18,000 feet but for one minute or less at 30,000 feet. Exercise would obviously shorten these times greatly.

On the other hand, human ability to adjust to higher environments over a period of time is truly phenomenal. It was reported (5) that a member of the 1924 British Mount Everest expedition reached an altitude of 28,126 feet without oxygen equipment. Since then other climbers have accomplished this feat.

The acclimatizing process can be accomplished by various systems of physical conditioning and at progressively higher altitudes if possible. If altitude cannot be increased systematically, a progressive conditioning program at the *game altitude* is undertaken in which cardiorespiratory endurance is gradually improved by progressively increasing demands.

Altitudes below 3,000 feet probably require no acclimatization, the problem is slight up to about 5,000 feet, and the problem of altitude is only academic above 10,000 feet since no serious competition occurs above that level. The area of concern for physical education and athletics in the United States is really for altitudes between 5,000 and 10,000 feet.

D. B. Dill (14) has provided evidence that suggests that the physiological adaptation to altitude occurs in four phases:

1. The *acute phase*—In the first thirty minutes of exposure to the altitudes of concern here the loss in maximal O_2 consumption and consequently in performances that depend on aerobic power is less than 10%.

2. The *second phase*—Decrements may be from 20% to 30% (in one to three days).

3. The *third phase*—Adaptation to the decrements of phase two requires several weeks.

4. The *fourth phase*—Adaptation depends on the increase of red blood cell volume, which reaches a maximum in about a year or more.

Over a period of years it is eventually possible to achieve sea level performance up to as high as 13,200 feet. Above 17,500 feet there is only deterioration, and no adaptation seems to occur. This represents a schema (fig. 28.4) that varies widely from individual to individual with respect to both rate and capacity for adaptation to altitude.

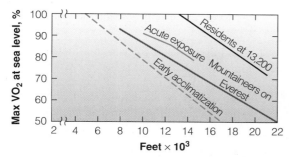

Figure 28.4   Decrement in capacity for supplying oxygen to tissues, $\dot{V}O_2$ max, at four stages of acclimatization. (From Dill, D. B., in *Journal of the American Medical Association* 250:753. © 1968 American Medical Association. Reprinted by permission.)

Thus the coach whose athletes will compete at a site such as Mexico City at an altitude of 7,350 feet is faced with the choice of timing his or her trip to compete within minutes of arrival (impossible) or to arrive several weeks early to allow time for acclimatization (also usually impossible, except for the fortunate few in Olympic competition). Possibly the only real solutions are for flatlanders to limit their interscholastic competitions to other flatlanders or to accept the alternative of a predictable loss of performance in aerobic events.

The physiological mechanisms that bring about acclimatization have been well demonstrated, at least in part. Increases of 10% to 50% in the number of erythrocytes and in the hemoglobin content of the blood have been reported. Ability to increase the maximum ventilation rate has also been demonstrated, and there is a possibility that vascularization of lung and muscle tissue is also improved.

Administration of Oxygen to Improve Performance

There seems to be no evidence that breathing enriched mixtures of O_2 *before* an athletic event has a significant effect on the subsequent performance. Use of O_2 *during* work at high altitudes, however, is not only advantageous but absolutely necessary—at 18,000 to 20,000 feet—for most people without a long acclimatization period. (This, of course, is of no practical value for athletics.)

One use of O_2 for athletes that rests on sound theoretical and experimental bases is for shortening recovery times at altitude. In sports that involve rest periods between heavy endurance workouts, such as basketball and soccer, repayment of the O_2 debt can be hastened in unacclimatized athletes who have competed at an altitude substantially higher than the altitude they are used to.

Summary

1. Constant human body temperature is maintained by striking a balance between heat gain and heat loss. Heat gain is due to metabolism and also to gains from radiation and convection when environmental temperatures are above skin temperature (92° F). Heat loss occurs by *conduction, radiation, convection,* and *evaporation* at temperatures below skin temperature, and by *evaporation* only when the environmental temperature is greater than skin temperature.

2. In vigorous athletic events metabolic heat maintains an athlete's *core temperature* in all but the most severe cold.

3. The most serious problem for athletes in cold environments is having enough flexibility in dress to bring about heat retention during warm-up and rest periods and yet allow heat dissipation during competitive periods.

4. Cold acclimatization is probably brought about through a combination of physiological and psychological factors. The most important physiological factors seem to be an increased metabolic rate and a greater

temperature gradient between core and skin temperatures.

5. In hot, dry environments the ability to adjust to the severely increased cardiovascular load is most critically limited by *dehydration.*

6. In hot, wet environments the ability to adjust to the severely increased cardiovascular load is most critically limited by rising body core temperature due to inability to dissipate heat by evaporation.

7. For both hot and dry and hot and wet environments, acclimatization can be brought about by progressively increasing workouts in an artificial hot room over four or five days. This acclimatization will persist at least three weeks in cold weather.

8. Water replacement schedules should be set up to achieve both early replacement and overhydration to maintain performance at its highest level.

9. Exercise or competitive sport performance at altitudes higher by 3,000 feet or more than the home environment will be noticeably impaired by hypoxia if the activity depends largely upon aerobic energy (of one minute or greater duration).

10. Physiological adaptation to altitude appears to follow a time course of four phases: a) during the acute phase of up to thirty minutes, performance is not greatly affected (up to 10% at 10,000 feet); b) in one to three days performance falls off more severely; c) over several weeks, acclimatization brings performance back to that of phase one; d) red blood cell volume increases over a period of months, reaching its maximum after a year or more, with commensurate improvement in performance and eventual return to

sea level performance at altitudes up to 13,200 feet.

11. Administration of oxygen to athletes at high altitudes should result in faster recovery times, but its use before an event cannot be expected to bring about large changes in performance.

References

1. ACSM position stand on prevention of thermal injuries during distance running. *Med. Sci. Sports Exer.* 16(5):IX–XIV, 1984.

2. Adolph, E. F. *Physiology of Man in the Desert.* New York: Interscience Publishers, 1947.

3. Astrand, P-O. Physiological aspects of cross-country skiing at the high altitudes. *J. Sports Med. Phys. Fitness* 3:51–52, 1963.

4. Avellini, B. A., Kamon, E., and Krajewski, J. T. Physiological responses of physically fit men and women to acclimation to humid heat. *J. Appl. Physiol.* 49:254–61, 1980.

5. Balke, B. Work capacity at altitude. In *Science and Medicine of Exercise and Sports,* ed. W. R. Johnson, chap. 18. New York: Harper & Row, 1960.

6. Bar-Or, O., Dotan, R., Inbar, O., Rotshtein, A., and Zonder, H. Voluntary hypohydration in 10–12-year-old boys. *J. Appl. Physiol.* 48:104–8, 1980.

7. Bergh, U., and Ekblom, B. Physical performance and peak aerobic power at different body temperatures. *J. Appl. Physiol.* 46:885–89, 1979.

8. Botsford, J. H. A wet globe thermometer for environmental heat measurement. *Am. Ind. Hyg. Assoc. J.* 32:1–10, 1971.

9. Cohen, J. S., and Gisolfi, C. V. Effects of interval training on work-heat tolerance of young women. *Med. Sci. Sports Exer.* 14:46–52, 1982.

10. Costill, D. L. Fluids for athletic performance: Why and what should you drink during prolonged exercise. In *Toward Understanding Human Performance,* ed. E. J. Burke. Ithaca, N.Y.: Mouvement Publications, 1977.

11. Costill, D. L., Cote, R., Miller, E., Miller, T., and Wynder, S. Water and electrolyte replacement during repeated days of work in the heat. *Aviat. Space Environ. Med.* 46:795–800, 1975.

12. Costill, D. L., and Saltin, B. Factors limiting gastric emptying during rest and exercise. *J. Appl. Physiol.* 37:678–83, 1974.

13. Coyle, E. F., Costill, D. L., Fink, W. J., and Hoopes, D. G. Gastric emptying rates for selected athletic drinks. *Res. Q.* 49:119–24, 1978.

14. Dill, D. B. Physiological adjustments to altitude changes. *J.A.M.A.* 205:123–30, 1968.

15. Dressendorfer, R. H., Wade, C. E., Keen, C. L., and Scaff, J. H. Plasma mineral levels in marathon runners during a 20-day road race. *Physician and Sportsmed.* 10 (June):113–18, 1982.

16. Drinkwater, B. L., and Horvath, S. M. Heat tolerance and aging. *Med. Sci. Sports* 11:49–55, 1979.

17. Drinkwater, B. L., Kupprat, I. C., Denton, J. E., Crist, J. L., and Horvath, S. M. Response of prepubertal girls and college women to work in the heat. *J. Appl. Physiol.* 43:1046–53, 1977.

18. Fox, E. L., Mathews, D. K., Kaufman, W. S., and Bowers, R. W. Effects of football equipment on thermal balance and energy cost during exercise. *Res. Q.* 37:332–39, 1966.

19. Gisolfi, C. V. Exercise, intestinal absorption, and rehydration. *Gatorade Sports Sci. Exch.* 4(32), 1991.

20. Gisolfi, C. V., and Cohen, J. S. Relationships among training, heat acclimatization and heat tolerance in men and women: The controversy revisited. *Med. Sci. Sports* 11:56–59, 1979.

21. Haymes, E. M. Physiological responses of female athletes to heat stress: A review. *Physician and Sportsmed.* 12 (March):45–59, 1984.

22. Haymes, E. M., Buskirk, E. R., Hodgson, J. L., Lundegren, H. M., and Nicholas, W. C. Heat tolerance of exercising lean and heavy prepubertal girls. *J. Appl. Physiol.* 36:566–71, 1974.

23. Haymes, E. M., Dickinson, A. L., Malville, N., and Ross, R. W. Effects of wind on the thermal and metabolic responses to exercise in the cold. *Med. Sci. Sports Exer.* 14:41–45, 1982.

24. Haymes, E. M., McCormick, R. J., and Buskirk, E. R. Heat tolerance of exercising lean and obese prepubertal boys. *J. Appl. Physiol.* 39:457–61, 1975.

25. Hughson, R. L., Staudt, L. A., and Mackie, J. M. Monitoring road racing in the heat. *Physician and Sportsmed.* 11 (May):94–105, 1983.

26. Kang, B. S., Song, S. H., Suh, C. S., and Hong, S. K. Changes in body temperature and basal metabolic rate of the ama. *J. Appl. Physiol.* 18:483–88, 1963.

27. Kaufman, W. C. Cold-weather clothing for comfort or heat conservation. *Physician and Sportsmed.* 10 (Feb.): 71–75, 1982.

28. ———. The hand and foot in the cold. *Physician and Sportsmed.* 11 (Feb.):156–68, 1983.

29. Kissen, A. T., Reifler, C. B., and Thaler, V. H. Modification of thermoregulatory responses to cold by hypnosis. *J. Appl. Physiol.* 19:1043–50, 1964.

30. Kotze, H. F., van der Walt, W. H., Rogers, G. G., and Strydom, N. B. Effects of plasma ascorbic acid levels on heat acclimatization in man. *J. Appl. Physiol.* 42:711–16, 1977.

31. LeBlanc, J. Local adaptation to cold of Gaspé fishermen. *J. Appl. Physiol.* 17:950–52, 1962.

32. Milan, F. A., Hannon, J. P., and Evonuk, E. Temperature regulation of Eskimos, Indians, and Caucasians in a bath calorimeter. *J. Appl. Physiol.* 18: 378–82, 1962.

33. Minard, D. Prevention of heat casualties in Marine Corps recruits. *Milit. Med.* 126:261–72, 1961.

34. Nadel, E. R. Control of sweating rate while exercising in the heat. *Med. Sci. Sports* 11:31–35, 1979.

35. Nadel, E. R. New ideas for rehydration during and after exercise in hot weather. *Gatorade Sports Sci. Exch.* 1(3), 1988.

36. Nadel, E. R. Limits imposed on exercise in a hot environment. *Gatorade Sports Sci. Exch.* 3(27), 1990.

37. Pandolf, K. B. Effects of physical training and cardiorespiratory physical fitness on exercise-heat tolerance: Recent observations. *Med. Sci. Sports* 11:60–65, 1979.

38. Pate, R. R. Special considerations for exercise in cold weather. *Gatorade Sports Sci. Exch.* 1(10), 1988.

39. Pugh, L.G.C.E. Tolerance to extreme cold at altitude in a Nepalese pilgrim. *J. Appl. Physiol.* 18:1234–38, 1963.

40. Reeves, J. T., Wolfel, E. E., Green, H. J., Mazzeo, R. S., Young, A. J., Sutton, J. R., and Brooks, G. A. Oxygen transport during exercise at altitude and the lactate paradox: Lessons from Operation Everest II and Pikes Peak. In *Exercise and Sport Sciences Reviews,* ed. J.O. Holloszy, Baltimore: Williams and Wilkins, pp. 275-96, 1992.

41. Roberts, M. F., and Wenger, C. B. Control of skin circulation during exercise and heat stress. *Med. Sci. Sports* 11:36–41, 1979.

42. Saltin, B. Circulatory response to submaximal and maximal exercise after thermal dehydration. *J. Appl. Physiol.* 19:1125–32, 1964.

43. Sawka, M. N., and Young, A. J. Acute polycythemia and human performance during exercise and exposure to extreme environments. In *Exercise and Sport Sciences Reviews,* ed. K. B. Pandolf, Baltimore: Williams and Wilkins, pp. 265-93, 1989.

44. Senay, L. C. Effects of exercise in the heat on body fluid distribution. *Med. Sci. Sports* 11:42–48, 1979.

45. Shapiro, Y., Pandolf, K. B., Avellini, B. A., Pimental, N. A., and Goldman, R. F. Physiological responses of men and women to humid and dry heat. *J. Appl. Physiol.* 49:1–8, 1980.

46. Shoenfeld, Y., Udassin, R., Shapiro, Y., Ohri, A., and Sohar, E. Age and sex differences in response to short exposure to extreme dry heat. *J. Appl. Physiol.* 44:1–4, 1978.

47. Squires, R. W., and Buskirk, E. R. Aerobic capacity during acute exposure to simulated altitude, 914 to 2286 meters. *Med. Sci. Sports Exer.* 14:36–40, 1982.

48. Sutton, J. R. Exercise and the environment. In *Exercise, Fitness, and Health,* ed. C. Bouchard, R. J. Shepard, T. Stephens, J. R. Sutton, and B. D. McPherson, Champaign, IL: Human Kinetics Books, pp. 165–83, 1990.

49. West, J. B., Lahiri, S., Gill, M. B., Milledge, J. S., Pugh, L.G.C.E., and Ward, M.P. Arterial oxygen saturation during exercise at high altitude. *J. Appl. Physiol.* 17:617–21, 1962.

50. Williams, C. G., Bredell, G. A. G., Wyndham, C. H., Strydom, N. B., Morrison, J. F., Peter, J., Fleming, P. W., and Ward, J. S. Circulatory and metabolic reactions to work in the heat. *J. Appl. Physiol.* 17:625–38, 1962.

51. Yaglou, C. P. Temperature, humidity and air movement in industries: The effective temperature index. *J. Ind. Hyg.* 9:297–309, 1927.

52. Young, A. J. Energy substrate utilization during exercise in extreme environments. In *Exercise and Sport Sciences Reviews,* ed. K. B. Pandolf, Baltimore: Williams and Wilkins, pp. 65–117, 1990.

29

Nutrition for Athletes

Long-Term Dietary Considerations and
    Requirements
  Caloric Intake
  Proportion of Macronutrients
    (Carbohydrate, Protein, and Fat)
    in the Diet
  Dietary Carbohydrate Intake for
    Athletes
  Dietary Protein Intake for Athletes
  Dietary Fat Intake for Athletes
  Vitamins
  Minerals

Suggested Training Rules for Good
    Nutrition
Effect of Exercise on the Function of the
    Stomach
Pre-Event Objectives
Pregame Procedure
  The Pregame Meal
Glycogen Supercompensation
    (Carbohydrate Loading) for
    Endurance Events

In recent years, with ever-improving levels of competition, athletes and coaches have developed considerable interest in nutrition. Unfortunately, this is an area in which the scientific efforts of trained nutritionists (and biochemists, who are the experts in this field) have often been obscured by clouds of misinformation generated by faddists and self-proclaimed experts.

Furthermore, athletes seem to be too easily influenced by the success of other athletes whose training regimens include such dietary fads as royal honey, kelp, blackstrap molasses, or other substances thought to have miraculous properties for improving athletic performance. More often than not, when these potions are tested by scientific methods in controlled experiments, it turns out that an athlete's success was achieved in spite of— not because of—his or her unusual dietary modifications.

Let it be clearly stated from the outset: *There is no scientific evidence at the present time to indicate that athletic performance can be improved by modifying a basically sound diet.* Furthermore, there are many different ways in which a nutritious diet can be obtained, and the best diet for one athlete will seldom be the best diet for all athletes. Individual differences exist in our senses of taste as well as in our enzyme systems, which are so necessary for digestion and absorption. In other words, one person's meat may be another person's poison.

It should also be recognized that for explosive or short-duration events skill is the all-important factor. Even in endurance events where the total energy supply and the rate of energy supply are very important, the role of conditioning is infinitely more important than diet (if a diet is nutritionally sound). Still, in all athletic events, psychological as well as physiological factors affect performance, and there is no way to evaluate the psychological

importance of eating steak when less expensive protein foods are just as nutritious. When ego and prestige enter the picture, science may fade into the background.

Although we may not be able to modify a sound diet to improve performance, athletes can go downhill very rapidly if their diet is less than optimum. Thus diet is still a very important consideration.

Long-Term Dietary Considerations and Requirements

Caloric Intake

Table 29.1 provides the recommended daily caloric intake by males and females of various ages (56). These recommendations were designed for the maintenance of good nutrition for healthy persons in the United States. It should be recognized, however, that these caloric intake values would not be sufficient for athletes involved in heavy training.

Because caloric intake was discussed in chapter 17, it is enough to say that athletes must consume enough food daily to meet the energy demands of their training program. If they eat less than this, they will burn body tissues to make up the deficit and will approach "staleness" more rapidly. If they consume more food than they need, the result will be an increase in body weight with its accompanying mechanical disadvantages.

Proportion of Macronutrients (Carbohydrate, Protein, and Fat) in the Diet

A typical American diet contains approximately 46% carbohydrate, 12% protein, and 42% fat (22). These proportions are not considered optimal and it has been suggested that a healthful diet for nonathletes should be composed of 58% carbohydrates, 12% protein, and 30% fat (22). Furthermore, it is recommended

Table 29.1	Recommended Caloric Intake for Healthy Persons in the United States	
Age (years)	**Males**	**Females**
11–14	2,700	2,200
15–18	2,800	2,100
19–22	2,900	2,100
23–50	2,700	2,000
51–74	2,400	1,800
75+	2,050	1,600

Values expressed in kilocalories
Table adapted from Nutritive Value of Foods. United States Department of Agriculture, Science and Education Administration. U.S. Government Printing Office, Washington, D.C., 1981, p. 32.

that saturated fat should make up no more than 10% of total calories (20% of total calories from mono- and polyunsaturated fats) (22, 43), and the carbohydrate component of the diet should consist of approximately 48% starches and 10% simple sugars (15).

Abrahams (1) reported that Schenck, who studied the diet of 4,700 competitors in the 1936 Olympic games, found an average daily consumption of over 7,000 kcal. Interestingly, the macronutrient proportions included 46% carbohydrate, 19% protein, and 35% fat. Recently, Coleman (15) recommended that "athletes in heavy training will need to consume 70% of calories from carbohydrate, which means that fat will need to be reduced to 20% of total calories. Simple carbohydrate intake may be increased to meet overall caloric needs, but at least 50% of the calories should come from complex carbohydrates." These general guidelines (15) should be considered by coaches, trainers, and allied health professionals when making dietary recommendations for athletes in training.

Dietary Carbohydrate Intake for Athletes

(Recommendation for athletes: heavy training for several hours per day, 70% of total calories from carbohydrates with approximately 10% in the form of simple sugars; light training for less than or equal to one hour per day, 60% of total calories from carbohydrates with approximately 10% in the form of simple sugars (15).)

Carbohydrates have been called the "master fuel" because of their importance to energy metabolism and potential in preventing diseases (15, 59). Dietary carbohydrates contribute to energy production during exercise in the form of blood glucose and stored muscle glycogen. As will be discussed later in this chapter, manipulation of carbohydrate intake and exercise can result in larger than normal stores of muscle glycogen and increased endurance time for moderate-intensity, long-duration activity.

Although fat produces more than twice as much energy per gram as carbohydrate (4 kcal per gram of carbohydrate and 9 kcal per gram of fat) (59), it requires more oxygen for each calorie (213 ml per kcal of fat compared to 198 ml per kcal of carbohydrate). In any athletic event where energy production per unit of oxygen consumed is an important factor, there would seem to be an advantage of some 7.5% in favor of carbohydrate. As long ago as 1920, increased overall muscular efficiency of up to

10% had been shown experimentally for high carbohydrate diets (37).

Simple and Complex Carbohydrates

Complex carbohydrates (such as starches) are a combination of three or more glucose molecules, while simple carbohydrates (sugars) contain only one or two sugar molecules joined together (59). Simple carbohydrates can be further subdivided into monosaccharides (such as glucose, fructose, and galactose) and disaccharides (such as sucrose, lactose, and maltose). Disaccharides are two simple sugar molecules in combination (for example, glucose plus fructose form sucrose).

As stated earlier in this chapter, it is generally recommended that only approximately 10% of total caloric intake should be in the form of simple sugars. It is interesting to note, however, that diets high in both simple and complex carbohydrates have been shown to increase muscle glycogen stores (17, 49). Presently it is unclear whether simple or complex carbohydrates are most effective for increasing muscle glycogen stores. It should be recognized, however, that complex carbohydrates are nutrient dense and provide more B vitamins, fiber, and iron than simple sugars (15).

High-Carbohydrate Supplements

Some athletes have difficulty eating enough food to account for the energy demands of very high volumes of training (15). Inadequate total caloric intake often results in less than optimal carbohydrate consumption. Coleman (15) has identified three reasons athletes can have difficulty consuming enough carbohydrates:

1. The stress of hard training can decrease appetite.
2. Consuming a large volume of food can cause gastrointestinal distress and interfere with training.
3. The athlete may be spending so much time training that there are few rest hours available for replenishment.

If, for these or other reasons, an athlete does not consume enough carbohydrates, it would probably be beneficial to supplement his or her normal diet with commercial high-carbohydrate products. These products however, should not be used as a replacement for carbohydrate from a nutritionally sound diet (15).

Carbohydrate Intake Prior to Exercise

Traditionally, it has been recommended that athletes avoid eating large amounts (200 to 300 kcal) of sugar thirty to forty-five minutes prior to an endurance event (16, 24). Consuming sugar results in an increase in blood glucose, which stimulates the release of insulin into circulation from the pancreas. Over a period of time, the combination of elevated insulin and exercise facilitates glucose removal from the blood and can result in hypoglycemia (depressed blood glucose), which may hinder performance.

Hargreaves and coworkers (29), however, reported that 300 kcal of glucose ingested forty-five minutes prior to an exhaustive bout of cycle ergometry had no effect on endurance time. A recent study by Calles-Escandon and colleagues (12) also reported that ingestion of 260 kcal of fructose thirty minutes prior to exercise had no effect on endurance time at 70% of $\dot{V}O_2$ max during cycle ergometry. In addition, Gleeson, Maughan, and Greenhaff (26) reported that ingestion of 284 kcal of carbohydrate forty-five minutes before cycle ergometry exercise at approximately 70% of maximal aerobic power resulted in a 12% increase in endurance time.

It is important to emphasize at this point that there are substantial interindividual differences in the response of athletes to pre-exercise ingestion of sugar (15). That is, consuming sugar shortly before an endurance event may hinder performance in some athletes but not affect the performance of others. In this regard, Sherman (51) has recommended that "Every athlete should initially test the effectiveness of pre-exercise meals on exercise capacity during training and not during an important competition." Coaches recommendations regarding sugar intake prior to exercise should be based on personalized data regarding the response of each individual athlete.

Carbohydrate Intake during Exercise

Ingestion of high-carbohydrate food or drink increases endurance time during long duration (greater than approximately ninety minutes) exercise. Studies by Coyle and coworkers (18, 19) demonstrated that the ingestion of 100 to 200 kcal of carbohydrate every one-half hour resulted in an increase in the time to exhaustion of greater than 25% during cycling. Recent studies by Murray and colleagues (42) and Fielding and colleagues (23) have also reported enhanced cycling performance from carbohydrate feeding during exercise. Carbohydrates ingested during exercise help to maintain blood glucose levels and provide a source of glucose for energy metabolism when muscle glycogen stores are reduced or depleted. In addition, it has been suggested that maintenance of blood glucose by carbohydrate feeding helps to attenuate the perception of fatigue during prolonged exercise (8). Coleman (15) has recommended that to improve endurance performance "athletes should take in 25 to 30 g of carbohydrate (100 to 200 cal) every one-half hour. This amount can be obtained through either carbohydrate-rich foods or fluids. Drinking 8 oz of a sports drink containing 5% to 8% carbohydrate (Gatorade, Exceed or Bodyfuel 450) every 15 minutes provides this amount of carbohydrate and also aids in hydration."

Carbohydrate Intake after Exercise

Consuming carbohydrates after strenuous exercise helps to replenish muscle glycogen stores. Restoration of glycogen stores is very important for athletes involved in heavy training or competition on a daily basis. Failure to replenish muscle glycogen stores can result in premature fatigue and performance that is less than expected.

The rate of glycogen synthesis following exercise is, in part, dependent on when the carbohydrates are consumed. Ivy and colleagues (34) found that muscle glycogen synthesis was greater when carbohydrate intake occurred immediately after exercise. The greater the time delay between the end of exercise and carbohydrate feeding, the slower the rate of muscle glycogen synthesis. Coleman (15) has suggested three potential explanations for the greater rate of glycogen synthesis immediately following exercise:

1. Greater blood flow to the muscle.
2. The muscle fiber is more likely to take up glucose.
3. The muscle fiber is more sensitive to the effects of insulin.

Based on the work of Ivy and colleagues, Coleman recommends "taking in 100 g of carbohydrate (400 cal) within 15 to 30 minutes of exercise and additional 100-g feedings every 2 to 4 hours thereafter." Often, athletes do not want to eat immediately following a strenuous workout. Therefore, the first post-exercise feeding may include a high-carbohydrate drink or fruit juice with subsequent feedings consisting of beverages or solid food.

Dietary Protein Intake for Athletes

(Recommendation for athletes in general: 10% to 15% of total calories from proteins; for endurance athletes, 1.2 to 1.5 gram per kilogram of body weight per day; for strength athletes, 1.5 gram per kilogram of body weight per day (33, 39).)

For many years it was believed that protein metabolism did not contribute significantly to energy production during exercise. More recent information, however, suggests that under normal dietary conditions, approximately 5% to 15% of energy production during exercise comes from protein sources (39, 59).

Under conditions of reduced muscle glycogen stores, protein catabolism may be even greater.

Several factors affect protein catabolism during exercise including the mode, frequency, intensity, and duration of exercise as well as the training status of the individual.

Effect of Mode of Exercise on Protein Metabolism

In general, it appears that high-intensity anaerobic activities derive less energy production from protein sources than continuous aerobic exercise. For example, Williams (59) has stated that strenuous weight training derives less than 5% of the energy needs from protein, while 15% of the energy needed for prolonged endurance exercise comes from protein catabolism.

Effect of Frequency of Exercise on Protein Metabolism

It is commonly believed that the frequency of training affects protein degradation and synthesis (33). Training that is too frequent may result in "overtraining" and reduced gains in strength and muscle mass, possibly due to increased protein catabolism (39). Unfortunately, it is not presently possible to recommend an optimal frequency of exercise based on the available evidence regarding protein metabolism.

Effect of Intensity of Exercise on Protein Metabolism

Lemon (38) examined the effect of one hour of treadmill exercise at 41.6%, 55.4%, and 67.3% of maximal aerobic capacity on protein metabolism. There was evidence of increased protein catabolism (28% to 36%) at 55% and 67% of $\dot{V}O_2$ max but not (-1%) at 42% of $\dot{V}O_2$ max. These findings suggest that very low-intensity exercise is not characterized by substantial energy production from protein sources. However, measurable protein catabolism is evident during continuous exercise with an intensity as low as 55% of $\dot{V}O_2$ max.

Effect of Duration of Exercise on Protein Metabolism

Haralambie and Berg (28) examined data from several laboratories and found a dramatic increase in protein degradation after approximately one hour of continuous exercise. It has been suggested (33) that this increase in amino acid oxidation is related to a decrease in carbohydrate availability. Lemon and Mullen (41) provided compelling data to support this hypothesis by demonstrating a twofold (10.4% versus 4.4% of total energy expenditure) greater protein contribution to energy production when muscle glycogen stores were low compared with when glycogen stores were high.

Effect of Training Status on Protein Metabolism

There is a transient increase in protein degradation at the beginning of an exercise program in previously untrained subjects (9, 11). Recent studies by Friedman and Lemon (25) and Tarnopolsky, MacDougall, and Atkinson (55) have also reported increased protein requirements in trained subjects. Apparently, there is an increase in dietary protein requirements during an exercise program for both trained and untrained individuals. Lemon (40) has suggested that, in athletes, the additional dietary protein may contribute to energy production and repair of muscle tissue, while in untrained subjects, it may reduce the loss of blood proteins.

Quality of Protein

We have so far concerned ourselves only with the total quantity and with the proportions of the basic foodstuffs within that total. In regard to protein, the quality is also very important. All proteins break down to amino acids during the digestive processes, so these may be considered the units or building blocks for the synthesis of the proteins found in the human body. Of the twenty-three amino acids normally present in animal protein, only thirteen can be synthesized in the cells. The other ten must be supplied in the diet and are therefore called *essential amino acids.*

Supplying the essential amino acids is no problem for those who eat meat and animal products. The use of complete proteins (those that include all the essential amino acids) from milk and eggs and a generous and varied use of meat solve the problem quite easily. For those who do not eat animal products, the problem is more complicated. But vegetarians can be well nourished if they include all the essential amino acids in their diet. This can be done by including a diversity of vegetable products such as leaves, seeds, roots, and fruits (60). It is also encouraging for vegetarians to note that a recent study by Richter and co-workers (48) found that there was no difference in the effect of a meat-rich versus lacto-ovo vegetarian diet on the function of specific immune parameters.

Dietary Fat Intake for Athletes

(Recommendation for athletes: 30% of total calories from fat with no more than 10% of total calories in the form of saturated fat (22, 43).)

Fatty acids are energy rich (9 kcal per gram) and are used as the primary energy source during low-intensity activity. As the intensity of exercise increases the contribution of carbohydrates to energy production also increases. This can be clearly demonstrated by monitoring the respiratory quotient (RQ) during incremental exercise (see chapter 12 for a discussion of the respiratory quotient). An RQ value of 0.7 to 0.8 indicates a primary reliance on fatty acid oxidation for energy production. As the intensity approaches maximum, the RQ will reach 1.0 or greater indicating an almost total reliance on carbohydrates for energy production.

At the initiation of exercise there is a decrease in the circulating level of free fatty acids (10). After a few minutes of continuous ex-ercise, there is mobilization of fatty acids stored in adipose tissue, which results in an increase in circulating free fatty acids (10). Thus, the fatty acids used for energy metabolism initially (at the beginning of an exercise bout) come from existing circulatory sources while those which contribute to energy production during prolonged exercise are derived from stored sources. During continuous submaximal exercise, the RQ peaks at approximately five to ten minutes into the workout (46, 47) and declines thereafter, which indicates an increase in the contribution of fat metabolism to energy production as the duration of exercise increases.

Phinney and coworkers (45) examined the effect of a high fat diet (85% of total calories) on endurance time during cycle ergometry. The results of this investigation indicated that there was no difference in endurance time whether the subjects had eaten a high fat or moderate carbohydrate (57% of total calories in carbohydrates) diet. Presently, there is no conclusive data for humans that indicate whether a high fat diet enhances or hinders endurance exercise performance.

Endurance training improves the ability to metabolize both fats and carbohydrates (10). Furthermore, training results in an increase in the utilization of fatty acids at a given absolute submaximal exercise intensity but not when the workload is expressed as a percent of maximal aerobic power (32, 50). That is, as a result of metabolic adaptations, the RQ is lower at the same submaximal (absolute) workload in a trained state when compared to an untrained state. The enhanced ability to metabolize fats during submaximal exercise may result in a sparing of carbohydrate stores and thereby increase the duration of moderate to high-intensity activity.

Vitamins

Table 29.2 includes the recommended daily intake, dietary sources, major body functions, and possible roles important during exercise for common vitamins and minerals. The need

Table 29.2   Vitamins and Minerals

Vitamin or Mineral	RDA for Healthy Adult Men and Women (mg)*	Dietary Sources	Major Body Functions	Possible Roles Important during Exercise
Water-soluble vitamins				
B₁ (thiamine)	1.5 1.1	Pork, organ meats, whole grains, legumes	Coenzyme (thiamine pyrophosphate) in reactions involving removal of carbon dioxide	Energy release from carbohydrate; formation of hemoglobin; proper nervous system functioning
B₂ (riboflavin)	1.7 1.3	Widely distributed in foods	Constituent of two flavin nucleotide coenzymes involved in energy metabolism (FAD and FMN)	Energy release from carbohydrate and fat
Niacin	19 15	Liver, lean meats, grains, legumes (can be formed from tryptophan)	Constituent of two coenzymes involved in oxidation-reduction reactions (NAD and NADP)	Energy release from carbohydrate, both aerobic and anaerobic; inhibition of FFA release from adipose tissue
B₆ (pyridoxine)	2.0 1.6	Meats, vegetables, wholegrain cereals	Coenzyme (PLP) involved in amino acid metabolism	Energy release from carbohydrate; formation of hemoglobin and oxidative enzymes; proper nervous system functioning
Pantothenic acid	4–7 4–7	Widely distributed in foods	Constituent of CoA, which plays a central role in energy metabolism	Energy production from carbohydrate and fat

Continued

Table 29.2   Vitamins and Minerals (*Continued*)

Vitamin or Mineral	RDA for Healthy Adult Men and Women (mg)*	Dietary Sources	Major Body Functions	Possible Roles Important during Exercise
Folacin	0.2 0.18	Legumes, green vegetables, whole-wheat products	Coenzyme (reduced form) involved in transfer or single-carbon units in nucleic acid and amino acid metabolism	Red blood cell production
B_{12}	0.002 0.002	Muscle meats, eggs, dairy products (not present in plant foods)	Coenzyme involved in transfer of single-carbon units in nucleic acid metabolism	Red blood cell production
Biotin	0.10–0.20 0.10–0.20	Legumes, vegetables, meats	Coenzyme required for fat synthesis, amino acid metabolism, glycogen (animal starch) formation	Carbohydrate and fat synthesis
C (ascorbic acid)	60 60	Citrus fruits, tomatoes, green peppers, salad greens	Maintains intercellular matrix of cartilage, bone, dentine; important in collagen synthesis	Antioxidant; increased absorption of iron; formation of epinephrin; promotion of aerobic energy production; formation of connective tissue
Fat-soluable vitamins A (retinol)	1.0 0.8	Provitamin A (β-carotene) widely distributed in green vegetables; retinol present in milk, butter, cheese, fortified margarine	Constituent of rhodopsin (visual pigment); maintenance of epithelial tissues; role in mucopolysaccharide synthesis	Antioxidant; prevention of red blood cell damage

Vitamin or Mineral	RDA for Healthy Adult Men and Women (mg)*	Dietary Sources	Major Body Functions	Possible Roles Important during Exercise
D	0.005–0.010 0.005–0.010	Cod-liver oil, eggs, dairy products, fortified milk, margarine	Promotes growth and mineralization of bones; increases absorption of calcium	Calcium transport in muscle
E (tocopherol)	10 8	Seeds, green leafy vegetables, margarines, shortenings	Functions as antioxidant to prevent cell membrane damage	Antioxidant; prevention of red blood cell damage; promotion of aerobic energy production
K (phylloquinone)	0.070–0.080 0.060–0.065	Green leafy vegetables; small amounts in cereals, fruits, and meats	Important in blood clotting (involved in formation of active prothrombin)	None determined
Minerals				
Calcium	800–1200 800–1200	Dairy products, dark green leafy vegetables, dried legumes	Bone and tooth formation; blood clotting; nerve transmission	Muscle contraction; glycogen breakdown
Phosphorus	800–1200 800–1200	Milk, cheese, meat, poultry, grains	Bone and tooth formation; acid-base balance	Formation of ATP and creatine phosphokinase; release of oxygen from red blood cells
Potassium	1875–5625	Meats, milk, many fruits	Acid-base balance; body water balance; nerve function	Nerve impulse transmission; muscle contraction; glycogen storage

Continued

Table 29.2   Vitamins and Minerals (*Continued*)

Vitamin or Mineral	RDA for Healthy Adult Men and Women (mg)*	Dietary Sources	Major Body Functions	Possible Roles Important during Exercise
Sodium	1100–3300	Common salt	Acid-base balance; body water balance; nerve function	Nerve impulse transmission; muscle contraction; water balance
Magnesium	350 280–300	Whole grains, green leafy vegetables	Activates enzymes; involved in protein synthesis	Muscle contraction; glucose metabolism in muscle cells
Iron	10 15	Eggs, lean meats, legumes, whole grains, green leafy vegetables	Constituent of hemoglobin and enzymes involved in energy metabolism	Oxygen transport by red blood cells; oxygen utilization in muscle cells
Zinc	15 12	Widely distributed in foods	Constituent of enzymes involved in digestion	Energy production in muscle cells
Chromium	0.05–0.20	Fats, vegetables, oils, meats	Involved in glucose and energy metabolism	Glucose and energy metabolism; normal blood sugar metabolism
Copper	2 2	Meats, drinking water	Constituents of enzymes associated with iron metabolism	Oxygen transport and utilization; close work with iron
Selenium	0.070 0.050–0.055	Seafood, meat, grains	Functions in close association with Vitamin E	Antioxidant

*First values are for men.

Reprinted from *Sports Nutrition for the 90s,* by J. R. Berning and S. N. Steen, pp. 136–39, with permission of Aspen Publishers, Inc., © 1991

Data from Scrimshaw, NS, Young, VR.
The requirements of human nutrition. *Sci. Am.,* 235:50, 1976; *Recommended Dietary Allowances,* revised, Washington, DC, Food and Nutrition Board, NAS-NRC, 1989 (from the National Dairy Council); Williams, M. H. *Beyond Training,* Human Kinetics Publishers, 1989; Anderson, R. A., Guttman, H. N. Trace minerals and exercise, in: *Exercise, Nutrition and Energy Metabolism,* Macmillan, 1988.

for vitamins in the human diet is well established (6) but a question of recurring interest is whether athletes need vitamin supplements in addition to their normal diet. It was thought at one time that the requirements for vitamins increased much more rapidly than the increase in metabolism due to exercise. But more recent work (7) indicates that vitamin needs increase only in approximate proportion to metabolic activity. Thus ingestion of larger amounts of food as daily workout levels increase automatically provides the needed increase in vitamins (if the diet is sound to begin with).

Some investigators have claimed that vitamin supplementation has improved athletic performance in their subjects. However, when the proper controls are instituted, assuring that subjects are on an adequate diet *before starting the experiment,* these improvements in performance can no longer be demonstrated. Thus in all likelihood the reported improvements in performance because of vitamin supplementation were the result of having improved previously inadequate diets (4, 36, 58).

Since athletes (and the general population as well) do not always have optimal nutritional habits, table 29.3 offers the best available knowledge concerning vitamin and mineral supplementation, when that seems desirable (60).

One point should be made before we leave this subject. Trace quantities of mineral elements seem to be intimately connected with the body's proper use of certain vitamins (60). Furthermore, it seems likely that many unknown factors affect nutrition. Therefore, it is important to recognize that obtaining the daily requirement of a specific vitamin from food sources, rather than the individual purified form, will likely result in simultaneously obtaining other important vitamins and minerals. There is no benefit, however, to so-called "organic" vitamins versus synthetic vitamins since they have the same chemical structure.

Minerals

As with vitamins, there is no evidence that the need for minerals is increased in exercise (in comfortable climates) beyond the increase brought about by the increased daily food consumption needed for metabolic demands.

Iron Deficiency—Sports Anemia

One important exception to the above statement must be emphasized. While a normal diet usually provides sufficient mineral constituents, several groups of athletes may require iron supplementation (under medical guidance) including male and female endurance athletes, adolescent athletes, athletes who lose weight for competition, and vegetarian athletes (21, 27, 30, 54). It has been known for at least thirty years that highly trained distance runners are likely to have low hemoglobin and hematocrit values. The term *sports anemia* was coined to describe this anemia that occurs in response to heavy endurance training in the absence of any recognizable disease process.

Iron deficiency is commonly divided into three stages. The earliest stage is referred to as *prelatent iron deficiency* and is characterized by a decrease or absence of storage iron (iron is stored as ferritin and hemosiderin in the liver, bone marrow, and spleen). Following exhaustion of the body's iron stores, the iron supply to the developing red cells is diminished and iron deficient erythropoiesis occurs. This second stage of iron deficiency is known as *latent iron deficiency* and is characterized by an increased total iron binding capacity and reduced serum iron. In these first and second stages of iron deficiency, hemoglobin level remains essentially in the normal range. Only in the third stage of iron deficiency is there a significant drop in hemoglobin level below normal values. Thus the detection of anemia represents an advanced stage of iron deficiency. Clement and Sawchuk (14) have concluded that even the early stages of iron deficiency

Table 29.3	Recommended Vitamin and Mineral Supplementation		
Vitamins		**Minerals**	
Vitamin A	10,000 units	Calcium	300.0 mg
Vitamin D	500 units	Phosphate	250.0 mg
Ascorbic acid	100 mg	Magnesium	100.0 mg
Thiamine	2 mg	Cobalt	0.1 mg
Riboflavin	2 mg	Copper	1.0 mg
Pyridoxine	3 mg	Iodine	0.1 mg
Niacinamide	20 mg	Iron	10.0 mg
Vitamin B_{12}	5 mcg	Manganese	1.0 mg
Pantothenic acid	20 mg	Molybdenum	0.2 mg
Tocopherols (vitamin E)	5 mg	Zinc	5.0 mg
Inositol	100 mg		
Choline	100 mg		

From R. J. Williams. *Physician's Handbook of Nutritional Science* 1975. Courtesy of Charles C Thomas, Publisher, Springfield, Ill.

without anemia can substantially reduce an athlete's ability to maximize performance and constitute a clearly undesirable condition. In the third stage of *frank anemia,* the evidence is clear that optimal energy release is impossible because of the combined effects of inefficient cell metabolism and decreased O_2 transport.

The level of plasma ferritin has been shown to reflect iron storage levels. Clement and Asmundson (13) found that of fifty-two middle distance and distance runners at Simon Fraser University, 29% of the men and 82% of the women had plasma ferritin concentrations that showed them to be at risk for iron deficiency. Subsequent work has supported their findings (44).

A diet high in iron sources such as meat, poultry, and fish (heme iron) and non-heme iron foods such as dried peas and beans, nuts, whole grain breads and cereals, leafy vegetables, eggs, and dried fruits should prevent iron deficiency problems. But it is very difficult to correct the iron deficiency by diet alone once

it has been established (14). On the other hand, iron supplements should not be given routinely to athletes without medical supervision because of the possibility of inducing deficiencies of other trace minerals such as copper and zinc. Also, a high iron intake can produce an iron overload (hemochromatosis) in some people. An excellent review of the literature regarding iron status and sports performance has been provided by Clement and Sawchuk (14).

Suggested Training Rules for Good Nutrition

It is obviously impossible, as well as undesirable, to belabor athletes with the specifics of diet. It is also unnecessary because a relatively simple set of rules will result in good nutrition without making a dietitian (and possibly a hypochondriac) of each athlete. deVries has found the following rules to be workable and effective, not only for good athletic conditioning but also for forming sound, lifelong dietary habits.

1. Distribute the daily consumption of food over three regularly spaced meals. If weight gain (or prevention of weight loss) is desirable, an evening snack can be added.

2. Eliminate from the diet as much as possible the foods that furnish only calories without contributing their share of vitamins and minerals (candy, cake, carbonated beverages, and so on). Use fruit and fruit juices for desserts and snacks.

3. Eliminate tea, coffee, and alcohol. Not only do these drinks usurp the place of more nutritious food, they may cause undesirable pharmacological effects such as decreased muscular efficiency.

4. Avoid fatty foods—they slow peristalsis and therefore gastric emptying.

5. Eat two servings daily of fresh fruit (one should be citrus fruit or tomatoes).

6. Eat four servings daily of vegetables, including leafy green vegetables (salads) and roots and tubers (turnips, beets, potatoes).

7. Eat at least three slices of whole-grain bread daily.

8. Eat enough butter or fortified margarine to supplement the bread in item 7.

9. Drink at least three glasses of low-fat (1% to 2%) milk daily.

A study of twenty-eight athletes from varsity teams of three Big Ten universities (7) showed that only ten of the athletes followed sound diets. The foods most commonly omitted were the green and yellow vegetables, citrus fruits, eggs, and milk. This indicated that their diets were probably low in vitamins A and C as well as calcium. If these dietary habits can be accepted as typical of American athletes,

then coaches would be well advised to provide vitamin supplements for their athletes in the form of a multiple vitamin and mineral pill, in spite of the earlier comment that athletes on a well-balanced diet do not require vitamin or mineral supplements because of heavy workouts. Table 29.4 provides a simple and quick means for evaluating athletes' diets, which deVries used for many years with swimmers, divers, and water polo teams (20).

In situations that involve mature athletes, coaches may have to compromise their principles in the case of firmly held dietary beliefs. But, individual differences being what they are, it is conceivable that some individuals will thrive on diets that would be totally unsatisfactory for most athletes. Furthermore, it is all important to maintain harmonious relationships and undisturbed psychological equilibrium for successful athletic efforts.

Effect of Exercise on the Function of the Stomach

The digestive functions of the stomach can be divided into two components: secretory and motor. The secretory function consists of the elaboration and discharge into the stomach of hydrochloric acid, digestive enzymes, and alkaline mucus. The motor function consists of the maintenance of a degree of tonus plus the peristaltic contractions found during digestive processes. In some individuals there are, in addition, muscular contractions related to hunger pangs. Any factor that interferes with either secretory or motor functions may cause nausea.

The most definitive work on the effects of exercise on the functions of the stomach in the human was done some time ago by Hellebrandt and Hooper (31). For the secretory cycle, it was found that severe exercise results in inhibition of the secretory response and that the resulting hypoacidity lasted as long as one hour. In mild activity, the acidity (secretory

Table 29.4   Evaluation of Daily Food Selection

Food Group	Amount	Scores		Daily Score
				S M T W T F S
1. Milk	4 cups or more (1 cup = 8 oz)	4 cups = 3 cups = 2 cups = 1 cup =	10 8 6 4	
2. Meat* (also fish, poultry, eggs, legumes)	2 servings or more, including at least one of meat, poultry, or fish	2 servings, including 1 of meat, poultry, or fish = 1 serv. as above = 1 serv. eggs, legumes =	10 8 6	
3. Citrus fruit (also tomatoes, raw cabbage, salad greens)	1 serving or more (1 piece of fruit or ½ cup juice)	1 serving =	10	
4. Leafy green or yellow vegetable	1 serving or more (½ cup)	1 serving =	10	
5. Potatoes and other fruits and vegetables	2 servings or more (1 serving = ½ cup)	2 servings = 1 serving =	10 6	
6. Whole-grain or enriched cereals and breads†	2 servings or more	2 servings = 1 serving =	10 6	
7. Butter or fortified margarine	2 pats or 2 tbsp	2 pats = 1 pat =	10 6	
8. For *not* eating any candy, cake, pastry, or other sweets			10	
9. For *not* eating any food fried in deep fat			10	
10. For *not* drinking any cola, carbonated soft drinks, coffee, tea, or imitation fruit drinks Total			10 100	

*1 serving = 2–4 oz lean cooked meat, poultry, or fish (not counting bone)
 1 serving = 2 eggs
 1 serving = 1 cup of cooked dry beans, peas, or lentils
 1 serving = ½ cup peanuts or other nuts
†1 serving = 1 slice bread
 1 serving = 1 oz ready-to-eat cereal
 1 serving = ½ cup cooked cereal, etc.

From *Health Science: A Positive Approach,* by Herbert A. deVries. Copyright © 1979 by Scott, Foresman & Co. Reprinted by permission.

activity) was either unchanged or only slightly increased.

In respect to stomach motility, they found that mild exercise during the digestion of a meal seemed advantageous in hastening the final emptying time. Violent or exhaustive exercise, however, was found to inhibit gastric peristalsis, although this inhibition was followed (after exercise was ended) by augmented activity that resulted in little alteration of the final emptying time of the stomach.

There was some evidence of a psychic effect in their series of experiments, in that repetition generally decreased a subject's response to the same exercise stressor.

Experimental evidence for the effects of exercise on the other portions of the digestive tract is lacking, inconclusive, or has been performed only on animals under conditions that do not justify extrapolation of the conclusions to humans.

Pre-Event Objectives

The objectives to be attained in the twenty-four- to forty-eight-hour period preceding competition are as follows:

1. Attaining the largest possible storage of carbohydrate in the liver and musculature.

2. Entering competition with the smallest possible stomach volume, so that the diaphragm can descend as far as possible in inhalation.

3. Preventing gastric disturbances from occurring during a competition.

4. Maintaining an optimum psychological attitude in the athlete while accomplishing the first three items.

Pregame Procedure

Liver and muscle glycogen can be increased by the methods to be discussed.

Breakfast on the day of competition can be relatively larger if the event is scheduled for the afternoon, and breakfast and lunch can be larger if the event is in the evening.

In any event the pre-event meal should be light, and the two meals that immediately precede competition should be high carbohydrate meals: cereals such as oatmeal, toast with jam, honey, and so on.

The final pre-event meal usually precedes competition by three or four hours. But there is evidence that if it consists of cereal and milk of no more than 500 kcal, no adverse effects are suffered if it is taken up to thirty minutes before competition (2, 3, 53, 57).

The Pregame Meal

Theory and common sense dictate that the following precautions be observed for the pregame meal.

1. Avoid foods that are even mildly distasteful to an individual athlete— no matter how well they may serve nutritional objectives. An athlete may get sick even though the food is excellent.

2. Avoid irritating foods, such as highly spiced foods and roughage.

3. Avoid gas-forming foods: onions, cabbage, apples, baked beans.

4. Avoid fatty foods—they slow peristalsis and therefore gastric emptying.

5. Hold protein foods to a minimum because their metabolism results in fixed acids. In large quantities, this could result in an undesirable acidosis.

6. Fluid can best be supplied by bouillon (which supplies sodium, which is excreted in perspiration during an event). Many athletes will prefer milk or juices, and if experience shows no ill effects it is probably wise to accede to this preference.

Glycogen Supercompensation (Carbohydrate Loading) for Endurance Events

The theoretical basis for the importance of glycogen storage in endurance-type exercise was discussed in chapter 3. When work loads greater than about 70% of aerobic capacity must be borne for thirty to sixty minutes or more, the *rate* of work is limited by aerobic power, but the *duration* over which the load can be maintained depends very largely on the level of glycogen storage in the involved muscles. Apparently the muscle cell cannot use other energy substrates to any great extent at high levels of work. When glycogen depletion occurs, work can be continued on other energy substrates (such as fat) but only at work loads considerably below 70%.

Karlsson and Saltin (35) demonstrated this effect quite clearly when they had ten subjects run the same 30-km race twice, three weeks apart, once after a carbohydrate-enriched diet and once after a mixed diet. They found the muscle glycogen level in the quadriceps for the high carbohydrate diet to be double that for the mixed diet, and every subject turned in the best performance after the high carbohydrate diet. Interestingly, identical pace was maintained after both diets in the early part of the race when glycogen content was high, but pace fell off earlier after the mixed diet as glycogen depots were emptied.

The classic work of the original investigators in this area, Bergstrom and colleagues (5), also provided clear-cut data for modifying the diet to best prepare for prolonged endurance-type events. To achieve the highest possible level of muscle glycogen for such events, the athlete was to work the same muscles to exhaustion about one week prior to the event. For the next three days, the diet was to be made up almost exclusively of fat and protein, since it was shown that low carbohydrate diet followed by high carbohydrate diet results in the greatest possible glycogen storage. About three days were to be left for a carbohydrate-rich diet with only very light workouts to produce the maximum possible glycogen storage in the muscles. The low carbohydrate diet consisted of 1,500 kcal protein and 1,300 kcal fat for a total daily energy expenditure estimated at 2,800 kcal. The high carbohydrate diet made up the same total with 2,300 kcal of carbohydrate and 500 kcal of protein (5).

More recent work by Sherman and his co-workers has modified the classic method, which was both physically and psychologically taxing for the athlete (52). Their group of runners consumed three different trial diets in preparation for three separate 13-mile performance runs. In preparation for each performance run, the runners all ran on a treadmill at 73% $\dot{V}O_2$ max for 90, 40, 40, 20, and 20 minutes and then rested one day of the six days before each of the 13-mile performance runs. The diet for the first trial was from the classic regimen: 15% carbohydrate for the first three days and 70% for the last three. The second trial diet was 50% carbohydrate for the first three days and 70% for the last three. The third trial diet was an average diet (50% carbohydrate for all six days). Muscle biopsies showed that the low/high carbohydrate regimen (15% to 70%) elevated muscle glycogen to 207 mM/kg; the second regimen of average-high carbohydrate (50% to 70%) yielded 203 mM/kg; and the normal regimen (50% on all six days) produced only 160 mM/kg. Thus it appears that this much more moderate regimen can accomplish the same supercompensation as the difficult classic approach. It should be noted that this procedure, which relies heavily on the declining level of training in the six days before competition for its glycogen storage effect, is not greatly different from what knowledgeable coaches have recommended for many decades past.

References

1. Abrahams, A. The nutrition of athletes. *Br. J. Nutr.* 2:266–69, 1948.

2. Asprey, G. M., Alley, L. E., and Tuttle, W. W. Effect of eating at various times on subsequent performances in the 440-yard dash and half-mile run. *Res. Q.* 34:267–70, 1963.

3. ———. Effect of eating at various times upon subsequent performance in the one-mile run. *Res. Q.* 35:227–30, 1964.

4. Belko, A. Z. Vitamins and exercise—An update. *Med. Sci. Sports Exerc.* 19 (Supplement): S191–S196, 1987.

5. Bergstrom, J., Hermansen, L., Hultman, E., and Saltin, B. Diet, muscle glycogen and physical performance. *Acta Physiol. Scand.* 71:140–50, 1967.

6. Bicknell, F., and Prescott, F. *The Vitamins in Medicine.* New York: Grune & Stratton, 1953.

7. Bobb, A., Pringle, D., and Ryan, A. J. A brief study of the diet of athletes. *J. Sports Med.* 9:255–62, 1969.

8. Burgess, M. L., Robertson, R. J., Davis, J. M., and Norris, J. M. RPE, blood glucose, and carbohydrate oxidation during exercise: Effects of glucose feeding. *Med. Sci. Sports Exerc.* 23:353–59, 1991.

9. Butterfield, G. E. Whole-body protein utilization in humans. *Med. Sci. Sports Exerc.* 19 (Supplement): S157–S165, 1987.

10. Butterfield, G. E. Fat as a fuel for exercise. In *Sports Nutrition for the 90s,* eds. J. R. Berning and S. N. Steen, Gaithersberg, MD: Aspen Publishers, Inc., 1991.

11. Butterfield, G. E., and Calloway, D. H. Physical activity improves protein utilization in young men. *Br. J. Nutr.* 51:171–84, 1984.

12. Calles-Escandon, J., Devlin, J. T., Whitcomb, W., and Horton, E. S. Pre-exercise feeding does not affect endurance cycle exercise but attenuates post-exercise starvation-like response. *Med. Sci. Sports Exerc.* 23:818–24, 1991.

13. Clement, D. B., and Asmundson, R. C. Nutritional intake and hematological parameters in endurance runners. *Physician and Sportsmed.* 10 (March):37–43, 1982.

14. Clement, D. B., and Sawchuk, L. L. Iron status and sports performance. *Sports Med.* 1:65–74, 1984.

15. Coleman, E. Carbohydrates: The master fuel. In *Sports Nutrition for the 90s,* eds. J. R. Berning and S. N. Steen, Gaithersburg, MD: Aspen Publishers, Inc., 1991.

16. Costill, D. L., Coyle, E., Dalsky, G., Evans, W., Fink, W., and Hoopes, D. Effects of elevated plasma FFA and insulin on muscle glycogen usage during exercise. *J. Appl. Physiol.* 43:695–99, 1977.

17. Costill, D. L., Sherman, W. M., Fink, W. J., Maresh, C., Witten, M., and Miller, J. M. The role of dietary carbohydrates in muscle glycogen resynthesis after strenuous running. *Am. J. Clin. Nutr.* 34:1831–36, 1981.

18. Coyle, E. F., Coggan, A. R., Hemmert, M. K., and Ivy, J. L. Muscle glycogen utilization during prolonged strenuous exercise when fed carbohydrate. *J. Appl. Physiol* 61:165–72, 1986.

19. Coyle, E. F., Hagberg, J. M., Hurley, B. F., Martin, W. H., Ehsani, A. A., and Holloszy, J. O. Carbohydrate feeding during prolonged strenuous exercise can delay fatigue. *J. Appl. Physiol* 55:230–35, 1983.

20. deVries, H. A. *Health Science: A Positive Approach.* Glenview, IL: Scott, Foresman & Co., 1979.

21. Eichner, E. Sports anemia: Poor terminology of a real phenomenon. *Gatorade Sports Sci. Exch.* 1(6), 1988.

22. Falls, H. B., Baylor, A. M., and Dishman, R. K. *Essentials of Fitness.* Philadelphia: Saunders College/Holt, Rinehard and Winston, 1980.

23. Fielding, R. A., Costill, D. L., Fink, W. J., King, D. S., Hargreaves, M., and Kovaleski, J. E. Effect of carbohydrate feeding frequencies and dosage on muscle glycogen use during exercise. *Med. Sci. Sports Exerc.* 17:472–76, 1985.

24. Foster, C., Costill, D. L., and Fink, W. J. Effects of preexercise feedings on endurance performance. *Med. Sci. Sports* 11:1–5, 1979.

25. Friedman, J. E., and Lemon, P. W. R. Effect of chronic endurance exercise on retention of dietary protein. *Int. J. Sports Med.* 10:118–23, 1989.

26. Gleeson, M., Maughan, R. J. and Greenhaff, P. L. Comparison of the effects of pre-exercise feeding of glucose, glycerol and placebo on endurance and fuel homeostasis in man. *Eur. J. Appl. Physiol.* 55:645–53, 1986.

27. Grandjean, A. C. The vegetarian athlete. *Phys. Sportsmed.* 15:191–94, 1987.

28. Haralambie, G., and Berg, A. Serum urea and amino nitrogen changes with exercise duration. *Europ. J. Appl. Physiol.* 36:39–48, 1976.

29. Hargreaves, M., Costill, D. L., Fink, W. J., King, D. S., and Fielding, R. A. Effect of pre-exercise carbohydrate feedings on endurance cycling performance. *Med. Sci. Sports Exerc.* 19:33–36, 1987.

30. Haymes, E. M. Nutritional concerns: Need for iron. *Med. Sci. Sports Exerc.* 19 (Supplement): S197–S200, 1987.

31. Hellebrandt, F. A., and Hooper, S. L. Studies in the influence of exercise on the digestive work of the stomach. *Am. J. Physiol.* 107:348, 355, 364, 370, 1934.

32. Holloszy, J. O., and Coyle, E. F. Adaptations of skeletal muscle to endurance exercise and their metabolic consequences. *J. Appl. Physiol.* 56:831–38, 1984.

33. Houck, J., and Slavin, J. Protein nutrition for the athlete. In *Sports Nutrition for the 90s,* eds. J. R. Berning and S. N. Steen, Gaithersburg, MD: Aspen Publishers, Inc., 1991.

34. Ivy, J. L., Katz, A. L., Cutler, C. L., Sherman, W. M., and Coyle, E. F. Muscle glycogen synthesis after exercise: Effect of time of carbohydrate ingestion. *J. Appl. Physiol.* 64:1480–85, 1988.

35. Karlsson, J., and Saltin, B. Diet, muscle glycogen, and endurance performance. *J. Appl. Physiol.* 31:203–6, 1971.

36. Kris-Etherton, P. M. The facts and fallacies of nutritional supplements for athletes. *Gatorade Sports Sci. Exch.* 2(18), 1989.

37. Krogh, A., and Lindhard, J. The relative value of fats and carbohydrates as sources of muscular energy. *Biochem. J.* 14:290, 1920.

38. Lemon, P. W. R. Effect of intensity on protein utilization during prolonged exercise. *Med. Sci. Sports Exerc.* 16:151 (Abstract), 1984.

39. Lemon, P. W. R. Protein and exercise: Update 1987. *Med. Sci. Sports Exerc.* 19 (Supplement): S179–S190, 1987.

40. Lemon, P. W. R. Influence of dietary protein and total energy intake on strength improvement. *Gatorade Sports Sci. Exch.* 2, 1989.

41. Lemon, P. W. R., and Mullin, J. P. Effect of initial muscle glycogen levels on protein catabolism during exercise. *J. Appl. Physiol.* 48:624–29, 1980.

42. Murray, R., Paul, G. L., Seifert, J. G., and Eddy, D. E. Response to varying rates of carbohydrate ingestion during exercise. *Med. Sci. Sports Exerc.* 23:713–18, 1991.

43. National Research Council. *Diet and Health, Implications for Reducing Chronic Disease Risk.* Washington, D.C.: National Academy Press, 1989.

44. Nickerson, H. J., and Trip, A. D. Iron deficiency in adolescent cross country runners. *Physician and Sportsmed.* 11 (June):60–66, 1983.

45. Phinney, S. D., Bistrian, B. R., Evans, W. J., Gervino, E., and Blackburn, G. L. The human metabolic response to chronic ketosis without caloric restriction: Preservation of submaximal exercise capability with reduced carbohydrate oxidation. *Metabolism* 32:769–76, 1983.

46. Reybrouck, T., Ghesquiere, J., Cattaert, A., Fagard, R., and Amery, A. Ventilatory threshold during short-and long-term exercise. *J. Appl. Physiol.* 55:1694–1700, 1983.

47. Ribeiro, J. P., Hughes, V., Fielding, R. A., Holden, W., Evans, W., and Knuttgen, H. G. Metabolic and ventilatory responses to steady state exercise relative to lactate thresholds. *Eur. J. Appl. Physiol.* 55:215–21, 1986.

48. Richter, E. A., Kiens, B., Raben, A., Tvede, N., and Pedersen, B. K. Immune parameters in male athletes after a lacto-ovo vegetarian diet and a mixed Western diet. *Med. Sci. Sports Exerc.* 23:517–21, 1991.

49. Roberts, K. M., Noble, E. G., Hayden, D. B., and Taylor, A. W. Simple and complex carbohydrate-rich diets and muscle glycogen content of marathon runners. *Eur. J. Appl. Physiol.* 57:70–74, 1988.

50. Scrimgeour, A. G., Noakes, T. D., Adams, B., and Myburgh, K. The influence of weekly training distance on fractional utilization of maximum aerobic capacity in marathon and ultramarathon runners. *Eur. J. Appl. Physiol.* 55:202–9, 1986.

51. Sherman, W. M. Pre-event nutrition. *Gatorade Sports Sci. Exch.* 1(12), 1989.

52. Sherman, W. M., Costill, D. L., Fink, W. J., et al. Effect of exercise-diet manipulation on muscle glycogen and its subsequent utilization during performance. *Int. J. Sports Med.* 2:114–17, 1981.

53. Singer, R. N., and Neeves, R. E. Effect of food consumption on 200-yard free style swim performance. *Res. Q.* 39:355–60, 1968.

54. Steen, S. N. Nutritional concerns of athletes who must reduce body weight. *Gatorade Sports Sci. Exch.* 2(20), 1989.

55. Tarnopolsky, M. A., MacDougall, J. D., and Atkinson, S. A. Influence of protein intake and training status on nitrogen balance and lean body mass. *J. Appl. Physiol.* 64:187–93, 1988.

56. United States Department of Agriculture. *Nutritive Value of Foods.* Washington, D.C.: U.S. Government Printing Office, 1981.

57. White, J. R. Effects of eating a liquid meal at specific times upon subsequent performances in the one-mile run. *Res. Q.* 39:206–10, 1968.

58. Whitmire, D. Vitamins and minerals: A perspective in physical performance. In *Sports Nutrition for the 90s,* eds. J. R. Berning and S. N. Steen, Gaithersberg, MD: Aspen Publishers, Inc., 1991.

59. Williams, M. H. *Nutrition for Fitness and Sport,* 3d ed. Dubuque, IA: Wm. C. Brown Publishers, 1992.

60. Williams, R. J. *Physician's Handbook of Nutritional Science.* Springfield, IL: Charles C. Thomas, 1975.

30

Special Aids to Performance

Alkalinizers

Phosphate Loading

Amphetamines (Benzedrine)

Anabolic Steroids

Aspartates

Blood Doping (Erythrocythemia)

Blood Doping with Erythropoietin

Caffeine

Carbohydrate Feeding (Glucose, Fructose, and Glucose Polymer)

Improving Lactate Tolerance by Lactate Ingestion

Oxygen and Vitamins

Wheat-Germ Oil

Very small improvements in athletic performance can make the difference between mediocre and championship achievement. Differences of 1% or 2% can be very meaningful. For example, an improvement of only 2% in a four-minute mile brings the time down to 3:55.2.

Because of the importance of small improvements, which are very difficult to obtain by normal training methods when performance approaches record times or championship levels, coaches and athletes have tried to identify special aids to performance, sometimes called *ergogenic aids* (ergo=work, genics=producing). Manipulation of diet, use of various drugs, and use of "miracle" foods have all been areas of interest at times. This search for methods to improve athletic achievement can be considered wholesome as long as: 1) special aids are used to supplement, not to supplant, excellence in training and conditioning, 2) the special aids constitute no hazard to the athletes, and 3) the aids are not illegal or banned by sanctioning bodies.

Ergogenic aids can function in one of two ways: 1) by improving the capacity of the muscles and/or the O_2 transport system to do work or 2) by removing or reducing inhibitory mechanisms to allow use of previously untapped reserves. The first function must be considered the sounder approach because the second function must inevitably reduce the safety factor with which the organism has been provided.

In general, the use of drugs falls into the second category. Furthermore, the use of any drugs to improve athletic performance is cause for disqualification by the International Amateur Athletic Federation, the Amateur Athletic Union, and the U.S. Olympic Association as contrary to the highest ideals of sportsmanship. Even more important, some drugs that have reportedly been used by athletes (such as the amphetamines) can be habituating and can have other harmful effects. Although the ergogenic effects of some drugs are discussed in this chapter, this should in no way be construed as support for their use. This discussion is included for academic purposes only.

Alkalinizers

Over the years it has been thought that the amount of O_2 debt (recovery O_2) attainable by an athlete is a very important factor during anaerobic or heavy endurance work. The size of the O_2 debt achievable was thought to be limited by the blood and tissue pH. For these reasons pharmacological interventions that improve the buffering of the fixed acids such as lactic acid produced by anaerobiosis were considered potential ergogenic aids. Modification of pH is now even more attractive because changes in pH are known to exert metabolic effects by influencing enzyme activity. Anaerobic glycolysis is associated with the production of H^+ (drop in pH), and the change in pH in turn may lead to other metabolic effects tending to impair muscle performance by reducing aerobic glycolysis or fatty acid oxidation.

Early workers in this area established the feasibility of displacing the pH of the blood upward (prior to exercise) by the ingestion of alkaline salts, so that a heavy workout resulted only in a return to the normal pH value instead of the displacement toward more acidic values that usually occurs (64). Dennig and associates (24), working at the Harvard Fatigue Laboratory, demonstrated a decreased ability to accumulate O_2 debt in acidosis brought about by ingestion of acid salts. It was inferred from this that alkalosis should improve the possibility for buffering an increased O_2 debt. Dill and coworkers (26) demonstrated this increased O_2 debt capability. A runner in an alkaline state ran 6:04 minutes to exhaustion (on a treadmill), compared with 5:22 minutes from a normal state. The O_2 debt was about 20% greater in the first case, which agrees roughly with the increased time of running.

Dennig (25) continued this line of experimentation in Germany with a well-controlled study on ten subjects who worked to exhaustion on a treadmill and cycle ergometer. In all cases, his subjects were able to increase their endurance by 30% to 100% when they started in an alkaline state. His procedure, after many experiments, consisted of ingestion of a mixture of sodium citrate (5.0 gm), sodium bicarbonate (3.5 gm), and potassium citrate (1.5 gm) in two to four doses per day taken after mealtime (this started two days before an event and ceased at least five hours before the event). Dennig pointed out that the effect will be lost over longer periods because the organism adjusts to the artificial alkalinization (it would also be undesirable from a health standpoint). Some of his subjects experienced moderate side effects, such as stomach gas and loose bowels.

More recently, a well-controlled study by Jones and colleagues (44) has shown clearly improved endurance performance on a cycle ergometer at 95% $\dot{V}O_2$ max after ingestion of sodium bicarbonate. Acting as their own controls, subjects showed a 41% decrement in performance after taking ammonium chloride to acidify blood reaction (lowered pH) and a 62% improvement after alkalinizing with bicarbonate, which was administered in small portions over a three-hour period for a total dose of 0.3 gm/kg body weight. Such a dose would amount to four to five level measuring teaspoonfuls of bicarbonate for an average-sized male. Their subjects apparently tolerated this amount well, but in some people the amount might induce symptoms such as diarrhea and vomiting. Interestingly, bicarbonate loading has been shown to decrease the rating of perceived exertion (RPE) during exercise at intensities above approximately 60% of $\dot{V}O_2$ max (63, 74, 83) but has no effect at lower intensities (49, 63). In view of the large benefits reported, this procedure would seem worthy of further investigation, especially for application to athletes whose events require high fractions of $\dot{V}O_2$ max for periods of time up to four to five minutes.

McCartney and coworkers (59), working in the same laboratory with the same protocol, found no significant change in performance on short-term (thirty-second) maximal performance. This is in agreement with findings of German investigators who also found no improvement in the 400-meter run as the result of alkalinization (47). A recent investigation using a similar protocol found significant improvement of 2.9 seconds in 800-meter run times of trained track athletes (79). Thus it is tempting to conclude that alkalinization is effective only in events that are two minutes or more in duration. It has been suggested that the difference in findings is best explained on the basis that alterations in blood pH had little influence on muscle pH. It is well established that the pH of resting muscle is unaltered by variations in plasma pH above 7.5. Thus the resting muscle pH just before the start of exercise may not have been altered, and the short duration of the exercise would not have allowed full expression of the effect of the blood pH changes (59).

A recent review by Williams (83) indicates that while the results of research investigations are equivocal, bicarbonate loading using approximately 0.3 grams of sodium bicarbonate per kilogram of body weight consumed one to two hours prior to exercise appears to:

1. Decrease the acidity of the blood at rest and following high-intensity exercise.

2. Reduce the psychological perception of effort during high-intensity exercise.

3. Have no effect on performance in very high-intensity exercise bouts that last less than thirty seconds.

4. Have no effect on performance in endurance events lasting longer than ten minutes, although additional research is merited.

5. Enhance performance in high-intensity exercise bouts lasting approximately one to seven minutes.

6. Enhance performance in the later stages of high-intensity exercise bouts that are interspersed with rest periods.

Phosphate Loading

Oral administration of sodium phosphate has been used as an ergogenic aid. The procedure normally involves ingesting approximately 600 to 1,000 milligrams of sodium phosphate, four to six times per day for three to six days prior to exercise (1, 11, 27, 50, 73, 76). Kreider and coworkers (50) have identified six potential mechanisms through which phosphate supplementation may affect human performance:

1. Elevations in serum and intracellular phosphate promoting phosphate-stimulated glycolysis.

2. Increased availability of phosphate for oxidative phosphorylation and creatine phosphate synthesis.

3. An increased red cell anaerobic glycolysis and efficiency.

4. An elevation in red cell 2,3-diphosphyglycerate (2,3-DPG) promoting a reduced oxyhemoglobin affinity at a given oxygen tension.

5. An enhanced myocardial and cardiovascular efficiency.

6. A possible attenuation in anaerobic threshold.

There is conflicting evidence concerning the ergogenic effects of phosphate loading. While some investigations have reported increases in $\dot{V}O_2$ max (11, 50, 73) and anaerobic threshold (50), in general, phosphate loading has not been shown to significantly improve endurance performance during running (27, 50), bicycling (50, 76), or isokinetic leg extension activities (27). Stewart and colleagues (73), however, reported 10% to 25% increases in the time to exhaustion during an incremental cycle ergometer test as a result of phosphate loading compared to placebo or control situations. Because of the lack of consistent findings among investigations, Williams (82) has stated "Whether or not phosphate salt supplementation confers an ergogenic effect is still questionable." Considerable additional research is necessary before phosphate loading should be considered an effective ergogenic aid to performance.

Amphetamines (Benzedrine)

An amphetamine, in all its various forms (primarily d-amphetamine sulfate and its European relative Pervitin), is a sympathomimetic amine, and it is used by the medical profession as a central nervous system stimulant. Pharmacology texts warn against its use as a remedy for sleepiness or fatigue or to increase capacity for work because: 1) there is a danger of addiction, 2) it removes the warning of impending overstrain, 3) its vasopressor effects are undesirable, and 4) cases of collapse have been reported. Obviously, this discussion is academic, as the use of such drugs by athletes is to be strongly discouraged.

The literature provides evidence that amphetamine sulfate inhibits fatigue as measured by voluntary contractions on an ergograph (3), improves hand and arm coordination (56), improves the strength of forearm flexion (40) and handgrip (40, 56), and improves the athletic performance of swimmers, runners, and weight throwers (71). Pervitin was found to increase work output on a cycle ergometer (53).

On the other hand, some investigators have been unable to verify these results (15, 37, 45, 84), and we must conclude that the ergogenic effects are—at best—debatable and that the dangers involved are considerable.

The only recent study in this area, by Chandler and Blair (12), confirms the fact that these drugs have no consistent effect in all people nor even a reproducible effect on any one subject. They also confirmed the cardiovascular hazards of the drugs.

Anabolic Steroids

Evidence provided some years ago suggested that administering testosterone (a male sex hormone) to animals (61) and humans (70) results in an increase in muscle weight (hypertrophy) and strength. Testosterone is a steroid that has both androgenic (producing masculine characteristics) and anabolic (nitrogen retention–protein building) qualities. Steroids have been synthetically developed that are chemically related to testosterone but have structural changes at the molecular level that increase the anabolic effects while decreasing the androgenic effects. Various commercial preparations of the *anabolic steroids* are in vogue among strength athletes. This, again, is a drug of considerable physiological potency, with many undesirable side effects, and thus it must be prescribed by a physician.

The health hazards incurred by the use of the anabolic steroids are such that the American College of Sports Medicine (4) has issued the position statement given in table 30.1.

The position statement by the ACSM was not made lightly. It must be realized that while the benefits to muscle strength, body mass, and performance are questionable at best, the health hazards are very real and can be extremely serious. Alterations of normal liver function have been found in as many as 80% of sixty-nine patients treated with oral anabolic-androgenic steroids, and five reports document the occurrence of hepatitis in seventeen patients treated with these steroids, of whom seven died of liver failure (4). In the male athlete, endogenous hormone production is suppressed, and the production of sperm cells may be reduced to the point of sterility. In the female, these steroids may cause masculinization, disruption of normal growth pattern,

voice changes, acne, hirsutism, and enlargement of the clitoris (4). The trade-off of real health hazards for scientifically unproven performance benefit seems imprudent.

The ACSM position stand (4) on the use of anabolic-androgenic steroids in sports includes a comprehensive literature review and 115 references. The interested reader is referred to this source.

Aspartates

Aspartic acid is a dicarboxylic amino acid that is known to form one of the links between protein and carbohydrate metabolism. Its conversion to oxaloacetic acid places it in the citric acid cycle, which provides energy from carbohydrate breakdown (chap. 3). It has been shown that the respiration of a minced pigeon breast muscle can be increased by the addition of aspartic acid.

These well-known facts of biochemistry led to experimentation by the medical profession with aspartic acid salts for the relief of fatigue. In a group of 200 patients, all of whom complained of fatigue (postinfluenza, neurosis, gastrointestinal problems, menopause, old age, and so on), administration of potassium and magnesium aspartates resulted in subjective relief in a large percentage of cases (51). A more objective study on rats showed that the swim time to complete exhaustion was increased 15% in a group of thirty-six on aspartates, compared with a similar control group (65). It is of interest that in this experiment the improvement was seen most clearly in the low-endurance group of rats; the performance of "athletic" rats was altered very little.

In an investigation of fatigue in 163 subjects that included a blind study (subjects did not know whether they were on aspartates or placebo) and a double-blind crossover trial (neither subjects nor investigator knew, and

Table 30.1	American College of Sports Medicine Position Stand on the Use of Anabolic-Androgenic Steroids in Sports (4)

1. Anabolic-androgenic steroids in the presence of an adequate diet can contribute to increases in body weight, often in the lean mass compartment.
2. The gains in muscular strength achieved through high-intensity exercise and proper diet can occur by the increased use of anabolic-androgenic steroids in some individuals.
3. Anabolic-androgenic steroids do not increase aerobic power or capacity for muscular exercise.
4. Anabolic-androgenic steroids have been associated with adverse effects on the liver, cardiovascular system, reproductive system, and psychological status in therapeutic trials and in limited research on athletes. Until further research is completed, the potential hazards of the use of the anabolic-androgenic steroids in athletes must include those found in therapeutic trials.
5. The use of anabolic-androgenic steroids by athletes is contrary to the rules and ethical principles of athletic competition as set forth by many of the sports governing bodies. The American College of Sports Medicine supports these ethical principles and deplores the use of anabolic-androgenic steroids by athletes.

each group had a course of aspartates and placebo), subjective and objective evidence of relief of fatigue was presented (69).

On the other hand, Consolazio and his co-workers (14, 58) at the U.S. Army Medical Research and Nutrition Laboratory were unable to verify these results on animals or on men. Fallis and associates (32) ran an experiment on twenty-six penitentiary-inmate weight lifters who regularly engaged in athletic activities, and they reported no significant differences in eight different measures that involved weight lifting and endurance. It is of interest, however, that in six of the seven events that could be considered as having a muscular endurance factor, the results favored the aspartate trials. The lack of statistical significance of the differences could conceivably be the result of a real difference, which was obscured by a large variability and the small number of subjects.

Since the aspartic acid salts can be considered foods rather than drugs, there would be no danger (with sensible doses) in further experimentation. This seems advisable in view of the lack of agreement.

Blood Doping (Erythrocythemia)

Blood doping usually involves removing approximately two pints of blood, eight to twelve weeks prior to an endurance competition (18). The red blood cells (RBC) are then separated and frozen. The athlete continues to train as usual and the body restores the RBC count to normal levels through a process called hemopoiesis. During the week prior to competition, the RBCs are reinfused (18). This process results in an increase in RBC concentration and thus, oxygen transport capability (35, 81).

In two different studies, Ekblom and co-workers (29, 30) showed that drawing 800 to 1,200 ml of blood and then reinfusing subjects with their own red blood cells three to four weeks later resulted in 8% to 9% increases in $\dot{V}O_2$ max. Although some other investigators have had difficulty reproducing this phenomenon (20, 75, 80), the only other group that verified an increase of blood O_2-carrying capacity was able to find similar improvements in $\dot{V}O_2$ max (8), thus corroborating the work of the Ekblom group.

More recent work has shown conclusively that $\dot{V}O_2$ max and endurance performance can be significantly improved by blood doping, more properly called *erythrocythemia* because of the resulting increase in hemoglobin level and consequently enhanced O_2 transport (8, 35, 36, 81). Previous work that failed to find significant improvement was flawed by: 1) inadequate reinfusion volumes, 2) premature reinfusion before subjects had recovered from the anemia following blood withdrawal, or 3) blood being improperly stored.

Unfortunately, there is an ethical dilemma. The Medical Commission of the International Olympic Committee defines doping as the administration of, or the use by a competing athlete of, any substance foreign to the body or of any physiological substance taken in abnormal quantity or taken by an abnormal route of entry into the body with the sole intention of increasing in an artificial and unfair manner his or her performance in competition. On the other hand, it might be argued that blood doping offers only the same advantage in enhancing hemoglobin concentration that some athletes enjoy by training at high elevation to compete at sea level. Blood doping appears to be an effective method of improving distance running performance but has been banned by the International Olympic Committee and the National Collegiate Athletic Association (18).

Blood Doping with Erythropoietin

The drug erythropoietin has been approved by the Food and Drug Administration for use, primarily, in patients with various forms of anemia and/or kidney disease. The function of erythropoietin is to stimulate bone marrow to produce red blood cells (RBC). Erythropoietin is also a naturally occurring hormone produced by the kidneys that responds to low blood hemoglobin levels (18).

Exogenous administration of erythropoietin can, theoretically, improve endurance exercise performance in the same way as conventional blood doping procedures. In essence, erythropoietin is a drug that mimics the results of blood doping by increasing hematocrit (percentage of RBCs) and thereby enhances oxygen transport to the working muscles (18).

To date there is little evidence with regard to the performance-enhancing effect of exogenous erythropoietin administration although anecdotal evidence has suggested that endurance performance may be improved by as much as 19% (9). Ekblom (28) has reported that seven weeks of erythropoieten injections increased endurance performance by a minimum of 10%. A recent study by Schena and associates (66) found that blood levels of endogenous erythropoietin were increased by 15% to 24% following endurance running and bicycle races. These changes were transient, however, with no change reported in basal erythropoietin levels.

There are potentially dangerous side effects associated with the drug erythropoietin. Elevation of hematocrit above 55% is generally considered risky, and theoretically, excessive doses of erythropoieten could elevate hematocrit to 80%. In addition, hematocrit is generally increased as a result of long-duration endurance activity such as the marathon due to fluid loss. The thickened blood clots more quickly and can increase the risk of heart attack, stroke, and pulmonary edema (18). It has been suggested that competitive athletes may have died as a result of erythropoietin abuse (9). Because of the potential health hazards, the International Olympic Committee has recently banned the use of artificial erythropoietin (72).

Caffeine

Caffeine is used in medicine as a central nervous system stimulant, particularly for psychical functions. It is also used as a diuretic. Medicinal dosage ranges from 100 to 500 mg. A cup of coffee usually contains 100 to 150 mg, and tea contains slightly less.

Graf (38) has reported on experiments in Germany during World War II to find stimulants suitable for improving physical and mental efficiency in combatting the stressful conditions of war. It was found that, although caffeine was a strong mental stimulant, it resulted in a very undesirable impairment of motor coordination (in target shooting, writing, and simulated auto driving). There was also a hangover effect, in which mental efficiency, after having been improved, fell off below normal values from one to three hours after the stimulant was taken.

More recent data have provided conflicting results with respect to the ergogenic effects of caffeine. Theoretically, during heavy endurance exercise caffeine should shift energy consumption toward a greater utilization of fat (free fatty acids) with a concomitant glycogen sparing effect (chap. 3), thus improving endurance performance. Interestingly, however, Wilcox (78) has indicated that "the majority of the studies evaluating substrate utilization during a fixed interval (ranging from 60 to 120 minutes) of running or cycling find no evidence of enhanced fat utilization following caffeine consumption." Thus the theoretical effect of caffeine on fatty acid utilization during exercise has not been conclusively supported by the empirical evidence.

Ivy and coworkers (41, 42) and Costill, Dalsky, and Fink (17) conducted some of the original controlled studies with regard to the effect of caffeine on endurance performance using trained cyclists riding for one to two hours. In one experiment (42), they found that 250 mg caffeine (two to three cups of coffee) ingested one hour prior to the ride, followed by ingestion of an additional 250 mg taken at fifteen-minute intervals over the first ninety minutes of exercise, increased work output by 7.4% and $\dot{V}O_2$ by 7.3% compared with control. Since the perceived exertion remained unchanged, it is possible that at least part of the improvement is related to the psychological effects of caffeine. It is important to note, however, that more recent investigations (6, 10) have failed to demonstrate improved endurance performance following caffeine ingestion. Based on the conflicting evidence, Wilcox (78) in a recent review stated "caffeine intake does not appear to jeopardize athletic performance, but there is not sufficient evidence at this time to support an expectation of improved performance."

It is possible that caffeine has a direct effect on muscle contraction. The work of Lopes and coworkers (55) suggests that 500 mg caffeine has a significant direct effect on skeletal muscle response. The effect observed was an improvement in force of 8% to 10%. Since this was produced in response to electrical stimulation of the muscles' motor nerve the effect could not have been psychogenic. Thus there are several routes by which caffeine may aid performance and additional research is necessary to clearly delineate the ergogenic effects of caffeine ingestion.

Caffeine is one of a number of stimulants banned by the International Olympic Committee (IOC). The IOC allows urinary concentrations of caffeine up to 12 micrograms per milliliter (82). A five ounce cup of coffee contains approximately 100 milligrams of caffeine (range equals 40 to 150 milligrams) and results in 1.5 micrograms per milliliter of caffeine in the urine within two to three hours (78). Thus, the caffeine equivalent of six to eight cups of coffee could exceed the IOC legal limit.

Carbohydrate Feeding (Glucose, Fructose, and Glucose Polymer)

As was discussed in chapters 3 and 29, the duration of moderately intense work that can be sustained depends on the initial level of glycogen stored in the working muscle and its rate of utilization. When the glycogen reserves in the active muscles are depleted, work can be continued only at a lower power output, which allows utilization of free fatty acids as energy substrate. On this basis one would not expect glucose feeding to improve performance in athletic events of short to moderate duration. However, if exogenous glucose (that fed orally) could substitute for some of the energy substrate requirement normally provided by muscle glycogen, then the point of depletion of endogenous muscle glycogen should be delayed, with a consequent enhancement of performance in the later stages of endurance events such as cross-country running, marathons, and cross-country skiing.

Both animal studies and human investigations have shown that skeletal muscle can take up large amounts of glucose and that when it is supplied from an external source it can exert a glycogen sparing effect on the liver and the working skeletal muscles, thus delaying the onset of fatigue (2, 5, 19, 39, 43, 52).

It has also been shown that the ergogenic effect of glucose feeding is not seen until at least 20 to 30 minutes after ingestion (16, 42, 62) and probably reaches its maximum between 60 and 120 minutes later. If the event lasts four hours, about 100 gm of glucose may be utilized. This may represent as much as 55% of the overall carbohydrate metabolism, with peak utilization occurring after ninety minutes (62). Therefore it would be advisable to repeat glucose intake every sixty to ninety minutes or, even better, in smaller amounts administered more frequently.

Glucose feeding has been shown to improve endurance time by 19% and efficiency by 6% in a simulated bicycle road race of 100 miles that elicited 67% of the $\dot{V}O_2$ max in eight trained racing cyclists (7).

The most recent work suggests that fructose (fruit sugar), a monosaccharide sugar closely related to glucose, has a considerable advantage over glucose. It has been observed that glucose ingestion before exercise results in increased insulin secretion that in turn causes an exercise-induced hypoglycemia (lowering of blood sugar) and therefore an earlier depletion of muscle glycogen. The practical effect of this phenomenon has been demonstrated in decreased endurance performances of up to 25% (33, 46). Fructose, on the other hand, does not cause this hypoglycemic response but still furnishes the same amount of carbohydrate energy (48, 54, 60).

The problem grows more complex when the athlete faces the dual problems of exhaustion from muscle glycogen depletion and the loss of body water in endurance exercise in a hot environment that ultimately results in hyperthermia. While the use of glucose or fructose could be advantageous in a cool environment, they are both small molecules and therefore raise the osmotic pressure in the gastro-intestinal tract. This slows the movement of both water and carbohydrate into the tissues where it is needed. For this reason more complex molecules of carbohydrate in which several units of glucose are joined together to create a larger molecule (glucose polymer) have been used in athletic drinks. Such a polymer represents a molecule that may be three to four times larger. Therefore it creates only one-third to one-fourth the osmotic pressure when dissolved in the stomach, for the same amount of sugar provided. It has been shown by several investigators that this can be an effective approach in events where both fluid and carbohydrate delivery are important (endurance events in the heat) (34, 43, 67). At carbohydrate concentration comparable to that frequently used in athletic drinks (5% or less), Foster and coworkers found that glucose polymer simultaneously delivered 69% more fluid and 33% more carbohydrate than glucose (34).

Improving Lactate Tolerance by Lactate Ingestion

It has recently been suggested that since removal of the lactate generated by exercise constitutes one limit of physical fitness, performance might be augmented by a diet that would induce the enzymes necessary for lactate clearance through gluconeogenesis (57). Preliminary studies have suggested that both fitness and the rate of clearance of blood lactate were augmented by feeding lactate in humans, but the experiments provided no evidence as to whether these effects resulted from a change in membrane transport of lactate or from the induction of some limiting enzyme in gluconeogenesis (57). This hypothesis has interesting implications, but much more investigation is needed.

Oxygen and Vitamins

The use of oxygen to improve athletic performance was discussed in chapter 9. Vitamin supplementation as an ergogenic aid has also been discussed (chap. 29).

Wheat-Germ Oil

Wheat-germ oil (WGO) contains several factors that seem to have biological activity: 1) vitamin E (alpha, beta, and gamma tocopherols), 2) fatty acids, such as linoleic acid, and

3) octacosanol, an alcohol that can be synthetically prepared. Cureton (21, 23) has provided evidence of an improved training effect on middle-aged men when the physical training was supplemented by WGO. However, a later study by Cureton (22) on young men showed only statistically nonsignificant differences.

In a dietary study on guinea pigs that lasted twenty-eight days and ended with a swim test to exhaustion, it was found that all animals on a natural (control) diet drowned within ten minutes; 25% to 33% of those on a corn-oil (vitamin E) supplemented diet were still swimming at sixty minutes; and 60% of those fed WGO were still swimming at sixty minutes. Weanling rats who were fed on WGO showed no difference in swimming ability from those supplemented with corn oil (31).

In another study on swimming rats, no differences in performance were observed between those on WGO, vitamin E, or octacosanol as compared with controls (13).

Well-controlled studies on adolescent human swimmers have also shown no effect due to vitamin E supplementation (68).

It must be concluded that neither an ergogenic principle in WGO nor an ergogenic effect of the whole oil has been conclusively established. Cureton's early work (21, 23) is persuasive, and the failure to achieve significant differences in the later work might be explained on the basis of age differences in the subject populations. Further experimentation seems justified.

Summary

1. A survey of the literature on ergogenic aids leaves the distinct impression that even if "doping" with drugs were legal, ethical, and nonhazardous, the practice would be difficult to justify on the basis of experimental evidence. On the other hand, use of some proposed ergogenic aids that are nonhazardous and that can be considered normal hygienic

procedures to help an athlete gain an extra 1% or 2% improvement in performance can be justified if every effort has been exerted to bring training and conditioning to a peak.

2. A further disadvantage of ergogenic aids is that an athlete may become psychologically addicted, and a decrement from normal performance can occur if at a critical moment the aid is unavailable.

3. In interpretation of research data, the finding of no positive results can never be conclusive because a single experiment is never capable of seeing all the possible changes that may occur. For example, an investigator using a simple magnifying glass might deny the existence of bacteria, which are clearly seen under a high-powered microscope. Similarly, a research design is not all-encompassing.

4. In some experiments the differences that favor the working hypothesis were disregarded because they did not achieve statistical significance. This is as it should be, but the rigor of our method must not obscure the fact that even a real difference may remain statistically nonsignificant if: a) the difference is small, b) the number of subjects is small, and c) the variability within or between subjects on the parameter of interest is large.

   This concept was clearly demonstrated in a study that showed the advantage of using expert swimmers instead of nonexperts for evaluation of the effects of ergogenic aids (77). Obtaining as much precision with nonexperts as was obtained with fifteen experts would have necessitated (because of greater intrasubject variability) an increase of the nonexpert sample size from fifteen to about eighty.

5. In view of the experiments cited, it seems that further experimentation is justified for such ergogenic aids as the alkalinizers, aspartates, caffeine, glucose, and wheat-germ oil. Used judiciously, none of these should be hazardous.

References

1. Ahlberg, A., Weatherwax, R. S., Deady, M., Perez, H. R., Otto, R. M., Cooperstein, D., Smith, T. K., and Wygand, J. W. Effect of phosphate loading on cycle ergometer performance. *Med. Sci. Sports Exerc.* 18 (supplement):S11, 1986.

2. Ahlborg, G., and Felig, P. Influence of glucose ingestion on fuel-hormone response during prolonged exercise. *J. Appl. Physiol.* 41:683–88, 1976.

3. Alles, G. A., and Feigen, G. A. The influence of benzedrine on work decrement and patellar reflex. *Am. J. Physiol.* 136:392–400, 1942.

4. American College Sports Medicine. Stand on the use of anabolic-androgenic steroids in sports. *Sports Med. Bull.* 19:13–18, 1984.

5. Bagby, G. J., Green, H. J., Katsuta, S., and Gollnick, P. D. Glycogen depletion in exercising rats infused with glucose, lactate or pyruvate. *J. Appl. Physiol.* 45:425–29, 1978.

6. Berglund, B., and Hemmingsson, P. Effects of caffeine ingestion on exercise performance at low and high altitudes in cross-country skiers. *Int. J. Sports Med.* 3:234–36, 1982.

7. Brooke, J. D., Davies, G. J., and Green, L. F. The effects of normal and glucose syrup work diets on the performance of racing cyclists. *J. Sports Med. Phys. Fitness* 15:257–65, 1975.

8. Buick, F. J., Gledhill, N., Froese, A. B., Spriet, L., and Meyers, E. C. Effect of induced erythrocythemia on aerobic work capacity. *J. Appl. Physiol.* 48:636–42, 1980.

9. Burke, E., Coyle, E. F., Eichner, E. R., Nadel, E. R., and Williams, M. H. Blood doping and plasma volume expansion: Benefits and dangers. *Gatorade Sports Sci. Exch.* (Roundtable) Spring, 1991.

10. Butts, N. K., and Crowell, D. Effect of caffeine ingestion on cardiorespiratory endurance in men and women. *Res. Q. Exerc. Sport* 56:301–5, 1985.

11. Cade, R., Conte, M., Zauner, C., Mars, D., Peterson, J., Lunne, D., Hommen, N., and Packer, D. Effects of phosphate loading on 2,3-diphosphoglycerate and maximal oxygen uptake. *Med. Sci. Sports Exerc.* 16:263–68, 1984.

12. Chandler, J. V., and Blair, S. N. The effect of amphetamines on selected physiological components related to athletic success. *Med. Sci. Sports Exer.* 12:65–69, 1980.

13. Consolazio, C. F., Matoush, L. O., Nelson, R. A., Isaac, G. J., and Hursh, L. M. Effects of octacosanol, wheat germ oil, and vitamin E on performance of swimming rats. *J. Appl. Physiol.* 19:265–67, 1964.

14. Consolazio, C. F., Nelson, R. A., Matoush, L. O., and Isaac, G. J. Effects of aspartic acid salts (Mg + K) on physical performance of men. *J. Appl. Physiol.* 19:257–61, 1964.

15. Cooter, G. R., and Stull, G. A. The effect of amphetamine on endurance in rats. *J. Sports Med. Phys. Fitness* 14:120–26, 1974.

16. Costill, D. L., Bennett, A., Branam, G., and Eddy, D. Glucose ingestion at rest and during prolonged exercise. *J. Appl. Physiol.* 34:764–69, 1973.

17. Costill, D. L., Dalsky, G. P., and Fink, W. J. Effects of caffeine ingestion on metabolism and exercise performance. *Med. Sci. Sports* 10:155–58, 1978.

18. Cowart, V. S. Erythropoietin: A dangerous new form of blood doping? *Phys. Sportsmed.* 17:115–18, 1989.

19. Coyle, E. F., Hagberg, J. M., Hurley, B. F., Martin, W. H., Ehsani, A. A., and Holloszy, J. O. Carbohydrate feeding during prolonged strenuous exercise can delay fatigue. *J. Appl. Physiol.* 55:230–35, 1983.

20. Cunningham, K. G. The effect of transfusional polycythemia on aerobic work capacity. *J. Sports Med. Phys. Fitness* 18:353–58, 1978.

21. Cureton, T. K. Effects of wheat germ oil and vitamin E on normal human subjects in physical training programs. *Am. J. Physiol.* 179:628, 1954.

22. ———. Improvements in physical fitness associated with a course of U.S. Navy underwater trainees with and without dietary supplements. *Res. Q.* 34:440–53, 1963.

23. Cureton, T. K., and Pohndorf, R. Influence of wheat germ oil as a dietary supplement in a program of conditioning exercises with middle-aged subjects. *Res. Q.* 26:391–407, 1955.

24. Dennig, H., Talbot, J. H., Edwards, H. T., and Dill, D. B. Effect of acidosis and alkalosis upon capacity for work. *J. Clin. Invest.* 9:601–13, 1931.

25. ———. Über Steigerung der korperlichen Leistungsfahigkeit durch eingriffe in den Saurebasenhaushalt. *Dtsch. Med. Wochenschr.* 63:733–36, 1937.

26. Dill, D. B., Edwards, H.T., and Talbott, J.H. Alkalosis and the capacity for work. *J. Biol. Chem.* 97:58–59, 1932.

27. Duffy, D. J., and Conlee, R. K. Effects of phosphate loading on leg power and high intensity treadmill exercise. *Med. Sci. Sports Exerc.* 18:674–77, 1986.

28. Ekblom, B. Effects of iron deficiency, variations in hemoglobin concentration and erythropoietin injections on physical performance and relevant physiolgoical parameters. *Proceedings of First I.O.C. World Congress on Sports Sciences* pp. 9–11, 1989.

29. Ekblom, B., Goldbarg, A. N., and Gullbring, B. Response to exercise after blood loss and reinfusion. *J. Appl. Physiol.* 33:175–80, 1972.

30. Ekblom, B., Wilson, G., and Astrand, P-O. Central circulation during exercise after venesection and reinfusion of red blood cells. *J. Appl. Physiol.* 40:379–83, 1976.

31. Erschoff, B. H., and Levin, E. Beneficial effect of an unidentified factor in wheat germ oil on the swimming performance of guinea pigs. *Fed. Proc.* 14:431–32, 1955.

32. Fallis, N., Wilson, W. R., Tetreault, L. L., and La Sagna, L. Effect of potassium and magnesium aspartates on athletic performance. *J.A.M.A.* 185:129, 1963.

33. Foster, C., Costill, D. L., and Fink, W. J. Effects of pre-exercise feedings on endurance performance. *Med. Sci. Sports* 11:1–5, 1979.

34. ———. Gastric emptying times characteristic of glucose and glucose polymer solutions. *Res. Q.* 51:299–305, 1980.

35. Gledhill, N. Blood doping and related issues: A brief review. *Med. Sci. Sports Exer.* 14:183–89, 1982.

36. ———. The ergogenic effect of blood doping. *Physician and Sportsmed.* 11 (Sept.):87–90, 1983.

37. Golding, L. A., and Barnard, J. R. The effects of d-amphetamine sulfate on physical performance. *J. Sports Med.* 3:221–24, 1963.

38. Graf, O. Increase of efficiency by means of pharmaceutics (stimulants). In *German Aviation Medicine, W.W. II,* vol. 2, p. 1080. Washington, D.C.: U.S. Government Printing Office, 1950.

39. Hargreaves, M., Costill, D. L., Coggan, A., Fink, W. J., and Nishibata, I. Effect of carbohydrate feedings on muscle glycogen utilization and exercise performance. *Med. Sci. Sports Exer.* 16:219–22, 1984.

40. Hurst, P. M., Radlow, R., and Bagley, S. K. The effects of d-amphetamine and chlordiazepoxide upon strength and estimated strength. *Ergonomics* 11:47–52, 1968.

41. Ivy, J. L., Costill, D. L., Fink, W. J., and Lower, R. W. Role of caffeine and glucose ingestion on metabolism during exercise. Abstract in *Med. Sci. Sports* 10:66, 1978.

42. ———. Influence of caffeine and carbohydrate feedings on endurance performance. *Med. Sci. Sports* 11:6–11, 1979.

43. Ivy, J. L., Miller, W., Dover, V., Goodyear, G., Sherman, W. M., Farrell, S., and Williams, H. Endurance improved by ingestion of a glucose polymer supplement. *Med. Sci. Sports Exer.* 15:466–71, 1983.

44. Jones, N. L., Sutton, J. R., Taylor, R., and Toews, C. J. Effect of pH on cardiorespiratory and metabolic responses to exercise. *J. Appl. Physiol.* 43:959–64, 1977.

45. Karpovich, P. V. Effect of amphetamine sulfate on athletic performance. *J.A.M.A.* 170:558–61, 1959.

46. Keller, K., and Schwarzkopf, R. Pre-exercise snacks may decrease exercise performance. *Physician and Sportsmed.* 12 (April):89–91, 1984.

47. Kinderman, W., Keul, J., and Huber, G. Physical exercise after induced alkalosis (bicarbonate or Tris-buffer). *Eur. J. Appl. Physiol.* 37:197–204, 1977.

48. Koivisto, V. A., Karonen, S. L., and Nikkila, E. A. Carbohydrate ingestion before exercise: Comparison of glucose, fructose and sweet placebo. *J. Appl. Physiol.* 51:783–87, 1981.

49. Kostka, C., and Cafarelli, E. Effect of pH on sensation and vastus lateralis electromyogram during cycling exercise. *J. Appl. Physiol.* 52:1181–85, 1982.

50. Kreider, R. B., Miller, G. W., Williams, M. H., Somma, C. T., and Nasser, T. A. Effects of phosphate loading on oxygen uptake, ventilatory anaerobic threshold, and run performance. *Med. Sci. Sports Exerc.* 22:250–56, 1990.

51. Kruse, C. A. Treatment of fatigue with aspartic acid salts. *Northwest Med.* 60:597–603, 1961.

52. Krzentowski, G., Jandrain, B., Pirnay, F., Mosora, F., Lacroix, M., Luyckx, A. S., and Lefebvre, P. J. Availability of glucose given orally during exercise. *J. Appl. Physiol.* 56:315–20, 1984.

53. Lehman, G., Straub, H., and Szakall, A. Pervitin als Leistungssteigerndes Mittel. *Arbeitsphysiologie* 10:680–91, 1939.

54. Levine, L., Evans, W. J., Cadarette, B. S., Fisher, E. C., and Bullen, B. A. Fructose and glucose ingestion and muscle glycogen use during submaximal exercise. *J. Appl. Physiol.* 55:1767–71, 1983.

55. Lopes, J. M., Aubier, M., Jardim, J., Aranda, V., and Macklem, P. T. Effect of caffeine on skeletal muscle function before and after fatigue. *J. Appl. Physiol.* 54:1303–05, 1983.

56. Lovingood, B. W., Blythe, C. S., Peacock, W. H., and Lindsay, R. B. Effects of d-amphetamine sulfate, caffeine and high temperature on human performance. *Res. Q.* 38:64–71, 1967.

57. Mann, G. V., and Garrett, H. L. Lactate tolerance, diet and physical fitness. In *Nutrition, Physical Fitness and Health,* eds. J. Pariskova and V. A. Rogozkin. Baltimore, MD: University Park Press, 1978.

58. Matoush, L. O., Consolazio, C. F., Nelson, R. A., Isaac, G. I., and Torres, J. B. Effects of aspartic acid salts (Mg + K) on swimming performance of rats and dogs. *J. Appl. Physiol.* 19:262–64, 1964.

59. McCartney, N., Heigenhauser, G. J. F., and Jones, N. L. Effects of pH on maximal power output and fatigue during short-term dynamic exercise. *J. Appl. Physiol.* 55:225–29, 1983.

60. McMurray, R. G., Wilson, J. R., and Kitchell, B. S. The effect of fructose and glucose on high intensity endurance performance. *Res. Q.* 54:156–62, 1983.

61. Papanicolaou, G. N., and Falk, E. A. General muscular hypertrophy induced by androgenic hormone. *Science* 82:238–39, 1938.

62. Pirnay, F., LaCroix, M., Mosora, F., Luyckx, A., and Lefebvre, P. Glucose oxidation during prolonged exercise evaluated with naturally labeled (^{13}C) glucose. *J. Appl. Physiol.* 43:258–61, 1977.

63. Robertson, R., Falkel, J., Drash, A., Swank, A., Metz, K., Spungen, S., and LeBoeuf, J. Effect of blood pH on peripheral and central signals of perceived exertion. *Med. Sci. Sports Exerc.* 18:114–22, 1986.

64. Ronzoni, E. The effect of exercise on breathing in experimental alkalosis by ingested sodium bicarbonate. *J. Biol. Chem.* 67:25–27, 1926.

65. Rosen, H., Blumenthal, A., and Agersborg, H. P. K. Effects of the potassium and magnesium salts of aspartic acid on metabolic exhaustion. *J. Pharm. Sci.* 51:592–93, 1962.

66. Schena, F., Cevese, A., Guidi, G. G., Mosconi, C., and Pattini, A. Serum erythropoietin changes in runners and mountain-bikers after a 42 km race. *Med. Sci. Sports Exerc.* 22 (supplement):S135, 1990.

67. Seiple, R. S., Vivian, V. M., Fox, E. L., and Bartels, R. L. Gastric emptying characteristics of two glucose polymer-electrolyte solutions. *Med. Sci. Sports Exer.* 15:366–69, 1983.

68. Sharman, I. M., Down, M. G., and Sen, R. N. The effects of training and vitamin E supplementation on the performance of adolescent swimmers. *Br. J. Sports Med.* 7:27–30, 1973.

69. Shaw, D. L., Jr., Chesney, M. A., Tullis, I. F., and Agersborg, H. P. K. Management of fatigue: A physiologic approach. *Am. J. Med. Sci.* 243:758–69, 1962.

70. Simonson, E., Kearns, W. M., and Enzer, N. Effect of methyl testosterone treatment on muscular performance and central nervous system of older men. *J. Clin. Endocrinol. Metab.* 10:528–34, 1944.

71. Smith, G. M., and Beecher, H. K. Amphetamine sulfate and athletic performance. *J.A.M.A.* 170:542–57, 1959.

72. Spriet, L. L. Blood doping and oxygen transport. In *Ergogenics, Enhancement of Performance in Exercise and Sports,* eds. D. R. Lamb and M. H. Williams. Dubuque, IA: Brown and Benchmark, 1991.

73. Stewart, I., McNaughton, L., Davies, P., and Tristram, S. Phosphate loading and the effects on $\dot{V}O_2$ max in trained cyclists. *Res. Quart. Exerc. Sport* 61:80–84, 1990.

74. Swank, A., and Robertson, R. Effect of induced alkalosis on perception of exertion during intermittent exercise. *J. Appl. Physiol.* 67:1852–57, 1989.

75. Videman, T., and Rytomaa, T. Effect of blood removal and autotransfusion on heart rate response to a submaximal workload. *J. Sports Med. Phys. Fitness* 17:387–90, 1977.

76. Weathermax, R. S., Ahlberg, A., Deady, M., Otto, R. M., Perez, H. R., Cooperstein, D., and Wygand, J. Effects of phosphate loading on bicycle time trial performance. *Med. Sci. Sports Exerc.* 18(supplement):S11–S12, 1986.

77. Weitzner, M., and Beecher, H. K. Increased sensitivity of measurements of drug effects in expert swimmers. *J. Pharm.* 139:114–19, 1963.

78. Wilcox, A. R. Caffeine and endurance performance. *Gatorade Sports Sci. Exch.* 3(26), 1990.

79. Wilkes, D., Gledhill, N., and Smyth, R. Effect of acute induced metabolic alkalosis on 800-M racing time. *Med. Sci. Sports Exer.* 15:277–80, 1983.

80. Williams, M. A., Goodwin, A. R., Perkins, R., and Bocrie, J. Effect of blood reinjection upon endurance capacity and heart rate. *Med. Sci. Sports* 5:181–86, 1973.

81. Williams, M. H. Blood doping: An update. *Physician and Sportsmed.* 9 (July):59–64, 1981.

82. Williams, M. H. Ergogenic aids. In *Sports Nutrition for the 90s,* eds. J. R. Berning and S. N. Steen. Gaithersburg, MD: Aspen Publishers, Inc., 1991.

83. Williams, M. H. Bicarbonate loading. *Gatorade Sports Sci. Exch.* 4(36), 1992.

84. Williams, M. H., and Thompson, J. Effect of variant dosages of amphetamine upon endurance. *Res. Q.* 44:417–22, 1973.

31

The Female in Athletics

Structural Gender Differences

Physiological Gender Differences
Blood Constituents
Microcirculation
Metabolic Rate and Efficiency
Oxygen Pulse
Maximum O_2 Consumption
Cardiac Output
Phenomenal Success of Young Girl Swimmers
Neuromuscular Functions

Female Limitations in Athletics

Physiological Adaptations to Training in Females
Adaptations in $\dot{V}O_2$ Max
Nature of the Cardiovascular Adaptations
Adaptation to Distance Running

Adaptations to Strength Training in Females
Socio-Psychological Considerations for Strength Training

Physiological Considerations for Strength Training

The Menstrual Cycle and Athletics
Onset of Menarche
Participation in Sports and Exercise during Menstruation
Athletic Menstrual Cycle Irregularity (AMI)
Effects of the Menstrual Cycle on Performance

Pregnancy, Childbirth, and Athletics
Effects of Heavy Exercise Programs on Labor and Delivery
Effects of Pregnancy and Childbirth on Subsequent Athletic Performance

Athletic Injuries

Emotional Factors

Athletic competition for women at the higher levels is a fairly recent development. It awaited the emancipation of women from antiquated social concepts and from clothes that were unsuited for comfortable movement, let alone athletic performance. It is indeed amusing to attempt to visualize present-day swimming or running performance in the athletic costumes of the nineteenth century. Women's athletics worthy of the name did not exist prior to World War I, and women began Olympic competition only in 1928.

As a consequence we are only beginning to learn the specialized physiology involved in the reaction of females of different ages to the various stressors in athletic competition. Furthermore, women's athletics have developed around modifications of existing men's sports, and whether these activities are best suited to the unique interests and the physiological, psychological, and sociological needs of girls and women has not really been investigated. Nevertheless, participation by girls and women in competitive athletics is increasing, and every physical educator and coach should be aware of the available knowledge about the special problems of the female in competitive sports.

Another aspect of gender differences in performance has recently become important. There is the question of the physical ability of girls and women to participate with (compete with?) boys and men at all levels of physically demanding work. This issue has been most clearly defined when related to military duty, police work, and fire fighting.

Structural Gender Differences

One of the most obvious and important differences between the genders in regard to sports performance is the ratio of strength to weight, which after puberty is normally much greater in males. This factor is most important in activities in which the weight is supported by the relatively smaller muscles of the arms and shoulder girdle, as in gymnastics. It is also a consideration when the mass of the body must be accelerated rapidly, as in jumping.

The reason for the poorer strength-weight ratio is, of course, the smaller proportion of muscle in relation to the considerably larger amount of adipose tissue in females (chap. 17). The larger stores of fatty tissue are not an unmitigated disadvantage, however; in swimming, for example, this results in better buoyancy and less heat loss to cold water.

Differences in average height and weight are well known. The differences in height and weight between the genders are quite small until the start of the girls' adolescent period. At about age eleven girls surge ahead, but within a couple of years the adolescent spurt of boys pushes them ahead and establishes their adult advantage in this respect.

In general, from adolescence on girls have narrower shoulders and broader hips than the boys (16). In the preadolescent years, the differences in mean leg lengths of boys and girls of the same age are not significant. Yet in adults the leg lengths of males relative to body length are greater than for females. During adolescence, the major gain in height is due to growth of the legs and not so much to lengthening of the trunk (16). The arms of boys are consistently longer than the arms of girls, due largely to longer forearms in boys. Unlike most other physical differences between genders, this difference is already established at two years of age (16). The longer forearm of boys would theoretically be an advantage in the third-class lever system involved in throwing.

Not only are the proportions of various tissues different in females, but the chemical constituents within each tissue are different. The female tissues, for example, contain much greater amounts of sulfur (23% more in skeletal muscle), and the creatinine coefficients are also different. More research is required to establish the significance of these facts.

A structural difference that has very significant physiological implications for athletic performance is the difference in the ratio of heart weight to body weight between the genders. From the age of ten to the age of sixty, the average value for women is only 85% to 90% of the value for men (13). After age sixty, however, the ratio is similar for men and women.

Physiological Gender Differences

Although there are many physiological differences that have general significance, only those that apply directly to athletic performance will be considered here.

Blood Constituents

On the average, twenty- to thirty-year-old men have approximately 15% more hemoglobin per 100 ml of blood and about 6% more erythrocytes (red blood cells) per cubic millimeter (13) than women in the same age group. The combination of these two factors should mean greater oxygen-carrying capacity for men.

Microcirculation

When the reddening of skin in reaction to ultraviolet radiation was used as a measure of capillary function, men were found to be less vulnerable through the entire age range (13). The resistance of the capillary wall to breakdown from mechanical manipulation was also found to be greater in males. This very likely is the reason for the greater susceptibility to bruises in females.

Metabolic Rate and Efficiency

From just before puberty through the rest of the life span, basal metabolic rate (BMR), as customarily measured and normalized for body surface area, is higher for males than for females. When BMR is evaluated in relation to muscle mass instead of surface area, however, the gender difference disappears (13).

Recent evidence has shown that the O_2 cost of running was lower in male than in female runners of college age. This difference was significant in comparisons of trained as well as untrained groups and existed at all speeds at which comparisons could be made (10). However, factors other than gender, such as level of training or mechanics of running, could have influenced the findings. These findings were supported in a recent review by Daniels and Daniels (24) concerning gender differences in the running economy of elite male and female runners.

Oxygen Pulse

This is a widely used measure of the efficiency of the heart as a respiratory organ, and it is calculated as the O_2 consumption in milliliters per heartbeat. For equal work loads, boys and girls are about equal on this measure for ages twelve to fifteen. However, there is a rapid improvement in O_2 consumption in males to a value about twice as high at ages twenty-one to twenty-five, while the oxygen pulse of females remains constant at the twelve to fifteen age value (54). This has implications that will be discussed in the following paragraphs.

Maximum O_2 Consumption

The classic work of Astrand (4) has shown that girls reach a high point in their maximum O_2 per unit weight between eight and nine years of age. This figure declines slowly until about age fifteen, after which it remains constant through young adulthood. Boys reach their peak later, at about fifteen or sixteen years of age, and maintain this peak through young adulthood.

Thus in the younger age groups (seven to thirteen) gender differences grow larger with each increasing year. At ages seven to nine the differences are small and probably not significant. By age twelve or thirteen, however, differences favoring boys of 13% to 16% in maximal O_2 consumption normalized for body weight have appeared (72). McNab, Conger, and Taylor (47) have shown in a direct comparison of twenty-four male and twenty-four female college physical education majors that the difference at this age has grown to 32% when measured as maximal O_2 per kilogram weight, as in the data above. Even when the increasing adiposity of the female is taken into consideration by expressing the data as O_2 per unit of fat-free weight the difference still favors the male by 18%. These differences were, of course highly significant. More recent data from Dill and colleagues (25) on high school age boys and girls provide similar findings, with $\dot{V}O_2$ max being 15% lower in the girls even when expressed as $\dot{V}O_2$ per unit of fat-free weight.

Cardiac Output

In view of the smaller O_2-carrying capacity of the blood in females due to lower levels of hemoglobin and red blood cells, one would expect that females would have to provide more cardiac output at any given level of O_2 consumption at submaximal workloads. This does turn out to be the case for young women (5, 7, 32). However, for women beyond childbearing age this difference is no longer significant (7). The physiological basis for this change with age remains to be elucidated.

With respect to maximal cardiac output, the best available data shows a value of 18.5 liters/min for young women compared with 24.1 liters/min for men (6). Thus there appears to be a 30% difference between genders, but it is unlikely that levels of training were equal, and therefore the true gender difference may not be quite that large.

Phenomenal Success of Young Girl Swimmers

In the light of the foregoing facts about O_2 pulse and maximum O_2 consumption, the success of young American girl swimmers in national and international competition becomes understandable. It would seem that all physiological functions essential to competitive swimming have achieved peak values by age twelve to fourteen in females, whereas these are delayed in males to late high school and college age. When we add to this the factors of: 1) very early commencement of training and 2) absence of social pressures, the accomplishment of our young girl swimmers is entirely comprehensible.

Neuromuscular Functions

Thus far we have discussed the physiology of endurance-type sports, and it is time to consider some of the factors that collectively make up the skill of motor performance. It has been reported from Germany that women generally have greater manual skill and dexterity than men (40). In the United States, Pierson and Lockhart (60) have shown there is no significant gender difference in reaction time to a visual stimulus, although men have faster movement times.

A review of the literature in this area seems to indicate that there are probably no real gender differences in either motor learning rate or capacity, unless strength is a factor.

Female Limitations in Athletics

Table 31.1 shows a comparison of male and female world records in various activities. Among other things, the table shows the undesirability of competition between the genders. Most important, however, is the comparison of how close women come to men in

| Table 31.1 | Comparison of World Records for Men and Women as of September, 1991 |

Event	Women	Men	Ratio of Performance 1991, %	Ratio of Performance 1978, %	Ratio of Performance 1963, %
Swimming (meters)					
100 freestyle	54.73	48.42	88	89	90
200 freestyle	1:57.55	1:46.69	91	93	90
400 freestyle	4:03.85	3:46.95	93	94	89
800 freestyle	8:16.22	7:50.64	95	94	90
1500 freestyle	15:52.10	14:50.30	94	93	91
100 breaststroke	1:07.91	1:01.49	91	89	86
200 breaststroke	2:26.71	2:10.60	89	89	89
100 butterfly	57.93	52.84	91	91	86
200 butterfly	2:05.96	1:56.24	90	92	86
100 backstroke	1:00.31	54.51	90	90	88
200 backstroke	2:08.60	1:57.30	91	90	88
Running (meters)					
100	10.49	9.86	94	91	89
400	47.60	43.29	91	89	85
800	1:53.28	1:41.73	89	90	86
1500	3:52.28	3:29.46	90	90	—
3000	8:22.62	7:29.45	89	89	—
Marathon	2:21.06	2:06.50	93	83	—
Field events					
High jump (meters)	2.096	2.45	86	82	84
Long jump (meters)	7.55	8.98	84	79	80
Powerlifting					
(82.5 kg weight class)					
Squat (kg)	230.0	379.5	61	—	—
Bench press (kg)	150.0	240.0	63	—	—
Dead lift (kg)	227.5	357.5	64	—	—
Total (kg)	577.5	952.5	61	—	—

the various types of activity. For lack of better information at this time, it can be inferred from table 31.1 that those activities in which women approach men's records most closely are those in which women and men are the most "physiologically" similar.

Gender differences are most evident in events that require strength and explosive power such as powerlifting, high jump, and long jump. For all other events listed in table 31.1, the ratios of female to male world records (as of 1991) ranged from 88 to 95 percent. The events where the genders were most similar in terms of performance (ratio of ≥ 93 percent) were 400, 800, and 1,500 meter freestyle swimming, the 100 meter dash, and the marathon.

The percentage ratios of performance for men and women are also given in table 31.1 for 1963 and 1978 to allow comparisons with 1991. Over this period of time, great changes occurred in the involvement of women in high-level competition. It is interesting to note that in many events (200 meter freestyle, 400 meter freestyle, 800 meter freestyle, 100 meter butterfly, 200 meter butterfly, and 800 meter run) there was a relatively large increase in the ratio of performance between females and males between 1963 and 1978 with very little additional improvement thereafter. This trend likely reflects the dramatic increase in the number of females choosing to participate in athletics during the 1960s and 1970s. This stability in performance between females and males from 1978 and 1991 in these events likely reflects what may be considered true gender differences. This may also be the case for the marathon, where the ratio increased by ten percentage points (from 83 to 93 percent) between 1978 and 1991 when females began to regularly compete at this distance. On the other hand, it is interesting to note that in several events (100 meter breaststroke as well as 100 and 400 meter dashes) the ratio of performance increased (by at least two percentage points) for females relative to males between 1963 and 1978 as well as 1978 and 1991. Apparently, in some events, females continue to improve in performance relative to males and have not as yet reached levels that reflect the true gender differences.

Wells and Plowman (69) have furnished an excellent review of the data concerning the basic question of gender differences in athletic performance and the related question of whether observed differences are biological or behavioral in nature. They conclude that the differences in performance that can be explained on the basis of body dimensions must be considered biological and are the natural result of boys' longer growth period and higher androgen levels at puberty. They believe that the biological gender differences must be accepted, while differences that are merely behavioral, given time and appropriate effort, will change. Table 31.1 supports this view.

Physiological Adaptations to Training in Females

The physiological adjustments to training in girls and women have only recently gotten the attention they deserve. Astrand and his co-workers (6) in Stockholm studied thirty girl swimmers, twelve to sixteen years of age, for one year. The girls trained from 6,000 to 71,500 yards (six to twenty-eight hours) per week and were examined extensively—medically and physiologically—during this period. It was shown that large differences existed in such important measures as maximal O_2 consumption when these girls were compared with average, untrained girls. Furthermore, the differences were highly correlated to the volume of training for each girl. More recently, Brown and associates (11) studied the effects of training for competitive cross-country running on preadolescent girls. They found maximal O_2 consumption increased by 18% at six weeks and 26% at twelve weeks. Heart rates at submaximal loads declined, and no detrimental effects were seen.

For endurance, the experiments of Klaus and Noack (40) on physical education students showed that at the end of an eighteen-week training program, the men's capacity was about one-third better than that of the women. This is to be expected in the light of the physiological measurements discussed earlier. More recent work (14), however, showed no significant difference in the responses of males and females to endurance training with respect to either aerobic power or O_2 pulse.

Kilbom (38) studied the effects of conditioning on mature females with the bicycle or walking routines using work loads that represented 52% to 77% of maximal O_2. In the young group (nineteen to thirty-one years), aerobic power improved 12% and cardiac output 11%; in the middle-aged, the improvements were 11% and 10%; and in the older women (fifty-one to sixty-four), 8% and 10%. Systolic blood pressure dropped by 15 mmHg in the older group, and serum cholesterol declined by 10%. They saw no orthopedic training complications since they used the bicycle and walking-type exercise. However, they did find that serum iron levels declined by 25% in all groups. This finding was thought to be due to greater iron usage in the enhanced erythropoiesis that accompanies vigorous exercise.

More recent work does not support the need of iron supplementation for women in moderately heavy training such as basketball (19) or cycling workouts at 70% $\dot{V}O_2$ max for twenty-five to thirty minutes three times per week (73).

The recommended daily allowance (RDA) of iron for females is 15 milligrams per day for ages eleven to fifty years and 10 milligrams per day after fifty years of age (17, 70). These values are appropriate for active as well as sedentary females, and Whitmire (70) has stated "Research to determine whether iron status changes with training has yielded somewhat contradictory results and no conclusive evidence for an increase in iron requirements in exercising individuals."

As discussed in chapter 29, there are three stages (listed from least to most serious) of iron deficiency (17):

1. Iron depletion (also called prelatent iron deficiency).
2. Iron-deficiency erthropoiesis (latent iron deficiency).
3. Iron deficiency anemia.

Iron depletion usually does not affect exercise capacity, but iron deficiency anemia can severely compromise athletic performance. Clarkson (17) has stated "There is little basis to suggest iron supplementation for individuals without iron deficiency anemia will have any ergogenic effect." In the case of iron deficiency anemia, however, iron supplementation can contribute to improved performance (17). Because of the potential for iron toxicity, iron supplementation should occur under a physician's supervision (70).

Adaptations in $\dot{V}O_2$ Max

As pointed out earlier, the physiological functions necessary for success in competitive swimming are well established in young girls twelve to fifteen. But the question may be raised: "Are girls also capable of better training adaptation at this age?" A well-controlled study of eight girls (twelve to thirteen) compared with eight young women (eighteen to twenty-one) showed that not only did the two age groups increase in $\dot{V}O_2$ max by a similar magnitude, but they also demonstrated similar rates of change in $\dot{V}O_2$ max during the training period (29). A recent study by Cress and coworkers (20) has also shown that septuagenarian women can increase in $\dot{V}O_2$ max as a result of training. Clearly endurance exercise can increase aerobic power in females of all ages from adolescence through older adulthood.

Data from Krahenbuhl, Archer, and Pettit (43) suggest that the magnitude of the training adaptation with respect to $\dot{V}O_2$ max is related to the level of serum testosterone. More data on endocrine function in relation to training parameters are badly needed.

Nature of the Cardiovascular Adaptations

A summary by Rowell (61) suggests that in the young, unfit male, training produces improved $\dot{V}O_2$ max by a combination of improvements in stroke volume and arteriovenous O_2 difference. However, in the young, unconditioned female, it appears that the initial changes over a period of some nine weeks are almost entirely due to central changes (stroke volume and cardiac output), with peripheral adaptations occurring only after the early central changes have taken place (21, 42). The increased left ventricular dimension at the end of diastolic filling, which is a typical training response in the young male, is also seen in the young female (76).

Adaptation to Distance Running

Using an experimental paradigm in which weight is added to male runners to match the greater amount of fat carried by female runners, Cureton and Sparling (23) showed a reduction in the gender difference in performance on an endurance treadmill test and on a twelve-minute run test by about 30%. This agreed with earlier work reported from the same laboratory (22). Their findings suggest that the greater level of body fat of the female is one, but not the only, important characteristic that contributes to a lower level of performance in endurance-type athletic events.

A comprehensive review of the pertinent literature in 1979 (2) resulted in the conclusion that males and females adapt to endurance training in a similar manner. Female distance runners are characterized by having a large $\dot{V}O_2$ max and low body fat (relative to the norms for females). The challenges of heat stress seem to be well tolerated by females, as discussed in chapter 28.

Based on the available evidence, the American College of Sports Medicine (2) issued the following opinion statement: "It is the opinion of the American College of Sports Medicine that females should not be denied the opportunity to compete in long-distance running. There exists no conclusive scientific or medical evidence that long-distance running is contraindicated for the healthy, trained female athlete. The American College of Sports Medicine recommends that females be allowed to compete at the national and international level in the same distances in which their male counterparts compete."

The data of table 31.1 seem to indicate that endurance per se is not gender related, since in freestyle swimming events, where power (strength) is not a large factor, females do relatively as well (or better) at 1,500 meters as at 100 meters. In running events, a drop in relative performances is seen between the sprints and the middle distances but in the marathon, the ratio of performance for women is 93% that of men. In any event, the pure strength and power events (power lifting, high jump, and long jump) show the greatest gender difference, which undoubtedly is a reflection of the lower strength to body weight ratio in females.

Adaptations to Strength Training in Females

In relation to strength, the early work of Hettinger (35) suggested that females are much less responsive to training than males. At the age of greatest trainability, twenty to thirty, women responded to training with only 50% the rate of improvement of men. However, Wilmore (71) found similar relative gains in strength for males and females in a well-controlled study using weight training. More recent work (55) supports Wilmore's findings.

Occasionally females are concerned that heavy training may result in increased growth rates, or that cessation of activity will lead to substantial increases in body weight. No real evidence has been found to substantiate these fears.

Another great concern to young females contemplating athletic participation is developing larger or more bulky muscles. The observation that some female athletes are very muscular is undoubtedly due to the fact that muscular females are more apt to be successful in such sports as track and field and therefore are more likely to elect to participate in such competition.

Recently three different investigations have shown that even heavy resistance weight training does not result in any substantial hypertrophy of the exercised muscles in women, although strength gains are similar on a relative basis to those of men (12, 51, 71). Wilmore (71) showed that when men and women used the same weight training techniques and worked to the same fraction of maximum capacity, the degree of muscle hypertrophy was substantially greater in the men than in the women. Muscle hypertrophy in the women was less than one-quarter inch for the upper body girths, which must be considered an insignificant amount for all practical purposes. Wilmore also showed that, whereas the correlation between strength and girth for the men was strong ($r = .63$ to .77), there was virtually no real relationship between strength and girth for the women ($r = .09$ to .42). Brown and Wilmore (72) showed that while women responded to maximum resistance training with large and significant strength gains, their subjects showed only 0.4% and 2.9% increases in thigh and arm girth, respectively, after six months of training. Indeed these gains were no greater than the controls who did no weight training. Thus it would seem that even the heaviest of weight training programs does not bulk up the female athlete! The explanation for this gender difference in adaptation to heavy resistance training probably lies in the fact that serum testosterone levels and production rates are from twenty to thirty times less in females, and therefore females are unable to achieve the same degree of hypertrophy as males.

Throughout adulthood, muscular strength tends to decrease with age in females. Sandler and coworkers (62) reported significant negative correlations ranging from $r = -0.29$ to -0.54 between age and various measures of strength in 620 women from twenty-five to seventy-three years of age. In addition, however, strength was positively correlated with physical activity ($r = 0.12$ to 0.35) indicating that the decline in strength across age can be minimized by an active life-style (62).

Recent studies (20, 50, 56) have examined the effects of resistance weight training on strength, bone mineral density, lipoprotein profiles, and muscle fiber cross-sectional area in middle-aged and older adult females. While muscular strength increased as a result of training in each of the studies, there was no significant change in bone mineral density (56) or blood lipid parameters (50). In septuagenarian women who participated in a combined aerobic plus resistance training program for fifty weeks, there was a 6.5% increase in strength and a 26% increase in type IIb (fast-twitch glycolytic) muscle fiber cross-sectional area (20). Thus, it appears that older females are capable of substantial hypertrophy as a result of physical training; particularly with respect to type IIb muscle fibers.

The National Strength and Conditioning Association (NSCA) has prepared a position paper entitled *Strength Training for Female Athletes* (52). Based on a thorough review of the literature, the NSCA has endorsed the following statements: "It appears that proper strength and conditioning exercise programs may increase athletic performance, improve physiological function and reduce the risk of injuries. These effects are as beneficial to female athletes as they are to males. The question that has to be addressed is whether female athletes require different training modalities, programs or personnel than those required by male athletes."

"Due to similar physiological responses, it appears that males and females should train for strength in the same basic way, employing similar methodologies, programs and types of exercises. Coaches should assess the needs of each athlete, male or female, individually, and train that athlete accordingly. Coaches should keep in mind that there may be more differences between individuals of the same gender than between males and females. Still, there may be psychological and/or physiological considerations that should be taken into account in training female athletes."

Socio-Psychological Considerations for Strength Training

The NSCA position paper (52) also discusses the following important socio-psychological and physiological aspects of strength training in female athletes:

1. Cultural and sociological stigmas may significantly affect the pursuit of strength training by females in western societies. These stigmas are manifested by concerns about femininity, appearance, aggression, self-esteem, self-concept, and appropriateness of behavior.

2. The learned belief systems of females differ significantly from those of males in western societies in regard to physical expressions and body image. These belief systems can affect training intensities and maximum expressions of strength.

3. Despite a degree of social stigma, females who participate in strength-power conditioning programs have good feelings about themselves. This may be due to the positive impact strength training has on self-concept.

4. Female role models in the weight room may play an essential part in the initial adjustment to training and in the long-term success of female athletes' strength training programs. Female role models appear to be especially important during adolescence and young adulthood. The support and example of male athletes are also important in the development of female athletes. Therefore, coeducational coaching staffs for strength and conditioning, as well as coeducational weight rooms, can greatly aid in providing the communication and role models necessary to make strength training accepted as positive, rewarding, and appropriate for females.

5. Strength and conditioning personnel, both male and female, need to examine their own belief systems regarding strength training of females. These personnel, through verbal and nonverbal cues, may communicate lesser expectations of female athletes than they do of males. As a result, groundless fears about strength training for females are perpetuated, and the female athlete may be inhibited from reaching her genetic potential.

Physiological Considerations for Strength Training

1. Data at this time suggest that in untrained individuals, the absolute total body strength of females is approximately two-thirds that of males, although this difference is not consistent for all muscle groups. Absolute lower body strength ranges from 60% to 80% that of males, and absolute upper body strength from 35% to 79% that of males. It should be noted that these differences are based on studies involving nonathletic subjects; the studies primarily involved tests of static strength. Studies assessing the relative and absolute strength of highly trained female athletes are needed. Strength differences in the studies to date are largely attributable to the greater body size of males and their higher lean body mass to fat ratio.

2. When the gender differences in body size and lean body mass are taken into

consideration, relative strength differences are considerably less appreciable. In the lower body, in fact, the relative strength (strength to lean body mass) of untrained women appears to be approximately equal to that of males. Researchers who have examined the ability to generate force per unit of cross-sectional muscle have found no significant gender differences.

3. The role of the hormone testosterone in strength expression is not clearly understood at this time. Although it is known that the rate of secretion for males is 5 to 10 milligrams per day and less than 0.1 milligrams per day for females, studies have yet to demonstrate that higher testosterone levels alone (in either males or females) correlate with greater strength values. Both empirical and some objective evidence suggests, however, that the exogenous administration of testosterone does positively affect strength expression in both males and females who practice weight training.

4. Little statistical evidence is available to document the existence of anabolic steroid use by female athletes. (Anabolic steroids are synthetic derivatives of the male hormone testosterone.) Because success in many competitive sports results in part from greater physical size and strength, however, the temptation for females to use anabolic steroids appears to be as great as for males. Furthermore, there is a growing body of anecdotal evidence that suggests that a large number of women athletes have already experimented with these drugs. Strength and conditioning coaches should help athletes pursue excellence through improved training methods and nutritional counseling. This approach should help coaching staffs avoid endangering the health of women athletes or compromising the ethics of sport.

5. Short-term studies and empirical evidence to date have shown that females hypertrophy as a consequence of resistance exercise. The relative degree of hypertrophy as a result of resistance training is equal to that of males, although the absolute degree is smaller. The genetic predisposition to hypertrophy and/or exogenous androgen use most likely play significant roles in determining the degree of hypertrophy achieved.

6. Female athletes appear to have similar fiber-type distributions to their male counterparts, although the fibers of females appear to be smaller in cross-sectional area. Whether this is genetically determined or training-induced is not clear at this time. Heavy resistance training has been demonstrated to increase fiber cross-sectional area, with corresponding increases in strength and power.

7. Little research evidence suggests that the onset of normal menstrual periods affects athletic performance. There is tremendous variability, however, in the physical and psychological ways in which women respond to their menses. If circumstances permit individualized strength programs, the monthly onset of menstruation should be considered during program design. It is to be hoped that discussions of the menstrual cycle will be handled with tact and sensitivity by strength and conditioning personnel. Athletes who experience extreme difficulty before and/or during menstruation should seek advice from their gynecologists regarding proper medical intervention.

8. Irregular menstrual cycles (oligomenorrhea) and/or the cessation

of the menses (amenorrhea) may pose health risks to female athletes. Amenorrheic athletes have an increased likelihood of developing musculoskeletal injuries (especially stress fractures and osteoporotic fractures) due to the weakening of the bones from reduced estrogen levels. It is strongly urged that all athletes experiencing amenorrhea or other menstrual irregularities consult a gynecologist. Proper nutritional intakes (such as calcium and iron) also must be evaluated. Finally, resistance training utilizing multijoint and structural exercises is recommended to induce sufficient stresses on the skeletal system and to enhance calcium storage in the bone.

9. Little data exist at this time regarding weight training and pregnancy. Anecdotal evidence suggests, however, that women may safely weight train during pregnancy. Of course, common sense should be employed when selecting training intensities, exercises, and loads during critical stages of pregnancy. Due to the influx of the hormone relaxin, which softens the tendons and ligaments in preparation for delivery, caution is warranted in performing heavy multijoint free weight exercises (squats, deadlifts, snatches, and cleans) after the first trimester. Also, the potential for hyperthermia (increase in body temperature) in pregnant women warrants the use of precautions in dress and environmental conditions during all types of exercise. Following childbirth, many women have returned to successful athletic careers.

10. Some have raised the question of whether the relatively narrow shoulder width of females may pose problems in certain overhead lifts. Thus far no data have been found to substantiate this concern. Coaches should pay close attention to hand spacing and to the carrying angle at the elbow. In the lower body, the greater pelvic width and the Q-angle (quadriceps angle) of the knee may pose problems for female weight trainers. The Q-angle is the angle formed between the longitudinal axis of the femur that represents the pull of the quadriceps muscles and a line that represents the patellar ligament. Again, although this has been raised as a point of concern, no data at this time support it. Coaches who are concerned about this condition may wish to caution female weight trainers with large Q-angles to squat with a toe-forward stance. Development of quadriceps strength can act as a strong deterrent of injuries in female athletes.

11. Considerable variation in body fat percent occurs among athletes of different sports. It is important to understand that the performance and health of the individual must be carefully considered before attempting to alter body composition. Furthermore, athletes and coaches need to be aware of societal norms regarding body image and the implications this has for the development of eating disorders. Finally, resistance training has demonstrated favorable changes in body composition with minimal change in body weight.

12. Proper nutrition is an important consideration in strength training for female athletes.

The Menstrual Cycle and Athletics

Onset of Menarche

The effects of strenuous exercise programs on the sexual and reproductive functions of females have been a matter of some concern in the past, although not on the basis of scientific evidence. Observations of 729 Hungarian female athletes showed there was no disturbance of the onset of menarche (30). Nor was there evidence of dysmenorrhea of any consequence as the result of athletic participation, much less moderate physical exercise (6, 30).

More recent data on American girls showed menarche occurring significantly later in athletes (13.58 years) compared with nonathletes (12.23 years) (48). A study by Malina and coworkers (49) corroborates this difference in the onset of menarche and also suggests significant differences related to the type of sport and intensity of training. They also found that the athletes reported a greater incidence of dysmenorrhea and menstrual irregularity, although the difference was not statistically significant.

On the other hand, Astrand and associates (6) reported a slightly earlier onset of menarche in highly trained, young Swedish swimmers compared with a Swedish reference group. Since swimmers do not typically reduce body fat to the extent that athletes involved in heavy running activity do (71), it is interesting to hypothesize a relationship between early onset of menarche and body fat, but much further investigation is needed.

A recent review by Loucks (45) addressed whether athletic participation during childhood delays the onset of menarche. There is compelling evidence that biased sampling procedures have led to the spurious conclusion that the exercise training associated with athletic participation causes a delay in menarche. After a thorough review of the available evidence, Loucks has concluded that "At present, it is correct to say that the average age of menarche is later in athletes than non-athletes, but there is no experimental evidence that athletic training delays menarche in anyone."

Participation in Sports and Exercise during Menstruation

At present there is no conclusive evidence that participation in exercise or sporting events during menstruation is harmful. In addition, it is unclear whether menstruation per se and/or the discomfort associated with primary dismenorrhea (pain from uterine contractions or ischemia during menstruation) affect performance (15). Surveys of athletes (30, 75) have indicated a diversity of opinion regarding the effect of menstruation on athletic performance with 17% to 48% believing that performance is adversely affected, 13% to 15% indicating improved performance, and 37% to 48% believing that performance is unaffected.

Although there is no consensus regarding the effect of menstruation on athletic performance or the effect of regular exercise on the symptoms associated with premenstrual syndrome (PMS) or menstruation (15), the most prudent course of action is to allow participation on a voluntary basis, without undue concern about undesirable consequences.

Athletic Menstrual Cycle Irregularity (AMI)

Regular, asymptomatic menstruation is usually considered a measure of general good health in females after a regular rhythm has been established. Conversely, medical authorities had felt that any deviation from the normal rhythmic pattern may be one of the first indications of overtraining (30, 39).

Menstrual irregularities seem to be reported with greater frequency as women become more involved in high-intensity, year-round training programs. Indeed, one review of this literature (9) lists fifteen studies that have shown a relatively high incidence of athletic menstrual cycle irregularity (AMI) associated with heavy training in various activities. These findings have also been confirmed in more recent reviews (15, 45). This problem could arise from physical or psychological stress (overtraining?), from changes in hormonal function or body composition, or a combination of these factors.

In a study of teenage swimmers training two to four hours daily, Bonen and coworkers (8) found that in the follicular phase of the cycle the swimmers' luteinizing hormone (LH) was elevated and their follicle-stimulating hormone (FSH) concentration was depressed compared with nonexercising controls. They concluded that the corpora lutea in the swimmers were not functioning properly and that even though menstruation occurred it was probably anovulatory. It was suggested that heavy endurance training can impair follicular development or maturation through the repeated elevation of circulating androgen concentration brought about by exercise (66). Unfortunately, little is yet known about how exercise stimulates changes in the cycle to cause AMI.

In a study of ballet dancers, AMI was related to both strenuous physical activity and to diminished body weight. The condition was found to be reversible, often disappearing with significant weight gain or intervals of less intense exercise (18).

It is not yet known whether AMI constitutes a threat to health or future reproductive function, or whether it is simply a normal variation in function that is reversible. In any event it would be wise for those involved with women's athletics and their sports medicine counseling to maintain a conservative approach. A woman should not be led to believe that this is a normal response and advised just to continue training. She should see a gynecologist and have a workup done to determine if she has a gynecological problem unrelated to her training regimen (15).

It would be good practice for coaches and physical educators of women to advise the members of their teams and classes to maintain accurate records of their menstrual cycles, and they should encourage consultation whenever deviations occur. This practice should result in better health and performance for the athletes.

Effects of the Menstrual Cycle on Performance

In spite of the widespread impression that performance is impaired during certain periods of the menstrual cycle, there is no agreement among the investigators who have attacked this problem (33). Some have found no effect of the menstrual cycle on motor performance (1, 26, 46, 57, 58, 59, 64, 65); others report that performance is best in the postmenstrual phase or intermenstrual phase, and at its worst in the two or three days preceding menstruation (30, 40, 53) or during menstruation (68).

One of the most definitive studies was performed by Jurkowski and coworkers (37) who measured hormonal levels to confirm the occurrence of ovulation and thus were able to compare performance in midfollicular phases to performance in midluteal phases. This is a more sensitive comparison than comparing pre- and postmenstrual periods. They found that maximal oxygen consumption was the same in the follicular and luteal phases, as were the cardiorespiratory responses to exercise. However, they found that during heavy exhaustive exercise (90% max) the time to exhaustion in the luteal phase was double that of the follicular phase, and blood lactate was significantly lower. This work strongly suggests that best performances in high-intensity efforts lasting up to three minutes may occur in the luteal (postovulatory) phase when progesterone and estradiol levels are at their highest point. For a review of this topic, see Carlberg, Peake, and Buckman (15).

Pregnancy, Childbirth, and Athletics

It was formerly suggested that participation in athletic competition, training, or vigorous sports should be forbidden during pregnancy.

The reasons for this are discussed by Klaus and Noack (40), who point out that the work of the right heart is increased threefold and the work of the left heart increased twofold, even in the nonpregnant female, by a moderate work load. During pregnancy, such an increase—with the demands of fetal circulation—could be considered hazardous for the right heart and for lung circulation. The danger would be especially great if unrecognized heart defects are present. In addition, it should be recognized that the kidneys and liver function with very little reserve capacity during pregnancy.

However, more recent findings do not seem to support this reasoning. Knuttgen and Emerson (41) studied thirteen normal pregnant women during rest and moderate exercise. They found no evidence of ventilatory impairment or dyspnea and concluded that exercise does not constitute a more severe physiological stress during pregnancy, if lifting work and possible encumbrance of the fetal tissues are minimized.

Erkkola (31) investigated sixty-two healthy young women in their first pregnancy beginning in the tenth or fourteenth week of pregnancy and lasting until term. One-half of the group was encouraged to exercise with strenuous physical exertion. The increase in physical work capacity during pregnancy was 17.6% greater in the training group, who showed no negative effects from the training program.

Dressendorfer (27) measured $\dot{V}O_2$ max in one healthy young woman during the course of two of her pregnancies and subsequent lactation periods over a period of four years. Training mileage averaged only five to ten miles per week in the first trimester because of nausea, but thereafter the subject was able to run an average of fifteen miles a week up to delivery. Training was gradually increased to twenty miles per week at four months postpartum. It was concluded that during normal pregnancy and lactation, $\dot{V}O_2$ max and endurance performance cannot only be maintained but even improved by physical training without harmful effects on the mother or child. The most recent findings from three laboratories support this conclusion (3, 28, 36).

Wolfe and coworkers (74) reviewed the available literature concerning the interaction between pregnancy and aerobic exercise and concluded as follows:

1. The metabolic cost of standard submaximal exercise is not greatly affected by pregnancy, but heart rate and pulmonary ventilation are significantly increased. Effects of pregnancy on ratings of perceived exertion are not well documented.

2. During mild or moderate submaximal exertion stroke volume and cardiac output are augmented progressively until late gestation. Depending on maternal posture, venous return, stroke volume, and cardiac output are reduced to varying degrees in late gestation as a result of compression of the inferior vena cava by the gravid uterus. Cardiovascular adaptations to more strenuous exertion may differ from mild or moderate exercise and remain for future investigation.

3. Physical conditioning appears to reduce both heart rate and ratings of perceived exertion during strenuous steady-state exercise. The usual increase in submaximal exercise stroke volume may be obscured since pregnancy effects on venous return appear to dominate the influences of aerobic conditioning, particularly at low exercise intensities.

4. Effects of pregnancy on $\dot{V}O_2$ max are poorly documented because of concerns related to the safety of maximal exercise testing during gestation. Reductions in both maximal heart rate and $\dot{V}O_2$ max have been postulated, but have yet to be confirmed by serial studies of maximal exercise performance. Effects of physical conditioning on both maximal aerobic

and anaerobic power also remain for clarification.

5. Studies of fetal heart rate during acute maternal exertion suggest that the fetus may be exposed to moderate transient hypoxia. Apparently, this is well tolerated by the fetus in the absence of uteraplacental insufficiency, maternal metabolic and cardiovascular diseases, environmental stresses, or other complicating factors. Further research concerning fetal adaptability to maternal exercise is definitely needed.

6. Studies of laboratory animals and human epidemiological studies suggest that pregnancy outcome can be altered by chronic exertion, especially if exercise is excessively strenuous or accompanied by occupational, nutritional, or other environmental stresses. On the other hand, the bulk of available evidence suggests that carefully prescribed fitness training promotes maternal physical and psychological health without compromising fetal well-being. Additional research is needed urgently to properly test this hypothesis.

The results of a meta-analysis by Lokey and colleagues (44), which simultaneously evaluated the results of eighteen studies involving 2,314 pregnant women, indicated that "Overall, an exercise program using any of a variety of exercise modes that is performed for an average of 43 minutes per day, 3 times per week, at a heart rate of up to 144 beats per minute, does not appear to be associated with adverse effects to the mother or fetus in a healthy normal pregnancy. However, these findings should be cautiously applied owing to the nature of the currently available data base. Recommendations or precautions for programs of greater intensities cannot be made at this time."

Effects of Heavy Exercise Programs on Labor and Delivery

Although it was once believed that athletic women developed tense (unyielding) abdominal walls that hindered normal delivery, the results of many investigations in more recent years indicate that athletic women have quick and easy deliveries (40). Erdelyi (30), who has studied many Hungarian women athletes, found a smaller incidence of complications (especially toxemia) during pregnancy and 50% fewer cesarean sections performed in women athletes when compared with controls. It was also found that the duration of labor was shorter than the average in 87.2% of the women athletes.

It would therefore appear that there is no need for concern about the effects of strenuous exercise on subsequent pregnancies or childbirth. Indeed, physical conditioning seems to be a valuable prophylactic procedure.

Effects of Pregnancy and Childbirth on Subsequent Athletic Performance

Noack (53) took histories of fifteen German champion women athletes who bore children during their athletic careers. Of the fifteen, five gave up sports because of their new responsibilities. Of the remaining ten, two maintained equal performance and eight made definite objective improvements after childbirth. All of the women agreed that after childbirth they were "tougher" and had more strength and endurance.

It has been pointed out that pregnancy, far from being an illness, should be considered an intensive, day and night, nine-month period of physical conditioning because of the increased demands on metabolism and the entire cardiovascular system (40).

Athletic Injuries

Even a cursory study of anatomy reveals a considerable difference in the locomotor structures of females compared with males. On the average, bones, muscles, tendons, and ligaments are somewhat less substantial, although body weight is not decreased proportionately because of the greater percentage of fatty tissue in the female. On this basis, a gender difference in incidence of athletic injuries might be expected.

It had been shown in studies involving comparable groups of men and women that the overall incidence of athletic injuries in women was almost double that in men (39). Furthermore, the incidence of injuries involving overstrain—such as contractures, inflammations of tendons, tendon sheaths, bursae, foot deficiencies, and periosteal injuries—was almost four times more common in women than in similarly trained men.

The distribution of injuries according to the sport activity is of interest. In women, by far the greatest percentage of all injuries is found in sports that require explosive efforts: short runs (53%) and the long jump (31%).

However, more recent investigations do not entirely support the earlier work. In a study of Seattle high school athletes, the type and frequency of injuries were comparable in boys and girls when contact sports were eliminated from consideration (34). During the 1978–79 school year, the Oklahoma injury registry collected information from seventy-nine Oklahoma high schools in which similar sports were paired for boys and girls, so that gender comparisons could be made. They reported 165 injuries in 6,478 boys and 132 injuries in 4,807 girls, with remarkably similar overall injury rates of 25.4 and 27.4 injuries per 1,000 participants, respectively (63). However, the girls had a significantly greater number of major injuries (defined as altering play for seven days or more). Girls also had a significantly greater number of knee and major ankle injuries.

Emotional Factors

The female is often said to be less well suited to competitive sport than males because of a more emotional nature that might produce unfavorable responses in highly competitive situations. There is no acceptable scientific evidence to support this assertion. Ulrich (67), who used eosinophil count and cardiorespiratory response to measure the stressfulness of various competitive situations, found that measurable stress reactions occurred not only in response to participation in class, intramural, and interscholastic basketball games but in written test situations as well! She concluded that stress was much more closely related to the psychological than the physiological components of a situation. It is of interest that her study showed lesser levels of stress as the result of experience, which suggests that females successfully adjust to the stress of competition.

Astrand and associates (6), in a year-long study of girl swimmers age twelve to sixteen (a supposedly emotional, labile period), could not find a single case of demonstrable nervous symptoms that could be attributed to training or to participation in competitive events.

Summary

1. One of the most important structural gender differences is the better strength to weight relationship in the male, which is greatest with respect to the upper body and becomes almost negligible with respect to leg strength.

2. Among the many physiological gender differences, the most important in athletics relate to the larger ratio of heart weight to body weight and the better O_2 carrying capacity of the blood in males.

3. Adaptations to athletic training are more similar than different between the

genders, but important differences do exist. The capacity for muscular hypertrophy in response to strength training is much greater in males, although strength increments are similar if compared on a relative basis. The only difference in response to distance running appears to be related to the greater amount of fat carried by the average female.

4. Gynecological problems relating to athletic participation are rare and probably of no real importance in otherwise healthy females.

5. It is not yet known whether athletic menstrual cycle irregularity (AMI) constitutes a threat to health or future reproductive function, or whether it is simply a normal variation in function that is reversible. In any case it seems wise to maintain a conservative approach: women should not be led to believe that AMI is a normal response and advised simply to continue training. Rather they should be advised to seek medical advice to rule out gynecological problems unrelated to the training.

6. The best available evidence suggests that the best time for performance of heavy exhaustive exercise may be during the luteal phase of the menstrual cycle. Other lighter levels of work load are probably unaffected by the phases of the menstrual cycle.

7. There is no evidence to suggest that moderate aerobic exercise during pregnancy is in any way harmful to either mother or fetus if both are healthy and normal. However, this should be done under medical supervision to assure the good health of both.

8. Contrary to earlier research, there appears to be little difference in the incidence of athletic injuries to boys and girls, although a somewhat greater incidence of knee and ankle injuries has been reported for girls.

References

1. Allsen, P. E., Parson, P., and Bryce, G. R. Effect of the menstrual cycle on maximum oxygen uptake. *Physician and Sportsmed.* 5:53–55, 1977.

2. American College of Sports Medicine. Opinion statement on the participation of the female athlete in long distance running. *Med. Sci. Sports* 11:IX–XI, 1979.

3. Artal, R., and Wiswell, R. A. *Exercise in Pregnancy.* Baltimore: Williams and Wilkins, 1986.

4. Astrand, P-O. *Experimental Studies of Physical Working Capacity in Relation to Sex and Age.* Copenhagen: E. Munksgaard, 1952.

5. Astrand, P-O., Cuddy, T. E., Saltin, B., and Stenberg, J. Cardiac output during submaximal and maximal work. *J. Appl. Physiol.* 19:268–74, 1964.

6. Astrand, P-O., Engstrom, L., Eriksson, B., Karlberg, P., Nylander, I., Saltin, B., and Thoren, C. Girl swimmers—with special reference to respiratory and circulatory adaptation and gynecological and psychiatric aspects. *Acta Paediatr.* (Stockholm), suppl. 147, 1963.

7. Becklake, M. R., Frank, H., Dagenais, G. R., Ostiguy, G. L., and Guzman, C. A. Influence of age and sex on exercise cardiac output. *J. Appl. Physiol.* 20:938–47, 1965.

8. Bonen, A., Belcastro, A. N., Ling, W. Y., and Simpson, A. A. Profiles of selected hormones during menstrual cycles of teenage athletes. *J. Appl. Physiol.* 50:545–51, 1981.

9. Bonen, A., and Keizer, H. A. Athletic menstrual cycle irregularity: Endocrine response to exercise and training. *Physician and Sportsmed.* 12:78–94, 1984.

10. Bransford, D. R., and Howley, E. T. Oxygen cost of running in trained and untrained men and women. *Med. Sci. Sports* 9:41–44, 1977.

11. Brown, C. H., Harrower, J. R., and Deeter, M. R. The effects of cross-country running on preadolescent girls. *Med. Sci. Sports* 4:1–5, 1972.

12. Brown, C. H., and Wilmore, J. H. The effects of maximal resistance training on the strength and body composition of women athletes. *Med. Sci. Sports* 6:174–77, 1974.

13. Burger, M. Zur pathophysiologie der Geschlechter. *Munch. Med. Wochenschr.* 97:981–88, 1955.

14. Burke, E. J. Physiological effects of similar training programs in males and females. *Res. Q.* 48:510–17, 1977.

15. Carlberg, K., Peake, G. T., and Buckman, M. T. Exercise and the menstrual cycle. In *Sports Medicine* (3d ed.), ed. O. Appenzeller. Baltimore: Urban and Schwarzenberg, pp. 161–80, 1988.

16. Clarke, H. H. Physical and motor sex differences. *Phys. Fitness Res. Digest* 9, #4, October 1979. The President's Council on Physical Fitness and Sports, Washington, D.C.

17. Clarkson, P. M. Tired blood: Iron deficiency in athletes and effects of iron supplementation. *Gatorade Sports Sci. Exch.* 3(28), 1990.

18. Cohen, J. L., Kim, C. S., May, P. B., and Ertel, N. H. Exercise, body weight and amenorrhea in professional ballet dancers. *Physician and Sportsmed.* 10:92–101, 1982.

19. Cooter, G. R., and Mowbray, K. Effect of iron supplementation and activity on serum iron depletion and hemoglobin levels in female athletes. *Res. Q.* 49:114–18, 1978.

20. Cress, M. E., Thomas, D. P., Johnson, J., Kasch, F. W., Cassens, R. G., Smith, E. L., and Agre, J. C. Effect of training on $\dot{V}O_2$ max, thigh strength, and muscle morphology in septuagenarian women. *Med. Sci. Sports Exerc.* 23:752–58, 1991.

21. Cunningham, D. A., and Hill, J. S. Effect of training on cardiovascular response to exercise in women. *J. Appl. Physiol.* 39:891–95, 1975.

22. Cureton, K. J., Hensley, L. D., and Tiburzi, A. Body fatness and performance differences between men and women. *Res. Q.* 50:333–40, 1979.

23. Cureton, K. J., and Sparling, P. B. Distance running performance and metabolic responses to running in men and women with excess weight experimentally equated. *Med. Sci. Sports Exerc.* 12:288–94, 1980.

24. Daniels, J., and Daniels, N. Running economy of elite male and elite female runners. *Med. Sci. Sports Exerc.* 24:483–89, 1992.

25. Dill, D. B., Myhre, L. G., Greer, S. M., Richardson, J. C., and Singleton, K. J. Body composition and aerobic capacity of youth of both sexes. *Med. Sci. Sports* 4:198–204, 1972.

26. Doolittle, T. L., and Engebretsen, J. Performance variations during the menstrual cycle. *J. Sports Med.* 12:54–58, 1972.

27. Dressendorfer, R. H. Physical training during pregnancy and lactation. *Physician and Sportsmed.*, vol. 6, February 1978.

28. Dressendorfer, R. H., and Goodlin, R. C. Fetal heart rate response to maternal exercise testing. *Physician and Sportsmed.* 8:91–96, 1980.

29. Eisenman, P. A., and Golding, L. A. Comparison of effects of training on $\dot{V}O_2$ max in girls and young women. *Med. Sci. Sports* 7:136–38, 1975.

30. Erdelyi, G. J. Gynecological survey of female athletes. *J. Sports Med.* 2:174–79, 1962.

31. Erkkola, R. The influence of physical training during pregnancy on physical work capacity and circulatory parameters. *Scand. J. Clin. Lab. Invest.* 36:747–54, 1976.

32. Freedson, P., Katch, V. L., Sady, S., and Weltman, A. Cardiac output differences in males and females during mild cycle ergometer exercise. *Med. Sci. Sports* 11:16–19, 1979.

33. Garlick, M. A., and Bernauer, E. M. Exercise during the menstrual cycle: Variations in physiological baseline. *Res. Q.* 39:533–42, 1968.

34. Garrick, J. G., and Requa, R. K. Girls' sports injuries in high school athletics. *J.A.M.A.* 239:2245–48, 1978.

35. Hettinger, T. *Physiology of Strength.* Springfield, IL: Charles C. Thomas, 1961.

36. Hutchinson, P. C., Cureton, K. J., and Sparling, P. B. Metabolic and circulatory responses to running during pregnancy. *Physician and Sportsmed.* 9:55–61, 1981.

37. Jurkowski, J. E. H., Jones, N. L., Toews, C. J., and Sutton, J. R. Effects of menstrual cycle on blood lactate, O_2 delivery and performance during exercise. *J. Appl. Physiol.* 51:1493–99, 1981.

38. Kilbom, A. Physical training in women. *Scand. J. Clin. Lab. Invest.* vol. 28, suppl. 119, 1971.

39. Klaus, E. J. The athletic status of women. In *International Research in Sport and Physical Education,* eds. E. Jokl and E. Simon, Springfield, IL: Charles C. Thomas, 1964.

40. Klaus, E. J., and Noack, H. *Frau und Sport.* Stuttgart: Georg Thieme Verlag, 1961.

41. Knuttgen, H. G., and Emerson, K. Physiological response to pregnancy at rest and during exercise. *J. Appl. Physiol.* 36:549–53, 1974.

42. Kollias, J., Barlett, H. L., Mendez, J., and Franklin, B. Hemodynamic response of well-trained women athletes to graded treadmill exercise. *J. Sports Med. Phys. Fitness* 18:365–72, 1978.

43. Krahenbuhl, G. S., Archer, P. A., and Pettit, L. L. Serum testosterone and adult female trainability. *J. Sports Med. Phys. Fitness* 18:359–64, 1978.

44. Lokey, E. A., Tran, Z. V., Wells, C. L., Myers, B. C., and Tran, A. C. Effects of physical exercise on pregnancy outcomes: A meta-analytic review. *Med. Sci. Sports Exerc.* 23:1234–39, 1991.

45. Loucks, A. B. Effects of exercise training on the menstrual cycle: Existence and mechanisms. *Med. Sci. Sports Exerc.* 22:275–80, 1990.

46. Loucks, J., and Thompson, H. Effect of menstruation on reaction time. *Res. Q.* 39:407–8, 1968.

47. MacNab, R. B. J., Conger, P. R., and Taylor, P. S. Differences in maximal and submaximal work capacity in men and women. *J. Appl. Physiol.* 27:644–48, 1969.

48. Malina, R. M., Harper, A. B., Avent, H. H., and Campbell, D. E. Age at menarche in athletes and nonathletes. *Med. Sci. Sports* 5:11–13, 1973.

49. Malina, R. M., Spirduso, W. W., Tate, C., and Baylor, A. M. Age at menarche and selected menstrual characteristics in athletes at different competitive levels and different sports. *Med. Sci. Sports* 10:218–22, 1978.

50. Manning, J. M., Dooly-Manning, C. R., White, K., Kampa, I., Silas, S., Kesselhant, M., and Ruoff, M. Effects of a resistive training program on lipoprotein-lipid levels in obese women. *Med. Sci. Sports Exerc.* 23:1222–26, 1991.

51. Mayhew, J. L., and Gross, P. M. Body composition changes in young women with high resistance weight training. *Res. Q.* 45:433–40, 1974.

52. National Strength and Conditioning Association. *Position paper on strength training for female athletes.* Lincoln, NE: NSCA, 1990.

53. Noack, H. Die sportliche Leistungsfähigkeit der Frau im Menstrualzyklus. *Dtsch. Med. Wochenschr.* 79:1523–25, 1954.

54. Nocker, J., and Bohlau, V. Abhangigkeit der Leistungsfähigkeit vom Alter und Geschlecht. *Much. Med. Wochenschr.* 97:1517–22, 1955.

55. O'Shea, J. P., and Wegner, J. Power weight training and the female athletes. *Physician and Sportsmed.* 9:109–20, 1981.

56. Peterson, S. E., Peterson, M. D., Raymond, G., Gilligan, C., Checovich, M. M., and Smith, E. L. Muscular strength and bone density with weight training in middle-aged women. *Med. Sci. Sports Exerc.* 23:499–504, 1991.

57. Petrofsky, J. S., LeDonne, D. M., Rinehart, J. S., and Lind, A. R. Isometric strength and endurance during the menstrual cycle. *Eur. J. Appl. Physiol.* 35:1–10, 1976.

58. Phillips, M. Effect of the menstrual cycle on pulse rate and blood pressure before and after exercise. *Res. Q.* 39:327–33, 1968.

59. Pierson, W. R., and Lockhart, A. Effect of menstruation on simple reaction and movement time. *Br. Med. J.* 1:796–97, 1963.

60. ———. Fatigue, work decrement, and endurance of women in a simple repetitive task. *Aerospace Med.* 35:724–25, 1964.

61. Rowell, L. B. Human cardiovascular adjustments to exercise and thermal stress. *Physiol. Rev.* 54:75–159, 1974.

62. Sandler, R. B., Burdett, R., Zaleskiewicz, M., Sprouls-Repcheck, C., and Harwell, M. Muscle strength as an indicator of the habitual level of activity. *Med. Sci. Sports Exerc.* 23:1375–81, 1991.

63. Shively, R. A., Grana, W. A., and Dennis, E. High school sports injuries. *Physician and Sportsmed.* 9:46–50, 1981.

64. Sloan, A. W. Effect of training on physical fitness of women students. *J. Appl. Physiol.* 16:167–69, 1961.

65. ———. Physical fitness of college students in South Africa, U.S.A., and England. *Res. Q.* 34:244–48, 1963.

66. Sutton, F. R., Coleman, M. J., Casey, J., and Lazarus, L. Androgen responses during physical exercise. *Br. Med. J.* 1:520–23, 1973.

67. Ulrich, C. Measurement of stress evidenced by college women in situations involving competition. Ph.D. diss., Physical Education, University of Southern California, 1956.

68. Wearing, M. P., Yuhasz, M. D., Campbell, R., and Love, E. I. The effect of the menstrual cycle on tests of physical fitness. *J. Sports Med.* 12:38–41, 1972.

69. Wells, C. L., and Plowman, S. A. Sexual differences in athletic performance: Biological or behavioral? *Physician and Sportsmed.* 11:52–63, 1983.

70. Whitmire, D. Vitamins and minerals: A perspective in physical performance. In *Sports Nutrition for the 90s,* eds. J. R. Berning and S. N. Steen. Gaithersburg, MD: Aspen Publishers Inc., pp. 129–51, 1991.

71. Wilmore, J. H. Alterations in strength, body composition, and anthropometric measurements consequent to a 10-week weight training program. *Med. Sci. Sports* 6:133–38, 1974.

72. Wilmore, J. H., and Sigerseth, P. O. Physical work capacity of young girls, 7–13 years of age. *J. Appl. Physiol.* 22:923–28, 1967.

73. Wirth, J. C., Lohman, T. G., Avallone, J. P., Shire, T., and Boileau, R. A. The effect of physical training on the serum iron levels of college age women. *Med. Sci. Sports* 10:223–26, 1978.

74. Wolfe, L. A., Ohtake, P. J., Mottola, M. F., and McGrath, M. J. Physiological interactions between pregnancy and aerobic exercise. In *Exercise and Sport Sciences Reviews,* ed. K. B. Pandolf. Baltimore: Williams and Wilkins, pp. 295–351, 1989.

75. Zaharieva, E. Survey of sportswomen at the Tokyo Olympics. *J. Sports Med. Phys. Fitness* 5:215–19, 1965.

76. Zeldis, S. M., Morganroth, J., and Rubler, S. Cardiac hypertrophy in response to dynamic conditioning in female athletes. *J. Appl. Physiol.* 44:849–52, 1978.

Index

A

AAHPER Youth Fitness Test
Battery, 281–82
Abdominothoracic pump, 124
Accelerator nerve, 98
Accelerator tone, 98
Accessory muscles, 134
Accumulation fatigue hypotheses,
415–17
Acid-base balance
buffer systems in, 162–64
performance limiting factor, 165
physiological regulation of, 164
Acids
respiratory gasses, liquids,
158–59
See also Acid-base balance
Actin, 17–18, 21, 53
Active warm-up, 531
Actomyosin, 22
Actomyosin adenosine-
triphosphatase (actomyosin
ATPase), 21, 35
Actomyosin ATPase. *See*
Actomyosin adenosine-
triphosphatase (actomyosin
ATPase)
Acute exercise, 522
Acute inflammation theory, delayed
onset muscle soreness
(DOMS), 513–14
Adenosine diphosphate (ADP),
contractile process and, 18,
29–30
Adenosine triphosphate (ATP)
anaerobic metabolism and, 37, 39
carbohydrate metabolism and,
30–33, 35
contractile process and, 18, 22,
29–30
fat and protein metabolism and,
33–34
fatigue and, 415–17
glucose metabolism and, 36
muscle contraction speed and,
485–86
strength, power training and, 40

ADP. *See* Adenosine diphosphate
(ADP)
Adrenal cortex
glucocorticoids released by, 178,
181–82
hormones produced by, 178–79
hypothalamus-pituitary-adrenal
axis and, 180–82
training effects on, 179–80
Adrenal medulla, catecholamine
effects, 182–84
Adrenergic fibers, 121, 178
Adrenocorticotrophic hormone
(ACTH), 178, 181–82
Aerobic efficiency, 470
Aerobic exercise, exercise-induced
asthma (EIA) and, 147
Aerobic metabolism, 29–30, 32–33,
35–37
Aerobic power, 254
See also Physical working
capacity (PWC)
Aerobic training
age factors and, 365–68, 385–87
circulorespiratory endurance and,
455
endurance performance and,
367–68
exercise and, 365–67
limits of, and oxygen, 167–69
long-distance running and, 368
prescription of exercise, 293–95,
297, 300
respiratory muscle fatigue and,
146
Aerobic work, 365–68, 470
Afferent neurons, 69–70
Age factors
aerobic training and, 365–68,
385–87
anaerobic training and, 369–71
athletic training and, 6–7
blood pressure and, 123
body composition and, 363–64,
392

cardiovascular system and,
387–88, 394
conditioning
effects of, 392–96
programs, components of,
396–400
fiber atrophy, hypertrophy and,
384–85
flexibility affected by, 507–508
force-velocity curve and, 384
heart rate affected by, 105
heat stress and, 550
height, body weight patterns of,
362–63
long-distance running and, 368
maximal oxygen consumption
and, 389–91
muscular efficiency and, 391
muscular endurance and, 384,
452
nervous system and, 391–92
physical education implications
of, 381–83, 400–402
physical fitness and, 282
physical working capacity
(PWC) and, 389–91,
393–96
prescription of exercise and, 305
pulmonary function changes and,
388–89
running efficiency and, 470
strength and, 371, 374, 383–84
weight training and, 371–76
Air pollution, breathing affected by,
150–51
Airway resistance, 142–44
Alactacid, in oxygen debt, 218–20
Aldosterone, 178
Alkaline reserve
acid-base balance and, 165
training and, 130
Alkalinizers, 584–86
Allergies, PC corticoids and, 178
All-or-none law, 49
Alpha system, muscle control, 78–81
Altitude, running efficiency and, 471
Alveolar ducts, 137

American Association for Health, Physical Education, and Recreation (AAHPER)
  Health-Related Physical Fitness Test, 282
  Youth Fitness Test, 281
American College of Sports Medicine (ACSM)
  aerobic recommendation, 293–95
  exercise duration recommendation, 297–300
  exercise frequency recommendation, 300–301
  exercise intensity recommendation, 295
  exertion range recommendation, 297
  heart rate range recommendation, 295–96
  heat injury prevention, running recommendation, 552–53
  making weight and, 364–65
  metabolic equivalent range recommendation, 297
  participation referral form, 254, 255
  steroid use recommendation, 587–88
  strength training recommendation, 438
  target oxygen consumption rate range recommendation, 295
  weight reduction recommendation, 347–48
Amphetamines, 5, 586–87
Anabolic steroids, 787
Anaerobic efficiency, 470
Anaerobic fitness
  circulorespiratory endurance and, 455
  effect of, 369–71
  Margaria Step-running Anaerobic Power Test, 273–74
  Wingate Anaerobic Test, 274–75
Anaerobic metabolism
  ATP energy from carbohydrate food, 32–33
  muscle contraction and, 29–30
  recovery oxygen and, 221
  sprint training and, 37–38
Anaerobic power, 221

Anaerobic threshold concept
  importance of, 224–25
  issues in, 225–26
  lactate threshold as, 226
Anaerobic work, 368–71, 470
Anatomical dead space, 142–44
Anemia, sports, 130, 573–74
Angina pectoris, 314
Angle of pull, muscle contraction and, 52
Annulo spiral ending, 75, 78–81
Anoxia, 141
Anterior pituitary, 181
Anthropometric flexibility measurement, 502
Antibodies
  antibody dependent cell-mediated cytotoxicity (ADCC) and, 197–98
  classification of, 196–98
  exercise and, 200–201
Antigens, immune system, 196
Anti-inflammatory corticoids (AC), 178–79
Anti-inflammatory drugs, muscle soreness, 522
Anxiety, neuromuscular system and, 244
Army/Air Force Physical Fitness Test, 281
Arterial blood pressure, 124
  exercise and, 125–26
Arteriovenous anastomoses (AVA), 119–20
Aspartates, performance improvement, 587–88
Association neuron, 70
Astrand-Rhyming Nomogram, 262–67
Athletes. *See* Athletic training
Athletic menstrual cycle irregularity (AMI), 611–12
Athletic training
  aerobic metabolism and, 35–37
  anaerobic metabolism and, 37–38
  cellular response overview of, 34–35
  conditioning and physiology of, 9
  energetics application to, 29
  female limitations in, 602
  gender, age differences in response to, 6–7
  glycogen depletion and, 39–42

heart affected by, 109
  making weight, 364–65
  neuromuscular fatigue and, 411
  over life span, 400–402
  overtraining and, 418
  performance improvement in, 4–5
  pregnancy and, 7
  professionalism in, 5–6
  pulmonary function and, 146
  strength, power training, 38–39
  sympathicotonics and, 180
  vagotonics and, 180
  See also Exercise; Physical fitness; Prescription of exercise; Weight training
ATP. *See* Adenosine triphosphate (ATP)
Autogenetic governors, 75
Autonomic nervous system, 69
Autorhythmicity, heartbeat, 94
Axon, of motor neuron, 69

B

Balance, nervous system and, 84
Ballistic method, range of motion, 503–7
Basal metabolic rate (BMR), 177
  with age, 392
Bases
  respiratory gasses, liquids, 158–59
  See also Acid-base balance
B cells, humoral immunity, 196
Bench-stepping, 210–11
Benzedrine, 586–87
Beta oxidation, 345
Bioelectrical impedance analysis (BIA), 341–42
Blood
  coefficient of oxygen utilization, 162
  hemoglobin of, 159–60
  muscle tissue supply of, 23
  oxygen dissociation curve and, 160–62
  oxygen levels and, 166–67
  total blood volume (TBV) of, 241
  See also Hormones; Immune system

Blood distribution, 120–21
  chemical regulation, 121
  nervous regulation, 121
  rest vs. exercise measurement,
    121–22
Blood doping, 588–89
Blood pressure
  age factors and, 394
  arterial, exercise effects on,
    125–26
  arterial blood pressure, 124
  diurnal variation and, 124
  exercise and, 240
  measurement of, 122–24
  norepinephrine and, 176
  PC corticoids and, 178
  posture and, 124
  sex differences and, 123
  systolic/diastolic, 123
  venous blood pressure, 124
Blood supply, cardiac output and,
    103–5
Blood volume, age factors and, 394
Blowing off, carbon dioxide, 164
Body composition
  age factors and, 392
  bioelectrical impedance analysis
    (BIA), 341–42
  body volume measurement, 340
  growth patterns of, 363–64
  hydrometric method, 340
  near-infrared spectrophotometry
    (NIR) of, 342–45
  skinfold measures, 340–45
  underwater weighing, 338–39
Body fluid
  erythrocyte count and, 129
  hemoconcentration and, 129
  training effects on, 129–31
Body mass index (BMI), 335
Body mechanics
  running speed, 489–90
  swimming speed, 490
Body temperature, heart rate
    affected by, 106
Body temperature, warm-up and,
    529–30
Body volume measurement, 340
Boyle's Law, 157
Brain
  extrapyramidal system, 83, 86
  proprioceptive cerebellar system,
    83
  pyramidal system of, 86

Break point, breath-holding and, 149
Breath-holding, 148–50
Breathing. See External respiration;
    Internal respiration; Lungs;
    Pulmonary function
Bronchi, bronchioles, 137

C

Cable tension strength tests, 433
Caffeine, performance, 590
Calorimetry
  direct, 214
  indirect, 214–16
Canadian Home Fitness Test, 268
Cancer, exercise and, 243–44
Carbohydrate feeding, 563–66, 578,
    591–92
Carbohydrate metabolism, 30–35
  exercise and, 563–66, 578
  Krebs cycle and, 33–35
  thyroid hormones and, 177
  weight control and, 337
Carbon dioxide
  blowing off, 164
  breath-holding and, 149–50
  diffusion gradients of, 158
  gas transport by blood, 160
  hyper/hypoventilation and, 148
  indirect calorimetry
    measurement of, 215–16
  lung ventilation and, 141
  respiratory quotient and, 223–24
  See also External respiration;
    Internal respiration
Carbonic anhydrase, 160
Carbon monoxide, 150
Cardiac cost concept, 108–9
Cardiac cycle
  heartbeat, 94
  output of, 95–103
  pressure relationships in, 94–95
Cardiac muscle, 11
Cardiac output
  age factors and, 387, 394
  blood supply and, 103–5
  heart rate control, 98–101
  measurement of, 95–98
  nervous system control of,
    98–101
  nervous system heart rate
    control, 98–101
  sex differences in, 602

Starling's law, 101–2
  stroke volume, 109
  stroke volume control, 101–2
  venous return importance,
    102–103
  See also Cardiovascular system;
    Heart
Cardiac rehabilitation
  exercise prescription for, 324–25
  exercise testing in, 320–24
  program development of, 326–28
  weight training for, 325–26
  See also Coronary heart disease
    (CHD); Exercise testing
Cardiac reserve capacity, 110
Cardiorespiratory fitness. See
    Prescription exercise
Cardiovascular system
  age factors and, 394
  exercise and, 237–41
  sex differences and, 605–6
  of women in athletics, 601–2
Catecholamines
  adrenal medulla and, 182–84
  leukocytosis and, 200
  muscle contraction and, 176
Cell. See Muscle tissue
Cell-mediated immunity, 198–99
Cells, of the immune system, 198–99
Central nervous system, 69
Childbirth, sports participation and,
    612–14
Cholesterol
  coronary heart disease and, 315
  exercise effects on, 241–42
Cholinergic fibers, 121, 178
Chronic exercise training, 520–21
Circulation
  muscular endurance and, 452–53
  norepinephrine and, 176
Circulatory system
  age factors and, 388
  alkaline reserve and, 130
  blood distribution
    control of, 120–21
    rest vs. exercise, 121–22
  blood flow, 116–18
    during exercise, 126–31
  blood volume, exercise and, 129
  hemodynamics, 116–18
  hemoglobin and, 130
  microcirculation, 118–20
  peripheral circulation and, 240

postural effects on, 130–31
sports anemia and, 130
See also Blood pressure;
      Hemodynamics
Circulorespiratory endurance
   aerobic vs. anaerobic work and,
      455
   distance event training and,
      457–62
   energy substrate and, 456
   genetic factor and, 456–57
   lactate threshold in training and,
      459
   marathon running and, 462
   maximum oxygen consumption
      and, 456
   motivation and, 457
   training effects and, 457
   warm-up effect on, 533
Closed-circuit method, indirect
      calorimetry, 214
Cocontractions, dynamogenic effect
      of, 87
Coefficient of oxygen utilization, 162
Cold environment
   acclimatization to, 543
   exercise in, 542–43
   limitations in, 543–44
   performance and, 544
   wind chill factor and, 544
Complement proteins, 194–95
   antibodies and, 197
Concentric muscle contraction,
      51–52
Conditioning programs, for elderly,
      392–400
Congestive heart failure, 315
Connective tissue, exercise effects
      on, 242–43
Contractile mechanism, 17–22
   See also Muscular contraction
Contraction phase of muscle
      contraction, 47
   See also Muscular contraction
Contracture, 50
   See also Muscular contraction
Controlled frequency breathing
      (CFB), 461
Cooling down, 131
Cooper Twelve-Minute Run-Walk
      Test, 268–70
Core temperature, cold environment,
      543

Coronary arteries
   age factors and, 387
   anatomy, physiology of, 313–14
Coronary heart disease (CHD)
   angina pectoris, 314
   causative theories of, 315–17
   congestive heart failure, 315
   exercise and, 179, 237–40,
      317–19
   myocardial infarction, 314
   PC corticoids and, 178
   risk factor concept in, 317
   serum cholesterol and, 315
   sudden death, 314–15
   Type A personality and, 316
   See also Cardiac rehabilitation
Corpus striatum, 83
Corrected effective temperature
      (CET), 547
Corticoids, 181
Corticotropin-releasing factor
      (CRF), 180–81
Cortisol, 181
Costal breathing, 144
Crista, 72
Critical Power Test, 275–78
Crossed extensor reflex, 70
Cross-education effect
   muscle strength and, 427–28
   muscular endurance and, 452
Cycle ergometer, 211–14
   anaerobic power measurement
      by, 221
   physical working capacity
      (PWC) measurement by,
      257
Cycling
   efficiency of, 473–74
   glycogen depletion and, 40
   muscle temperature and, 529–30
   negative work, 227
   prescription of exercise, 293–95

D

Death, sudden (heart), 314–15
Dehydrogenase, 33
Delayed onset muscle soreness
      (DOMS)
   acute inflammation theory of,
      513–14
   local ischemia theory of, 514–15
   mechanical trauma theory of,
      512–13 .

spasm theory of, 515–18
   static stretching and, 519, 521
   warm-up prevention of, 535
   See also Muscle soreness
Dendrites, 69
Depletion fatigue hypotheses,
      415–17
Desoxycorticosterone, 178
Development. *See* Growth
Diaphragmatic breathing, 144
Diastasis, heartbeat, 95
Diastolic blood pressure, 123
Diet, efficiency of, 351–52, 475
Dieting, 351–52
Diffusion gradients, respiratory
      gasses, 158
Direct calorimetry, 214
Disaccharides, 32
Dissociation curve, oxygen, 160–62
Distance training, circulorespiratory
      endurance and, 457–62
Disuse phenomena, nervous system
      and, 85
Disynaptic reflex, 70
Diurnal variation, blood pressure
      and, 124
Dose-response data, for elderly,
      397–98
Douglas bag, 214–15
Drag, running efficiency and, 476
Dynamic constant external
      resistance (DCER), 51
Dynamic flexibility, 500–502
Dynamic strength, 489

E

Eccentric muscle contraction, 51–52
Edema, 124
Effective temperature, corrected
      (CET), 547
Effective temperature (ET), 546–47
Efferent neurons, 23, 69–70, 78–81
Efficiency
   aerobic vs. anaerobic, 470
   age factors and, 391
   definition of, 210, 468
   diet and, 475
   drag and, 476
   elastic energy storage, 474
   of electrical activity (EEA), 59
   fatigue effect on, 475
   heart, 104–5

improvement guidelines, 479–80
looseness factor in, 476
measurement of, 468–70
obesity effects on, 476
pace and, 477–78
positive, negative work and,
    478–79
running economy, 470–72
smoothness of movement and,
    476–77
speed effects on, 472–74
speed force-velocity relationship,
    486–87
temperature effects on, 475
wind effects in running, 475–76
work rate effect on, 474
Effort impulse value, muscle tension,
    58
Elastic energy storage, 474
Elastic resistance, 142–44
Electrocardiography, 56
Electrolyte replacement, heat,
    554–55
Electromyography, resting tonus,
    63–65
Electromyography (EMG)
    bilateral strength deficit
        measurement by, 428–29
    efficiency of electrical activity
        (EEA) and, 59
    effort impulse value of, 58
    endurance measurement by,
        59–61
    fatigue causes measured by,
        414–15
    hypertrophy and, 385
    hyperventilation and, 62
    interference pattern of, 57–58
    muscle action potential (MAPs)
        and, 56–57
    muscle fatigue, 417–18
    muscles soreness measured by,
        516–17
    muscle tension estimation and,
        58
    muscle tonus and, 62–65
    muscular endurance and, 384,
        452
    physical working capacity
        (PWC) at fatigue threshold,
        278–80

planimetry of, 57
qualitative, quantitative
    measurements of, 56
second wind and, 147
shivering response and, 62
strength, endurance, fatigue
    estimation and, 58–59, 61
strength estimation, 58–59
tension estimation by, 58
EMG. See Electromyography
    (EMG)
Emotional factors
    blood pressure and, 123–24
    heart rate affected by, 105–6
    performance and, 86–87
    of women athletes, 615
Endocrine system
    adrenal cortex, training and,
        179–80
    adrenocortical axis and, 177–80
    catecholamine effects and,
        182–84
    exercise effects on, 180–82
    general adaptation syndrome
        (GAS), 177–78
    gonadal hormones, 176–77,
        184–85
    hypothalamus-pituitary-adrenal
        axis and, 180–82
    pancreatic hormones, 184
    performance related effects,
        176–77
    pituitary-adrenocortical axis and,
        177–80
    See also Hormones
Endolymph, 72
Endomysium, 12
Endurance
    aerobic fitness and, 367–68
    blood doping and, 588–89
    electromyography (EMG)
        measurement of, 59–61
    glycogen supercompensation and,
        578
    muscular, 384
    performance and, 448
    See also Circulorespiratory
        endurance; Endurance
        training; Muscular
        endurance; Performance;
        Strength; Strength training

Endurance training
    aerobic fitness and, 367–68
    aerobic metabolism and, 35–37
    air pollution and, 150–51
    immunoglobulins and, 200–201
    oxygen debt and, 221
    pulmonary function and, 146–47
    second wind and, 147
    strength training, 437–38
Energy
    activity requirements of, 352–53
    consumption measurement,
        214–16
    definition of, 210
    efficiency measurement and,
        468–70
    elastic energy storage, 474
    fat used for, 34
    food source, 210
    kinetic, 210
    law of conservation of, 210
    metabolic energy exchange,
        335–37
    potential, 210
    protein used for, 34
Energy consumption measurement
    direct calorimetry, 214
    gas analysis, 216
    indirect calorimetry, 214–16
Energy substrate
    circulorespiratory endurance and,
        456
    glycogen-sparing effect and, 42
    overshoot phenomenon, 41–42
    pancreatic hormones and, 176
Environmental factors, 4
    adaptations to temperature,
        physiology, 541–42
    cold environment exercise,
        542–44
    heart rate affected by, 106
    high altitudes, 555–57
    hot environment acclimatization,
        551–55
    hot environment exercise, 544–51
Epimysium, 11–13
Epinephrine (E), 182–84
Ergogenic aids. See Performance
Ergography
    isotonic testing by, 450–51
    muscular endurance
        measurement, 411–14

Erythrocyte count, 129
Erythrocythemia, 588–89
Erythropoietin, 589
Esophagus, 137
Exercise
    adrenal cortex and, 179–80
    adrenocorticotropin (ACTH)
        and, 181–82
    aerobic fitness and, 365–68
    anaerobic fitness and, 368–71
    antibodies and, 200–201
    blood flow during, 121–22,
        126–29
    blood pressure and, 240
    blood properties and, 240–41
    body fluids during, 129–31
    breathing pattern affected by,
        144
    cancer and, 243–44
    carbohydrate food intake and,
        563–66, 578
    cardiac rehabilitation and,
        320–24
    cold environment and, 542–44
    complement proteins and, 201
    cooling down after, 131
    coronary circulation and,
        103–5, 239–40
    coronary heart disease (CHD)
        and, 179, 237–39, 317–19
    endocrine system affected by,
        180–82
    epinephrine (E), norepinephrine
        (NE) and, 182–84
    exercise-induced asthma (EIA)
        and, 147–48
    fat food intake and, 563–64, 568
    genetic effects on respiration and,
        147
    glucagon and, 176
    gonadal hormones and, 184–85
    heart rate affected by, 101–2,
        106–9
    high altitudes and, 556–57
    hormones affecting, 175–76
    in hot environment, 544–51
    in hot environment,
        acclimatization to, 551–55
    immune system affected by,
        199–203
    insulin and, 176, 184
    interferon and, 202
    joint angle specificity during,
        strength and, 430–31

    leukocytosis and, 199–200
    life expectancy and, 236–37
    lipid metabolism and, 241–42
    long-distance running and, 368
    lung diffusion and, 165–66
    lymphocytosis and, 200
    metabolic aftereffects of, 350
    ovarian hormones and, 185
    oxygen levels and, 145, 166–67,
        242
    parathyroid hormone (PATH)
        and, 184
    peripheral circulation and, 240
    physical fitness and, 236–37
    physiology overview of, 8–9
    protein food intake and, 563–64,
        566–68
    psychiatric state and, 245–46
    pulmonary function and, 242,
        531
    resting muscle tonus and, 64
    skeletal system affected by,
        242–43
    stomach function affected by,
        575–77
    stress and, 179, 240–41
    tranquilizer effect of, 244–45
    upper respiratory infections and,
        202–3
    weight reduction and, 349–50
    wind chill factor and, 544
    See also Age factors; Exercise
        loads; Exercise metabolism;
        Exercise testing;
        Prescription of exercise
Exercise-induced asthma (EIA),
    147–48
Exercise intensity
    cardiac rehabilitation and,
        324–25
    heart rate response and, 295–96,
        302–4
Exercise loads
    bench-stepping, 210–11
    cycle ergometer, 211–14
    energy consumption
        measurement, 214–15
    measurement of, 210–14
    treadmill, 211
    watts units, 209–10
    See also Exercise; Exercise
        intensity; Exercise loads;
        Exercise metabolism;
        Exercise testing

Exercise metabolism
    anaerobic power measurement
        and, 221
    anaerobic threshold concept,
        224–26
    efficiency definition of, 210
    energy consumption
        measurement, 214–15
    energy definition of, 210
    increasing work load, 222–23
    intermittent work and, 221–22
    load measurement, 210–14
    maximal oxygen consumption
        and, 222–23
    negative work, 226–27
    oxygen deficit and, 216–18
    power definition of, 208–10
    recovery oxygen and, 216–20
    respiratory quotient, 223–24
    work definition of, 208
    See also Exercise; Exercise
        intensity; Exercise loads;
        Exercise testing
Exercise prescription. See
    Prescription exercise
Exercise testing
    abnormal responses to, 321
    metabolic equivalents (METs) as
        measured in, 322
    oxygen cost calculation, 321–22
    parameters measured, 322–23
    principles of, 320–21
    rate-pressure product of, 322–23
    safety, litigation experience,
        323–24
    See also Exercise; Exercise
        intensity; Exercise loads;
        Exercise metabolism
Exocrine glands, 173, 176
External respiration
    air pollution and, 150–51
    anatomy of, 137
    breath-holding, 148–50
    breathing pattern importance,
        142–44
    control of, 139–42
    costal breathing, 144
    diaphragmatic breathing, 144
    exercise and breathing pattern,
        144
    exercise and oxygen
        consumption, 145–46,
        166–67, 242

exercise-induced asthma (EIA)
    and, 147–48
hyperventilation and, 148, 164
hypoventilation and, 148
nasal breathing, 145
oral breathing, 145
oxygen cost of breathing, 145–46
performance and breathing, 146
rate vs. depth of, 142–44
second wind phenomena, 147
smoking and, 151
stitch in the side phenomena, 147
training effects on, 146
Valsalva maneuver, 150
ventilation, lung, 145
    See also Lungs; Pulmonary
        function
Extrafusal fibers, 79–80
Extrapyramidal system, 86
Extrapyramidal system, muscular
    control, 83

F

Fartlek training, circulorespiratory
    endurance, 461
Fasciculus, 11–12, 23
Fast twitch fibers
    age factors and, 384–87
    arterial blood pressure and, 126
    catecholamine and, 176
    description, discussion of, 15–17
    endurance training and, 36
    hypertrophy and, 427
    muscle contraction speed and,
        485–86
    respiratory muscle fatigue and,
        146
    running efficiency and, 470
    sprint training and, 37–38
    strength, power training and, 39
    training and, 34
Fat cell theory, obesity, 348–49
Fatigue
    accumulation vs. depletion
        hypotheses, 415–17
    basic nature of, 413–14
    central vs. peripheral causes of,
        414–15
    cocontractions effect on, 87
    efficiency affected by, 475
    electromyography (EMG)
        measurement of, 59–61,
        417–18

historical perspective on, 410–11
muscle temperature effect on,
    417
muscular, 50–51
nervous system and, 88
psychological effect of, 410
recovery from, 450
    See also Neuromuscular fatigue
Fat metabolism, 33–34
    exercise and, 563–64, 568
    weight control and, 337
Feedback, nervous system, 85
Feedback, respiration and, 142
Feed forward, respiration, 142
Females. *See* Women in athletics
Fiber atrophy, 385
Fiber hypertrophy, 385
Fiber types
    running efficiency and, 470
    training and, 34
    See also Fast twitch fibers; Slow
        twitch fibers
Fick principle, 98
Flexibility
    anthropometric measurement
        issue, 502
    ballistic method to improve,
        503–7
    connective tissue and, 499–500
    dynamic measurement of, 502
    goniometric measurement of,
        501–2
    limits of, 499
    proprioceptive neuromuscular
        facilitation (PNF), 506–7
    speed and, 489
    static measurement of, 501–2
    static stretching method to
        improve, 503–7
    static vs. dynamic, 500–501
    stretching theory of, 500
    stretch reflexes and, 501
    variables affecting, 507–8
    weight training and, 507
    Yoga method of improvement,
        503
Flexion reflex, 70
Flexometer, range of motion, 502
Flower spray ending, 75, 79
Fluid replacement, heat, 554–55
Force-Velocity Curve, 55, 384
Force-velocity relationship, speed,
    486–87

Free fatty acids (FFA), 176
    energy substrate,
        circulorespiratory
        endurance, 456
Fructose, 32

G

Galactose, 32
Gamma system, muscular control,
    81
Gases
    analysis of, 218
    indirect calorimetry
        measurement of, 214–16
    properties of, 157–58
    transport by blood, 159–60
Gay-Lussac's Law, 157
General adaptation syndrome
    (GAS), 177–78
Glottis, 137
Glucagon, 176
Glucocorticoids, 178–79, 181
Glucose, 30–33
    endurance training and, 36
    glucose-alanine-glucose cycle, 36
Glycogen
    depletion of, 40
    glycogen-sparing effect and, 42
    glycolytic enzymes and, 36
    muscle contraction and, 32
    overshoot phenomenon, 41–42
    supercompensation, 578
    training effects on, 40–42
Glycogenolysis, 30
    See also Carbohydrate
        metabolism
Glycolysis, 30, 33, 36–38
Golgi tendon organ, 77
    kinesthesis, 80
Gonadal hormones, 176–77, 184–85
Goniometry, joint angle movement,
    501–2
Growth
    body composition and, 363–64
    definition of, 361
    height, body weight patterns of,
        362–63
    infancy, childhood, adolescence,
        361–62
    puberty, 362
    See also Age factors
Growth hormone (GH), 38, 182

H

Handane apparatus, procedure, 216
Harvard Step Test, 268
Health, Selye theory of stress and, 177–78
Heart
  athletic training effecting, 109
  cardiac cost concept, 108–9
  cardiac cycle, 94–95
  cardiac output, 95–103
  cardiac reserve capacity of, 110
  catecholamine and, 176
  coronary artery physiology, 313–14
  coronary circulation and, 103–4
  efficiency of, 104–5
  exercise and
    blood pressure, 240
    cardiac rehabilitation, 320–24
    coronary circulation, 103–5, 239–40
    coronary heart disease (CHD), 17–19, 179, 237–39
    heart rate, 101–2, 106–9
  heartbeat, 94
  murmurs of, 110–11
  pressure relationships within, 95
  rate
    age factors and, 387, 394
    control of, 98–101
    during/after exercise, 106–9
    factors affecting, 105–6
    prescription of exercise, 295–96, 302–4
    See also Physical working capacity (PWC)
  size, 109
  warm-up effect on, 535
  See also Cardiac output; Cardiac rehabilitation; Cardiac reserve; Cardiovascular system; Coronary Heart Disease (CHD)
Heat. *See* Hot environment
Heat stress, 546–51
Heavy water, 338–39
Height, growth patterns of, 362–63
Helper T cells, 198
Hemoconcentration, 129

Hemodynamics, 116–18
  blood flow velocity, 116–18
  hydrostatic pressure, 118
  Poiseuille's Law, 118
  pressure gradient and, 116
  resistance to flow, 118
  sport variations and, 127–29
Hemoglobin
  exercise and, 130
  oxygenation of, 159–60
Hemopoiesis, 588
Henry's Law, 158
Hexokinase, 32, 37
High altitudes
  acclimatization to, 556–57
  oxygen administration at, 557
  performance limitations at, 556
High density lipoprotein (HDL), 241–42, 315
Homeostasis, 94
Hormones
  catecholamine effects, 176, 182–84
  corticotropin-releasing factor (CRF), 180–81
  cortisol level, 181
  exercise, sports and, 175–76
  exercise effects and, 184–85
  glucagon, 176
  gonadal hormones, 176–77, 184–85
  growth hormone (GH), 38, 182
  nature of, 173–75
  norepinephrine (NE), 176, 182–84
  pancreatic hormones, 184
  parathyroid hormones, 184
  protein hormones, 173
  steroid hormones, 173
  stress reaction, general adaptation syndrome (GAS), 177–78
  thyroid hormones, 177, 184
Hot environment
  acclimatization to, 551
  age factors, 550
  corrected effective temperature (CET), 547
  effective temperature (ET), 547
  fluid/electrolyte replacement and, 554–55
  hot/dry, 544–45
  hot/humid, 545–46

  limitations in, 546–50
  obesity and, 550–51
  sex difference, 550
Humoral immunity, 196–98
Hydrocarbons, air pollution, 150
Hydrometric method, body composition, 340
Hydrostatic pressure, 118
Hypercapnia, 147–48, 461
Hyperplasia
  in strength, power training, 38
  strength and, 426–27
Hypertension, weight lifting, 375
Hyperthyroidism, 177
Hypertrophy
  age factors and, 384–85
  electromyography (EMG) evaluation of, 59
  in strength, power training, 38
  strength and, 426–27
Hyperventilation, 62, 148, 164
Hypnosis, performance and, 86–87
Hypoinsulinemia, 176
Hypothalamus
  corticotropin-releasing factor (CRF) of, 180–81
  performance and, 86–87
  stress syndrome and, 178
Hypothalamus-pituitary-adrenal axis, 180–82
Hypothyroidism, 177
Hypoventilation, 148
Hypoxia, 147
Hypoxic training, swimming, 461

I

Immune system
  antigens and, 196
  cell-mediated immunity, 198–99
  complement proteins of, 194–95
  exercise effects on, 199–203
  functional overview of, 193
  humoral immunity, 196–98
  interferon and, 196, 198
  leukocytes of, 193
  natural killer (NK) cells of, 194
  nonspecific mechanisms of, 193–96
  phagocytosis and, 194
  specific mechanisms of, 196–99
Immunoglobulins
  exercise and, 200–201
  types of, 196–97

Indirect calorimetry, 214–16
Infancy, 361–62
Inferior vena cava, shortening/
        lengthening of, 124
Injuries
        musculoskeletal, elderly, 399–400
        warm-up prevention and, 535
        weight training, 374–75
        to women, 615
Insulin, 38
        carbohydrate metabolism and,
                176
        exercise and, 184
Interference pattern, of
        electrocardiography
        (EMG), 57–58
Interferon, 196, 198
Intermittent work, oxygen
        consumption, 221–22
Internal respiration
        acid-base balance of, 162–65
        aerobic power capacity and,
                167–69
        exercise and lung diffusion,
                165–66
        gas transport by blood, 159–60
        oxygen
                aerobic power capacity and,
                        167–69
                blood transport of, 160
                dissociation curve of, 160–62
                performance improvement
                        and, 166–67
                utilization coefficient of, 162
        respiratory gasses composition,
                157–58
        upper respiratory infections,
                202–3
Internuncial neuron, 70
Intersegmental reflex, 71–72
Interval training, 221–22
        circulorespiratory endurance,
                459–60
        vs. continuous exercise, 292–93
Intrafusal muscle fibers, 76, 78–81
Inverse myotatic reflex, 77
Iron deficiency, sports anemia,
                573–74
Ischemia
        flexibility affected by, 508
        local ischemia theory of DOMS,
                514–15
Ischemic heart disease, 315

Islets of Langerhans, 176
Isokinetic muscle contraction, 51
Isokinetic training, 435–37
        muscular endurance and, 451–52
Isometric muscle contraction, 51,
                433
Isometric training
        advantages of, 433
        glycogen depletion and, 40
        isometric tension, 450
        measurement of, 432–33
Isotonic muscle contraction, 51
Isotonic training
        ergographic measurement of,
                450–51
        measurement of, 435
        methods using, 434

K

Killer T cells, 198
Kinesthesis
        free nerve endings and, 73, 78
        Golgi tendon organ in, 73, 77, 80
        muscle spindles in, 73, 75
        pacinian corpuscle and, 73, 77
        Ruffini receptors and, 73, 77
        voluntary movement and, 84–85
Kinetic energy, 210
Krebs cycle, 33–35

L

Lactacid, in oxygen debt, 218–20
Lactate threshold, 226
        circulorespiratory endurance and,
                459
Lactate tolerance, 592
Lameness, 512
Latent period, muscle contraction,
                47
Law of conservation of energy, 210
Length of muscle, 52–53
Leukocytes, 193
        leukocytosis and, 199–200
Life expectancy, exercise and,
                236–37
Lipid metabolism, exercise and,
                241–42
Liquids, respiratory, 157–59
Local ischemia theory, delayed onset
        muscle soreness (DOMS),
                514–15

Long, slow distance (LSD) training,
                458
Looseness factor, efficiency, 476
Low density lipoprotein (LDL),
                241–42, 315
Lower motor neurons, 82
Lungs
        anatomy of, 137–39
        capacities of, 388
        exercise and, 242
        oxygen consumption during
                exercise, 145
        volumes, capacities of, 139, 388
        See also External respiration;
                Internal respiration
Luteinizing hormone (LH), 185
Lymphatics
        lymphocytosis, 200
        lymphotoxins, 198
        muscle tissue and, 23

M

Macrophages, 198
Making weight, 364–65
MAP. See Muscle action potential
        (MAP)
Marathon running,
        circulorespiratory
        endurance, 462
Marathon running, training, 462
Margaria Step-running Anaerobic
        Power Test, 273–74
Maturation. See Growth
Maximal oxygen consumption
        age factors and, 365–68, 389–91
        alkalinizers and, 585
        anaerobic threshold controversy
                and, 224–25
        blood doping and, 588–89
        circulorespiratory endurance and,
                456
        cycle ergometer, 257
        exercise and, 242
        exercise testing and, 323
        fatigue and, 412–13
        at high altitudes, 555–56
        increased work load and, 222–23
        long slow distance (LSD)
                training and, 458
        measurement of, 211–12
                data extrapolation, 260
                end of test criteria, 260

environmental considerations, 258–59
exercise protocol, 257–58
informed consent, 254
parameters measured, 259–60
personnel, equipment needed, 254, 257
muscle soreness and, 515
negative work and, 227
oxygen pulse, 223
phosphate loading and, 586
prescription of exercise and, 295–96
running efficiency and, 470
sex differences in, 601–2, 605
speed efficiency and, 472–73
warm-up and, 530–31
warm-up physiology and, 528
Maximal voluntary contraction (MVC)
endurance, fatigue and, 61
isokinetic training and, 437
muscular endurance and, 61, 384, 449–50
sex differences and, 452
strength gain and, 430
Mechanical trauma theory, delayed onset muscle soreness (DOMS), 512–13
Memory B cells, 198
Memory drum theory, 88
Memory T cells, 199
Menstrual cycle
athletic menstrual cycle irregularity (AMI) and, 611–12
onset of menarche, 610–11
performance affected by, 612
sports participation and, 611
MET. See Metabolic equivalents (METs)
Metabolic equivalents (METs), 297–99, 322
Metabolism
basal metabolic rate (BMR) and, 177
fats, carbohydrates, protein, 337
thyroid hormones and, 184
weight gain, loss physiology and, 335–37
See also Energy; Exercise metabolism
Metarterioles, 119

Microcirculation, blood flow, 118–20
Mineralocorticoids (MC), 178–79
Minerals, 569–74
Mitochondrial enzymes, 35, 37, 39
Monosaccharides, 32
Monosynaptic reflex, 70
Motivation, circulorespiratory endurance and, 457
Motor fitness, 253
Motor fitness tests
AAHPER Youth Fitness Test Battery, 281–82
Army/Air Force Physical Fitness Test, 281
Motor neurons, 23, 69–81
Motor set, 88
Motor unit, 69–70
Movement time, 87–88
Multisynaptic reflex, 70
Murmurs, heart, 110–11
Muscle action potential (MAPs)
electromyography (EMG) of, 56–57
resting muscle tonus and, 63–65
Muscle soreness
cramping, 50
delayed onset muscle soreness (DOMS), 512–18
immediate, 512
practical aspects for coach and athlete, 518–19
prevention of, 520–21
relief of, 521–22
severe, 522
static stretching and, 519, 521
See also Delayed onset muscle soreness (DOMS)
Muscle spindles, 78–81
intrafusal muscle fibers (IF) in, 76
kinesthesis and, 73, 75
muscle tonus and, 62
Muscle strength. See Strength
Muscle tissue
blood supply to, 23
cell structure of, 12–15
contractile mechanism of, 18
endurance training and, 35–37
glycogen levels in, 40–42
gonadal hormones and, 176–77
growth hormone (GH) and, 182
lymphatics and, 23
myofibril structure, 17–18, 21–22

nerve supply and, 23
of skeletal muscles, 11–12
sprint training and, 37–38
strength, power training and, 38–39, 438–39
types of, 11
See also Electromyography (EMG)
Muscle tonus
definition of, 62–63
electromyography (EMG) and, 62–65
exercise and, 64
physiology of, 64
postural, 64
resting, 63–65
Muscular contraction
aerobic metabolism, 29–30, 32–33, 35–37
all-or-none law of, 49
anaerobic metabolism and, 32–33
angle of pull of, 52
carbohydrate metabolism and, 29–33
catecholamine effects on, 176
concentric, 51–52
contractile mechanism of, 17–22
contraction phase of, 47
eccentric, 51–52
efficiency of electrical activity (EEA) and, 59
electromyography (EMG) and, 56–58
endurance training and, 35–37
energetics overview of, 29–30
energy substrate, 40–42
fat and protein metabolism and, 33–34
fatigue and, 50–51
gradation of response of, 49–50
intrinsic speed of, 485–86
isokinetic, 51
isometric, 51
isotonic, 51
length of muscle and, 52–53
mechanism of, 29
muscle shortening, 55
myogram of, 47–48
relaxation phase of, 47–48
size principle of, 50
speed and, 492–93
sprint training and, 48
static, 51

strength/power training and, 38–39
strength estimation of, 58–59
stretching muscles and, 55
summation of contractions and, 48
temperature effects on, 48–49, 417
tension estimation of, 58
tetanus and, 48
twitch myogram of, 47–48
types of, 51–52
velocity of, 55
work output measure, 55
See also Efficiency
Muscular control. *See* Nervous system
Muscular endurance
accumulation fatigue hypothesis, 415–16
age factors and, 384, 452
central vs. peripheral fatigue causes, 414–15
depletion fatigue hypothesis, 416–17
electromyography (EMG) and, 414–18, 452
improvement of, 453–54
isokinetic tests of, 451–52
measurement of, 450–52
muscle temperature and, 417
strength and, 449–50
strength-decrement index and, 451
warm-up and, 533, 535
See also Circulorespiratory endurance; Fatigue; Neuromuscular fatigue
Myocardial infarction, 314
Myofibril, 12
contractile mechanism, 17–22
structure of, 17–18, 21–22
Myoglobin, 35
Myogram of muscular contraction, 47–48
Myosin, 17–18, 21, 53
Myositis, muscle soreness, 512
Myotatic reflex, 62, 70

N

Nasal breathing, 145
National Children and Youth Fitness Study (NCYFS), 288

Natural killer (NK) cells, immune system, 194
Near-infrared spectrophotometry (NIR), body composition, 342–45
Negative work, 211, 226–27, 478–79
Nervous system
age factors and, 391–92
alpha system of muscle control, 78–81
balance and, 84
blood flow control by, 121
cocontractions, dynamogenic effect of, 87
cross-education effect and, 427–28, 452
emotional response and performance, 86–87
extrapyramidal system, 83, 86
fatigue and, 88
gamma system of, 81
heart rate control by, 98–101
involuntary movement of, 70–71
kinesthesis, 84–85
kinesthesis by, 73, 75, 77–78
motor/sensory set and, 88
motor unit of, 69–70, 73
perception of effort and, 85
posture and, 84
proprioception by, 72
proprioceptive-cerebellar system, 83
proprioceptive neuromuscular facilitation (PNF) and, 87
pyramidal system, 82–83, 86
rate coding, recruitment by, 50
reaction/movement time and, 87–88
reflex arc, 70–71
strength gain and, 427
use-disuse phenomena, 85
vestibular receptors of, 72–73
viscerosomatic reflexes, 86
voluntary movement and, 84
Neuromuscular fatigue
anxiety, tension and, 244
athletic performance affected by, 411
industrial workers affected by, 412–13
reflexes, coordination affected by, 412
strength loss and, 411–12

Neurons
afferent, 69–70
association, 70
motor (efferent), 23, 69–70, 78–81
of muscle tissue, 23
Neurons. *See* Nervous system
Nitrogen oxides, air pollution, 150
Norepinephrine (NE), 176, 182–84
Nutrition, 5
caloric intake, 563
carbohydrates and, 563–66, 578
efficiency affected by, 475
fats and, 563–64, 568
glycogen supercompensation, endurance events, 578
iron deficiency, 573–74
minerals and, 569–74
muscle contraction and, 29
pregame nutrition, 577
proteins and, 563–64, 566–68
training guidelines for, 564–76
vitamins and, 568–73
See also Weight control; Weight reduction

O

Obesity
definition of, 338
disadvantages of, 335
efficiency affected by, 476
etiology of, 348
fat cell theory of, 348–49
heat stress and, 550–51
Open-circuit method, indirect calorimetry, 214–15
Oral breathing, 145
Oro-nasal-breathing-shift (ONBS), 145
Osteoporosis, 242–43
Otolith organ, of vestibule, 73
Ovarian hormones, exercise and, 185
Overload
muscular endurance improvement and, 453–54
warm-up, 532
Overshoot phenomenon, 41–42
Overtraining, "staleness" and, 418
Oxygen
aerobic power capacity and, 167–69
by altitude, 157–58

anaerobic power measurement
and, 221
arterial blood pressure and, 127
before, during, after exercise,
166–67
blood transport of, 160
breath-holding and, 149–50
coefficient of utilization of, 162
conductance equation of, 167–69
deficit of, 216–18
diffusion gradients of, 158
dissociation curve of, 160–62
exercise and consumption of,
145–46
gas transport by blood, 159–60
high altitude administration of,
556–57
indirect calorimetry
measurement of, 214–16
lung ventilation and, 141
maximal oxygen consumption
and, 222–23
oxygen debt, 217–20
performance and, 592
performance improvement and,
166–67
recovery oxygen, 218–20
transport affected by exercise,
242
See also Internal respiration
Oxygenation, 160
Oxygen debt, 217–18
lactacid-alactacid in, 218–20
lactic acid and, 217
Ozone, air pollution, 150–51

P

Pace, efficiency affected by, 477–78
Pacinian corpuscle, 77
Pancreatic hormones
energy substrates and, 176
exercise effects of, 184
Parasympathetic division, nervous
system, 69
Parathyroid hormones, 184
Partial pressures, Law of, 157
Particulate matter, air pollution, 150
Passive warm-up, 531
Performance
acid-base balance and, 165
air pollution and, 150–51
alkalinizers and, 584–86
amphetamines and, 586–87

anabolic steroids and, 587
aspartates and, 587–88
blood doping and, 588–89
breathing and, 146
caffeine, 590
carbohydrate feeding, 591–92
cold environment effects on, 544
emotional response and, 86–87
endocrine system and, 176–77
endurance factor in, 448
hypnotic effect on, 87
lactate tolerance and, 592
menstrual cycle effects on, 612
motor/sensory set and, 88
oxygen administration and, 557
oxygen and, 166–67, 592
phosphate loading and, 586
vitamins and, 592
wheat-germ oil and, 592
Perimysium, 11–12, 23
Periodization, strength training,
434–35
Peripheral circulation, 240
Peripheral nervous system, 69
pH
alkalinizers, performance and,
584–85
lung ventilation and, 141
respiratory gasses, liquids,
158–59
See also Acid-base balance
Phagocytosis, 194, 197
Phosphatase, 32
Phosphate loading, performance
improvement, 586
Physical education
physical working capacity
(PWC) and, 253–54
professionalism in, 5–6
Selye theory of stress and,
177–78
Physical fitness
age factor and, 282
Critical Power Test, 275–78
life expectancy and, 236–37
maximal oxygen consumption
and, 222–23
reason for, 4
See also Athletic training;
Exercise; Physical working
capacity (PWC);
Prescription of exercise;
Weight control; Weight
reduction

Physical working capacity (PWC)
age factors and, 389–91, 393–96
cardiac rehabilitation and,
319–20
concept of, 253–54
fatigue and, 416
at fatigue threshold
from submaximal power
outputs, 279–80
from supramaximal power
outputs, 278–79
measurement of
Astrand-Rhyming
Nomogram, 262–67
Canadian Home Fitness Test,
268
Cooper Twelve-Minute Run-
Walk Test, 268–70
Harvard Step Test, 268
maximal oxygen consumption
measurement, 254–60
PWC-170 test, 261–62
Rockport Walking Test,
272–73
Treadmill Walking Test,
270–72
Twelve-Minute Swimming
Test, 270
See also Motor fitness tests
Physicochemical properties, of blood,
240–41
Pituitary-adrenocortical axis,
177–82
Pituitary gland
growth hormone (GH) secretion
by, 182
stress syndrome and, 178
Planimetry, electromyography, 57
Plasma cells, 196–98
Plyometric training, 437
Poiseuille's Law, 118
Polygraph, 123–24
Polymer, 32
Positive energy balance, 347
Positive work, 211, 226, 478–79
Post-tetanic-twitch potentiation
(PTP), 87
Postural muscle tonus, 64
Posture
blood pressure and, 124
circulation and, 130–31
heart rate affected by, 105
nervous system and, 84
vagal rebound phenomenon,
130–31

Potential energy, 210
Power
    definition, measurement of,
        208–10
    speed force-velocity relationship,
        486–87
    warm-up effect on, 533
Power training, 38–39
Precapillary sphincter, 119
Precentral gyrus, 82
Preferential channels, 119
Pregnancy, sports participation and,
        612–14
Premotor cortex, 83
Prescription of exercise
    age factors and, 305
    for cardiac rehabilitation, 324–25
    daily workout plan, 302
    for elderly, 397–98
    elements of, 302–4
    evaluation prior to, 289–92
    exercise duration, 297–300
    exercise frequency, 300–301
    exercise intensity, 295
    exercise modality in, 293–95
    exertion range recommendation,
        297
    heart rate range, 295–96
    interval training and, 292–93
    metabolic equivalent range, 297
    need for, 288
    physiological changes from, 305
    scientific principles involved in,
        289
    specificity of, 305
    as stressor, 306
    target oxygen consumption rate
        range, 295
    training curves and, 292
President's Council on Physical
        Fitness and Sports
        (PCPFS), 288
Pressure gradient, 116
    internal respiration and, 157
Pressure relationships, cardiac cycle,
        94
Prior exercise (PE)
    maximal oxygen consumption
        and, 530–31
    warm-up physiology and, 528
Progressive resistance exercise
        (PRE), 289
Pro-inflammatory corticoids (PC),
        178–79

Proprioception, 72
    heart rate impulses, 99
    kinesthetic receptors, 73, 75–78,
        85
    lung ventilation and, 141–42
    vestiular receptors, 72–73
    See also Kinesthesis
Proprioceptive cerebellar system,
        muscular control, 83
Proprioceptive neuromuscular
        facilitation (PNF), 87,
        506–7
Protein hormones, 173
Protein metabolism, 33–34
    exercise and, 563–64, 566–68
    weight control and, 337
Proteins
    complement proteins, 194–95
    food intake, 563–64, 566–68
    testosterone and, 176–77
P substance, muscle soreness, 516
Psychiatric state, exercise and,
        245–46
Psychological factors, strength and,
        440
Puberty, 362
Pulmonary function
    age factors and, 388–89
    exercise effects on, 242
    pulmonary diffusion, 389
    See also External respiration;
        Internal respiration; Lungs
Pulmonary ventilation. See External
        respiration
PWC-170 test, 261–62
Pyramidal system, muscular control,
        82–83, 86, 428

R

Range of motion, improvement
        methods, 503–7
Rate coding by nervous system, 50
Rating of Perceived Exertion (RPE),
        85, 585
Reaction time, 87–88, 391–92
Reactive hyperemia, 129
Reciprocal inhibition, 70, 501
Recovery oxygen
    anaerobic metabolism and, 221
    exercise metabolism and, 216–18
    interval training and, 221–22
    lactacid, alactacid in, 218–20
    processes used, 218–20

Recruitment by nervous system, 50
Rectal temperature, 529–30
Red nucleus, 83
Reflex, myotatic, stretch, 75
Reflexes
    crossed extensor, 70
    disynaptic, 70
    fatigue and, 88
    intersegmental, 71–72
    inverse myotatic, 77
    monosynaptic, 70, 78–81
    multisynaptic, 70
    myotatic, 70, 84
    neuromuscular fatigue and, 412
    reflex arc, 70–71
    righting reflex, 84
    stretch reflexes, 501
    suprasegmental, 71–72, 84
    viscerosomatic reflexes, 86
Related warm-up method, 531
Relaxation phase of muscle
        contraction, 47–48
Renshaw cell, 80
Repetition (REP) training,
        circulorespiratory
        endurance, 460–61
Respiration. See External
        respiration; Internal
        respiration; Lungs;
        Pulmonary function
Respiratory bronchioles, 137
Respiratory quotient, 223–24
Rheumatoid arthritis, PC corticoids
        and, 178
Ribosomal RNA, 176–77
Righting reflex, 84
Risk factor concept, coronary heart
        disease (CHD), 317
Rockport Walking Test, 272–73
Ruffini receptors, 77
Running
    air pollution and, 150
    body mechanics in speed, 489–90
    breath-holding and, 149–50
    breathing patterns and, 144
    complement proteins and, 201
    efficiency of, 470–72
    energy efficiency and, 477–78
    exercise-induced asthma (EIA)
        and, 148
    glycogen depletion and, 40
    heat injury prevention, running,
        552–53
    long-distance, 368

marathon running and, 462
Margaria Step-Running
    Anaerobic Power Test,
    273–74
muscle stretching and, 55
oxygen supplementation and, 166
prescription of exercise, 293–95
recovery between events in,
    534–35
secretory immunoglobulins and,
    201
sex differences and, 605–6
vs. swimming, speed, 492
track design, psychological
    factors, 490
upper respiratory infection and,
    202
wind effects on, 475–76

S

Saccule, of vestibule, 72–73
Sarcolemma, 12, 32
    MAP and, 56
Sarcomere, 17, 21, 53
Sarcoplasm, 12, 35
Scalene muscles, 134
Scholander apparatus, 216
Scientific method, 5–8
Second wind phenomena, 147
Secretory immunoglobulins, 201
Selye theory of stress, 177–80
Semicircular canals, 72
Sensory end organ, 70
Sensory neurons, 69
Sensory set, 88
Servomechanism, 80
Sex differences, 305
    athletic training and, 6–7
    blood pressure and, 123
    flexibility affected by, 507
    heart rate affected by, 105
    heat stress and, 550
    muscular endurance affected by,
        452
    running efficiency and, 471–72
    speed of movement, 490–91
    See also Women in athletics
Shivering response, 62
Sinoatrial (SA) node, heartbeat, 94,
    98
Size principle, muscle contraction,
    50

Skeletal muscle
    cardiac output and, 103–5
    catecholamine effect on, 176
    classification, characteristics of,
        16
    exercise and, 240
    gross structure of, 11
    growth hormone (GH) and, 182
    microscopic structure of, 11–12
    muscle tonus of, 62–63
Skeletal system, exercise effects on,
    242–43
Skinfold measures, 340–45
Slow, oxidative (SO) fibers, 16
Slow twitch fibers
    age factors and, 384–87
    arterial blood pressure and, 126
    catecholamine and, 176
    definition, description of, 15–17
    endurance training and, 36
    hypertrophy and, 427
    muscle contraction speed and,
        485–86
    running efficiency and, 470
    sprint training and, 37–38
    strength, power training and, 39
    training and, 34
Smoking
    breathing affected by, 151
    coronary heart disease (CHD)
        and, 316–17
    heart rate affected by, 106
SO fibers. See Slow, oxidative (SO)
    fibers
Somatic nervous system, 69
Spasm theory, delayed onset muscle
    soreness (DOMS), 515–18
Speed
    body mechanics, running, 489–90
    body mechanics, swimming, 490
    coaching for, 494–95
    efficiency and, 472–74, 486–87
    flexibility and, 489
    force-velocity relationship of,
        486–87
    gross motor movements, 493–94
    muscle contraction intrinsic
        speed, 485–86
    running track design, 490
    sex differences, 490–91
    single muscle contractions and,
        492–93
    specificity of, 487

sprint speed improvement, 494
    strength and, 488–89
    variations, swimming and
        running, 492
    warm-up effect on, 532
Sphygmomanometer, 122
Sports anemia, 130, 573–74
Sports training. See Athletic
    training; Physical fitness
Spot reducing, weight reduction, 354
Sprint speed improvements, 494
Sprint training
    anaerobic metabolism, 37–38
    summation of contractions in, 48
Staleness, psychological effect of,
    418
Starling's Law, heart stroke volume,
    101–2
Static contraction, 51
Static flexibility, 501
    measurement of, 500–502
    stretching method, 503–7
Static strength, 488
Static stretch, 503
    muscle soreness and, 519, 521
Stature, age factors and, 392
Sternocleidomastoid muscles, 134
Steroids, 587–88
    steroid hormones, 173
Stitch in the side phenomena, 147
Strength
    age factors and, 383–84, 439
    bilateral deficit in, 428–29
    cross-education effect and,
        427–28
    diurnal variation and, 439
    electromyography (EMG)
        measurement of, 58–59
    gain in, 427, 430
    gender differences in, 439
    hypertrophy and, 59
        versus hyperplasia, 426–27
    joint angle specificity during
        exercise and, 430–31
    mechanical factors in, 429–30
    muscular endurance and, 449–50
    neuromuscular fatigue and,
        411–12
    vs. power, 208–9
    psychological factors and, 440
    seasonal effects on, 439
    speed and, 488–89
    static, 488

strength decrement index (SDI),
    451
temperature effects on, 439–40
warm-up effect on, 532
See also Endurance;
    Performance; Strength
    training
Strength-decrement index, of
    muscular endurance, 451
Strength training
    age factors and, 371, 374
    cable tension strength tests, 433
    concurrent strength, endurance
        training, 437–38
    generality vs. specificity, 438
    isokinetic training and, 435–37
    isometric training and, 432–33
    isotonic training, 433–35
    joint angle and exercise, 430–31
    maximal voluntary contraction
        (MVC) and, 430
    muscle tissue quality/quantity
        and, 38–39
    muscle tissue quantity, quality,
        438–39
    periodization, 434–35
    plyometric training and, 437
    sex differences and, 606–10
    time course of, 431–32
    variability in, 438
    women and, 606–10
Stress
    adrenocorticotropin (ACTH)
        and, 181–82
    blood properties and, 240–41
    coronary heart disease (CHD)
        and, 317
    exercise and, 179, 240–41
    general adaptation syndrome
        (GAS) and, 177–78
    heart rate affected by, 108–9
    Selye theory of, 177–78
    stress syndrome, 177–78
    training as stressors, 306
Stretching
    bouncing stretch, 519
    improvement of force and work,
        55
    proprioceptive neuromuscular
        facilitation (PNF) and, 87
    static stretching method,
        503–7
    stretching theory, 500

stretch reflex, 70
stretch reflexes and, 501
See also Flexibility
Stroke volume reserve, 110
Substantia nigra, 83
Sudden death, 314–15
Summation of muscle contractions,
    48
Suppressor T cells, 198
Suprasegmental reflexes, 72, 84
Sweat, 545
Swimming
    body mechanics in, 490
    breath-holding and, 148–50
    breathing patterns and, 144
    energy efficiency and, 477–78
    exercise-induced asthma (EIA)
        and, 148
    glucagon levels and, 184
    Hypoxic training and, 461
    lung diffusion capacity and, 165
    oxygen supplementation and, 166
    prescription of exercise, 293–95
    recovery between events in,
        534–35
    vs. running, speed, 492
    secretory immunoglobulins and,
        201
    Twelve-Minute Swimming Test,
        270
    warm-up effect on, 534
    young girl swimmers and, 602
Sympathetic division, nervous
    system, 69
Sympathicotonics, 180
Synapses, 69
Syncytium, 11
Système International (SI) units,
    208–9
Systolic blood pressure, 123

T

T cells, 198–99
    exercise and, 200
Temperature effects
    efficiency and, 475
    flexibility affected by, 508
    lung ventilation and, 142
    muscular contraction and, 48–49
    muscular endurance, 417, 452
    rectal vs. muscle, 529–30
    thyroid hormones and, 177
    See also Environmental factors;
        Thermal balance

Tension
    muscular, 58
    neuromuscular system and, 244
Tension-time index, heart rate,
    104–5
Terminal bronchioles, 137
Testosterone
    exercise and, 176–77, 184–85
    strength, power training and, 38
Tetanus, muscle contractions, 48
Thermal balance, 541–42
Throwing, warm-up and, 533
Thyroid hormones, 184
    metabolic rate and, 177
Thyroxine, 177
Tonus. *See* Muscular contraction
Trachea, 137
Track. *See* Running
Training curves
    prescription of exercise and, 292
    strength training and, 431–32
Training effects. *See* specific subjects
Tranquilizer effect, of exercise,
    244–45
Treadmill, 211
    physical working capacity
        (PWC) measurement by,
        257
    Treadmill Walking Test, 270–72
Treppe effect, 50–51
Triglycerides, 34
    exercise effects on, 242
Triiodothyronine, 177
Tropomyosin, 17–18, 21–22
Troponin, 18, 21–22
True capillaries, 119
Turbinates, 137
Twelve-Minute Swimming Test, 270
Twitch. *See* Fast twitch fibers;
        Muscular contraction; Slow
        twitch fibers
Tying up, 86–87
Type A personality, coronary heart
    disease (CHD) and, 316

U

Underwater weighing, 338–39
Unrelated warm-up method, 531
Upper motor neurons, 82
Upper respiratory infection, 202–3
    exercise and, 202–3
    secretory immunoglobulins and,
        201

Use-disuse phenomena, nervous system and, 85
Utricle, of vestibule, 72–73

V

Vagal rebound phenomenon, 130–31
Vagotonics, 180
Valsalva effect, 125
Valsalva maneuver, 150
Velocity of muscle contraction, 55
Venous return, 102–3, 124
Ventilation equivalent, 145
Very low density lipoprotein (VLDL), 241–42, 315
Vestibular receptors, 72–73
Viscerosomatic reflexes, 86
Vitamins, 568–73
    performance and, 592
VO$_2$ max. *See* Maximal oxygen consumption
Volumes, lung, 139, 388
Voluntary movement, nervous system and, 84

W

Walking
    efficiency of, 473
    local ischemia and, 514
    prescription of exercise, 293–95
    Rockport Walking Test, 272–73
    Treadmill Walking Test, 270–72
Warm-up
    active, 531
    blood flow in lungs, 531
    circulorespiratory endurance and, 533
    duration of, 531–32, 534
    general vs. local heating, 529
    heart function and, 535
    intensity of, 531–32
    muscle injury and, 48–49
    muscle injury prevention and, 535
    muscular endurance and, 533
    overload, 532
    oxygen consumption and, 530–31
    passive, 531

physiology of, 528–31
    power and, 533
    recovery between events and, 534–35
    rectal vs. muscle temperature, 529–30
    related warm-up method, 531
    speed, 532
    strength and, 532
    swimming and, 534
    throwing and, 533
    unrelated warm-up method, 531
Warm-up processes, 520
Water retention, weight reduction, 353–54
Weight control
    age factors and, 392–93
    body composition estimation, 338–45
    body weight and health, 335
    gaining weight, 346
    long haul concept of, 354–55
    making weight, 364–65
    metabolism of carbohydrate, fat, protein, 337
    misconceptions of, 350
    normal weight and, 337–38
    See also Weight reduction
Weight gain, 346
    physiology of, 335–37
Weight reduction
    American College of Sports Medicine (ACSM) recommendations, 347–48
    dieting and, 351–52
    exercise and, 349–53
    obesity etiology, 348–49
    physiology of, 335–37
    protein metabolism and, 33
    spot reducing and, 354
    theory of, 346–47
    water retention in, 353–54
Weight training
    biochemical adaptations during, 38–39
    cardiac rehabilitation and, 325–26
    during pre/postpubescence, 372–74

flexibility and, 507
    gender differences in, 6–7
    hazards of, 374–75
    hypertrophy measured in, 59
    vs. lifting vs. body building, 371–72
    program of, 375–76
    strength improvement and, 432–33
    testosterone levels and, 185
Wet globe thermometer (WGT), 547–49
Wheat-germ oil, performance, 592
White blood cells. *See* Immune system
Wind, efficiency and, 475–76
Wind chill factor, 544
Wingate Anaerobic Test, 274–75
Women in athletics, 6
    cardiovascular adaptations of, 601–2, 605–6
    distance running adaptations by, 606
    emotional factors of, 615
    injuries to, 615
    limitations of, 602–4
    maximal oxygen consumption adaptations by, 605
    menstrual cycle and, 610–12
    pregnancy/childbirth and, 612–14
    running efficiency and, 471–72
    sex differences, 600–601
    speed and, 490–91
    strength training adaptations by, 606–10
    See also Sex differences; specific subjects
Work
    definition of, 208
    positive/negative, 211
Work load measurements
    bench-stepping, 210–11
    cycle ergometer, 211–14
    treadmill, 211
Work rate, efficiency and, 474

Y

Yoga, static stretching, 503